URGENT CARE MEDICINE

SECRETS

W0082161

URGENT CARE MEDICINE

SECRETS

ROBERT P. OLYMPIA, MD
Professor, Departments of Emergency Medicine & Pediatrics
Penn State College of Medicine
Assistant Director of Research, Department of Emergency Medicine
Attending Physician, Department of Emergency Medicine
Penn State Milton S. Hershey Medical Center/Penn State Children's Hospital
Hershey, PA, United States

RORY M. O'NEILL, DO
Owner & Chief Operating Officer
AllBetterCare Urgent Care Centers
Harrisburg, PA, United States

MATTHEW L. SILVIS, MD
Associate Chief Medical Officer, Primary Care, Penn State Hershey
Program Director, Penn State Primary Care Sports Medicine Fellowship,
    Hershey
Professor, Departments of Family and Community Medicine & Orthopedics
    and Rehabilitation
Penn State Milton S. Hershey Medical Center
Hershey, PA, United States

ELSEVIER

ELSEVIER

1600 John F. Kennedy Blvd.
Ste 1800
Philadelphia, PA 19103-2899

URGENT CARE MEDICINE SECRETS

ISBN: 978-0-323-46215-0

Library of Congress Cataloging-in-Publication Data

Names: Olympia, Robert, editor. | O'Neill, Rory, D.O., editor. | Silvis,
    Matthew, editor.
Title: Urgent care medicine secrets / [edited by] Robert Olympia, Rory
    O'Neill, Matthew Silvis.
Other titles: Secrets series.
Description: Philadelphia, Pa. : Elsevier, [2018] | Series: Secrets series |
    Includes bibliographical references and index.
Identifiers: LCCN 2017027311 | ISBN 9780323462150 (pbk.)
Subjects: | MESH: Ambulatory Care | Evidence-Based Medicine | Study Guide
Classification: LCC RA974 | NLM WB 18.2 | DDC 362.12--dc23 LC record available at
https://lccn.loc.gov/2017027311

Content Strategist: James Merritt
Content Development Specialist: Meghan Andress
Project Manager: Srividhya Vidhyashankar
Design Direction: Ryan Cook

 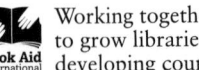

Working together
to grow libraries in
developing countries

www.elsevier.com • www.bookaid.org

Printed in United States of America.

Last digit is the print number: 9   8   7   6   5   4   3   2   1

To my parents, Manuel and Delia, for showering me with love and inspiring me to be the best person that I can be. Maraming salamat, Mahal kita. To Coco for making the ultimate sacrifice. Magbigay ng inspirasyon mo sa akin. To my sisters, Patricia and Catherine, for allowing me to be your "big brother" and keeping me grounded. To my mentors Drs. Magdy Attia, Steven Selbst, Waseem Hafeez, and Jeff Avner for being amazing role models and teaching me the art of being a professional. To my princesses, Abigail and Madelyn, for being my pillars of strength and knowing how to turn papa's frown upside down with just one laugh. Lastly, to my wife, Jodi, Mo Chuisle (my blood, my pulse), for being my partner in life, for showing me unconditional love, and for allowing me to pursue my professional dreams. Matthew 19:4-6.

—Robert Olympia

To Carina, Padraig, and Finn, who make my life truly special and to Greg, Marlys, and Peter, who bear responsibility for my life in urgent care.

—Rory O'Neill

To my parents who instilled in me a passion for lifelong learning and to my wife (Christine) and children (Nicholas, Benjamin, and Emory) who fill my life with love.

—Matthew Silvis

CONTRIBUTORS

Ayesha Abid, MD
Resident Physician, PGY-3 Department of
    Family and Community Medicine Penn
    State Milton S. Hershey Medical Center
Hershey, PA, United States

Spencer A. Adoff, MD FACEP
Asst. Medical Director
St. Joseph's Hospital
Assistant Clinical Professor
Medical College of Georgia
Georgia Emergency Associates
Savannah, GA, United States

Tabassum F. Ali, MD
Comprehensive Ophthalmologist
Delaware Ophthalmology Consultants
Wilmington, DE, United States

Siraj Amanullah, MD, MPH
Associate Professor
Department of Emergency Medicine and
    Pediatrics
Alpert Medical School of Brown University,
    Hasbro Children's Hospital, Rhode Island
    Hospital
Providence, RI, United States

Adae Amoako, MD
Primary Care Sports Medicine Fellow
Drexel University Sports Medicine
Drexel University, Tenet, Hahnemann
    University Hospital
Philadelphia, PA, United States

Jennifer F. Anders, MD
Pediatric Emergency Medicine
Johns Hopkins Children's Center
Base Station Medical Director
Johns Hopkins Children's Center
Associate State Medical Director for Pediatrics
Maryland Institute of Emergency Medical
    Services Systems
Baltimore, MD

Nadine Aprahamian, MD, FAAP
Associate Director, In-House Pediatrics-
    Winchester Hospital
Site Director for Boston University Medical
    Students
Clinical Instructor, Harvard Medical School
Department of Emergency Medicine
Boston Children's Hospital
Boston, MA, United States

Jeffrey R. Avner, MD, FAAP
Chair, Department of Pediatrics
Maimonides Infants and Children's Hospital
    of Brooklyn
Brooklyn, NY, United States

Michael C. Bachman, MD, MBA
Regional Medical Director
PM Pediatrics
Lake Success, NY, United States

Richard G. Bachur, MD
Chief, Division of Emergency Medicine
Professor, Pediatrics and Emergency Medicine
Harvard Medical School
Boston Children's Hospital
Boston, MA, United States

Jennifer Bellis, MD, MPH
Clinical Fellow
Division of Pediatric Emergency Medicine
Icahn School of Medicine at Mount Sinai
New York, NY, United States

Craig F. Betchart, MD
Family Medicine/Primary Care Sports
    Medicine
Dartmouth-Hitchcock
Concord, NH, United States

Harsh Bhakta, DO
Staff PhysicianEmergency DepartmentBaylor
    Scott and White Healthcare SystemDallas,
TX, United States

Toral Bhakta, DO
Chief of Emergency Medicine,
Medical Director Clinical Decision Unit
    Baylor Scott and White All Saints Medical
    Center
Fort Worth, TX, United States

Lauren E. Borowski, MD
Adjunct Instructor
Family and Preventive Medicine
University of Utah School of Medicine
Salt Lake City, UT, United States

Jodi Brady-Olympia, MD
Assistant Professor of Pediatrics
Department of Pediatrics
Division of Adolescent Medicine
Penn State Children's Hospital
Hershey, PA, United States

Kathryn S. Brigham, MD
Instructor in Pediatrics
Department of Pediatrics
Division of Adolescent and Young Adult
    Medicine
Massachusetts General Hospital
Boston, MA, United States

Jeffrey I. Campbell, MD
Boston Medical Center and Boston Children's
    Hospital
Boston, MA, United States

Therese L. Canares, MD
Assistant Professor
Pediatric Emergency Medicine
Johns Hopkins University School of Medicine
Baltimore, MD, United States

Steven Chan, MD
Assistant Professor of Pediatrics
Department of Pediatrics, Division of
    Emergency Medicine
Cincinnati Children's Hospital Medical
    Center, University of Cincinnati School of
    Medicine
Cincinnati, OH, United States

Bradley Chappell, DO, MHA, FACOEP, FACEP
Medical Director, RME
Harbor-UCLA Medical Center
Assistant Professor of Emergency Medicine
David Geffen School of Medicine at UCLA
Torrance, CA, United States

Joel M. Clingenpeel, MD, MPH, MS, MEdL
Associate Professor & Fellowship Director
Pediatric Emergency Medicine
Eastern Virginia Medical School
Norfolk, VA, United States

Jeff Cloyd, MD
Assistant Professor
Department of Emergency Medicine
University of Tennessee Medical Center
Knoxville, TN, United States

Ariel Cohen, DO
Pediatric Emergency Medicine Fellow
Department of Pediatrics
Johns Hopkins University
Baltimore, MD, United States

Douglas Comeau, DO, FAAFP
Medical Director, Sports Medicine
Director, Sports Medicine Fellowship
Ryan Center for Sports Medicine
Boston Medical Center
Assistant Professor, Family Medicine
Boston University School of Medicine
Head Team Physician, Boston University
Team Physician, Boston College
Boston, MA, United States

Ryan Cudahy, MD
Resident Physician
Family Medicine
Mayo Clinic
Jacksonville, FL, United States

Kaynan Doctor, MD, MBBS, BSc
Assistant Professor of Pediatrics,
The Sidney Kimmel Medical College at
    Thomas Jefferson University
Philadelphia, PA, United States
Attending Physician
Division of Emergency Medicine
Nemours/Alfred I. duPont Hospital for Children
Wilmington, DE, United States

Jennifer Dunnick, MD, MPH
Resident Physician
Pediatrics
University of Utah
Salt Lake City, UT, United States

Michele J. Fagan, MD
Assistant Professor of Pediatrics
Division of Pediatric Emergency Medicine
    Albert Einstein College of Medicine
    Children's Hospital at Montefiore
Bronx, NY, United States

Daniel M. Fein, MD
Assistant Professor of Pediatrics
Albert Einstein College of Medicine
Children's Hospital at Montefiore
Bronx, NY, United States

Fidel Garcia Fernandez, MD, FAAP, FACEP
Medical Director
PM Pediatrics
Brooklyn, NY, United States

Jennifer Fishe, MD, FAAP
Assistant Professor
Department of Emergency Medicine
University of Florida - Jacksonville
Jacksonville, FL, United States

Sylvia E. Garcia, MD
Assistant Professor
Division of Pediatric Emergency Medicine
Icahn School of Medicine at Mount Sinai
New York, NY, United States

Timothy J. Gill, MD
Resident Physician
Drexel University Sports Medicine
Drexel University, Tenet, Hahnemann
    University Hospital
Philadelphia, PA, United States

Scott Goldstein, DO, FACEP, EMT-PHP
Clinical associate Professor of Emergency
    Medicine
Sidney Kimmel College of Medicine
Director, EMS/Disaster Medicine
Einstein Healthcare Network
Philadelphia, PA, United States

Bryan Greenfield, MD
Associate Instructor of Pediatrics
Department of Pediatrics
Eastern Virginia Medical School/Children's
    Hospital of the King's Daughters
Norfolk, VA, United States

Vernne W. Greiner, DO, FAAFP
Staff Physician
AllBetterCare Urgent Care Center
Mechanicsburg, PA, United States

Maya Haasz, MD
Assistant Professor of Pediatrics
Albert Einstein College of Medicine
Children's Hospital at Montefiore
Bronx, NY, United States

Selena Hariharan, MD, MHSA
Associate Professor of Pediatrics
Division of Emergency Medicine
Cincinnati Children's Hospital Medical
    Center
University of Cincinnati College of Medicine
Cincinnati, OH, United States

Kristin Herbert, DO, MPH
Fellow
Pediatric Emergency Medicine
Eastern Virginia Medical School/Children's
    Hospital of the King's Daughters
Norfolk, VA, United States

Bruce E. Herman, MD
Professor and Vice-Chair for Education
Department of Pediatrics
Pediatric Residency Program Director
University of Utah School of Medicine
Salt Lake City, UT, United States

Sixtine Valdelièvre Herold, MD
Associate Director
Pediatric Emergency Services
South Shore Hospital
Emergency Medicine
Boston Children's Hospital
Boston, MA, United States

Crystal M. Higginson, MD
Resident Physician
Family Medicine
Wake Forest Baptist Health
Winston-Salem, NC, United States

Toni Clare Hogencamp, MD
New England Regional Medical Director
PM Pediatrics
Dedham, MA, United States

Bret C. Jacobs, DO, MA
Assistant Professor
Department of Orthopaedic Surgery
Division of Primary Care Sports Medicine
NYU Langone Medical Center
New York, NY, United States

Leah Kaye, MD
Clinical Instructor
Section of Emergency Medicine/Network of
    Care
Children's Hospital Colorado
University of Colorado School of Medicine
Aurora, CO, United States

Abbie Kelley, DO
Sports Medicine Physician
OSS Health Orthopedic Care
York, PA

Alicia Kenton, MD
Attending Physician
Rutgers University Student Health
New Brunswick, NJ, United States

Brian Kipe, MD
Attending Physician
Cumberland Valley Emergency Associates
Chambersburg Hospital Emergency
    Department, Summit Health
Chambersburg, PA, United States
Assistant Professor of Emergency Medicine
Penn State Hershey Department of Emergency
    Medicine
Hershey, PA, United States

Steven J. Kleinman, DO
Assistant Ultrasound Director
Department of Emergency Medicine
Wellspan York Hospital
York, PA, United States

Atsuko Koyama, MD, MPH
Assistant Professor, Pediatrics
Attending Physician
Division of Pediatric Emergency Medicine
Emory University, School of Medicine
Atlanta, GA, United States

Karen Y. Kwan, MD
Assistant Professor, Pediatrics
University of Southern California Keck School
of Medicine
Attending Physician
Division of Emergency and Transport Medicine
Children's Hospital of Los Angeles
Los Angeles, CA United States

Mark E. Lavallee, MD, CSCS, FACSM
Director
York Hospital Sports Medicine Fellowship
Program
York, PA, United States
Assistant Clinical Professor, Pennsylvania
State University College of Medicine
Hershey, PA, United States
Adjunct Clinical Professor
Drexel University School of Medicine
Philadelphia, PA, United States
Head Team Physician
Gettysburg College
Gettysburg, PA, United States
Chairman
USA Weightlifting Sports Medicine Society
Colorado Springs, CO, United States
Medical Director
International Weightlifting Federation –
Masters World Championships
Budapest, Hungary

Duron A. Lee, MD
Primary Care Sports Medicine Fellow
Penn State Hershey Bone and Joint Institute –
State College
State College, PA, United States

Susannah Lichtenstein, DO
Primary Care Sports Medicine Fellow
Department of Family & Community Medicine
Wake Forest Baptist Medical Center
Winston-Salem, NC, United States

Laura J. Lintner, DO, CAQSM
Assistant Professor
Department of Family and Community
Medicine
Wake Forest University School of Medicine
Winston-Salem, NC, United States

Jayson Loeffert, DO
Assistant Professor
Family and Community Medicine &
Orthopedics and Rehabilitation
Penn State Health Milton S. Hershey Medical
Center
Hershey, PA, United States

Todd Mastrovitch, MD FAAP
Clinical Assistant Professor
Department of Pediatrics
Rutgers Robert Wood Johnson Medical School
New Brunswick, NJ
Director, Pediatric Emergency Medicine
Education
Attending, Pediatric Emergency Medicine
St. Peter's University Hospital
New Brunswick, NJ

Sarah D. Meskill, MD
Assistant Professor
Pediatric Emergency Medicine
Baylor College of Medicine/ Texas Children's
Hospital
Houston, TX, United States

Christopher M. Miles, MD
Associate Program Director
Primary Care Sports Medicine Fellowship
Assistant Professor
Department of Family and Community
Medicine
Wake Forest University School of Medicine
Winston-Salem, NC, United States

Mark H. Mirabelli, MD, FAAFP
Program Director, Primary Care Sports
Medicine Fellowship
Faculty, Sports Concussion Center, Hip and
Knee Arthritis Clinic
Associate Professor, Departments of
Orthopaedics, Family Medicine and Physical
Medicine and Rehabilitation
University of Rochester
Rochester, NY, United States

Ariella Nadler, MD
Pediatric Emergency Medicine Fellow
Albert Einstein College of Medicine
Children's Hospital at Montefiore
Bronx, NY, United States

Ariel Nassim, DO
Attending Physician
Internal Medicine/Sports Medicine
Nassim Medical, P.C.
Hospital Affiliation-North Shore University
Hospital
Great Neck, NY, United States

Yashas Nathani, MD
Chief Resident
Department of Pediatrics
Saint Peter's University Hospital
New Brunswick, NJ, United States

Chadd E. Nesbit, MD, PhD, FACEP
Assistant Professor
Department of Emergency Medicine
Penn State Milton S. Hershey Medical Center
Hershey, PA, United States

Anne M. O'Connor, MD, MSc
Assistant Professor
Emergency Medicine, Pediatric Emergency
    Medicine
Dartmouth Hitchcock Medical Center
Dartmouth Geisel School of Medicine
Lebanon, NH, United States

Robert P. Olympia, MD
Professor, Departments of Emergency Medicine
    & Pediatrics
Penn State College of Medicine
Assistant Director of Research,
    Department of Emergency Medicine
Attending Physician, Department of
    Emergency Medicine
Penn State Milton S. Hershey Medical Center/
    Penn State Children's Hospital
Hershey, PA, United States

Rory M. O'Neill, DO
Owner & Chief Operating Officer
AllBetterCare Urgent Care Centers
Harrisburg, PA, United States

Cayce Onks, DO, MS, ATC
Assistant Professor
Departments of Family and Community
    Medicine & Orthopaedics and
    Rehabilitation
Penn State Hershey Milton S. Hershey
    Medical Center
Penn State College of Medicine
Hershey, PA, United States

John A. Park, MD
Chief Resident
Department of Pediatrics
Penn State Children's Hospital
Hershey, PA, United States

Jay Pershad, MD, MMM, CPE
Professor
Pediatrics and Emergency Medicine
University of Tennessee Health Science
    Center and Le Bonheur Children's Hospital
Memphis, TN, United States

Nicholas Pfeifer, EdM, ATC
Athletic Trainer, Boston University
Department of Family Medicine, Sports
    Medicine Division
Ryan Center for Sports Medicine at Boston
    University
Boston Medical Center
Boston, MA, United States

Christopher M. Pruitt, MD, FAAP
Assistant Professor
Department of Pediatrics, Division of Pediatric
    Emergency Medicine
University of Alabama at Birmingham
Birmingham, AL, United States

George G.A. Pujalte, MD, FACSM
Senior Associate Consultant
Family Medicine and Sports Medicine
Assistant Professor
Mayo Clinic College of Medicine
Chair for Scholarship and Academics
Department of Family Medicine
Mayo Clinic
Jacksonville, FL, United States

Joni E. Rabiner, MD, FAAP
Associate Professor of Clinical Pediatrics
Division of Pediatric Emergency Medicine
Albert Einstein College of Medicine
Children's Hospital at Montefiore
Bronx, NY, United States

Eric Requa, DO
Sports Medicine Physician
Virtua Health
Marlton, NJ, United States

Lilia Reyes, MD, FAAP
Assistant Professor of Emergency Medicine and
    Pediatrics
Department of Emergency Medicine
Penn State Milton S. Hershey Medical Center
Hershey, PA, United States

Ruby F. Rivera, M.D.
Assistant Professor of Pediatrics
Program Director, Pediatric Emergency
    Medicine Fellowship Albert Einstein
    College of Medicine Children's Hospital at
    Montefiore
Bronx, NY, United States

Jeffrey A. Rixe, MD
Emergency Medicine Resident
Emergency Medicine
Boston University Medical Center
Boston, MA, United States

Emily Rose, MD, FAAP, FAAEM, FACEP
Assistant Professor of Clinical Emergency
Medicine
Keck School of Medicine of the University of
Southern California
Department of Emergency Medicine
Los Angeles County + USC Medical Center
Los Angeles, CA, United States

Jerri A. Rose, MD, FAAP
Attending Physician, Division of Pediatric
Emergency Medicine
Associate Professor of Pediatrics
Director, Pediatric Emergency Medicine
Fellowship
UH Rainbow Babies and Children's Hospital/
Case Western Reserve University School of
Medicine
Cleveland, OH, United States

Timothy Salkauskis, MD
Resident Physician
Family Medicine
Drexel University/Hahnemann University
Hospital
Philadelphia, PA, United States

Esther Maria Sampayo, MD, MPH
Assistant Professor
Pediatric Emergency Medicine
Baylor College of Medicine/Texas Children's
Hospital
Houston, TX, United States

Jennifer E. Sanders, MD
Assistant Professor
Division of Pediatric Emergency Medicine
Icahn School of Medicine at Mount Sinai
New York, NY, United States

Sandra K. Schumacher, MD, MPH, CTropMed
Pediatrician and Pediatric Infectious Diseases
Consultant
Boston Children's Hospital
Boston, MA, United States

Kara K. Seaton, MD
Attending Physician
Pediatric Emergency Medicine
Children's Hospitals and Clinics of Minnesota
Minneapolis, MN, United States

Peter H. Seidenberg, MD, FAAFP, FACSM, RMSK
Program Director
Penn State Primary Care Sports Medicine
Fellowship
Professor of Orthopaedics and Rehabilitation
Professor of Family and Community Medicine
Penn State Hershey Bone and Joint Institute –
State College
Team Physician, Penn State University
State College, PA, United States

Alexander Y. Sheng, MD
Assistant Residency Program Director
Assistant Professor of Emergency Medicine
Department of Emergency Medicine
Boston Medical Center/Boston University
School of Medicine
Boston, MA, United States

Matthew L. Silvis, MD
Associate Chief Medical Officer, Primary Care,
Penn State Hershey
Program Director, Penn State Primary Care
Sports Medicine Fellowship, Hershey
Professor, Departments of Family and
Community Medicine & Orthopedics and
Rehabilitation
Penn State College of Medicine
Hershey, PA, United States

Samantha F. Singer, PA-C
Lead Physician Assistant
AllBetterCare Urgent Care Centers
Harrisburg, PA, United States

Lindsay A. Smith, MD
Family Medicine Resident
Family Medicine
Wake Forest University School of Medicine
Winston Salem, NC, United States

Joseph Spinell, DO, FACEP
Emergency Medicine
Skyline Medical Center
Nashville, TN, United States

Ee Tein Tay, MD
Assistant Professor
Department of Emergency Medicine and
Pediatrics
Icahn School of Medicine at Mount Sinai
New York, NY, United States

Heath C. Thornton, MD
Associate Professor
Program Director, Primary Care Sports
Medicine Fellowship
Family and Community Medicine/Orthopedic
Surgery
Wake Forest School of Medicine
Winston-Salem, NC, United States

Thomas H. Trojian, MD
Professor, Chief, Division of Sports Medicine
Department of Family, Community &
Preventative Medicine
Drexel University, College of Medicine
Philadelphia, PA, United States

Peggy Tseng, MD
Resident Physician
Department of Emergency Medicine
LAC USC Medical Center
Los Angeles, CA, United States

Bryan D. Upham, MD, MSCE
Associate Professor
Division of Pediatric Emergency Medicine
Department of Emergency Medicine
University of New Mexico
Albuquerque, NM, United States

Michelle N. Vazquez, MD
Clinical Fellow
Division of Pediatric Emergency Medicine
Icahn School of Medicine at Mount Sinai
New York, NY, United States

Jeffrey A. Waskin, DO
Attending Physician
Emergency Medicine
Pinnacle Health Hospital
Harrisburg, PA, United States

Robert D. Wilkinson, DO
Fellow
Pediatric Emergency Medicine
University of New Mexico
Albuquerque, NM, United States

Robert B. Windsor, MD
Acting Assistant Professor
Anesthesia, Pain Medicine
Seattle Children's
Anesthesia Administration
Seattle, WA, United States

Daniel Ta Yo Yu, MB, BCh
Pediatric Emergency Medicine Fellow
Department of Pediatrics
Johns Hopkins Hospital
Baltimore, MD, United States

PREFACE

I have been a fan of the *Secrets Series* since medical school. I love the simplicity of the question and answer format and value the depth of medical knowledge each page holds. I remember using each of the *Secret Series* specialty books during every rotation of medical school, helping me to answer questions while on rounds, to research the diagnosis of an undifferentiated patient, or to prepare for in-training and board examinations. Throughout my career, the *Secrets Series* has been a large part of my professional life. I was blessed to be involved with the first, and subsequent, editions of *Pediatric Emergency Medicine Secrets* and, more recently, used *Pediatric Secrets* to successfully pass my recertification examination. Our department uses both the *Emergency Medicine Secrets* and *Pediatric Emergency Medicine Secrets* books as required reading for the medical student rotation.

Limited hours in primary health care offices and long wait times in emergency departments have fueled the economy for urgent care centers over the past decade. According to the American Academy of Urgent Care Medicine, there are currently over 9,300 walk-in, standalone urgent care centers in the United States, with 50 to 100 new centers expected to open every year. The establishment of urgent care medicine as a medical specialty, along with my affinity for the *Secret Series*, fueled a desire to orchestrate the first edition of *Urgent Care Medicine Secrets*. I was blessed to embark on this journey with two colleagues I admire and respect tremendously. Rory O'Neill is a board-certified emergency medicine physician, working both clinically and administratively in the arenas of emergency medicine and urgent care medicine. Matthew Silvis is board certified in both family medicine and primary care sports medicine, balancing his professional career with clinical medicine, education, administration, and research.

Rory, Matt, and I felt it was important to create a book that focused on evidence-based urgent care medicine, targeted toward health care providers from different levels of experience (graduate-level students to experienced providers) and different specialty backgrounds (medical, nursing, nurse practitioners, physician assistants). We searched far and wide for contributors who have demonstrated scholarship in their careers and are experts in their fields. Our contributors represent varied backgrounds, covering general pediatrics, emergency medicine, pediatric emergency medicine, family medicine, urgent care medicine, sports medicine, and anesthesiology.

We hope that the first edition of *Urgent Care Medicine Secrets* will provide a valuable tool for the health care provider and subsequently results in the best care delivered to each and every patient who walks into an urgent care center. The first edition is divided into five sections. The first and second sections focus on common chief complaints that may present to your urgent care center, divided into adult and pediatrics. The third section focuses on primary care sports medicine, covering common injuries and sport-related infections and illnesses. The fourth section focuses on procedures that may be performed in your urgent care center, including laceration repair, orthopedic reduction and splinting, incision and drainage, foreign body removal, and utilization of sedation and analgesia. The last section focuses on miscellaneous topics that may be of interest to the urgent care medicine health care provider, including the recognition and stabilization of adult and pediatric emergencies, office emergency and disaster preparedness, utilization of diagnostic ultrasound, mental health urgencies, travel medicine, and the business of urgent care medicine.

Robert P. Olympia, MD

CONTENTS

III   SPORTS-RELATED COMPLAINTS

TOP SECRETS IN URGENT CARE

1. All headaches can be treated with oxygen.

2. Bell palsy never involves the arms or legs, but does involve the forehead.

3. Benign positional vertigo (BPV) is usually in the posterior semicircular canal.

4. Stye and chalazion are single lesions, whereas blepharitis involves the entire eyelid.

5. Iritis causes pain with bright lights; glaucoma's pain comes in the dark.

6. Azithromycin and trimethoprim/sulfamethoxazole are no longer recommended for routine use for acute otitis media due to increased antibiotic resistance.

7. Otitis externa is five times more common in swimmers than in nonswimmers.

8. Approximately 90% of patients with a viral upper respiratory infection (URI) have sinus involvement.

9. Teeth sensitivity to hot or cold suggests pulp exposure or inflammation.

10. Teeth tenderness with pressure or eating suggests periodontal ligament injury.

11. With lost avulsed teeth, consider aspiration and obtain chest and/or abdominal x-rays.

12. Consider atypical infections, specifically *Mycobacterium tuberculosis*, in patients presenting with respiratory symptoms that are immunocompromised or have recently traveled to endemic areas.

13. The electrocardiogram (EKG or ECG) is the most important diagnostic tool in evaluating a patient with chest pain, but it only captures a moment in time and therefore may not be enough to rule out cardiac disease in patients with moderate to high-risk chest pain.

14. Be wary of the elderly patient with nonspecific abdominal pain, especially if it is described as a tearing/shearing pain with radiation to the back, or blood is present in the stool or urine. You should maintain a high index of suspicion for abdominal aortic aneurysm (AAA).

15. When evaluating right lower quadrant (RLQ) pain in a female, it is important to perform a bimanual exam to help differentiate between abdominal and pelvic origins of the pain as the imaging choices will vary.

16. Asymptomatic viral shedding is extremely common the first year after initial outbreak of genital herpes.

17. Fever occurs with acute pyelonephritis only about half of the time.

18. Nonbacterial prostatitis/chronic pelvic pain syndrome occurs in about 90% of cases of chronic prostatitis.

19. Of untreated gonococcal (most common cause in urban areas)/chlamydial (most common cause in college students) cervicitis, 10%–20% may progress to pelvic inflammatory disease (PID).

20. Patient older than 40 years of age who present with Bartholin abscess should be referred to a gynecologist to rule out Bartholin gland cancer.

21. Topical steroids for allergic contact dermatitis should not be given if systemic steroids are prescribed.

22. Elevation of an infected extremity is a key feature to outpatient management of cellulitis.

23. Corticosteroids do not reduce postherpetic neuralgia, but gabapentin and opiate treatment do.

24. Mothers of infant children commonly suffer from de Quervain tenosynovitis.

25. Trephination is contraindicated in patients with acrylic nails. The nails must be removed prior to procedure.

26. For the most definitive treatment removal of the entire lateral quarter to one third of the nail is recommended.

27. Erythema migrans if identified is an indication for treatment of Lyme disease without laboratory confirmation.

28. No one has ever contracted rabies from a dog, cat, or ferret who was observed for 10 days.

29. The height of the temperature is not an accurate marker of serious illness in otherwise healthy children and thus has limited use in determining management; other clinical features, especially the child's clinical appearance, are better predictors.

30. It is important to educate parents that fever is a symptom of their child's illness that will persist until the underlying illness has resolved. Fever itself is not dangerous to an otherwise healthy child and the specific temperature value is generally not important.

31. The most common cause of acute headaches in the pediatric patient is an upper respiratory infection with a fever.

32. With a normal neurological exam, pediatric headaches rarely warrant the use of emergent imaging.

33. The red, painful eye in a contact lens wearer is an ominous sign and warrants immediate referral for ophthalmological evaluation to assess for sight-threatening corneal ulcers.

34. Child abuse should be suspected in a *child* presenting with symptoms concerning for *N. gonorrhoeae* associated conjunctivitis.

35. Sinusitis is not a common diagnosis in early childhood and infancy. Don't jump the gun to treat children with viral symptoms (URI, cough) with antibiotics.

36. Acute otitis media and sinusitis share identical bacteriological etiologies (*Streptococcus pneumoniae*, nontypeable *Haemophilus influenzae,* and *Moraxella catarrhalis*). Hence, both are treated similarly. Amoxicillin is the first line drug of choice for both.

37. Routine chest x-rays are not recommended in the acute management of asthma, bronchiolitis, pneumonia, and croup. Consider if severe symptoms, significant hypoxemia, or persistent marked asymmetry present on lung exam.

38. Routine viral testing is not recommended in asthma, croup, or bronchiolitis.

39. Torticollis with neck pain after trauma (even minor) needs evaluation for C1–C2 subluxation.

40. A quick rule for lateral x-rays for retropharyngeal abscess is the soft tissue space should be less than half the width of the corresponding vertebral body.

41. Chest wall pain remains the most common etiology of chest pain in pediatric patients.

42. A good history and physical examination is sufficient to rule out serious pathology, without need for extensive workup.

43. All children with bilious emesis should be referred to an emergency department urgently for a workup for acute abdomen.

44. Always do a male genitourinary (GU) exam in male patients presenting with abdominal pain.

45. For young infants with symptoms of gastroenteritis, especially fever, consider testing for urinary tract infection.

46. Hyponatremic dehydration in infants is often caused by improper dilution of formula.

47. Children with hematuria and hypertension should be referred for emergent comprehensive evaluation.

48. Uncircumcised boys may present acutely with paraphimosis, a foreskin stuck in the retracted position. This is an emergency and requires urgent reduction.

49. Perform a pregnancy test in all females with primary or secondary amenorrhea.

50. Always consider the provision of emergency contraception, including pills or the copper intrauterine device (IUD).

51. The appearance of erythema migrans alone is sufficient to start antibiotic therapy in endemic areas.

52. There is no indication for a complete blood count or blood culture in the evaluation of cellulitis or erysipelas.

53. Brief resolved unexplained events (BRUE) (formerly known as apparent life-threatening events [ALTE]) rarely require further diagnostic evaluation.

54. Diagnostic testing for excessive crying should be guided by the history and physical exam.

55. Most serious causes of acute limp in afebrile, well-appearing children can be ruled out with plain radiographs and normal complete blood count (CBC), C-reactive protein (CRP), and erythrocyte sedimentation rate (ESR).

56. Back and pelvic causes of limp in children usually require emergent evaluation.

57. When evaluating a pediatric patient with head trauma, the goal should be to assess for clinically significant traumatic brain injury while minimizing unnecessary radiation exposure.

58. Neck injuries are uncommon in children, but the small size of the neck and the higher fulcrum of the cervical spine make injuries more likely to cause significant injury.

59. Abdominal bruising after a motor vehicle collision with a seatbelt is associated with increased risk of intraabdominal injury and should prompt emergency department transfer for further workup and evaluation.

60. Rib fractures in children require significant force and are associated with other injuries. Nonaccidental trauma should be suspected if present without a significant trauma history.

61. Consider nonaccidental trauma (NAT) if the fracture does not match the history or mechanism of injury. Fractures concerning for NAT include femur and spiral extremity fractures in preambulatory children, multiple fractures in various stages of healing, chip fractures of the metaphysis, and bucket handle fractures.

62. Torus, greenstick, and bowing fractures are often collectively referred to as "plastic fractures" and are unique to children as a result of the pliability of the pediatric skeleton.

63. Sports with the highest rate of acute cervical spine injuries include American football, wrestling, diving, ice hockey, skiing/snowboarding, and gymnastics.

64. Initial cervical spine injury management should be to establish ABCDE (airway, breathing, circulation, disability, and exposure) and then to maintain inline immobilization until serious injury can be cleared.

65. When concerned about Achilles tendonitis, it is important to rule out an Achilles tendon rupture. The Thompson test is performed to determine this.

66. The rectus femoris is the most commonly strained quadriceps muscle.

67. In lateral epicondylitis, the common extensor tendon origin is the area most involved and the extensor carpi brevis radialis is almost always the specific tendon affected.

68. Emergent/urgent causes of low back pain include cauda equina syndrome, fracture, infection, and malignancy.

69 Consider emergent/urgent causes of adipocyte lipid binding protein (ALBP) in a child who presents with self-imposed activity restrictions.

70. In the absence of red flags, do not image low back pain in the first 6 weeks.

71. If possible, always obtain *weightbearing* radiographs of the knee.

72. If septic arthritis is suspected, arthrocentesis for fluid analysis followed by parenteral antibiotics and urgent referral for surgical debridement is warranted.

73. Jersey fingers need urgent surgical referral.

74. Scaphoid fractures often have normal initial radiographs.

75. The scaphoid is the most common carpal bone fractured in a fall on outstretched hand (FOOSH) injury, but may have negative x-rays at initial evaluation.

76. Pediatric patients most commonly sustain a clavicle fracture after a FOOSH injury.

77 Utilization of validated imaging guidelines (i.e., Ottawa ankle/knee rules, Pittsburgh rules for knee trauma, Canadian C-spine rule) can reduce unnecessary imaging

78. In the skeletally immature athlete with injury and concern for growth plate injury, consider bilateral imaging for comparison views

79. Hypothermia is defined as body temperature <35°C (95°F) rectally, but can occur at higher temperatures, especially if clothing is wet

80. If patient is suspected to have heat stroke, access ABCs (airway, breathing, circulation), begin cooling with ice bags and/or fan mists, and alert emergency medical services for immediate transfer.

81. In evaluating the patient with acute shoulder pain, be sure to identify the mechanism of injury.

82. Imaging tests should be used to confirm a suspected diagnosis, and the imaging performed depends on the differential diagnosis.

83. Concussion is a disruption to the normal function of the brain secondary to a force to the head or body.

84. The symptoms and signs of concussion are divided into physical, cognitive, emotional, and sleep.

85. A person should not be returned to sports until resolution of concussion-related symptoms and a graded return to play.

86. Apophysitis should always be considered in adolescents with joint pain. These diagnoses can generally be managed conservatively, and will improve with a period of rest.

87. Radiographs rarely aid in the diagnosis and treatment of apophysitis; however, they can rule out avulsion fracture in some cases.

88. Use historical clues such as patient's age and onset of symptoms in addition to frog-leg radiographs to evaluate the acutely limping child.

89. If you suspect septic arthritis, urgent referral for aspiration followed by parenteral antibiotics is imperative.

90. The greatest risk factor for ankle sprain is a previous ankle sprain that has not been appropriately rehabilitated.

91. The Ottawa Ankle Rules are a set of guidelines that indicate when radiographs should be obtained for acute ankle sprains.

92. Gradual return to play may be started 3 weeks after an athlete is diagnosed with infectious mononucleosis, as long as asymptomatic with a normal examination and laboratory results (i.e., liver enzyme levels); however, typically contact and vigorous exercise is prohibited for the first 4 weeks after onset of symptoms.

93. Return to play guidelines are the same in general for most acute bacterial dermatoses: 48–72 hours of systemic antibiotics with no moist, oozing, or exudative lesions and no new onset of lesions in the last 48 hours. Athletes with "herpes gladiatorum" in general must complete oral antiviral treatment for at least 120 hours, have no new lesions for at least 72 hours, and remain free of systemic symptoms for 72 hours.

94. Decision making for all wounds including bites should be made based on the goals of establishing hemostasis, minimizing the risk of infection, optimizing cosmetic results, returning function to normal, and minimizing pain.

95. When in doubt, err on the side of caution: Consider antibiotic prophylaxis—unknown rabies status is treated to cover for possible exposure, etc.

96. Open wounds involving the metacarpophalangeal joints sustained from punching the mouth should be treated as human bites.

97. Absorbable sutures may be used for facial and scalp lacerations in young children.

98. Dislocations or fractures resulting in neurovascular compromise should be emergently reduced.

99. A patient with a history and physical findings compatible with a nursemaid's elbow does not require imaging prior to attempting reduction.

100. Contraindications to splinting include open fractures, fractures involving the joint, severe fractures (displaced, angulated, or overlapping fractures), Salter Harris V fractures, severe plastic fractures (greenstick, bowing), or evidence of compartment syndrome.

101. Ultrasound may help distinguish between cellulitis and abscess in soft tissue infections.

102. Incision and drainage is the treatment of choice for abscesses.

103. Firm immobilization and behavior management (e.g., pain control or anxiolysis) will aid in nasal or ear foreign body removal in children.

104. Button batteries in any location or two high-powered magnets ingested or across the nasal septum are medical emergencies and require immediate removal.

105. Suspect foreign body aspiration in a child who is toddler to preschool age; was last seen with a small, hard object; and has sudden onset of cough, choke, or wheeze.

106. Avulsion of a permanent tooth is a dental emergency and reimplantation should occur within the first 15 minutes for the best prognosis! Primary teeth should NOT be reimplanted.

107. When there is concern for facial cellulitis, buccal cellulitis, periorbital or orbital cellulitis, or systemic symptoms with a dental infection, the patient should be transferred to an emergency department or directly admitted to the hospital for definite care. Evidence has shown that early initiation of care for progressive dental infections improves outcomes.

108. Multimodal treatments should always be used to treat pain without opioids or to reduce the opioid to the minimum required dose.

109. In a true emergency, where delays can lead to increased risk of morbidity and mortality, the priorities of an urgent care facility are rapid recognition and disposition.

110. Stick to C-A-B (circulation, airway, breathing), according to Basic Life Support guidelines, when attempting to stabilize and support a sick patient as you enlist the help of paramedics by calling 911 for resuscitation and rapid transport to the nearest emergency department.

111. Hypotension is a late sign of shock in children.

112. Intramuscular epinephrine is the first line treatment for anaphylaxis, as well as a child with minimal air movement on examination (status asthmaticus), and doses can be repeated up to every 5 minutes.

113. Urgent care centers must be able to rapidly recognize, assess, stabilize, and transfer patients presenting to their center with medical and traumatic emergencies beyond the capability of the center.

114. Communication among staff, local EMS, and the receiving hospital is important when dealing with an office emergency and arranging patient transfer.

115. Point-of-care ultrasound is focused imaging performed and interpreted by clinicians with focused training to answer brief, important, clinical questions.

116. Ultrasound is useful in identifying all types of foreign bodies in soft tissue despite their composition.

117. In a child presenting with ongoing somatic complaints or change in school performance, clinicians must also consider a diagnosis of depression, anxiety, or other mood disorder.

118. A discussion of confidentiality is an essential component to obtaining a psychosocial history in an adolescent.

119. Visiting family and relatives (VFRs) tend to have a higher prevalence of travel-related infectious diseases than other tourists.

120. Many illnesses associated with travel can be prevented with pretravel medical guidance, often at a travel clinic.

121. Make sure to consider both upfront expenses and ongoing expenses that will occur after opening an urgent care center.

122. Make sure you have sufficient contingency funds before opening an urgent care center.

HEADACHE AND NEUROLOGIC COMPLAINTS

Scott Goldstein, DO, FACEP, FAAEM

CHAPTER 1

MIGRAINE HEADACHE

1. **What are the typical pain characteristics of migraine headache?**
   The migraine headache is unilateral and pulsatile in nature, ranging in severity from moderate to severe and usually worsened by physical activity.

2. **What is an aura?**
   Reversible cerebral dysfunction (abnormal smells, eye floaters, etc.) that develops over 5 (or more) minutes and lasts less than an hour.

3. **What is the classic presentation of a migraine headache *with* an aura?**
   A migraine headache, usually within 1 hour of an aura.

4. **What is the classic presentation of a migraine headache *without* an aura?**
   Unilateral, pulsatile headache that can last anywhere from 4 hours to 3 days. There is frequently associated nausea/vomiting and/or light/noise sensitivity.

5. **What is the treatment for a mild/moderate migraine headache?**
   Treatment can be done in a stepwise fashion. For headaches that are mild to moderate (without nausea/vomiting) nonspecific pain medications can be used (e.g., nonsteroidal antiinflammatory drugs [NSAIDs] and/or acetaminophen).
   Other nonspecific agents that can be used are dopamine antagonists (e.g., metoclopramide or chlorpromazine). Their greatest effect is in the treatment of nausea/vomiting.
   If available, the use of high flow oxygen can be a great adjunct to any treatment decision.

6. **What is the treatment for moderate/severe migraine headache?**
   Migraine-specific medications should be used, such as triptans. These can be given orally, subcutaneously, nasally, or intravenously; they work well alone or in conjunction with nonspecific agents.

7. **What are the different types of migraine headaches?**
   Hemiplegic, basilar, childhood periodic syndromes, retinal migraine, ophthalmologic, vertiginous, nocturnal.

TENSION HEADACHE

8. **What are the main causes of tension headaches?**
   Any stressor can lead to tension headaches, so it is not surprising that these are the most common type of headache. Other contributing factors are poor posture (especially weak neck extensors), depression, and anxiety.
   Any stressor that is not a direct cause of the headache can be a contributing factor by leading to spasm of the neck and scalp muscles.

9. **What is the best way to treat tension headaches?**
   Pharmacologic and stress reduction therapies work well together. In the fast-paced world of urgent care, stress reduction techniques are not a viable option. In the urgent care setting the use of NSAIDs, acetaminophen, and oxygen would be your best options.

10. **How can I differentiate a tension headache from other headaches?**
    If you were to guess a headache was tension type, you would be right most of the time as tension headaches are the most common type of headache.
    On physical exam you may also find diffuse scalp or trapezius tenderness.

CLUSTER HEADACHE

11. **What is the classic presentation of a cluster headache?**
    Cluster headaches present with unilateral pain (usually around the eye and temporal area) with cranial nerve autonomic dysfunction (tearing, facial pain, etc.).
    The cluster headache usually lasts 45 to 90 minutes and is episodic in nature, with these headaches lasting as long as 1 week.

12. **What is the best treatment for a cluster headache?**
    The same medications (triptans, NSAIDs, acetaminophen) for migraines are used to treat cluster headaches, with the best medication being triptans via the subcutaneous route. Unlike migraines, there is more of an emphasis on oxygen for the acute treatment.

FACIAL DROOP/BELL PALSY

13. **How can I differentiate Bell palsy from a stroke?**
    Bell palsy is an acute, unilateral, facial nerve paralysis. This results in weakness of the muscles of facial expression (including the forehead) and *never* any leg or arm involvement. There is always involvement of the unilateral forehead. If the forehead is spared, then this is an upper motor neuron lesion, not Bell palsy.

14. **What is the treatment for Bell palsy?**
    Symptomatic treatment with eye lubricant and an eye shield for sleep along with corticosteroids (prednisone is typically prescribed in a 10-day tapering course starting at 60 mg). Based on current literature antivirals are currently not recommended.

15. **How long does Bell palsy last?**
    It is dependent on the extent of nerve damage; therefore, it can range from weeks to never, but most patients recover completely by 2 months.

VERTIGO

16. **What is benign positional vertigo (BPV)?**
    It is a peripheral vestibular disorder involving the semicircular canals in the ear. There is no brain or central component.

17. **How can I differentiate BPV from central nervous system (CNS) causes?**
    History. Also positioning testing (e.g., Dix-Hallpike maneuver) helps establish the diagnosis of the origin being peripheral in nature.

18. **What is the Dix-Hallpike maneuver and how is it performed?**
    The patient starts in sitting position, facing forward with eyes open.
    Rapidly lie the patient backward with the head turned 45 degrees to the right and the neck extended over the end of the table for about 30 seconds. This is repeated on the left side.

19. **Why would I want to perform the Dix-Hallpike maneuver?**
    You may see nystagmus and reproduce the vertiginous symptoms that can lead to nausea/vomiting, which will force the patient to get out of the position. If the patient stays with the maneuver, this test is also the treatment, as repositioning the otoliths in the ear will aid in treatment.

20. **What is the initial workup/evaluation of vertigo?**
    If one cannot confidently say it is a peripheral cause, then a central lesion or nonneurologic cause must be considered. These tests can include computerized axial tomography (CAT) scan, magnetic resonance imaging (MRI), electrocardiogram (EKG), and blood work. These patients should probably be referred to the emergency department.

VASOVAGAL SYNCOPE

21. What is the definition of syncope?
Transient loss of consciousness due to hypoperfusion of the brain.
> The characteristics are rapid onset, brief duration, and spontaneous recovery.

22. What are the causes of vasovagal syncope?
Pain, prolonged standing, being in a hot and/or crowded area, emotional stress, urinating or defecating, seeing blood (if this is you, you may be in the wrong field).

23. Is there a prodrome to vasovagal syncope?
Yes. Symptoms may include yawning, lightheadedness, nausea, sweating, ringing in the ears, or visual changes.

24. How do you treat vasovagal syncope?
The main goal is to prevent injury from the actual physical event of falling.
> Most people will have completely resolved by the time you evaluate them. The key is to find out what the prodromal symptoms were to help decide if the episode was vasovagal or more concerning (cardiac, aortic, CNS, etc.).

25. What tests should I order?
1. EKG to evaluate for dysthymia or infarct
2. Human chorionic gonadotropin (HCG) for pregnancy status in women of childbearing age
   a. Which can cause hypovolemia
3. Urine dipstick to evaluate for ketones and/or glucose
   a. Ketones to evaluate for dehydration
   b. Glucose for possible poorly controlled diabetes
4. Blood glucose for glucose level

KEY POINTS

1. Migraine headaches are typically unilateral and pulsatile in nature.
2. The most common types of headaches are tension headaches.
3. Oxygen is a great adjunct to treat all types of headaches.
4. Bell palsy never involves the arms or legs.
5. Any stressor can precipitate a vasovagal syncopal episode.

BIBLIOGRAPHY

Bajwa Z, Smith J. Acute treatment of migraine in adults. The International Classification of Headache Disorders, 3 ed (beta version). *Cephalalgia*. 2013;33(July):629–808. http://www.uptodate.com/contents/acute-treatment-of-migraine-in-adults.

Becker W. Acute migraine treatment in adults. *Headache*. 2015;55(6):778–793. http://dx.doi.org/10.1111/head.12550.

Blanda M: Tension headache. Medscape. http://emedicine.medscape.com/article/792384-overview#a5.

Edvardsson B. Symptomatic cluster headache: a review of 63 cases. *SpringerPlus*. 2014;3:64. http://dx.doi.org/10.1186/2193-1801-3-64.

Fumal A, Schoenen J. Tension-type headache: current research and clinical management. *Lancet Neurol*. 2008;7(1):70–83.

Goroll AH, Mulley AG. *Primary Care Medicine: Office Evaluation and Management of the Adult Patient*. 6th ed. Philadelphia: Lippincott Williams & Williams; 2009.

Lockhart P, Daly F, Pitkethly M, Comerford N, Sullivan F. The neurologist dilemma. *Cochrane Database Syst Rev 4(October 7)*. 2009. CD001869.

Manjit M. Cluster headache. *BMJ Clin Evid* (February). 2010;1212. Fogan: A double-blind comparison of oxygen v air inhalation. *LArch Neurol*. 1985;42(4):362–363.

Moses S. *Dix-Hallpike maneuver*. FPnotebook (December). 2015.

Muhammet A, Tushar S, Wilke I, Willems S. Management and therapy of vasovagal syncope: a review. *World J Cardiol*. 2010;2(10):308–315.

Shukla GJ: Syncope. *Circulation*. 2006;113(16).

Ozkurt B, Cinar O, Cevik E. Efficacy of high-flow oxygen therapy in all types of headache: a prospective, randomized, placebo-controlled trial. *Am J Emerg Med*. 2012;30(9):1760–1764. http://dx.doi.org/10.1016/j.ajem.2012.02.010.

Walsh K, Hoffmayer K. Syncope: diagnosis and management. *Curr Probl Cardiol*. 2015;40(2):51–86.

CHAPTER 2

RED EYE, EYE PAIN, AND VISION LOSS

Jeff Cloyd, MD

1. **How does the anatomy of the eye affect the way a patient will present for an ophthalmologic emergency?**
   Although patients present for "eye pain" or "eye redness," it is important to differentiate between symptoms affecting the soft tissues surrounding the eye and those affecting the orbit specifically.

2. **How should the eye be examined?**
   Start with a visual acuity, followed by examination of the soft tissue around the eye. This is best performed in a dark room using a slit lamp, or at least an ophthalmoscope and a blue light (e.g., Wood lamp).

3. **How can you differentiate between periorbital and orbital cellulitis?**
   Periorbital cellulitis does not cause pain with eye movement and is treated with outpatient oral antibiotic therapy. Orbital cellulitis causes pain with eye movement and is treated as an inpatient.

4. **What is the treatment for a chalazion (cyst) and a hordeolum (stye) (Fig. 2.1)?**
   Both present with swelling, pain, and erythema of the affected eyelid. Neither require antibiotic treatment. Both are best treated with frequent warm compresses and antiinflammatory pain medication.

5. **What is blepharitis and how is management different from chalazion and hordeolum?**
   Blepharitis is an infection of the eyelash and can extend into the eyelid; it should be treated with topical antibiotic drops or ointment. Oral antibiotics are typically not indicated.

6. **Which method should be used to examine the underside of the eyelid for a foreign body?**
   Place a cotton-tip swab against the skin along the margin between the orbital and the superior orbital bone. Holding the patient's upper eyelashes, the lid can then be everted by rolling the skin over the cotton-tip swab. Repeat on the lower lid.

7. **How many places can a contact lens hide?**
   Careful examination of the cornea and sclera of a patient who has "lost" a contact lens in the eye may not reveal the missing contact. After anesthesia, evert the eyelid and sweep the upper fornix while the patient is looking down. Fluorescein stain can be used to help locate a missing lens in the eye, but staining of the lens is permanent.

8. **What are the characteristics of different corneal injuries with examination using fluorescein stain?**
   See Fig. 2.2 for the different characteristics.

9. **What options are there for removing a splinter caused by metal grinding?**
   After anesthetic drops are instilled in the eye, a cotton-tip swab typically removes most foreign bodies; however, a metal splinter can be removed using an electric bur drill, or if not available, a steady hand and an 18-gauge needle. Patient reassurance and compliance is important. Iron-containing foreign bodies will produce a rust ring within several hours that should be removed using a cotton-tip swab or bur drill.

10. **When is an appropriate time to use topical antibiotics with corneal injuries?**
    Most injuries to the cornea caused by a foreign body should be treated with topical antibiotics, especially if the injury is caused by an organic substance such as dirt. Antibiotics should be considered in simple corneal abrasions but are not considered standard of care. Drops and ointment

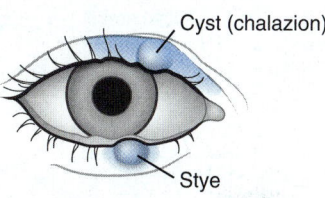

Fig. 2.1. Chalazion vs. Hordeolum. *(Adapted from Image 2. Styes and Chalazions Guide: Causes, Symptoms, and Treatment Options. [n.d.]. Available at:* https://www.drugs.com/health-guide/styes-and-chalazions.html. *Accessed 15.07.16.)*

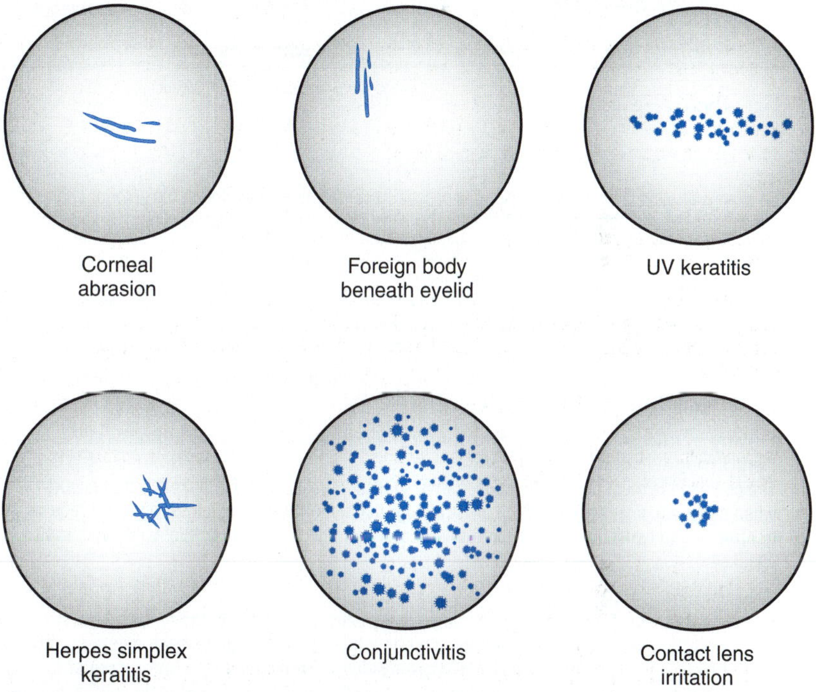

Corneal abrasion	Foreign body beneath eyelid	UV keratitis
Herpes simplex keratitis	Conjunctivitis	Contact lens irritation

Fig. 2.2. Pattern of Fluorescein Stain Uptake in Corneal Pain. *(Adapted from Roberts J, Hedges K: Clinical Procedures in Emergency Medicine, Philadelphia, 2010, Saunders Elsevier, p 1149, Fig. 63.11. Reprinted with permission.)*

have similar efficacy, and drops tend to be cleaner. Treatments for corneal injuries in patients wearing contact lenses should be chosen with *Pseudomonas* species in mind (e.g., ciprofloxacin).

11. Should conjunctivitis be treated with antibiotics?

Antibiotic therapy is not recommended in the treatment of acute conjunctivitis as the most common cause is viral. Allergic inflammation is another common cause of conjunctivitis and should be treated with standard allergy medications (e.g., histamine blockers, intranasal corticosteroids). Bacterial conjunctivitis treatment has not been shown to significantly reduce the number of days of symptoms, and most infections are self-limited. However, antibiotics should be considered in infants and immunocompromised patients.

12. How does iritis present differently from conjunctivitis?

Pain caused by iritis is not improved with topical anesthetics, and vision in the affected eye is often affected by inflammatory proteins in the aqueous humor of the anterior chamber. These proteins can

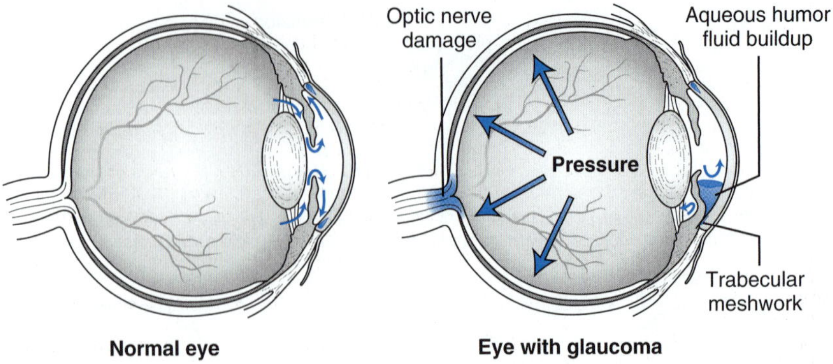

Fig. 2.3. Acute Angle Glaucoma. *(From Glaucoma, Garden City Eye Care. Available at:* http://gardencityeyecare.com/glaucoma/. *Accessed 15.07.16.)*

be seen with a slit lamp when the beam is passed from the lateral eye through the anterior chamber, known as "cell and flare." Conjunctival injection is typically adjacent to the iris, versus conjunctivitis, where the erythema is predominantly peripheral.

13. Why is iritis painful? How is it treated?

Iritis causes inflammation of the circular muscles of the iris, so when bright light stimulates pupillary constriction, pain is worsened. This inflammation can sometimes cause transient paralysis of the muscle, causing an asymmetric pupil. Iritis is treated with cycloplegic/parasympatholytic drops, which are always found in bottles with red caps (e.g., atropine, homatropine, cyclopentolate).

14. Do any studies need to be performed on a patient with a subconjunctival hemorrhage?

The condition is most commonly caused by a sudden increase in globe pressure that occurs when coughing, sneezing, vomiting, or straining; the hemorrhage is painless, does not require treatment, and typically resolves in 10 to 20 days. Patients taking warfarin should have levels checked.

15. What is hyphema?

Hyphema is bleeding into the anterior chamber, typically caused by trauma to the globe. The blood collection in the anterior chamber will form a fluid level that can be seen anterior to the iris. Patients with hyphema should remain in the sitting position. Hyphema that is greater than 33% of the iris, or any elevation of intraocular pressure, should be referred to an ophthalmologist as red blood cells can obstruct flow through the trabecular meshwork and elevate intraocular pressure.

16. Why is acute angle glaucoma made worse by the dark?

In patients with glaucoma, pupil dilation (mydriasis) blocks the canal of Schlemm, which drains the aqueous humor from the orbit. In turn, the pressure increase within the posterior chamber elicits pain (Fig. 2.3). Vision loss occurs when pressure from the fluid compresses the blood vessels surrounding the optic nerve, causing ischemia. Treatment of acute angle glaucoma should focus first on constricting the pupil (meiosis).

KEY POINTS

1. "Eye pain" should be carefully examined to determine if the problem is in the soft tissue or the orbit.
2. Visual acuity should be the first component of every eye exam.
3. Fluorescein stain is a helpful tool in most eye exams.

BIBLIOGRAPHY

Acute Angle Glaucoma. Glaucoma. Garden City Eye Care. <http://gardencityeyecare.com/glaucoma/>; Accessed 14.07.16.

Conjunctivitis Preferred Practice Patterns–2015. American Academy of Ophthalmology. <http://www.aao.org/summary-benchmark-detail/conjunctivitis-summary-benchmark–october-2012>; Accessed 23.05.16.

Garrity J: *Blepharitis.* Merck Manual Online, Professional Version. <http://www.merckmanuals.com/professional/eye-disorders/eyelid-and-lacrimal-disorders/blepharitis>; Accessed 15.06.16.

Garrity J: *Chalazion and hordeolum (stye).* Merck Manual Online, Professional Version. <http://www.merckmanuals.com/professional/eye-disorders/eyelid-and-lacrimal-disorders/chalazion-and-hordeolum-stye>; Accessed 15.06.16.

Garrity J: *Preseptal and orbital cellulitis.* Merck Manual Online, Professional Version. <http://www.merckmanuals.com/professional/eye-disorders/orbital-diseases/preseptal-and-orbital-cellulitis>; Accessed 01.07.16.

Knoop K, Dennis W, Hedges J. Ophthalmologic, otolaryngologic, and dental procedures. In: *Roberts and Hedges: Clinical Procedures in Emergency Medicine.* 5th ed. Philadelphia: Saunders Elsevier; 2010:1141–1177.

Oldham G: Hyphema. American Academy of Ophthalmology, EyeWiki. <http://eyewiki.aao.org/Hyphema>; Accessed 03.07.16.

Primary Angle Closure Summary Benchmark–2016. American Academy of Ophthalmology. <http://www.aao.org/summary-benchmark-detail/primary-angle-closure-summary-benchmark-october-2>; Accessed 12.07.16.

Styes and Chalazions Guide: Causes, Symptoms, and Treatment Options. <Drugs.com. https://www.drugs.com/health-guide/styes-and-chalazions.html>; Accessed 14.07.16.

CHAPTER 3

EAR, NOSE, AND THROAT

Samantha F. Singer, PA-C

1. What are the common causes of otalgia?

Common causes are otitis media, cerumen impaction, and otitis externa, as well as referred pain from the throat or temporal bone. Less common causes include foreign body in the ear canal, mastoiditis, perichondritis, external ear dermatitis/cellulitis, or ear tumors (such as eosinophilic granulomas or rhabdosarcomas).

2. How does otitis media typically present?

Ear pain, associated upper respiratory infection symptoms (including rhinitis and cough), constitutional symptoms (such as irritability, difficulty sleeping, or poor appetite in a child), and fever.

3. What are the common tympanic membrane findings with otitis media?

The tympanic membrane (TM) may be cloudy and opacified or appear red. There is often bulging, loss of landmarks (inability to see the umbo), and absent light reflex.

4. Which organisms typically cause otitis media?

Bacterial causes include *Streptococcus pneumoniae, Haemophilus influenzae,* and *Moraxella catarrhalis.* Viruses (including respiratory syncytial virus [RSV], adenovirus, rhinovirus, or influenza) account for less than 10% of otitis media; however, coinfection with bacteria is common in children.

5. What is the recommended treatment for otitis media?

Duration on first-line treatment may be 5–7 days; if recurrent otitis media, duration is recommended to be 7–10 days (Table 3.1). Azithromycin and trimethoprim/sulfamethoxazole are no longer recommended for routine use for acute otitis media due to increased antibiotic resistance.

6. What is mastoiditis?

A complication of acute otitis media, where the infection causes inflammation of the mastoid bone; subdivided into two categories: osteitis within the mastoid air-cell system and periosteitis of the mastoid process.

Table 3.1. Treatment of Otitis Media

RECOMMENDED FIRST-LINE TREATMENT	RECOMMENDED FIRST-LINE TREATMENT IF PENICILLIN ALLERGIC	SECOND-LINE TREATMENT, AFTER FAILURE TO FIRST-LINE ANTIBIOTIC
Amoxicillin 875 mg po bid	Cefdinir 300 mg po bid	Clindamycin 300 mg po tid/qid
Amoxicillin/clavulanate 875 mg/125 mg po bid	Cefuroxime 500 mg po bid	Levofloxacin 500 mg po qd
	Cefpodoxime 200 mg po bid	Moxifloxacin 400 mg po qd
	Ceftriaxone 2 g IM/IV qd x 1 or 3 days	May use amoxicillin/clavulanate or ceftriaxone IM/IV, if not used previously

Adapted from Harmes KM, Blackwood RA, Burrows HL, et al: Otitis Media: Diagnosis and Treatment. *Am Fam Physician* 89(5):318, 2014. Available at: http://www.aafp.org/afp/2013/1001/p435.html. Accessed 24.10.16; Natal BA: Acute Otitis Media Empiric Therapy. Medscape. Available at: http://emedicine.medscape.com/article/2012609-overview. Accessed 24.10.16.

7. How does mastoiditis present?

Pain located over the mastoid. Patients often complain of pain deep within the ear or behind the ear, with associated tenderness over the mastoid process. Mastoiditis can present at any age but is most common at age 2 years and younger, thus making localization of pain a difficult diagnostic indicator. There may also be a persistent fever (despite adequate antibiotic treatment for acute otitis media), mastoid erythema, or proptosis of the auricle.

8. What are the complications of mastoiditis?

Hearing loss, facial nerve palsy, cranial nerve involvement, osteomyelitis, labyrinthitis, sigmoid sinus thrombosis, and abscess formation.

9. What are the treatment recommendations for mastoiditis?

Subacute mastoiditis (mastoiditis without osteitis or periostitis) may be treated with purely medical management. Patients should be prescribed antibiotic coverage similar to otitis media with close follow-up. If worsening of pain or no significant improvement in 48 hours, patients should be referred to ENT as they will most likely require tympanoplasty (treatment and diagnostic for bacterial culture), imaging (CT scan or MRI for evaluation of extension of disease), and/or mastoidectomy.

10. What are the most common causes of a perforated tympanic membrane?

Trauma (including physical abuse, foreign body, or forceful ear irrigation), infection, and middle ear barotrauma (such as a blast trauma, scuba diving injury, or airplane ascent/descent).

11. How is a perforated tympanic membrane best managed in the urgent care setting?

The ear canal may be cleaned using gentle suction; do not irrigate the ear canal, as water in the middle ear may introduce bacteria and cause infection. Treat concurrent otitis media with antibiotic drops or oral antibiotics. In regard to antibiotic ear drops, avoid gentamicin, neomycin sulfate, or tobramycin, as they carry the risk of ototoxicity. May use ofloxacin otic, ciprofloxacin eye drops, or Ciprodex.[1] Prophylactic antibiotics (for perforated tympanic membrane in absence of acute infection) is only advised if the injury involved contamination with lake water, seawater, or a dirty object such as a tree branch. Advise patient to keep ear dry: use ear plugs for showering and avoid submerging head underwater. Recommend appropriate analgesia; oral nonsteroidal antiinflammatory drugs (NSAIDs) typically are sufficient.

12. What symptoms or physical exam findings warrant referral to an otolaryngologist?

The majority (80%–90%) of tympanic membrane perforations will heal spontaneously in 4–6 weeks. Referral to an otolaryngologist is advised for large or marginal perforations (as they may require surgery) and for patients with nystagmus, vertigo, profound hearing loss, or disruption of the ossicles.

13. How does otitis externa typically present?

Patients with otitis externa will often complain of ear pain, pruritus, otorrhea, and hearing loss. Pain may be exacerbated by chewing and other auricle movement. Inspection of otorrhea can act as a diagnostic indicator to the cause of otitis externa, as acute bacterial otitis externa will often have a white purulent drainage, whereas fungal otitis externa (otomycosis) will have a fluffy cottonlike grayish or black material.

14. What are the most common bacterial causes of otitis externa?

Staphylococcus aureus, Streptococcus pyogenes, Pseudomonas aeruginosa, and *Vibrio alginolyticus* are the bacteria most often associated with otitis externa.

15. How is otitis externa best treated?

Otitis externa is treated first with removal of the debris/purulent drainage with ear canal suctioning or ear irrigation, second with prescription ear drops specific to causative agent (Table 3.2), and third with management of pain either using topical analgesic agents such as Auralgan or tetracaine or oral analgesic agents such as NSAIDs. Often otitis externa will require placement of an ear wick to allow for medication penetration.

16. What are the recommendations for swimmers in regard to returning to the water?

Otitis externa is five times more common in swimmers than in nonswimmers. Conservative recommendation would be to avoid submersion for 7–10 days. To help prevent reoccurrence, advising use of ear plugs is a good idea.

Table 3.2. Treatment of Otitis Externa

UNCOMPLICATED BACTERIAL INFECTION	UNCOMPLICATED FUNGAL INFECTION
Neomycin-polymyxin B-hydrocortisone otic 4 drops in the affected ear tid or qid for 10 days	Acetic acid 2% with or without hydrocortisone otic 4 drops in the affected ear qid for 7 days
Ofloxacin 0.3% otic 10 drops in the affected ear once daily for 7 days	Clotrimazole 1% otic 4 drops in the affected ear qid for 7 days
Ciprofloxacin-hydrocortisone otic 3 drops in the affected ear bid for 7 days	

17. **How can otitis externa be prevented?**

Otitis externa is primarily caused by moisture and warmth in the ear canal, creating an environment conducive to bacterial growth. Preventative techniques include avoiding moisture from entering the canal (whether with tight-fitting swimming cap, ear plugs, etc.), drying the ear canal (such as with a hair dryer on lowest setting after bathing or swimming), or instilling one to two drops of otic acetic acid or aluminum acetate (Burrow solution) after bathing or swimming.

18. **What causes cerumen impaction?**

Cerumen, or earwax, is a naturally occurring substance in the ear canal, composed of secretions, sloughed epithelial cells, and hair. Typically, cerumen is naturally extruded, although sometimes it can accumulate and occlude the canal. Cerumen impaction can present with otalgia, hearing loss, clogged sensation, tinnitus, dizziness, and chronic cough (due to irritation of the auricular branch of the vagus nerve).

19. **How is cerumen impaction treated?**

Removal of cerumen can be performed with use of cerumenolytic agents (acetic acid, hydrogen peroxide, carbamide peroxide, or mineral oil), manual removal (using ear curette or forceps for large clumps of cerumen), and/or ear irrigation. Studies have shown no significant difference between effectiveness of varying cerumenolytic agents. Approximately 40% of patients with cerumen impaction can clear ear wax with use of a cerumenolytic agent alone (without irrigation).

20. **What are the most common ear/nose foreign bodies?**

Common ear foreign bodies include insects, plastic toys/beads, cotton such as tip from cotton swab/Q-tip, organic material such as popcorn kernels or candy, and small batteries. Organic material increases risk of bacterial infection, and batteries (especially button batteries) can be caustic.

21. **How do ear/nose foreign bodies typically present?**

Ear foreign bodies often present with ear pain, foreign body sensation, hearing loss/muffled hearing, and/or malodorous otorrhea. Nose foreign bodies often present with nasal pain, malodorous unilateral rhinorrhea, and/or epistaxis. Foreign bodies are more common in children, though not exclusively. Also, if foreign body is present in a child, ensure examination includes checking other orifices for additional foreign bodies, as multiple foreign bodies is not uncommon.

22. **Where is the most common location for an ear foreign body to become lodged/stuck?**

The narrowest portion of the external auditory canal is at the bony cartilaginous junction, which is the most common place for a foreign body.

23. **Where is the most common location for a nasal foreign body to become lodged/stuck?**

Nasal foreign bodies are most often located on the floor of the nasal passage just below the inferior turbinate or in the upper nasal fossa anterior to the middle turbinate.

24. **What is the best way to remove a foreign body from the ear?**

There are multiple techniques, and the choice is best determined by the clinical situation: type of foreign body, compliance of patient, associated factors (amount of associated edema/pain, concern for perforated TM, etc.). Options include ear irrigation, use of forceps (bayonet or alligator), cerumen loop, suction catheters, or magnet (for metal foreign bodies). Live insects should be killed prior to removal; you may place several drops of alcohol, 2% lidocaine, or mineral oil into the ear canal. Irrigation should not be used if foreign body is a battery due to concern for electrical current and/or battery contents causing tissue necrosis.

25. **What is the best way to remove a foreign body from the nose?**
As with ear foreign bodies, there are multiple techniques that can be utilized for nasal foreign body removal. Often before attempting removal, 0.5% phenylephrine or topical lidocaine can be used to reduce mucosal edema and to provide analgesia, respectively. First-line treatment should be to encourage the patient to expel the foreign body by blowing the nose while obstructing/blocking the opposite nostril. For young children, positive pressure ventilation can be delivered either using a small bag valve mask (BVM)—placed over the mouth with provider or parent using a finger to close the naris absent a foreign body—or having a parent blow a puff of air in the child's mouth while using a finger to close the naris absent a foreign body. For easily visualized and easily grasped foreign bodies, direct instrumentation (e.g., forceps, hook) is often preferred. Another technique is placing a thin, lubricated, balloon-tip catheter beyond the foreign body and inflating the balloon, then pulling the inflated catheter balloon forward. Gentle suction can also be utilized for foreign body removal.
   Sedation is typically not advised due to decreasing gag reflex and glottis closure, therefore increasing risk of choking/aspiration.

26. **When should a patient with an ear/nose foreign body be referred to an otolaryngologist?**
Success rates for removing the foreign body significantly decline after the first attempt; also, multiple attempts cause complications of increased pain and bleeding, thus limiting visualization and causing the foreign body to extend further into the canal. A patient should be referred to an otolaryngologist if there have been multiple unsuccessful attempts or if there is concern for trauma to the TM.

27. **What are common causes of epistaxis?**
Most cases of epistaxis are caused by direct trauma; however, epistaxis can also be caused by repetitive nasal mucosa irritation (such as with rhinitis), corticosteroid nasal sprays (such as Flonase or Nasonex), anticoagulant therapy (such as warfarin, Xarelto, Pradaxa), coagulopathy disorder, arteriovenous malformation, among others. A good history of present illness and medical history can help to determine if the epistaxis is benign or an indicator of a more serious condition.

28. **What is the most common site of bleeding for epistaxis?**
Anterior epistaxis is the most common etiology for nasal bleeds, accounting for more than 90% of bleeds. The most common site of anterior epistaxis is Little area, also known as Kiesselbach plexus.

29. **How is epistaxis best managed in the urgent care setting?**
Direct visualization of the bleed is beneficial; however, it can be difficult initially. Using phenylephrine or oxymetazoline nasal spray or soaking a cotton ball in topical tetracaine, epinephrine (adrenaline), and cocaine (TAC) solution or lidocaine epinephrine tetracaine and placing in naris for 10 to 15 minutes with associated 10–15 minutes of digital pressure anterior to the nasal bone occluding both nares may stop bleeding. Even if hemostasis is achieved with digital pressure alone, further measures should be considered to prevent rebleeding, such as electrocautery or silver nitrate cautery, application of a gel sponge (e.g., Gelfoam), and/or nasal packing. Patients who receive nasal packing should be placed on prophylactic antibiotics such as cephalexin (250–500 milligrams [mg] three times a day [tid]) or amoxicillin/clavulanate (875 mg/125 mg twice a day [bid]); for patients with a penicillin allergy, try clindamycin (150–450 mg four times a day [qid]) or sulfamethoxazole/trimethoprim (800 mg/160 mg). Packing should be removed 48 hours after placement.

30. **Which patients with epistaxis should not be managed in an outpatient setting?**
Patients who are not hemodynamically stable, have a coagulopathy disorder, have respiratory or cardiac compromise from the nasal bleeding, or have failed hemostasis attempts should be referred to the emergency department.

31. **How does rhinitis typically present?**
Rhinitis, inflammation of the nasal membranes, most commonly presents with nasal congestion, rhinorrhea, sneezing, and nasal pruritus. Rhinitis is most commonly allergic.

32. How is rhinitis treated?

First-line treatment for rhinitis includes oral antihistamines (such as first-generation H_1 blockers [diphenhydramine] or nonsedating/less sedation second-generation H_1 blockers [loratadine, fexofenadine, cetirizine]) along with intranasal corticosteroids (fluticasone or mometasone). Patients who fail to respond to first-line treatment can be referred to an allergist for consideration for immunotherapy.

33. How does sinusitis typically present?

Acute sinusitis or acute rhinosinusitis is one of the most common conditions that medical providers treat in the urgent care setting. Patients will complain of pain overlying frontal or maxillary sinuses, radiating pain to teeth and/or exacerbated with bending down, referred pain to temple or ear, postnasal drip, nasal congestion, and hyposmia.

34. What are the most common causes of rhinosinusitis?

Rhinosinusitis episodes are most commonly viral in origin, including rhinovirus, influenza, and parainfluenza. Viral upper respiratory tract infections (URIs) are the number one risk factor for development of acute bacterial sinusitis. Approximately 90% of patients with a viral URI have sinus involvement, and 5%–10% of these patients have bacterial superinfection requiring antibiotic treatment. The most common bacterial causes of rhinosinusitis are *Streptococcus pneumoniae, Haemophilus influenzae, Moraxella catarrhalis,* and *Staphylococcus aureus.* Fungal sinusitis is rare, but the most common fungal species associated with sinusitis are Aspergillus and Alternaria.

35. What are the indications that acute sinusitis is bacterial in origin and warrants antibiotic treatment?

Double sickening (initially got better, but then worsened), purulent rhinorrhea, purulent secretion in the nasal cavity, and elevated erythrocyte sedimentation rate increase the likelihood of bacterial etiology. Guidelines also suggest prescribing a patient an antibiotic if symptoms fail to improve within 7–10 days. Radiography is not recommended for evaluation of uncomplicated acute rhinosinusitis.

36. What are some alternative/adjunctive treatment options of sinusitis?

Patients may have symptom improvement with analgesics, oral decongestants, topical decongestants, mucolytics, intranasal corticosteroids, saline nasal irrigation, or oral antihistamines. There is limited evidence to suggest significant benefit from the aforementioned therapies.

37. What is the best antibiotic treatment for acute rhinosinusitis?

Antibiotic course should be prescribed for 10 days (Table 3.3).

Continued symptoms despite second-line treatment typically warrants computerized tomography (CT) of the sinuses (without contrast) for evaluation of possible complications or anatomic abnormalities and/or referral to an otolaryngologist.

38. How does pharyngitis typically present?

Pharyngitis most commonly presents with sore throat. Patients may also have low-grade fever, dysphagia, odynophagia, or hoarseness.

Table 3.3. Treatment of Rhinosinusitis

FIRST-LINE TREATMENT	SECOND-LINE TREATMENT
Amoxicillin 500 mg po tid or 875 mg po bid	Amoxicillin/clavulanate 875 mg/125 mg po bid
Clarithromycin 250–500 mg po bid	Cefuroxime 250–500 mg po bid
Azithromycin 500 mg po qd x 1 day, then 250 mg po qd x 4 days	Levofloxacin 500 mg po qd
	Trovafloxacin 200 mg po qd
	Clindamycin 300 mg po tid

39. What are the red flags associated with a sore throat?

Red flags with pharyngitis include associated unilateral sore throat pain, drooling/inability to swallow, trismus, muffled/"hot potato" voice, stridor/respiratory distress, or high fever.

40. What are the causes of pharyngitis?

Most common causes are viral or bacterial illness (including streptococcal pharyngitis). Sore throat can also be due to postnasal drip associated with upper respiratory infection or seasonal allergies or recurrent irritation from gastroesophageal reflux disease. Patients would then present with associated rhinorrhea, sneezing, nasal congestion, cough or eructation, epigastric discomfort, bloating, and so forth, respective to the disease process. Concerning causes of pharyngitis include peritonsillar abscess, Ludwig angina, foreign body, malignancy, epiglottitis, and diphtheria, among others.

41. How is streptococcal pharyngitis diagnosed?

On physical examination, a practitioner can use the modified Centor criteria: tonsillar exudate or erythema, anterior cervical lymphadenopathy, absent cough, present fever, and differential based on age (+1 point if age 3–14, 0 points if age 15–45, and −1 point if over age 45). Strep score of 4–5 warrants empiric treatment with antibiotics. Controversy exists in regard to empiric treatment. Rapid streptococcal antigen tests are frequently used for diagnostic purposes. Specificity and sensitivity vary based on test manufacturer; however, generally the tests are high in positive predictive values (90%–98%) but insufficient sensitivity to rule out group A beta-hemolytic streptococci (GABHS) infection (ranging from 79% to 95%). Negative rapid streptococcal antigen tests should be confirmed with culture. Culture for GABHS is 90%–95% sensitive and 94%–100% specific.

42. What are some caveats to streptococcal pharyngitis testing?

An estimated 15%–20% of the population are GABHS carriers, which will give a positive result on both the rapid streptococcal antigen tests and throat cultures, as neither test is specific for active infection. This results in overtreatment of a significant portion of patients. Also, an estimated 33% of patients with infectious mononucleosis and diphtheria have positive GABHS cultures, leading to misdiagnoses.

43. Does streptococcal pharyngitis require antibiotic treatment?

GABHS infection is a self-limited disease, often resolving in 3–5 days without treatment. However, streptococcal pharyngitis is treated for prevention of serious sequelae including rheumatic fever and glomerulonephritis.

44. What is the recommended treatment for streptococcal pharyngitis?

First line treatment for GABHS is penicillin, amoxicillin, or first-generation cephalosporin, clindamycin, or macrolide antibiotics (for patients allergic to penicillin). Other causes of pharyngitis such as candidal or herpetic should be treated appropriately based on causative agent, such as oral fluconazole, itraconazole or acyclovir, and famciclovir, respectively.

45. What is a peritonsillar abscess?

A peritonsillar abscess is the progression of a bacterial infection—exudative tonsillitis, to cellulitis, to abscess. The abscess generally forms in the Weber glands (group of salivary glands in the supratonsillar fossa). Presenting symptoms are similar to pharyngitis (fever, sore throat, dysphagia, odynophagia); however, on physical examination there may be trismus and/or a muffled/"hot potato" voice. Inspection of the oropharynx reveals edema and erythema of the anterior tonsillar pillar with tonsil displacement and contralateral deviation of the uvula.

46. What are the complications/concerns with a peritonsillar abscess?

The primary concern with a peritonsillar abscess is airway obstruction. However, there is also the possibility of aspiration pneumonitis, hemorrhage from erosion or septic necrosis into carotid sheath, or extension of the infection into the soft tissues of the deep neck or posterior mediastinum.

47. How is a peritonsillar abscess treated?

Treatment of choice for a peritonsillar abscess is needle aspiration or incision and drainage. Patients should then be placed on a broad spectrum antibiotic. In the outpatient setting oral options include amoxicillin/clavulanate (875 mg/125 mg bid), clindamycin (600 mg bid or 300 mg qid), or penicillin (500 mg qid) plus metronidazole (500 mg qid). Recent studies suggest an adjunctive corticosteroid can speed recovery. Patients with a peritonsillar abscess require close follow-up and should be reseen in 1–2 days.

48. How does mononucleosis present?

Mononucleosis, or Epstein-Barr virus, typically presents initially with mild flulike symptoms for a few days. Patients will then develop fever, sore throat, and lymphadenopathy; exudate tonsillitis and prominent cervical lymphadenopathy present in 97% of patients. Other common associated symptoms include fatigue, malaise, myalgias, and headache. Mononucleosis has highest incidence in the 15- to 24-year-old age group and increased frequency on college campuses and among military recruits (due to congested, confined spaces).

49. What are some diagnostic testing options for mononucleosis?

One of the most common tests is the mononuclear spot (monospot) test, which tests for heterophile antibody (Paul-Bunnell IgM). The monospot test has a high false-negative rate in the first week of symptoms (25%). Antibodies peak between weeks 2 and 5. The monospot test has a low false-negative rate by the third week of symptoms (5%). The test has low accuracy for children, as less than 50% of children under age 12 will develop the antibodies. Other testing includes a complete blood count (CBC) for reevaluation of lymphocyte count and predominance as well as lymphocyte atypia. Liver function tests are abnormal in 80% of mononucleosis patients. An Epstein-Barr virus antibody test can also be ordered; however, in an urgent care center this is expensive and is typically sent out to a lab, so it should only be ordered if the results would change management of the disease.

50. What is the best treatment for mononucleosis?

Most of the treatment for mononucleosis is symptomatic: rest (as patients tend to have fatigue), analgesic agents (NSAIDs or acetaminophen), and oral corticosteroid (such as prednisone or dexamethasone) for severe tonsillar enlargement/odynophagia. Approximately 75% of patients with mononucleosis have splenomegaly and should be advised limited exercise/athletics and no contact sport (due to risk of splenic rupture) for 4 weeks minimum, or longer if splenomegaly has not resolved.

KEY POINTS

1. Of tympanic membrane perforations, 80%–90% will heal spontaneously in 4–6 weeks.
2. Rhinitis is most commonly allergic.

REFERENCE

1. Caterino JM, Kahan S. *In a Page: Emergency Medicine*. Philadelphia: Lippincott Williams & Wilkins; 2003:226.

BIBLIOGRAPHY

Aghababian RV. *Essentials of Emergency Medicine*. Burlington, MA: Jones & Bartlett Learning; 2010:236–237.

Aring AM, Chan MM. Current concepts in adult acute rhinosinusitis. *Am Fam Physician*. 2016;94(2):97–105.

Block L, Harrison C. *Diagnosis and Management of Acute Otitis Media*. West Islip, NY: Professional Communications; 2005:90.

Brook I: Acute sinusitis. <http://emedicine.medscape.com/article/232670>; Accessed 24.10.16.

Caterino JM, Kahan S. *In a Page: Emergency Medicine*. Philadelphia: Lippincott Williams & Wilkins; 2003:226.

Devan PP: Mastoiditis. Medscape. <http://emedicine.medscape.com/article/2056657-overview>; Accessed 24.10.16.

DiMuzio J, Deschler DG. Emergency department management of foreign bodies of the external ear canal in children. *Otol Neurotol*. 2002;23:473–475.

Doern GV, Pfaller MA, Kugler K, et al. Prevalence of antimicrobial resistance among respiratory tract isolates of *Streptococcus pneumoniae* in North America: 1997 results from the SENTRY antimicrobial surveillance program. *Clin Infect Dis*. 1998;27(4):764–770.

Domino FJ, Baldor RA, Grimes JA, et al. *Griffith's 5 Minute Clinical Consult*. Philadelphia: Lippincott Williams & Wilkins; 2014:740.

Engelkirk PG, Duben-Engelkirk JL. *Laboratory Diagnosis of Infectious Diseases: Essentials of Diagnostic Microbiology*. Philadelphia: Lippincott Williams & Wilkins; 2015:458.

Fischer JI: Nasal foreign bodies. Medscape. <http://emedicine.medscape.com/article/763767-overview#a8>; Accessed 24.10.16.

Galioto NJ. Peritonsillar abscess. *Am Fam Physician*. 2008;77(2):199–202.

Hand C, Harvey I. The effectiveness of topical preparations for the treatment of earwax: a systematic review. *Br J Gen Pract*. 2004;54:862–867.

Heim SW, Maughan KL. Foreign bodies in the ear, nose, and throat. *Am Fam Physician*. 2007;76(8):1185–1189. <http://www.aafp.org/afp/2007/1015/p1185.html>; Accessed 24.10.16.

Hom D. *Essential Tissue Healing of the Face and Neck*. Shelton, CT: PMPH-USA; 2009:150.

Kalra MK, Higgins KE, Perez ED. Common questions about streptococcal pharyngitis. *Am Fam Physician*. 2016;94(1):24–31. <http://www.aafp.org/afp/2016/0701/p24.html>; Accessed 24.10.16.

Kaushik V, Malik T, Saeed SR. Interventions for acute otitis externa. *Cochrane Database Syst Rev 1*(January 20). 2010. CD004740. <https://www.ncbi.nlm.nih.gov/pubmed/20091565>; Accessed 24.10.16.

Kiger JR, Brenkert TE, Losek JD. Nasal foreign body removal in children. *Pediatr Emerg Care.* 2008;24(11):785–792.

Lieberthal AS, Carroll AE, Chonmaitree T, et al. The diagnosis and management of acute otitis media. *Pediatrics.* 2013;131(3):e964–e999.

Mahadevan SV, Garmel GM. *An Introduction to Clinical Emergency Medicine.* Cambridge, MA: Cambridge University Press; 2012:332.

Matz G, Rybak L, Roland PS, et al. Ototoxicity of ototopical antibiotic drops in humans. *Otolaryngol Head Neck Surg.* 2004;130(suppl 3):S79–S82. <https://www.ncbi.nlm.nih.gov/pubmed/15054365>; Accessed 24.10.16.

Moses S: Mononucleosis. Family Practice Notebook. <http://www.fpnotebook.com/ID/Virus/Mncls.htm>; Accessed 24.10.16.

Rovers MM, Schilder AG, Zielhuis, et al. Otitis media. *Lancet.* 2004;363:465–473. <http://www.aafp.org/afp/2007/1201/p1650.pdf>; Accessed 24.10.16.

Rutter P, Newby D. *Community Pharmacy ANZ: Symptoms, Diagnosis and Treatment.* Cambridge, MA: Elsevier Health Sciences; 2015:78.

Sanders MJ, Lewis LM, McKenn KD, et al. *Mosby's Paramedic Textbook.* Burlington, MA: Jones & Bartlett Publishers; 2012:730.

Schade J. *The Complete Encyclopedia of Medicine & Health.* Yardville, NJ: Foreign Media Group; 2006:339.

Sloane PD. *Essentials of Family Medicine.* Philadelphia: Lippincott Williams & Wilkins; 2008:292.

Togias AG. Systemic immunologic and inflammatory aspects of allergic rhinitis. *J Allergy Clin Immunol.* 2000;106(suppl 5):S247–S250.

Wolfson AB, Hendey GW, Ling LJ, et al. *Harwood-Nuss Clinical Practice of Emergency Medicine.* 5th ed. Philadelphia: Lippincott Williams & Wilkins; 2012:395.

Womack J, Jimenez M. Common questions about infectious mononucleosis. *Am Fam Physician.* 2015;91(6):372–376.

CHAPTER 4

DENTAL AND MOUTH PAIN

Spencer Adoff, MD

1. What is the anatomy of a tooth?
The crown is the visible portion of the tooth, which consists of three layers: The pulp (neurovascular supply of the tooth) is surrounded by dentin, which is covered by enamel. The root is the portion of the tooth that extends into the bone. It is covered by cementum, which adheres to the periodontal ligament.

2. How are teeth numbered? (Fig. 4.1)

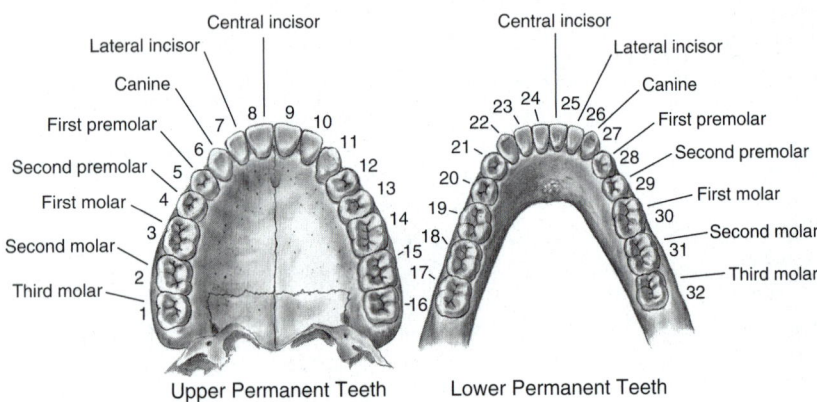

Fig. 4.1. Tooth identification using either name or American Dental Association numbering system; letters for deciduous teeth, numbers for permanent teeth. *(From* Mosby's Guide to Physical Examination, *2006.)*

3. Describe the types of dental fractures.
Ellis type I is a fracture of the enamel only and does not require treatment. Ellis type II fractures to the dentin are most common, and the tooth is usually sensitive to changes in temperature. Ellis type III (blood exposure) fractures expose the pulp. Types II and III require placement of a protective covering, such as calcium hydroxide base, as a delay in treatment increases the likelihood of pulpal necrosis. Patients need urgent referral to a dentist. Root fractures will have mobility of the crown (with or without Ellis fractures); radiographs will confirm. Alveolar fractures will allow multiple teeth to move together with palpation (Fig. 4.2).

4. Describe and define the different types of dental trauma.
See Table 4.1.

5. What is the treatment for an avulsed tooth?
The best way to transport the tooth is in the patient's tooth socket. Gently rinse (to remove debris) and replace it (only primary teeth should be reimplanted). Handle the tooth by the crown, as not to damage the periodontal ligament. It should be reimplanted within 2 hours, and stabilized with a dental dressing paste. If it cannot be reimplanted, use Hank salt-based solution or cold milk. The patient's saliva is less ideal, and do not place the tooth in the mouth due to risk of aspiration.

6. Which gum lacerations need to be sutured?
Gum lacerations that require suturing are those that are large, have flaps, or expose bone.

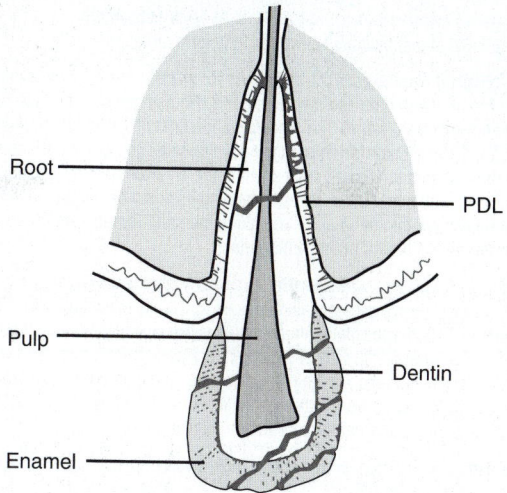

Fig. 4.2. Dental Tooth Fracture. *(From Curtis, Emergency and Trauma Care for Nurses and Paramedics, 2011.)*

Table 4.1. Types of Dental Trauma	
Concussion	Normal appearance, but will have pain with pressure (biting)
Subluxation	Loose tooth, without displacement; bleeding at the gumline
Intrusion	Tooth is driven upwards into the socket; bleeding at the gumline
Extrusion	Tooth is dislocated from the socket; bleeding at the gumline
Luxation	Tooth is displaced lateral, labial (toward lip), lingual (toward back/tongue)
Avulsion	Tooth is completely displaced from the socket

7. Describe the types of dental infections.

With dental caries, instruct patients to use fluoride mouth rinses and toothpastes to reduce occurrences. Irreversible pulpitis causes acute, severe pain and is a common cause for patients to seek nondental care. Gingivitis commonly has bleeding from the gums; and treatment consists of good brushing, flossing, warm saltwater rinses five times per day, and chlorhexadine (0.12%) rinses twice per day. Acute necrotizing ulcerative gingivitis (ANUG) consists of diffuse mouth pain, halitosis, and pain with chewing. Patients will have bleeding gums and sloughing of the gingiva with gray-white pseudomembrane, which will bleed when removed. Treatment consists of chlorhexadine or hydrogen peroxide rinses, pain control, debridement of the pseudomembrane (gauze), and antibiotics if extensive/systemic or lymphadenopathic. Periodontitis is a severe progression of gingival inflammation, loss of tooth attachment, and tooth loss/mobility. It generally affects young adults. Treat with chlorhexadine rinses and systemic antibiotics. Periapical abscesses have painful swelling at the buccal and gingival mucosa. The teeth may be sensitive and have pain with chewing. Treatment consists of incision and drainage and antibiotics.

8. Which antibiotics should I use for the dental infections described above?

Penicillin VK, amoxicillin-clavulanate, ampicillin-sulbactam, erythromycin, clindamycin, metronidazole. Beta-lactamase production within oral bacteria is becoming increasingly common; penicillin monotherapy may no longer be enough.

9. What are aphthous ulcers (canker sores)?

Canker sores are a chronic inflammatory and ulcerative disorder of unknown etiology. Patients will have painful, single, small, circular ulcerations. They are treated with topical anesthetics and cleansing rinses. They can be differed from oral herpes simplex virus 1 (HSV-1), which are small, painful, clustered vesicles. HSV-1 can be treated with topical acyclovir early in its course.

10. **What are the three main salivary glands that form stones?**
Parotid, submandibular, and sublingual salivary glands form stones.

11. **What are the clinical features that suggest a patient may have sialolithiasis?**
Patients typically present with pain and swelling of the affected gland, which will be exaggerated by anything that stimulates salivation. They may also present with painless swelling of the gland. Symptoms may be persistent or intermittent over days to weeks due to complete versus incomplete obstruction. You may be able to palpate stones within the Wharton duct by palpating on the floor of the mouth from a lingual to labial direction. Parotid gland stones may be palpated within the Stenson duct along the buccal mucosa within the mouth, and along the face from the earlobe along the mandible (place one finger within the mouth at the same time).

12. **When should you suspect sialadenitis and how should you treat it?**
Patients may have systemic symptoms such as fevers and chills in conjunction with pain, swelling, and erythema around the affected gland. Viral infections are typically bilateral, compared to bacterial infections, which are unilateral. You may see purulent drainage from the respective duct. Treatment consists of antibiotics, sialagogues, gentle heat, massage, and pain control. Consider clindamycin, amoxicillin-clavulanate, or cephalexin with metronidazole; 7 to 10 days should be effective. Lack of improvement or worsening of the patient's condition may suggest abscess formation.

13. **What are the most common presenting signs and symptoms of temporal mandibular disorder (TMD)?**
Facial pain triggered by jaw motions (chewing and speaking), limitation of jaw movements, temporal mandibular joint tenderness, popping sounds with jaw function, headaches, ear pain, neck stiffness, and pain.

14. **What treatment recommendations are there for TMD?**
Pharmacologic (NSAIDs and muscle relaxers for 14 days) and nonpharmacologic (patient education and behavioral modification) treatments are recommended.

15. **What does oral candidiasis look like?**
It is a white-cream, curdlike exudate; it could be scraped off, leaving raw or bleeding mucosa. It is most commonly on the tongue but may be present on the buccal mucosa, soft palate, and hypopharynx.

16. **What are the symptoms?**
Asymptomatic, pain with eating, loss of taste, change of sensation within the oral cavity.

17. **What patients are at risk for oral candidiasis?**
Infants, patients who wear dentures, patients on antibiotics or receiving chemotherapy, those getting radiation to the head/neck, all patients who are immunocompromised, such as those who have HIV/AIDS.

18. **What are the preferred treatment regimens for non-HIV- and HIV-induced oral candidiasis?**
Clotrimazole troches, miconazole buccal tablets, nystatin swish and swallow for 7 to 14 days. Failure of local therapy may require oral fluconazole. If patients wear dentures, they should remove them nightly, brush them, and soak them in chlorhexidine in addition to the local or oral therapies. If patients have HIV, you may try the above for mild disease, but for more serious or recurrent episodes, utilize fluconazole as first-line treatment.

KEY POINTS

1. The best way to transport an avulsed tooth is in the patient's tooth socket.
2. Gum lacerations that need to be repaired include large lacerations, flaps, and exposed bone.
3. Canker sores are treated with topical anesthetics and cleansing rinses.

BIBLIOGRAPHY

Andreasen JO, Andreasen FM. *Textbook and Color Atlas of Traumatic Injuries to the Teeth*. 4th ed. Munksgaard, Copenhagen: Wiley-Blackwell; 2007.

Cooper BC, Kleinberg I. Examination of a large patient population for the presence of symptoms and signs of temporomandibular disorders. *Cranio*. 2007;25:114.

Elluru RG. Inflammatory disorders of the salivary glands. In: Flint PW, Haughey BH, et al., eds. *Cummings Otolaryngology: Head and Neck Surgery*. 6th ed. Philadelphia: Mosby Elsevier; 2015 [chap 83].

Jackson NM, Mitchell JL, Walvekar RR. Inflammatory disorders of the salivary glands. In: Flint PW, Haughey BH, et al., eds. *Cummings Otolaryngology: Head and Neck Surgery*. 6th ed. Philadelphia: Mosby Elsevier; 2015 [chap 85].

Keels MA. Section on Oral Health, American Academy of Pediatrics. Management of dental trauma in a primary care setting. *Pediatrics*. 2014;133:e466.

Malmgren B, Andreasen JO, Flores MT, et al. International Association of Dental Traumatology guidelines for the management of traumatic dental injuries: 3. Injuries to primary dentition. *Dent Traumatol*. 2012;28:174.

Mujakperuo HR, Watson M, Morrison R, Macfarlane TV. Pharmacological interventions for pain in patients with temporomandibular disorders. *Cochrane Database Syst Rev*. 2010.

Pappas PG, et al. Clinical practice guideline for the management of candidiasis: 2016 update by the Infectious Diseases Society of America. *Clin Infect Dis*. 2016.

Selwitz RH, Ismail AI, Pitts NB. Dental caries. *Lancet*. 2007;369:51.

Slots J, Ting M. Systemic antibiotics in the treatment of periodontal disease. *Periodontaol*. 2000-2002;28:106.

CHAPTER 5

COUGH, SHORTNESS OF BREATH, AND CHEST PAIN

Jeffrey Waskin, DO

1. **What are the most common triggers for cough?**
Viruses, viruses, viruses! The majority of cases of acute cough are due to viral upper respiratory infections that lead to increased nasal secretions and subsequent postnasal drip. Other common triggers include asthma, chronic obstructive pulmonary disease (COPD), environmental or occupational exposures, gastroesophageal reflux disease (GERD), and congestive heart failure (CHF).

2. **What is the best way to treat a cough?**
The best management strategy depends on the specific problem that triggers the cough. For example, bronchospasm caused by asthma is best treated with corticosteroids and inhaled beta agonists. For cough associated with postnasal drip or viral bronchitis, symptomatic treatment may be achieved with over-the-counter antihistamines, decongestants, antitussives, or expectorants. More severe cough or bronchospasm sometimes responds to codeine-containing medications or to prescription antitussives such as benzonatate (Tessalon).

3. **What are some complications that may accompany severe or prolonged coughing?**
Common complaints in patients with persistent cough include musculoskeletal chest pain, pleurisy, posttussive emesis, sore throat, and headache. Rarely, more serious complications such as rib fractures, pneumothorax, or pneumomediastinum can occur with severe or prolonged bronchospasm.

4. **A patient presents with shortness of breath. What are the most important parts of the history?**
Age and history of known cardiac or pulmonary disease. Other key features of the history include associated symptoms such as diaphoresis or chest pain, presence of fever or cough, and status as a current or former smoker.

5. **What physical exam finding would be most concerning in a patient complaining of shortness of breath?**
Work of breathing! Vital signs and overall appearance are critical in determining how to manage these patients. Abnormal vital signs, accessory muscle use, and decreasing mental status are likely to have a more serious etiology as a cause of their difficulty breathing. Auscultating lung sounds, checking for lower extremity edema, and evaluating the nasopharynx, throat, and ears for signs of infection/inflammation are also important pieces of the clinical puzzle.

6. **Describe the relevance of wheezing, rales, rhonchi, and diminished breath sounds.**
Wheezing is generally associated with reactive airway disease such as COPD or asthma. It can also be heard in acute bronchitis, foreign body aspiration, or CHF. Rhonchi are generally coarse sounds heard in specific lobes that tend to correspond to underlying infection. Rales or crackles are wet sounds often heard at lung bases that usually are due to fluid accumulation. Diminished breath sounds can be due to diminished air movement, pleural effusion, pneumothorax, or prohibitive body habitus.

7. **What features of the history favor noncardiac etiology of chest pain?**
Younger patients without known cardiac risk factors are unlikely to have chest pain due to occlusive coronary artery disease. Pain that is very brief in duration, described as sharp or burning, does not radiate, is not associated with shortness of breath, Nausea/Vomiting (N/V), or diaphoresis, and that is not worse with exertion or improved with rest all decrease the chances of serious underlying disease as the cause of their symptoms.

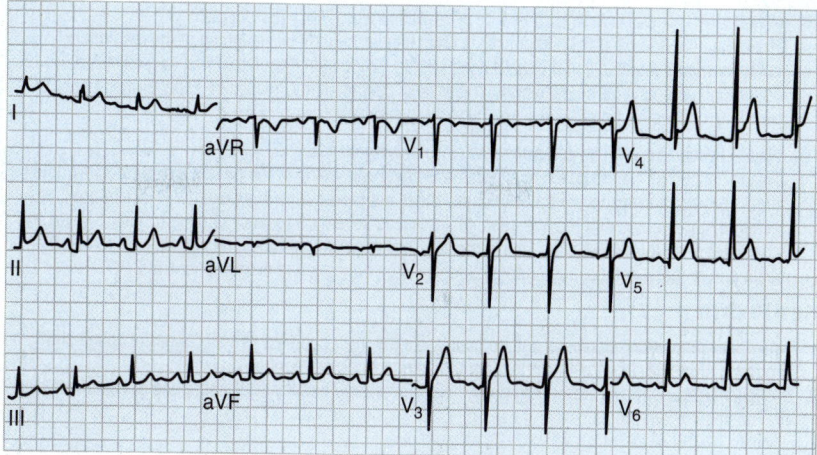

Fig. 5.1. Early EKG changes in pericarditis. This EKG shows typical EKG findings in early pericarditis, with J point changes and PR depression. Also noted are pronounced ST segment increases in II, aVF, V_2-V_6. *(Reprinted from Mann D: Braunwald's Heart Disease: A Textbook of Cardiovascular Medicine, ed 10, Philadelphia, 2014, Saunders, p 1639.)*

8. What are some common causes of chest pain in patients presenting to the urgent care setting?

Rib strains, costochondritis, pectoral muscle injury, and other variations of musculoskeletal pain are commonly found to be the cause of chest pain. GERD or chest discomfort associated with gastrointestinal (GI) illness, pleuritic discomfort in smokers or those suffering from acute bronchitis, and skin irritation including zoster rash in a thoracic dermatome can all present as a chief complaint of chest pain.

9. What tools are available in most urgent care settings that can help with your workup of chest pain or shortness of breath?

Electrocardiogram (EKG) and chest x-ray.

10. What features of the history favor cardiac etiology of chest pain?

History of prior coronary artery disease, diabetes, hypertension, hypercholesterolemia, and family history. Pressure, squeezing on chest, and diaphoresis with chest pain should raise the degree of suspicion of cardiac etiology as well.

11. If you are concerned that a patient is having cardiac chest pain, what should you do?

Call 911. Patient should be transported by ambulance to the nearest emergency department.

12. What is the treatment for patients with acute exacerbations of asthma or COPD?

Inhaled bronchodilators! These can be given as inhaled puffs from a metered dose inhaler, with or without a spacer, or as a nebulized solution. Patients may need to use these medications every 4 hours or even more frequently during an acute exacerbation. For moderate to severe symptoms, generally a course of steroids is recommended. Either a short 5-day burst course without a taper or a more prolonged course of 7–10 days with a taper is prescribed.

13. What is the typical presentation of acute pericarditis and the expected EKG findings?

Of patients who present, 95% will report chest pain. Usually the pain is described as "sharp and pleuritic," and classically sitting up and leaning forward improves the pain. Rarely, an audible pericardial friction rub can be appreciated. In the acute phase of disease, typical EKG findings include diffuse sinus tachycardia (ST) elevation that is usually concave upwards (Fig. 5.1). The PR segment may also be depressed below baseline, which is a more specific though less sensitive finding in acute pericarditis. These typical EKG changes may become much subtler or even normalize after the acute phase of the disease is over, typically within 1 week.

14. What are the common causes of a patient coughing up blood?

The most common cause of hemoptysis is bronchitis as superficial sloughing of the respiratory epithelium may result in some blood-tinged sputum production. Other common causes include pneumonia, bronchiectasis, autoimmune diseases, coagulopathy, neoplasm, expectorated upper GI bleeding, congestive heart failure, and pulmonary embolism.

15. How does one define an acute exacerbation of COPD?

This is defined as "an acute event characterized by a worsening of the patient's respiratory symptoms that is beyond normal day-to-day variations and leads to a change in medication."[1] There are generally three areas that may be affected: increased severity/frequency of cough, change in volume/character of sputum production, and increased shortness of breath beyond baseline. Generally, at least one of these criteria, and often all three, is seen during acute exacerbations of COPD.

KEY POINTS

1. Viral upper respiratory infections and bronchitis are the most common overall causes of cough and shortness of breath, and treatment is often directed at symptom control.
2. Be vigilant about not overprescribing antibiotics to otherwise healthy, well-appearing patients with clear viral etiology of symptoms.

REFERENCE

1. Anderson JL, Adams CD, Antman EM, et al. 2012 ACCF/AHA focused update incorporated into the ACCF/AHA 2007 guidelines for the management of patients with unstable angina/non-ST-elevation myocardial infarction: a report of the American College of Cardiology Foundation/American Heart Association Task Force on Practice Guidelines. *Journal of the American College of Cardiology.* 2013;61(23):e179.

BIBLIOGRAPHY

Anderson JL, Adams CD, Antman EM, et al. 2012 ACCF/AHA focused update incorporated into the ACCF/AHA 2007 guidelines for the management of patients with unstable angina/non-ST-elevation myocardial infarction: a report of the American College of Cardiology Foundation/American Heart Association Task Force on Practice Guidelines. *Journal of the American College of Cardiology.* 2013;61(23):e179.
Bohadana A, Izbicki G, Kraman SS. Fundamentals of lung auscultation. *New England Journal of Medicine.* 2014;370(8):744.
Dave BR, Sharma A, Kalva SP, Wicky S. Nine-year single-center experience with transcatheter arterial embolization for hemoptysis: medium-term outcomes. *Vascular and Endovascular Surgery.* 2011;45(3):258–268.
Fine MJ, Auble TE, Yealy DM, et al. A prediction rule to identify low-risk patients with community-acquired pneumonia. *New England Journal of Medicine.* 1997;336(4):243.
Global Strategy for the Diagnosis, Management and Prevention of COPD, Global Initiative for Chronic Obstructive Lung Disease (GOLD). <http://www.goldcopd.org>; Accessed 17.03.16.
Irwin RS, Boulet LP, Cloutier MM, et al. Managing a cough as a defense mechanism and as a symptom. A consensus panel report of the American College of Chest Physicians. *Chest.* 1998;114(suppl 2):133S.
Kwon NH, Oh MJ, Min TH, Lee BJ, Choi DC. Causes and clinical features of subacute cough. *Chest.* 2006;129(5):1142.
Troughton RW, Asher CR, Klein AL. Pericarditis. *Lancet.* 2004;363(9410):717.

CHAPTER 6

ABDOMINAL PAIN, NAUSEA, VOMITING, AND DIARRHEA

Bradley Chappell, DO, MHA, FACOEP, FACEP

1. **Why is abdominal pain so difficult to diagnose?**
   Pain in the abdomen is often referred based on the embryological development of the organs. There are two types of pain: visceral (diffuse crampy and achy pain from distention of the hollow organs) and somatic (localized constant pain from the parietal peritoneum).

2. **How should I approach a patient with right upper quadrant (RUQ) pain?**
   There are three main considerations:
   - Gallbladder (biliary colic, cholecystitis, choledocholithiasis, cholangitis)
   - Liver (hepatitis, Fitz-Hugh-Curtis syndrome)
   - Referred pain (renal colic, pyelonephritis, lower lobe pneumonia, colitis near hepatic flexure, duodenal ulcer)

3. **What workup is helpful in evaluating RUQ pain in the urgent care setting?**
   - Urinalysis (to look for pyelonephritis and assess pregnancy status when indicated)
   - Chest x-ray (if indicated)
   - Outpatient labs (complete blood count [CBC], metabolic panels, etc.) and a scheduled RUQ ultrasound (Note: If patient is ill appearing or in severe pain, these would need to be done acutely in an emergency department.)

4. **Why does the patient with abdominal pain also have pain in the shoulder?**
   This pain is called Kehr sign, an example of referred pain from diaphragmatic irritation that is transmitted through the phrenic nerve.

5. **Should I order an outpatient CT for my patient with RUQ pain?**
   Typically not. Ultrasound is the initial test of choice for gallbladder-related pathologies. There is no radiation exposure, computed tomography (CT) will often have a false appearance of gallbladder wall thickening, and other tests such as hepatobiliary iminodiacetic acid (HIDA) scan for gallbladder dysfunction or magnetic resonance cholangiopancreatography/endoscopic retrograde cholangiopancreatography (MRCP/ERCP) for intraductal stone confirmation and extraction are more appropriate. If there is concern for hepatic or biliary mass, then thin-slice CT may be indicated.

6. **My patient had a recent cholecystectomy and now is presenting with RUQ pain. What testing should I perform?**
   This patient will likely need to be evaluated in the emergency department. It is wise to have early consultation with the surgeon for postoperative management. Fever raises suspicion of complications, but local preference will vary between HIDA and CT to evaluate for postoperative biliary leak and abscess.

7. **What are commonly encountered causes of epigastric pain?**
   Esophagitis, esophageal foreign body, gastroesophageal reflux disease (GERD), peptic ulcer disease, pancreatitis.

8. **My patient has classic symptoms of peptic ulcer disease (PUD): gnawing, burning pain starting after eating. How do I differentiate between gastric and duodenal ulcers?**
   Gastric ulcers tend to worsen immediately after eating, whereas the duodenal ulcers tend to immediately improve after eating due to the bicarbonate production and ultimately cause pain several hours after a meal.

9. **What are some lifestyle modifications I can recommend to my patients with presumed PUD?**
Avoidance of contributing factors such as nonsteroidal antiinflammatory drugs (NSAIDs) or anything specific that worsens the pain; limit alcohol consumption.

10. **What is the medication regimen of choice for patients with PUD?**
   - Use proton pump inhibitors (PPIs) for 4 to 8 weeks.
   - Histamine H_2-receptor antagonists (H_2 blockers) are less effective than PPIs and do not have significant additive effect when combined with PPIs.
   - Sucralfate is most effective with duodenal ulcers.

11. **What are some potential complications of PUD?**
Hemorrhage (vomiting bright red blood or coffee-ground emesis, melena), perforation, scarring (resulting in gastric outlet obstruction).

12. **Should I order an electrocardiogram (EKG) on patients with epigastric pain?**
Patients with "atypical" chest pain often present with vague symptoms including nausea and epigastric pain. It is reasonable on patients over age 30 with vague symptoms or other risk factors (dyslipidemia, hypertension [HTN], diabetes mellitus [DM], smoker, family history, obesity) to use this as a screening exam for low-risk cardiac patients.

13. **What are some common causes of pancreatitis?**
Alcohol use (acute and chronic), biliary disease, triglyceridemia, medications, viral infections, pregnancy.

14. **What should be considered when evaluating left upper quadrant (LUQ) pain?**
Referred pain from myocardial infarction or lower lobe pneumonia, gastritis, splenomegaly, splenic infarct, or splenic laceration in the setting of trauma.

15. **What does mononucleosis have to do with abdominal pain?**
Because mono can cause splenomegaly, patients need to avoid contact sports or be evaluated after minor trauma for a minimum of 4 weeks after onset of illness. Mono can be confirmed using a monospot test or a CBC showing a lymphocytic predominance (>50%).

16. **How are patients with traumatic injury to the LUQ and stable vital signs managed?**
These patients should be referred to a trauma center for evaluation.

17. **What are some of the splenic complications associated with sickle cell anemia?**
Splenomegaly, sequestration crisis, splenic infarction, and abscesses.

18. **What common disease processes present with flank pain?**
   - Herpes zoster: often presents with a superficial burning sensation several days prior to the onset of rash. Be sure to carefully inspect for any lesions along a dermatomal distribution.
   - Nephrolithiasis: renal colic is typically severe and intermittent in nature. Posterior pain is associated with stones near the kidney, pain along the flank is typically referred as the stone transcends the ureter, and pelvic or scrotal pain is more prominent as the stone approaches the bladder.
   - Pyelonephritis: these patients often appear ill, have constant pain, and have had preceding urinary tract infections that may have been partially treated or untreated.

19. **What are significant causes of right lower quadrant (RLQ) pain?**
   - Appendicitis
   - Cecal diverticulitis
   - Referred pelvic causes such as ovarian cyst, ectopic pregnancy, ovarian or testicular torsion, sexually transmitted infections/pelvic inflammatory disease

20. **How should RLQ pain be approached?**
History and physical exam are key. Clinical components such as fever, anorexia, migration of pain to the RLQ, and leukocytosis increase the suspicion for appendicitis. A bimanual exam should be performed to help differentiate between RLQ and right pelvic pain. If the majority of pain appears to be in the pelvic region, ultrasound (US) to evaluate for torsion, cyst, or tubo-ovarian abscess (TOA) is a reasonable first step. If the pain is mainly in the RLQ, then CT is the test of choice. Depending on the degree of pain and what diagnosis you are expecting, the patient may need to be referred to the emergency department.

21. My patient states her last menstrual period (LMP) was 2 weeks ago. Do I really need a pregnancy test?

All females of childbearing age should receive a pregnancy test to rule out ectopic pregnancy.

22. What causes should be considered in lower left quadrant (LLQ) pain?

Diverticulitis, sigmoid volvulus, referred renal and pelvic causes (same as RLQ).

23. What are common symptoms that raise suspicion for diverticulitis?

Patients with diverticulitis often present with recurrent episodes, with previous diagnosis made by colonoscopy or CT. They are able to relate the current symptoms to previous ones, increasing the index of suspicion. Common symptoms include LLQ pain often worsened by food, change in bowel pattern (typically diarrhea), and occasional fever and urinary frequency. Rectal bleeding can be seen with diverticulitis, but frank bleeding (not occult, guaiac positive) does not typically have the inflammation associated with diverticulitis.

24. What are the current treatment recommendations for diverticulitis?

The current guidelines by the American Gastroenterological Association recommend selective use of antibiotics, as the current understanding is the disease is more inflammatory mediated than infectious. When antibiotics are used, several options exist, including ciprofloxacin plus metronidazole, trimethoprim-sulfamethoxazole plus metronidazole, amoxicillin-clavulanate, or moxifloxacin for 5 to 10 days.

25. Are there dietary changes for patients with diverticulosis?

Traditional teaching has been to avoid seeds, nuts, and popcorn; however, there is no statistically significant data to support the claims that this will decrease the incidence of flares through food avoidance. Newer recommendations include diets rich in fibrous foods, but there is little evidence that probiotics alter the course of disease.

26. How should pelvic tenderness be approached?

For females of childbearing age, pregnancy should be ruled out first. If there is a history of unprotected sex or vaginal discharge, the patient may need treatment for bacterial vaginosis or sexually transmitted infection. If significant pain is present on bimanual exam, the patient may need empiric treatment for pelvic inflammatory disease. When patients complain of severe intermittent or waxing/waning pain, consideration should be given to torsion (ovarian or testicular). For females with cyclical (monthly) ovarian pain, referral to gynecology may be warranted for fibroid or endometrial management. Although epididymitis is a clinical diagnosis, US should be performed to rule out torsion.

27. This patient has dysuria but a clean urine. What else could be the cause?

Be aware that chlamydia can present with dysuria as the major symptom.

28. Is there a role for observation in patients with abdominal pain?

There should be an effort toward shared decision making, especially given the potential cumulative effects of ionizing radiation. It is reasonable to have a patient with nonfocal abdominal pain of unclear etiology return for reevaluation in 8 to 12 hours. The concern for possible diagnosis and clear plan of follow-up should be documented, the patient should be tolerating orals, and vital signs must be stable.

29. What is the treatment of choice for pregnancy-induced vomiting?

- Eat small, frequent meals; avoid spicy, fatty, or other nausea-triggering foods
- Pyridoxine (25 mg q 6 hours)
- Doxylamine (12.5 mg q 12 hours)
- Metoclopramide (10 mg q 8 hours)

30. Which pregnant patients with hyperemesis need IV fluids?

When the urinalysis shows 3+ ketones or the patient has lost greater than 5% of her weight, administer IV fluids. If the patient has greater than 10% weight loss, she will likely require admission.

31. What are the best treatment options for patients with acute vomiting?

There is little evidence to suggest efficacy of one antiemetic over another. In fact, recent literature questions the efficacy of antiemetics in general. Multiple classes of medications including antihistamines (diphenhydramine, promethazine), dopamine receptor antagonists (prochlorperazine, metoclopramide), serotonin receptor antagonists (ondansetron), and glucocorticoids (dexamethasone—used in conjunction with chemotherapy) are used to treat nausea.

32. Should Gatorade be used for rehydration of patients with acute gastroenteritis?

The World Health Organization's (WHO's) recommended oral rehydration solution (ORS) varies significantly from most commercial athletic-targeted beverages. The excessive carbohydrate load may actually lead to osmotic diuresis, equating to increased diarrhea and further dehydration. The closest commercial product to the WHO-ORS available in the United States is Pedialyte.

33. How is hyperemesis from cannabis treated?

Discontinue all use of cannabis products for 1 to 2 weeks. Symptoms may temporarily improve with hot showers, and if symptoms persist after 2 weeks of no cannabis use, diagnosis of cyclical vomiting syndrome should be considered.

34. How should patients with chronic nausea from diabetic gastroparesis be managed?

- Dietary changes: blend food, tight glucose control
- Promotility agents
  - Metoclopramide (10 mg three times daily before meals)
  - Erythromycin (125 mg three times daily before meals)
- Antiemetics
  - Diphenhydramine
  - Ondansetron
  - Prochlorperazine

35. The patient is presenting with severe chest pain after multiple episodes of wretching and vomiting. How should this be evaluated?

Patients with severe vomiting will often have small Mallory-Weiss tears, often resulting in blood-tinged sputum. Sometimes, there can be rupture of the esophagus resulting in irritating and life-threatening mediastinitis. These have a high mortality rate, so clinical suspicion and early detection are essential. Approximately 90% of patients will have abnormalities on the chest x-ray.

36. What are common pathogens and sources for diarrhea?

- *Bacillus cereus:* reheated rice
- *Staphylococcus aureus:* mayonnaise
- *Salmonella*: eggs, poultry, pet reptiles
- *Shigella*: poor sanitation
- *Escherichia coli:* ground beef
- *Campylobacter*: untreated water
- *Vibrio parahaemolyticus:* shellfish
- *Yersinia*: pork
- *Clostridium botulinum:* honey

37. Do stool cultures need to be routinely sent on patients with diarrhea?

No. Cultures are expensive and have a low diagnostic yield (less than 5%). Antibiotics are not needed in most cases as the symptoms tend to be self-limited. However, high-risk populations such as the elderly, immunocompromised, those with fever, and those who travel to high-risk countries (refer to CDC website for guidance), have blood or mucus in the stool, or have greater than 10 stools in a 24-hour period may benefit from stool cultures.

38. What patients with diarrhea should receive antibiotics?

Empiric antibiotics (ciprofloxacin [500 mg] or trimethoprim-sulfamethoxazole [160/800 mg] twice daily for 3 days) may be considered for traveler's diarrhea, patients with associated fever, or symptoms greater than 2 weeks. In patients with recent hospitalization, consideration for *Clostridium difficile* should be given. Otherwise, antibiotics should be tailored to culture results. Those patients with bloody diarrhea should not receive antibiotics until cultures demonstrate it is not *E. coli O157:H7* due to the risk of precipitating hemolytic uremic syndrome. In either case, bismuth subsalicylate can be safely taken per label instructions, with caution to avoid use in HIV patients or overdose causing salicylate toxicity.

39. My patient states he feels a fishbone stuck in his throat. How quickly does he need to be seen by a gastroenterologist?

This patient should be referred for emergent endoscopy. Any sharp foreign body or button battery above the lower esophageal sphincter or any patient with a foreign body who is unable to handle his or her secretions should have it removed immediately due to risk of perforation. All other ingestions should be evaluated by endoscopy within 24 hours. Most objects that make it to the stomach will pass without intervention.

40. Can you clarify the terminology of gastrointestinal bleeding?
- Hematemesis—bright red blood or coffee-ground emesis
- Hematochezia—bright or dark red blood in stool; most commonly from lower gastrointestinal (GI) bleed, but can be from massive upper GI bleed
- Melena—black tarry stool, most frequently originates from the stomach or duodenum

41. A healthy young adult presents with reported small blood in stool or on toilet paper. Do I need to transfer this patient to the emergency department for evaluation?
If the heart rate and blood pressure are normal and the patient is not orthostatic and has normal appearing conjunctiva (no pallor) or normal hemoglobin, then the patient is likely stable for outpatient follow-up with gastroenterology. Be sure to perform a rectal exam looking for fissures or hemorrhoids.

42. A patient with atrial fibrillation had a colonoscopy last week and is now presenting with diffuse, severe abdominal pain. The abdominal x-ray did not show any free air, so perforation is less likely. What diagnosis should I be concerned about?
This is a classic presentation for mesenteric ischemia. The patient was likely off anticoagulants for the procedure and may have formed a clot with resultant bowel ischemia. These patients will appear ill (tachycardic, hypotensive), have nonfocal and unrelenting pain, and often have very abnormal labs (high leukocytosis, anion gap/lactic acidosis, base deficit). They should be transferred immediately for surgical evaluation and CT angiogram.

43. An elderly patient was brought in by family members for evaluation of a syncopal episode that was preceded by severe abdominal pain. The patient says the pain is tolerable and is declining analgesics but occasionally reports severe bouts of pain. There was blood in the UA, so is it safe to send the patient home with presumptive diagnosis of kidney stone?
First episodes on kidney stones should be imaged to confirm diagnosis. It is imperative to be mindful of other causes of painful hematuria, including critical items such as abdominal aneurysm. Unruptured abdominal aortic aneurysms are largely asymptomatic; however, once rupture occurs, the pain is often severe and can radiate to the back and groin. The classic pulsatile mass may not be appreciated in patients with a higher body mass index (BMI). Intermittent bouts of pain can be indicative of active shearing and enlargement of the rupture. This is a truly time-sensitive surgical emergency.

44. What recommendations can I give to the patient who is constipated?
- Increase daily fluid intake.
- Ingest adequate dietary fiber (fruits, vegetables, legumes, nuts, grains).
- Take bulk forming laxatives (psyllium or methylcellulose).
- Practice short-term use of osmotic agents such as polyethylene glycol to increase stool frequency.
- If related to short-term narcotic use, it will likely be transient, but use stimulant laxatives such as bisacodyl and senna to improve bowel function.

45. A patient presents with a large ventral hernia that had been intermittently protuberant for years but today does not slide back in. Does the patient require emergent surgery?
If it is truly incarcerated, the patient will require surgical evaluation. In most cases, however, with patience and proper positioning, most hernias are reducible. The first step is to have the patient lie in a supine or Trendelenburg position. Next, provide adequate analgesia and apply firm, direct pressure to the hernia. If this does not relieve the incarcerated hernia, the patient must be transferred. Incarcerated hernias can become strangulated, causing compromised blood supply to the herniated tissue, resulting in ischemic bowel. This can be diagnosed on CT or intraoperatively, but severe intractable pain is a clue toward this diagnosis.

46. How can I best manage the patient with painful hemorrhoids?
- Corticosteroids: topical or rectal suppositories
- Vasoactive agents (topical phenylephrine)
- Protectants: zinc oxide paste
- Bulk forming laxatives (psyllium or methylcellulose)
- Stool softeners (docusate)

KEY POINTS

1. Patients with an acute abdomen (guarding, rebound, or rigidity) need immediate transfer to an emergency department for surgical evaluation. Do not delay for lab testing or results.
2. Any female of childbearing age should have a pregnancy test performed.
3. Patients with abdominal trauma should be referred to a local trauma center to be evaluated for intraabdominal pathology, which can be present despite stable vital signs.
4. Elderly patients rarely have benign presentations of abdominal pain or vomiting. They have a high degree of suspicion for diagnoses such as bowel obstruction, cholangitis, ruptured appendicitis, abdominal aortic aneurysm, and mesenteric ischemia.

BIBLIOGRAPHY

Acute Colonic Diverticulitis. Medical Management. Available at: https://www.uptodate.com/contents/acute-colonic-diverticulitis-medical-management. Accessed July 31, 2016.

Al-Salem AH. Splenic Complications of Sickle Cell Anemia and the Role of Splenectomy. *ISRN Hematology 864257*, 2011.

Anderson BA, et al. A Systematic Review of Whether Oral Contrast is Necessary for the Computed Tomography Diagnosis of Appendicitis in Adults. *Am J Surg.* 2005;190(3):474.

Atilla R, Oktay C. Pancreatitis and Cholecystitis. In: Tintinalli J, ed. *Tintinalli's Emergency Medicine: A Comprehensive Study Guide.* 7th ed. China: The McGraw-Hill Companies, Inc; 2011: 558–566.

Backus BE, et al. A prospective validation of the HEART score for chest pain patients at the emergency department. *Int J Cardiol.* 2013 March 7;3.

Boerhaave Syndrome. Available at: http://emedicine.medscape.com/article/171683-overview. Accessed June 26, 2016.

Burgess BE. Anorectal Disorders. In: Tintinalli J, ed. *Tintinalli's Emergency Medicine: A Comprehensive Study Guide.* 7th ed. China: The McGraw-Hill Companies, Inc; 2011:587–601.

Chohan N, ed. *Nursing: Interpreting Signs and Symptoms.* 1st ed. Ambler, PA: Lipincott, Williams, and Wilkins; 2007:355.

Cohen SH, et al. Clinical Practice Guidelines for Clostridium Difficile Infection in Adults: 2010 Update by the Society for Healthcare Epidemiology of America (SHEA) and the Infectious Diseases Society of America (IDSA). *Infect Control Hosp Epidemiol.* 2010;31(5):431–455.

Cyclical Vomiting Syndromes. Available at: https://www.uptodate.com/contents/cyclic-vomiting-syndrome. Accessed July 31, 2016.

Egerton-Warburton D, Meek R, Mee MJ, Braitberg G. Antiemetic Use for Vomiting in Adult Emergency Department Patients: Randomized Controlled Trial Comparing Ondansetron, Metoclopramide, and Placebo. *Ann Emerg Med.* 2014;64(5):526.

Freedman SB, Thull-Freedman JD. Vomiting, Diarrhea, and Dehydration in Children. In: Tintinalli J, ed. *Tintinalli's Emergency Medicine: A Comprehensive Study Guide.* 7th ed. China: The McGraw-Hill Companies, Inc; 2011:830–839.

Graham A. Diverticulitis. In: Tintinalli J, ed. *Tintinalli's Emergency Medicine: A Comprehensive Study Guide.* 7th ed. China: The McGraw-Hill Companies, Inc; 2011:579–581.

Guss DA, Oyama LC. Disorders of the Liver and Biliary Tract. In: Marx JA, ed. *Rosen's Emergency Medicine: Concepts and Clinical Practice.* 7th ed. Philadelphia: Mosby Elsevier; 2010:1153–1171.

Hlibczuk V, et al. Diagnostic Accuracy of Non-contrast Computed Tomography for Appendicitis in Adults: A Systematic Review. *Ann Emerg Med.* 2010;55(1):51.

Kman NE, Werman HA. Disorders Presenting Primarily with Diarrhea. In: Tintinalli J, ed. *Tintinalli's Emergency Medicine: A Comprehensive Study Guide.* 7th ed. China: The McGraw-Hill Companies, Inc; 2011:531–540.

Management of Chronic Constipation in Adults. Available at: https://www.uptodate.com/contents/management-of-chronic-constipation-in-adults. Accessed August 1, 2016.

O'Brien MC. Acute Abdominal Pain. In: Tintinalli J, ed. *Tintinalli's Emergency Medicine: A Comprehensive Study Guide.* 7th ed. China: The McGraw-Hill Companies, Inc; 2011:519–527.

Peptic Ulcer Disease: Management. Available at: https://www.uptodate.com/contents/peptic-ulcer-disease-management?source=search_result&search=peptic+ulcer+disease%3A +management &selectedTitle=1%7E150. Accessed: July 28, 2016.

Salo JA, et al. Hematuria is an Indication of Rupture of an Abdominal Aortic Aneurysm into the Vena Cava. *J Vasc Surg.* 1990;12(1):41–44.

Selective Non-operative Management of Blunt Splenic Injuries. Available at: https://www.east.org/education/practice-management-guidelines/blunt-splenic-injury,-selective-nonoperative-management-of. Accessed June 25, 2016.

Stollman N; Smalley W, Hirano I. American Gastroenterological Association Institute Guideline on the Management of Acute Diverticulitis. *Gastroenterology.* 2015;149(7):1944–1949.

Treatment and Outcome of Nausea and Vomiting of Pregnancy. Available at: https://www.uptodate.com/contents/treatment-and-outcome-of-nausea-and-vomiting-of-pregnancy. Accessed July 31, 2016.

Treatment of Gastroparesis. Available at: https://www.uptodate.com/contents/treatment-of-gastroparesis. Accessed July 31, 2016.

Treatment of Hemorrhoids. Available at: https://www.uptodate.com/contents/treatment-of-hemorrhoids. Accessed August 1, 2016.

CHAPTER 7

GENITOURINARY COMPLAINTS

Vernne W. Greiner, DO, FAAFP

1. What organisms commonly cause epididymitis?

Sexually transmitted infections (*Neisseria gonorrhoeae* and *Chlamydia trachomatis*) are the most common in 16- to 30-year-old men, but *Escherichia coli, Klebsiella pneumoniae, Proteus mirabilis,* and *Pseudomonas aeruginosa* are a prevalent cause in the 51- to 70-year-old age group. Noninfectious inflammation of the epididymis is far less common, occurring mostly in prepubertal boys.

2. How does acute epididymitis typically present?

Several days to weeks of progressive dull aching pain of the epididymis and testes, often with swelling. Associated abdominal pain and fever are common, and urinary tract infection symptoms, such as dysuria, frequency, and hematuria, may also be present.

3. Are there risk factors associated with developing epididymitis?

Yes. Unprotected sexual activity, trauma from strenuous exercise, prolonged sitting, prostatic hypertrophy, and urologic instrumentation are potential risk factors for epididymitis.

4. What other urologic conditions can mimic epididymitis?

Scrotal pain and swelling can be caused by trauma, inguinal hernia, testicular torsion, torsion of the appendix epididymis (most common in prepubertal boys), Fournier gangrene, and testicular cancer may all cause genital pain and swelling of the scrotal contents.

5. What is the best exam approach to assess for scrotal pain?

A standing exam is helpful to differentiate epididymitis. Pain relief by elevation of the scrotum (Prehn sign) correlates highly with epididymitis, and presence of ipsilateral cremasteric reflex is reassuring that testicular torsion is not as likely. Tenderness and swelling of the epididymis, and often the adjacent testes, is palpable. A mass within the testes is not consistent with epididymitis and warrants further investigation. Supine abdominal examination is also integral to assess for an intraabdominal process radiating pain to the external genitalia.

6. What testing is indicated in the evaluation of suspected epididymitis?

Testing for sexually transmitted infections (STIs), especially gonorrhea and chlamydia, should be done for sexually active men, at least those under 35 years of age. A urine analysis with culture is indicated, particularly for older men and younger adolescents, as coliform bacteria are more likely causative in these age groups.

7. When is scrotal ultrasound indicated for a patient presenting with a scrotal complaint?

The loss of cremasteric reflex, a painless mass, uncertain diagnosis, or unexplained pain warrants further evaluation with an ultrasound.

8. With such variable bacterial causes, what treatment should be started for presumed epididymitis?

Treatment should be tailored to likely pathogens. Because sexually transmitted infection is the most common cause of epididymitis in younger men, standard treatment for *N. gonorrhoeae* and *C. trachomatis* should be given while studies are pending. For older men the same treatment may be appropriate given the clinical presentation, but coverage for typical urinary pathogens may be more appropriate. See Table 7.1 for drug and dosage details.

9. What are the adjunctive treatments for epididymitis?

Scrotal support and elevation, cold compresses, and antiinflammatory pain medication are helpful.

10. What tests should be considered for patients presenting with genital vesicles and/or ulcers?

By far, the most common cause of such genital lesions is herpes simplex virus (HSV), with or without systemic prodromal symptoms. Other ulcer-causing infectious agents include chancroid, granuloma

29

Table 7.1. CDC STD Treatment Guidelines

Epididymitis most likely STI with C or GC	Ceftriaxone 250 mg IM x 1 dose Doxycycline 100 mg bid x 10 days	
Epididymitis in MSM with enteric organism coverage	Ceftriaxone 250 mg IM x 1 dose Doxycycline 100 mg bid x 10 days OR ceftriaxone 250 mg IM x 1 dose + ofloxacin 300 mg bid x 10 days	
Epididymitis most likely enteric organism	Levofloxacin 500 mg/d x 10 days OR ofloxacin 300 mg/d x 10 days	
Urethritis, likely GU or NGU	Ceftriaxone 250 mg IM x 1 dose + azithromycin 1 g po x 1 dose	If ceftriaxone not available, cefixime 400 mg po x 1 dose + azithromycin 1 g po x 1 dose If cephalosporin allergy, gemifloxacin 320 mg po x 1 dose + azithromycin 1 g po x 1 dose OR gentamycin 250 mg IM x 1 dose + azithromycin 1 g po x 1 dose
NGU, confirmed chlamydia	Azithromycin 1 g po x 1 dose OR doxycycline 100 mg bid x 7 days	Erythromycin base 500 mg qid x 7 days Erythromycin ethyl succinate 800 mg qid x 7 days Levofloxacin 500 mg/d x 7 days Ofloxacin 300 mg bid x 7 days
NGU persistent/recurrent	Use the other treatment as above OR If *T. vaginalis* is highly prevalent, metronidazole 2 g po 1 dose	If failed on azithromycin, use moxifloxacin 400 mg/d x 7 days (active against *Mycoplasma genitalium*)
Trichomonas vaginalis	Metronidazole 2 g po 1 dose OR tinidazole 2 g po 1 dose	Metronidazole 500 mg bid x 7 days Consider sensitivities if treatment failure
Herpes simplex—genital first episode Episodic treatment	Acyclovir 400 mg tid x 7 days Valaciclovir 1 g bid x 7 days Famciclovir 250 mg tid x 7 days Acyclovir 400 mg tid x 5 days Valaciclovir 500 mg bid x 3 days Famciclovir 125 mg bid x 5 days	Acyclovir 200 mg 5 times a day x 7 days or 800 mg tid x 7 days Acyclovir 800 mg bid x 5 days or 800 mg tid x 2 days Valaciclovir 1 g/d x 5 days Famciclovir 1 g/bid x 1 day or 500 mg once + 250 mg bid x 2 days

C, *Chlamydia trachomatis*; GC, *Neisseria gonorrhoeae*; GU, gonococcal urethritis; MSM, men who have sex with men; NGU, nongonococcal urethritis; STD, sexually transmitted diseases.
Adapted from the United States Centers for Disease Control and Prevention, Sexually Transmitted Diseases. Summary of 2015 Treatment Guidelines. Available at: cdc.gov/std/treatment/default.htm. Accessed 10.04.16.

inguinale, lymphogranuloma venereum, and syphilis. There are less common noninfectious etiologies, including Behçet syndrome and trauma.

11. **Is viral culture better than polymerase chain reaction (PCR) testing, and better than serologic testing for genital herpes simplex?**
Viral culture is the diagnostic standard of care for genital infection. PCR testing currently has a higher rate of detection and may replace culture at some time. Serologic testing (antigen detection) by enzyme-linked immunosorbent assay (ELISA) and Western blot assay have high sensitivity and specificity for herpes simplex—that is, 96% to 100% and 97% to 100%, respectively.

12. Should the diagnosis be confirmed before initiating treatment?

No. Treat presumptively while cultures are pending. In addition to antiviral medication, pain management is important. Burrow solution or baking soda compresses (1 tsp to 1 quart of cool water) applied locally may provide significant relief.

13. How long is genital herpes contagious?

There is no clear-cut answer as asymptomatic viral shedding is quite common and the patient should be appropriately counseled. Abstinence from sexual contact during any prodromal symptoms or while there are active lesions should be maintained until there is complete healing. A barrier contraceptive method may be appropriate even when asymptomatic.

14. What are the antiviral treatment options for genital herpes?

See Table 7.1.

15. How is acute urethritis in men diagnosed?

History of penile discharge (with or without dysuria), urgency, or other typical urinary tract infection (UTI) symptoms with examination findings of urethral discharge, positive leukocyte esterase, or greater than 10 white blood cells (WBCs) per high-power field on urine analysis are diagnostic of acute urethritis.

16. Is acute urethritis in men always due to STIs?

Essentially yes. The incidence of reactive arthritis with urethritis subsequent to chlamydial nongonococcal urethritis (CNGU) is estimated to be 1% of presenting urethritis. For clinical purposes, urethritis can be categorized as gonococcal (GU) and nongonococcal (NGU). Gonorrhea and chlamydia are the most prevalent STIs. *Trichomonas* and *Ureaplasma urealyticum* are also common. *Mycoplasma genitalium* is a potential cause of NGU; however, specific testing for this is not currently available. Other less common causes include *Haemophilus influenzae,* adenovirus, and herpes simplex.

17. Do all patients with urethritis require diagnostic tests?

Remember that STIs are frequently coincident. In addition to symptom relief, preventing complications in the patient and sexual partner, and identifying and limiting transmission of additional STIs, testing should be done uniformly. For men who have sex with men, IV drug use, and other high-risk sexual behavior, hepatitis B, hepatitis C, human immunodeficiency virus (HIV), herpes (HSV), and syphilis should also be assessed.

18. What treatment is appropriate for urethritis?

Treatment should be given at the point of access to care (see Table 7.1). Expedited partner treatment, as advocated by the Centers for Disease Control and Prevention (CDC) and approved in many U.S. states, may be considered. Guidelines and legal status are available online through the CDC.

19. What populations get urinary tract infections?

UTIs are most common in women of childbearing age, but they are not uncommon in children with various urologic anatomic and functional problems. UTIs are less common in men, but with the onset of prostatic enlargement around age 50, they increase in frequency to equal the incidence in postmenopausal women.

20. What are the risk factors for getting a UTI?

Common risk factors include inadequate hydration and delayed or infrequent emptying of the bladder, all of which allow the infection to establish in the bladder epithelium. Coitus also is a risk factor for women as bacteria may be mechanically introduced into the distal urethra, and, due to the female anatomy, enteric bacteria are not uncommon in the bladder. Good hydration, regular emptying, and voiding shortly after coitus decrease the opportunity for infection. Anatomic abnormalities, including prostatic enlargement, increase the risk of UTI.

21. What defines a UTI as complicated?

There is some variation in definition, but practically, in the outpatient setting, pregnancy, urologic instrumentation (e.g., ureteral stent), and urolithiasis are complicating factors. A patient with a single kidney or other abnormal urologic anatomy requires careful management and follow-up. A UTI in the setting of an obstructing ureteral stone is a urologic emergency, as sepsis is common.

22. What are the most common symptoms of UTI?

Dysuria, frequency, and small amounts of urine voided are quite common. Dysuria alone is associated with UTI about 50% of the time; dysuria with another symptom (e.g., frequency) increases the likelihood of infection to 96%. Additional symptoms are commonly hematuria, nocturia, hesitancy, suprapubic pain, and mild nausea. Fever, vomiting, and back pain associated with dysuria are suggestive of upper tract infection. Dysuria as an isolated symptom has a high prevalence of STI in sexually active young adults.

23. What are the physical examination findings?
With uncomplicated UTI, there may be unremarkable or minimal findings on exam. Mild suprapubic and mild periumbilical pain on palpation are common; however, the presence of moderate to severe unilateral periumbilical pain on palpation or flank tenderness on percussion (Lloyd sign) should raise concern for pyelonephritis.

24. What findings on urine analysis confirm UTI?
The confirmatory test is a urine culture. The presence of leukocyte esterase on urine analysis has the best sensitivity and specificity. With the presence of leukocyte esterase and a high pretest probability, this may also be considered confirmatory. The presence of nitrite may support the diagnosis of UTI, but its absence does not rule out UTI because not all urinary pathogens form nitrite from nitrate.

25. What may commonly cause false-positive or -negative findings on urine analysis?
A false-positive leukocyte esterase is frequently caused by phenazopyridine and contamination (e.g., due to vaginal discharge, balanitis, urethritis, foreign body). A false-positive nitrite may be due to contamination, exposure to air, and phenazopyridine. A false-negative nitrite may be due to dilution secondary to aggressive hydration and frequent voiding.

26. Under what circumstances is it reasonable to treat for UTI based on history and exam alone?
A nonpregnant woman with urinary symptoms without gynecologic symptoms and consistent examination can self-diagnose and may be treated presumptively. A urine analysis may be omitted in this case.

27. Who should be cultured?
Patients who have dysuria with unrevealing dipstick, children, pregnant women, postmenopausal women, men, those with history of recurrent UTI, and those with single kidney/urologic anatomic problems all warrant urine culture with sensitivities.

28. Which antibiotics are not first line for empiric treatment of acute uncomplicated cystitis?
Due to the development of significant bacterial resistance, fluoroquinolones and beta lactam antibiotics are better held for complicated, resistant, or culture proven infection if there is treatment failure on a targeted antibiotic.

29. Does the absence of fever rule out pyelonephritis?
No, treat based on the presentation and physical findings, with supportive lab studies and probability assessment.

30. What are the recommended treatments for UTI?
See Table 7.2 for treatment of uncomplicated UTI/pyelonephritis in the outpatient setting.

31. What causes prostatitis?
Acute bacterial prostatitis (ABP) is thought to be caused by retrograde seeding of the prostate by bacteria and occurs in 2%–5% of episodes of diagnosed prostatitis. It occurs predominantly in men ages 20 to 40 years, often by typical gram-negative urinary tract pathogens, most often *E. coli*. Gonorrhea, chlamydia, and *Trichomonas* are not uncommon pathogens, especially in younger sexually active men, although those more commonly present as urethritis.

32. What differentiates acute from chronic prostatitis?
Chronic bacterial prostatitis (CBP) is a diagnosis made over time, involving repeated examinations for recurrent or persistent urologic symptoms of urogenital pain, dysuria, and urinary culture with the same organism. It accounts for about 10% of chronic prostatitis and is to be distinguished from nonbacterial prostatitis/chronic pelvic pain syndrome (NBP/CPPS).

33. What is NBP/CPPS?
Defining features of this condition are a chronic urologic condition with symptoms if UTI; and without, response to antibiotic treatment, variable organisms on culture, and often with associated sexual dysfunction and psychological symptoms.

Table 7.2. Treatment of Uncomplicated Urinary Tract Infections

URINARY TRACT INFECTION	MEDICATION	DOSAGE	LENGTH OF TREATMENT
	Cystitis		
Nitrofurantoin	100 mg	bid	5–7 days
TMP/SMS	160/800 mg	bid	3 days
Fosfomycin	3 g	1 dose	1 dose
Pivmecillinam	400 mg	bid	3–7 days
Fluoroquinolone	Variable	Variable	3 days
Beta-lactam	Variable	Variable	5–7 days
	Pyelonephritis		
Amoxicillin	500 mg	q8h	10–14 days
Amoxicillin	875 mg	q12h	10–14 days
Amoxicillin/clavulanate	875/125 mg	q12h	10–14 days
Ciprofloxacin	500 mg	q12h	10–14 days
Ciprofloxacin	1,000 mg	q12h	7 days
Levofloxacin	750 mg	q24h	5 days
TMP/SMS	160/800 mg	q12h	14 days

TMP/SMS, Trimethoprim/sulfamethoxazole.
From: Gupta K, Hooton TM, Naber KG, et al: International Clinical Practice Guidelines for the Treatment of Acute Uncomplicated Cystitis and Pyelonephritis in Women: A 2010 Update by the Infectious Disease Society of America and the European Society for Microbiology and Infectious Diseases. *Clin Infect Dis* 52:e103-e120, 2011; Meng MV: Infections of the Upper Urinary Tract. In Wessels H, editor: *Urologic Emergencies: A Practical Approach*, ed 2, New York, 2013, Springer Science & Business Media, pp 105-109. http://dx.doi.org/10.1007/978-1-62703-423-4_8.

34. What is the differential diagnosis of ABP?
Additional diagnoses include other urologic problems, such as acute cystitis, interstitial cystitis, STI, and gastrointestinal (GI) disease, including diverticulitis and proctitis. Prostate cancer may also cause outlet obstructive symptoms and needs to be considered.

35. How is ABP diagnosed?
As always, a good history and examination are the foundation and should include abdominal, genital, and digital rectal examinations. The diagnosis of ABP is clinical, and based on the findings of an enlarged, boggy, and tender prostate. Urine analysis should always be done to guide antibiotic choice and treatment of acute or chronic prostatitis.

36. What is the treatment?
For ABP in the outpatient setting without risk factors for admission, 10 to 14 days of levofloxacin (superior penetration of the prostate). Consider ceftriaxone + doxycycline if STI is a high probability. For CBP, initial levofloxacin (and guidance with culture) for 6 weeks is a good choice but may need to be repeated if symptoms recur. Reculture pre- and postprostatic massage to match the pathogen and confirm chronic infection may be appropriate.

37. What requires hospital care?
For patients with apparent prostatitis, reasons for hospital referral include urinary obstruction, inability to take oral medication, history of recent transurethral instrumentation, and systemic symptoms such as fever, chills, or signs of sepsis; all require admission with urologic consultation.

38. How is NBP/CPPS treated?
Antibiotics are appropriate initial treatment; however, with failed treatment, urology referral is appropriate. This will provide for diagnostic confirmation and additional treatment options, which may include alpha$_1$ blocker, pain management, urology physical therapy modalities, and psychological care.

39. **What causes kidney stones?**
Usually soluble mineral compounds, which precipitate when the saturation point is reached in the urine.

40. **What kind of stone is most common?**
Calcium compounds are most frequent at about 80%, along with uric acid and struvite as the common noninfectious stones. Stones formed due to genetic disorders include cysteine, xanthine, and 2,8-dihydroxyadenine. Stones associated with infectious etiology include magnesium ammonium phosphate, carbonate apatite, and ammonium urate.

41. **Who gets kidney stones?**
Urinary tract stones are common, occurring in up to 10% of the population. They occur predominantly in men. Causes are multifactorial, including nutritional and fluid issues, medical conditions, genetic predisposition, and less frequent causes, including infection and crystallized medication or supplements (e.g., vitamin C).

42. **What medical conditions predispose a patient to develop stones?**
Inadequate hydration, high dietary calcium, parathyroidism, and altered bone metabolism are frequently related. Gastrointestinal diseases such as malabsorption, chronic inflammatory bowel disease, and intestinal bypass surgery also have higher incidence of urinary stone formation. Common diseases including diabetes mellitus, hypertension, obesity, osteoporosis, gout, and chronic kidney diseases are also frequently associated.

43. **What is the typical presentation for a kidney stone?**
A stone in the ureter is generally quite symptomatic. When a stone dislodges from the renal collecting system and enters the ureter, it causes severe unilateral flank pain. There is often radiation into the abdomen or groin, associated nausea/vomiting, and urinary frequency may occur with a distal ureteral stone.

44. **What causes the pain?**
The average stone is 2.5 to 3 mm, which is larger than the lumen of the ureter. Scraping the lining of or obstructing the ureter causes the abrupt onset of symptoms. The pain is severe, independent of position or activity.

45. **What are the physical findings?**
The patient has severe pain and therefore cannot find a comfortable position and may be restless. There is often associated nausea/vomiting. The abdominal exam is generally soft without tenderness, although with longer duration of symptoms there may be flank or abdominal tenderness. The presence of fever with this presentation is concerning, and the patient must be thoroughly evaluated.

46. **What finding on urine analysis supports the diagnosis of a stone?**
Microscopic hematuria is usually present. The presence of leukocyte esterase or nitrate would suggest infection but does not rule out the possibility of a stone.

47. **Does ureterolithiasis always cause hematuria?**
No, while it is most common to have microscopic hematuria, an impacted stone may not permit passage of urine or blood.

48. **What imaging study is best for initial assessment of suspected urolithiasis?**
If available, an urgent retroperitoneal ultrasound is currently thought to be the best imaging study because it can confirm ureteral obstruction and may detect a stone, without a large radiation dose. If available, an abdominal plain film (kidney, ureter, and bladder [KUB]) may be helpful, but many ureteral stones are not radiopaque, and hydronephrosis is not detectable.

49. **When is noncontrast CT (NCCT) indicated for apparent renal colic?**
An NCCT of the abdomen and pelvis is appropriate when there is a presentation suggestive of urolithiasis but with a negative ultrasound, fever, or history of a solitary kidney or if the diagnosis is in question. One NCCT has the equivalent of about 30 times the radiation dose of one KUB.

50. **For a confirmed ureteral stone, what are the priorities in management?**
Immediate pain relief is imperative and allows for return to normal respiration and to facilitate return to normal activity. Ketorolac intramuscular (IM) has also been shown to be effective in the outpatient setting.

51. Which patients may be treated as outpatients?

Patients with a ureteral stone 4 mm or smaller and who have adequate pain control on oral medication and no infection or impairment of renal function may be given a chance to pass the stone. Pushing fluids, maintaining physical activity, and pain management promote stone passage, usually within several weeks.

52. Do alpha$_1$ blockers help with passing a stone in the short term?

Tamsulosin (0.4 mg) has the most evidence and does show benefit with increased percentage of stones passed and passed sooner than with placebo (one of three patients passed an average of 3 days sooner).

53. Of what value is stone analysis?

Recovery of a stone is important, and straining the urine should be done for the first diagnosed episode. Identification of the stone helps with prognosis, as recurrent stones are quite common. Additional metabolic evaluation of blood and urine tests (complete blood count [CBC], renal function, electrolytes, parathyroid hormone, calcium and urine creatinine, sodium, pH, oxalate, and citrate) should be considered to assess for underlying conditions.

54. What are the referral criteria?

Nonurgent urology referral would be appropriate for a large stone that may require lithotripsy or instrumentation, for a small stone that is not passed after a reasonable time as an outpatient, and if other concurrent urologic concerns are discovered.

Key Points

1. Treat acute epididymitis for STIs in men 35 years or younger and for typical urinary pathogens in older men.
2. Ultrasound is the preferred initial advanced imaging for suspected urolithiasis.
3. Absence of hematuria does not preclude the presence of urolithiasis.

Bibliography

Brill JR. Diagnosis and treatment of urethritis in men. *Am Fam Physician.* 2010;81(7):873–878.

Bultitude M, Smith D, Thomas K. Contemporary management of stone disease: the new EAU guidelines for 2015. *Eur Urol.* 2016;69(3):483–484. http://dx.doi.org/10.1016/jeurouro2015.08.010.

Campschroer T, Zhu Y, Duijvesz D, Grobbee DE, Lock MT. Alpha blockers as medical expulsive therapy for ureteral stones. *Cochrane Database Syst Rev.* 2014;4(April 2): CD008509.pub2. http://dx.doi.org/10.1002/14651858.

Centers for Disease Control and Prevention. Guidance on the Use of Expedited Partner Therapy in the Treatment of Gonorrhea. <http://www.cdc.gov/std/EPT/default.htm>, Accessed 10.04.10.

Crawford P, Crop J. Evaluation of scrotal masses. *Am Fam Physician.* 2014;89(May 1):723–727.

Curhan C. Nephrolithiasis. In: Kapser DL, Fauci AS, Jauser SL, Longo DL, Jameson JL, Loscalzo J, eds. *Harrison's Principles of Internal Medicine.* 19th ed. New York: McGraw-Hill; 2016:1866–1871.

Groves MJ. Genital herpes: a review. *Am Fam Physician.* 2016;93(11):928–934.

Gupta K, Hooton TM, Naber KG, et al. International clinical practice guidelines for the treatment of acute uncomplicated cystitis and pyelonephritis in women: a 2010 update by the Infectious Disease Society of America and the European Society for Microbiology and Infectious Diseases. *Clin Infect Dis.* 2011;52:e103–e120.

Gupta K, Trautner BW. Urinary tract infections, pyelonephritis and prostatitis. In: Kapser DL, Fauci AS, Jauser SL, Longo DL, Jameson JL, Loscalzo J, eds. *Harrison's Principles of Internal Medicine.* 19th ed. New York: McGraw-Hill; 2016: 861–868.

Hanno PM. Lower urinary tract infections in women and pyelonephritis. In: Hanno PM, Guzzo TJ, Malkowicz SB, Wein AJ, eds. *Penn Clinical Manual of Urology.* 2nd ed. Philadelphia: Saunders, an imprint of Elsevier, Inc.; 2014:114–116.

Ito S, Honaoka N, Shimata K, et al. Male non-gonococcal urethritis: from microbiological etiologies to demographic and clinical features. *Int'l Journal of Urology.* 2016;23(4):325–331.

Kodner C. Sexually transmitted infections in men. In: Heidelbaugh JJ, ed. *Men's Health in Primary Care* (electronic resource). 1st ed. Cham, Switzerland: Springer International Publishing; 2015:165–196.

Krieger JN. Bacterial infections of the male urinary tract. In: Bope E, Kellerman RD, eds. *Conn's Current Therapy.* Philadelphia: Elsevier; 2016:1005–1007.

Krieger JN, Nyberg Jr L, Nickel JC. NIH consensus definition and classification of prostatitis. *JAMA.* 1999;292(3): 236–237.

Legoff I, Pere H, Belec L. Diagnosis of genital herpes simplex virus infection in the clinical laboratory. *Virol J.* 2014;11:83.

Limpkin MW, Ferradino MN, Preminger GM. Evaluation and medical management of urinary lithiasis. In: McDougal WS, Wein A, Kavoussi LR, Partin AW, Peters CA, eds. *Campbell-Walsh Urology.* 11th ed. Philadelphia: Elsevier, 52; 2016:1200–1234, e7.

Malone M, Shiraz A. Testicular, scrotal & penile disorders. In: Heidelbaugh JJ, ed. *Men's Health in Primary Care* (electronic resource). 1st ed. Cham, Switzerland: Springer International Publishing; 2015:225–248.

Meng MV. Infections of the upper urinary tract. In: Wessels H, ed. *Urologic Emergencies: A Practical Approach* (electronic resource). 2nd ed. New York: Springer Science & Business Media; 2013:105–109. http://dx.doi.org/10.1007/978-1-62703-423-4_8.

Middlekoop SJ, van Pelt LJ, Kampinga GA, ter Maaten JC, Stegeman CA. Routine tests and automated urinalysis in patients with suspected urinary tract infection at the ED. *Am J Emerg Med.* (May 12), 2016; 16:30112– 30117. pii:S0735–S6757 http://dx.doi.org/10.1016/j.ajem.2016.05.005.

Rakel R, Rakel D, eds. *Textbook of Family Medicine.* 9th ed. Philadelphia: Saunders; 2015:213–215.

Ramakrishnan K, Salinas R. Prostatitis: acute and chronic. *Prim Care.* 2010;37(3):547–563.

Rees J, Abraham M, Doble A, Cooper A. Prostatitis Expert Reference Group (PERG). Diagnosis and treatment of chronic bacterial prostatitis and chronic prostatitis/chronic pelvic pain syndrome: a consensus guideline. *BJU Int.* 2015;116(4): 509–525.

Simerville JA, Maxted QC, Pahira JJ. Urinalysis: a comprehensive review. *Am Fam Phys.* 2005;71(6):1153–1162.

Smith-Bindman R, Aubin C, Bailitz J, et al. Ultrasonography versus computed tomography for suspected nephrolithiasis. *N Engl J Med.* 2014;71(12):1100–1110.

Tracy CR, Steer WD, Costabile R. Diagnosis and management of epididymitis. *Urol Clin N Am.* 2008;35(1):101–108, vii.

Trojian TH, Lishnak TS, Heiman D. Epididymitis and orchitis: an overview. *Am Fam Physician.* 2009;79(April 1):583–587.

Turk C, Petrik A, Sarica K, et al. EAU guidelines on diagnosis and conservative management of urolithiasis. *Eur Urol.* 2016;69(3):468–474. http://dx.doi.org/10.1016/jeurouro.2015.07.040.

Walker NA, Challacombe B. Managing epididymo-orchitits in general practice. *Practitioner.* 2013;257(1760):21–25.

CHAPTER 8

GYNECOLOGIC COMPLAINTS

Toral Bhakta, DO, Harsh Bhakta, DO

1. **What is vaginitis?**

   Vaginitis is the inflammation of vulvar and vaginal tissues. It is caused by a variety of etiologies such as infection, irritants, foreign bodies, and atrophy.

2. **What are common organisms that cause infectious vaginitis?**

   Infectious vaginitis can be caused by *Trichomonas vaginalis, Candida albicans, Gardnerella vaginalis,* and overgrowth of anaerobes.

3. **How does vaginitis present clinically?**

   Most common presenting symptoms of vaginitis are foul-smelling vaginal discharge and pruritus; however, depending on the cause, patients can also present with dysuria, dyspareunia, and pelvic pain.

4. **What are the CDC criteria for treatment of bacterial vaginosis?**

   Bacterial vaginosis can be diagnosed in the presence of three of the following four criteria: vaginal discharge, pH >4.5, positive amine test (emittance of a fishy odor upon addition of KOH to the vaginal discharge), and presence of clue cells on wet prep.

5. **How can vaginitis be treated?**

   The treatment of vaginitis involves treating the underlying etiology. Bacterial vaginosis is treated with antibiotics such as metronidazole (500 mg po bid for 7 days) or clindamycin (300 mg po bid for 7 days). For treatment of trichomoniasis, metronidazole (500 mg po bid for 7 days or a one-time 2-g dose) is indicated. Similarly, fungal (*Candida*) vaginitis can be treated with fluconazole (one dose, 150 mg po) or topical imidazole. Contact vaginitis is treated by removal of the foreign body or offending agent, whereas atrophic vaginitis is treated with topical estrogen creams.

6. **What is pelvic inflammatory disease?**

   Pelvic inflammatory disease (PID) is an ascending infection from the lower genital tract. It is a female disease and can include a variety of diseases such as salpingitis, endometritis, tuboovarian abscesses, and peritonitis.

7. **What are the risk factors for PID?**

   Multiple sexual partners, previous PID, adolescence, intrauterine device (IUD) use, recent menses, douching, cigarette smoking.

8. **What are the most common presenting signs and symptoms of PID?**

   The most common presentation of PID is lower abdominal pain. Other signs and symptoms include vaginal discharge, fever, nausea, vomiting, and dyspareunia. As the signs and symptoms are very nonspecific, PID should be considered in any female presenting with complaints of lower abdominal pain.

9. **How can PID be diagnosed?**

   In the urgent care setting, PID is a clinical diagnosis. Ancillary testing that can aid in making the diagnosis include urine analysis, urine pregnancy test, wet prep, and gonorrhea/chlamydia. If there is suspicion for tubo-ovarian abscess, pelvic sonography can be used as a definitive imaging study. Laparoscopy remains the most accurate test and the gold standard imaging test for diagnosing PID; however, this is not very useful in the urgent care setting.

10. **What are the clinical criteria for diagnosing PID?**

    The triad of minimal criteria for diagnosing PID includes lower abdominal tenderness, adnexal tenderness (usually bilateral) on pelvic exam, and cervical motion tenderness. Additional criteria include fever, vaginal discharge, elevated C-reactive protein (CRP) and erythrocyte sedimentation rate (ESR), leukocytosis, and laboratory evidence of gonococcal/chlamydia infection.

> **Box 8.1.** IM/Oral Treatment Regimens for PID
>
> 1. Ceftriaxone 250 mg IM in a single dose PLUS doxycycline 100 mg orally twice a day for 14 days WITH or WITHOUT metronidazole 500 mg orally twice a day for 14 days
>   OR
> 2. Cefoxitin 2 g IM in a single dose and probenecid 1 g orally administered concurrently in a single dose PLUS doxycycline 100 mg orally twice a day for 14 days WITH or WITHOUT metronidazole 500 mg orally twice a day for 14 days
>   OR
> 3. Other parenteral third-generation cephalosporin (e.g., ceftizoxime or cefotaxime) PLUS doxycycline 100 mg orally twice a day for 14 days WITH or WITHOUT metronidazole 500 mg orally twice a day for 14 days

Adapted from CDC.gov

> **Box 8.2.** Parenteral Treatment Regimens for PID
>
> 1. Cefotetan 2 g IV every 12 hours PLUS doxycycline 100 mg orally or IV every 12 hours
>   OR
> 2. Cefoxitin 2 g IV every 6 hours PLUS doxycycline 100 mg orally or IV every 12 hours
>   OR
> 3. Clindamycin 900 mg IV every 8 hours PLUS gentamicin loading dose IV or IM (2 mg/kg), followed by a maintenance dose (1.5 mg/kg) every 8 hours. Single daily dosing (3–5 mg/kg) can be substituted.

Adapted from CDC.gov

11. **What is the treatment for PID?**
    There are multiple outpatient and inpatient regimens recommended by the CDC for the treatment of PID. These are outlined in Boxes 8.1 and 8.2.

12. **What is defined as "normal" vaginal bleeding?**
    "Normal" vaginal bleeding can be defined as menses lasting less than 7 days, losing less than 60 mL of blood, and having greater than 21-day recurrence cycle.

13. **What is abnormal vaginal bleeding?**
    Abnormal vaginal bleeding can be defined as any bleeding that does not fall into the previous criteria: bleeding in between periods, bleeding after sex, spotting at any time in the menstrual cycle, bleeding heavier or for more days than normal, and bleeding after menopause.

14. **Name some causes of abnormal vaginal bleeding.**
    Abnormal vaginal bleeding can be caused by multiple etiologies. Some of the more common etiologies include:
    - Alterations in the endocrine system causing hormonal imbalance
    - Drugs: anticonvulsants and antibiotics (penicillin, tetracycline, trimethoprim/sulfamethoxazole [TMP-SMX]) are the most common causes of breakthrough bleeding
    - Pelvic infections
    - Neoplasm
    - Trauma
    - Bleeding dyscrasia

15. **What is the management of abnormal vaginal bleeding?**
    Treatment of abnormal vaginal bleeding in the urgent care setting is dictated by the patient's hemodynamic stability.
    - In the acute care setting the provider's first responsibility is to rule out life-threatening hemorrhage and pregnancy. If the patient has unstable vital signs, the first step is to stabilize the patient with intravenous (IV) fluids such as normal saline (NS) or lactated Ringer and blood products. Once the patient is stabilized, the next step is to initiate transfer immediately.
    - If the patient is hemodynamically stable, evaluation includes complete blood count (CBC), coagulation studies, pregnancy test, and pelvic ultrasound (US). Once the underlying cause is identified, a referral to gynecology is appropriate to provide further definitive treatment.

16. What are condyloma acuminata?
Genital warts that start as flesh-colored papules or cauliflower-like projections, caused by human papillomavirus (DNA virus) transmitted by direct contact.

17. How are they diagnosed and what is the treatment?
The diagnosis of genital warts is clinical. They can be treated with topical podofilox 0.5% applied bid for 3 days, followed by 4 days off and then repeating the cycle for up to 4 times. Alternatively, imiquimod 5% cream can be applied nightly at bedtime 3 times a week for 16 weeks.

18. What is the treatment for cases of condyloma acuminata that are resistant to topical therapy?
For those patients who fail topical treatment, cryotherapy in their physician's office is the best option.

19. What is a Bartholin abscess?
Bartholin glands are pea-sized glands located on the labia minora. This gland can sometimes form a fluid-filled cyst. When the cyst or the gland itself gets infected, it forms a Bartholin abscess.

20. What are the signs and symptoms of a Bartholin abscess?
A Bartholin abscess is most commonly present as a golfball-size swelling on the lateral aspect of the labia major. It is extremely painful, especially with walking and sitting.

21. Name the most common organisms that cause a Bartholin abscess.
Most common organisms are *Escherichia coli, Neisseria gonorrhoeae, Chlamydia,* or mixed organisms from the genital tract.

22. What is the treatment of a Bartholin gland abscess?
- Incision and drainage with Word catheter placement is the standard treatment of a Bartholin cyst or abscess. The Word catheter should subsequently be left in the wound for 2 to 4 weeks. If there is accompanying cellulitis, then antibiotics are indicated.
- Marsupialization is the definitive treatment. It involves opening the abscess or the cyst and suturing the edges, creating an open tract. This procedure is best performed by a gynecologist and is out of the scope of urgent care practice.

23. What is dysmenorrhea?
Dysmenorrhea can be defined as painful menses. About 55% of the women in the United States experience some degree of dysmenorrhea.

24. What is the difference between primary and secondary dysmenorrhea?
- Primary dysmenorrhea has no pelvic pathology. It is also known as spasmodic dysmenorrhea and is caused by an increase in prostaglandins.
- Secondary dysmenorrhea has pelvic pathology such as endometriosis or uterine fibroids. It is also known as congestive dysmenorrhea.

25. What are common risk factors associated with severe dysmenorrhea?
Early age at menarche, prolonged menses, heavy menses, smoking, family history.

26. How can dysmenorrhea be evaluated in the urgent care setting?
By abnormal findings on pelvic exam, and with the aid of ancillary tests such as a pelvic sonography.

27. What is the management of dysmenorrhea?
Mild to moderate dysmenorrhea can be managed with over-the-counter or prescription nonsteroidal antiinflammatory drugs (NSAIDs). For more severe cases, oral therapy with estrogens or progestins can also be implemented.

28. What is the most common age group that typically presents with a vaginal foreign body?
Vaginal foreign bodies are a common presentation across all age groups. Children may insert any object and not tell parents secondary to fear of being disciplined, whereas adults usually tend to forget objects such as tampons or pessaries.

29. How does a patient with a vaginal foreign body typically present?
Patients with a retained vaginal foreign body can complain of pelvic pain and/or foul-smelling vaginal discharge. In more severe and rare cases of retained tampons, patients may also have fever, rash, and leukocytosis from toxic shock syndrome.

30. How can you treat a vaginal foreign body?

Treatment of a vaginal foreign body involves removal of the foreign body itself, followed by a Betadine douche and outpatient follow-up with a gynecologist. In severe cases of toxic shock syndrome, treatment will also include IV antibiotics and IV fluids.

KEY POINTS

1. The most common cause of vaginal discharge or malodor is bacterial vaginosis.
2. PID during the first trimester may cause fetal loss; hence it is imperative to diagnose and treat during pregnancy.
3. In postmenopausal women, the most common causes of vaginal bleeding are exogenous estrogens, atrophic vaginitis, and endometrial lesions including cancers.

BIBLIOGRAPHY

American College of Obstetrics and Gynecology. <https://www.acog.org>.

Centers for Disease Control. <http://www.cdc.gov/std/tg2015/pid.htm>.

Dysmenorrhea Clinical Presentation. <http://emedicine.medscape.com/article/253812-clinical>.

Ma O, Cline D, Tintinalli J, Kelen G, Stapczynski O, eds. *Emergency Medicine: Just the Facts.* 2nd ed. New York: McGraw Hill Medical Publishing; 2005:207–212, 223–228.

Rivers C, Howell J, Barkin R, eds. *Preparing for the Written Board Exam in Emergency Medicine.* 5th ed. Milford, OH: Emergency Medicine Educational Enterprises Inc; 2006:534–549.

Tintinalli J, Kelen G, Stapczynski O, eds. *Emergency Medicine: A Comprehensive Study Guide.* 6th ed. New York: McGraw Hill Medical Publishing; 2004:647–653, 691–700.

CHAPTER 9

RASHES AND SKIN INFECTIONS

Brian Kipe, MD

CONTACT DERMATITIS

1. **Describe allergic contact dermatitis.**

   Allergic contact dermatitis (Fig. 9.1) is a very itchy eczematous rash with varying sizes of papules, vesicles, and bullae. It affects skin exposure sites and is associated with erythema and edema that can be oozing or crusting depending on the timing of presentation. These are immune-mediated, delayed hypersensitivity reactions and typically present 1–2 days after the exposure.

2. **What are some common precipitants of an allergic contact dermatitis?**

   Cosmetics, plants (poison ivy), detergents, soaps, lotions, antibiotic ointments and creams, metals, plastics, latex, rubber, various chemicals, tapes.

3. **Describe the treatment for an allergic contact dermatitis.**

   Avoidance or removal of identified allergen. Clean and wash skin with hypoallergenic soap. Symptom management with cold compresses and antihistamines. It is generally accepted that the mainstay of treatment is topical steroids for mild reactions and systemic steroids for severe reactions. It is key to appreciate any secondary infection and treat with appropriate antibiotics; however, antibiotics are only indicated if an infection is present.

4. **What is a common cause of treatment failure in contact dermatitis?**

   Short courses of steroids. Systemic corticosteroids such as prednisone or triamcinolone should usually consist of a higher dose for at least 5 days and then a prolonged taper in an effort to prevent rebound dermatitis. It is not necessary to provide both topical and systemic steroids. It should be noted that very potent topical steroids should be avoided for use on the face and genitals and fluorinated corticosteroids should be limited to 10–14 days, specifically on the face.

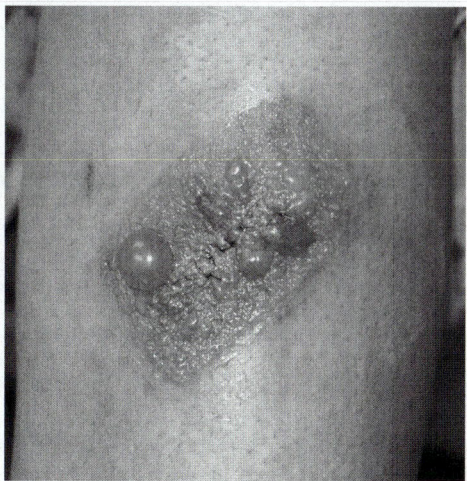

Fig. 9.1. Contact Dermatitis. *(From Nelson Essentials of Pediatrics, 2011. Fig. 191.2.)*

5. **Poison ivy, oak, and sumac all cause forms of allergic contact dermatitis. What is the typical duration of symptoms?**

Typical duration is 2 weeks untreated. If being treated with topical or oral steroids, duration may be shorter; however, treatment usually needs to be continued for 2 more weeks after resolution of symptoms or the dermatitis will reappear.

6. **A patient with small linear vesicles after exposure to poison ivy presents with severe itching that does not resolve with Benadryl cream or tablets. Why?**

This is a delayed immune-mediated reaction and not related to histamine release. Because of this, antihistamines may not provide much relief of symptoms. Initial treatment should include cool compresses and tepid baths with oatmeal colloid or baking soda. Small areas of involvement can be treated with topical steroids. Severe involvement or involvement of face, eyes, and genitalia may require oral steroids. This needs to be over a 2- to 3-week period or the patient will have rebound dermatitis.

7. **How can you tell the difference between allergic contact dermatitis and irritant contact dermatitis?**

In many cases, it is impossible to tell the difference by appearance, although you may be able to tell a difference with key parts of the history and timing of onset. Irritant contact dermatitis does not require previous sensitization and is not a delayed immune reaction, but it is a skin barrier disruption and may present within a few hours of exposure to an irritant. Many times there is repetitive exposure leading to skin breakdown.

8. **List some common irritants for irritant contact dermatitis and describe initial treatment.**

Anything that can cause a skin barrier disruption can lead to irritant contact dermatitis (ICD). This includes (but is not limited to) water, soaps, detergents, or repetitive trauma. Initial treatment is avoidance of the irritant and frequent moisturization of the skin. Since this is a barrier breakdown process and not related to an immune-mediated response, steroids are not always indicated. Topical steroids may be used to help with local inflammation, but only if necessary.

CUTANEOUS ABSCESSES

9. **What is the most accepted management for a simple cutaneous abscess?**

Simple abscess management is typically a bedside incision and drainage. Incision and drainage can be very painful and it is difficult to control pain and because the larger abscesses may require sedation for management.

10. **Why do people presenting with a cutaneous abscess think they have been bitten by a spider?**

Many abscesses will present with a central area of skin thinning with a dark necrotic center that does look similar to the erythematous lesion of a spider bite. A careful history can determine the patient's risk for a spider bite, although a confirmed bite typically requires a captured or recovered spider. If a bite is suspected, treatment is generally supportive care with immobilization, elevation, and cold compresses (avoid heat). Early excision or debridement is not recommended but should be delayed until the wound has stabilized. Other treatment strategies should be based on the type of spider involved.

11. **Should all cutaneous abscesses be incised and drained?**

In general, the standard treatment of an abscess is to drain it. There are times when a patient may present early in the formation of a simple abscess and the cavity may not be identified or yet present. For these patients, antibiotics with application of moist warm compresses and close follow-up in 24 hours is appropriate. The use of bedside ultrasound or attempted needle aspiration using aseptic technique to identify the abscess cavity is appropriate in these settings. Small pustules do not need large incisions but can be unroofed with an 18-gauge needle with aseptic technique and many times do not require any anesthesia.

12. **After incision and drainage of an abscess, should the cavity be packed with sterile or iodoform gauze?**

Recent literature has not shown a benefit to wound packing for simple cutaneous abscesses. In the past, it was taught that all drained abscesses should receive loose packing to allow for healing from the "inside out" and debridement of the wound bed with removal of packing. Unfortunately packing is difficult to keep in place and is associated with increased pain. It is now accepted that simple abscesses (not immunocompromised, smaller abscess size, nondiabetic patient) can be left unpacked. All drained abscesses should receive close follow-up as well as daily wound care with soap and water. Also, new commercially available products can be used to help keep an incision open for drainage, and new techniques can be used for larger abscess sizes (loop drainage).

13. Who should receive antibiotics after incision and drainage?

This is also a controversial question and has been changing over recent years. Based on recent literature, incision and drainage alone is adequate for management of simple abscesses (small size, nondiabetic, immunocompetent patients without surrounding cellulitis or systemic symptoms). When antibiotics are indicated they should be targeted to cover community-acquired methicillin-resistant *Staphylococcus aureus* (CA-MRSA) due to its increased prevalence. The provider should incorporate local antibiotic resistance patterns as well as stay current with the Infectious Diseases Society of America (IDSA) guidelines on management of skin and soft tissue infections.

14. Who would be considered higher risk or described as a complicated case in the management of a cutaneous abscess?

Immunocompromised patients, diabetic patients, large abscess size (>5 cm), patients who present toxic and febrile, significant associated cellulitis, infections on the hands or face.

15. What is the difference between a folliculitis, a furuncle, and a carbuncle?

Folliculitis (Fig. 9.2), a superficial infection of a hair follicle, can initially be treated with daily cleansing with soap and water, warm compresses, and topical mupirocin ointment. A furuncle is an extension of a folliculitis to subcutaneous tissue. Many times these require CA-MRSA antimicrobials and abscess drainage if indicated. A carbuncle represents interconnected furuncles, which are essentially multiseptate abscesses that require drainage with blunt dissection and antibiotic treatment.

CELLULITIS, ERYSIPELAS, IMPETIGO

16. What is the difference between erysipelas and cellulitis?

Both are soft tissue skin infections; however, cellulitis involves the deeper subcutaneous connective tissue. Erysipelas is typically bright red with very distinct, demarcated borders (Fig. 9.3). Cellulitis is also erythematous and red but has indistinctive borders and is more associated with systemic symptoms (Fig. 9.4). Both are warm to touch and tender upon palpation.

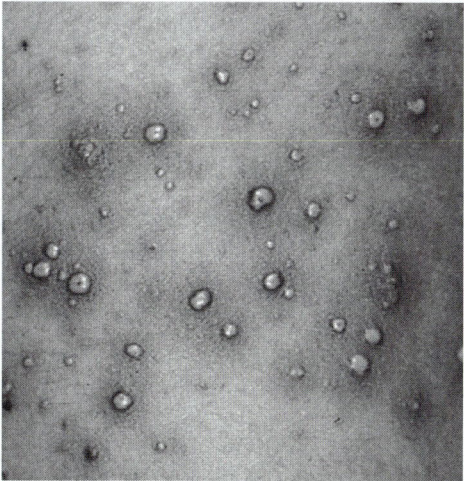

Fig. 9.2. Folliculitis. *(From* Clinical Dermatology, *2010, 1–74.)*

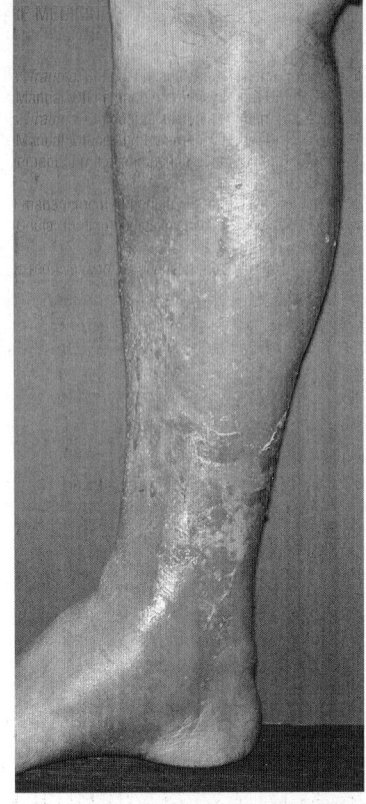

Fig. 9.3. Erysipelas. *(From Bacterial Infections.* Clinical Dermatology. *2010. Fig. 9.13.)*

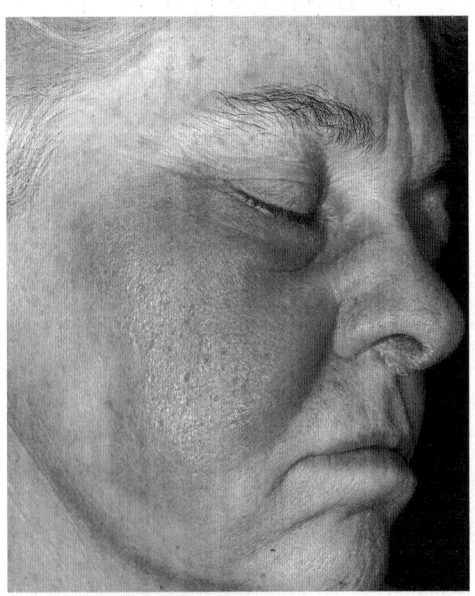

Fig. 9.4. Cellulitis. *(From Bacterial Infections.* Andrews' Diseases of the Skin: Clinical Dermatology. *Philadelphia, 2011, Saunders, pp 247–286. Fig. 14.17.)*

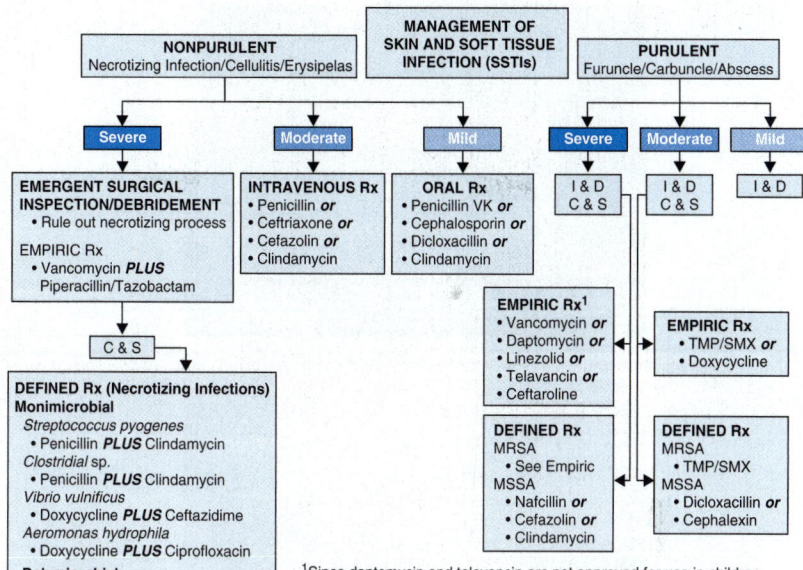

Fig. 9.5. Management of SSTIs. Purulent skin and soft tissue infections (SSTIs). Mild infection: for purulent SSTI, incision and drainage is indicated. Moderate infection: patients with purulent infection with systemic signs of infection. Severe infection: patients who have failed incision and drainage plus oral antibiotics or those with systemic signs of infection, such as temperature >38°C, tachycardia (heart rate >90 beats per minute), tachypnea (respiratory rate >24 breaths per minute), abnormal white blood cell count (<12 000 or <400 cells/μL), or immunocompromised patients. Nonpurulent SSTIs. Mild infection: typical cellulitis/erysipelas with no focus of purulence. Moderate infection: typical cellulitis/erysipelas with systemic signs of infection. Severe infection: patients who have failed oral antibiotic treatment or those with systemic signs of infection (as defined above under purulent infection), or those who are immunocompromised, or those with clinical signs of deeper infection, such as bullae, skin sloughing, hypotension, or evidence of organ dysfunction. Two newer agents, tedizolid and dalbavancin, are also effective agents in SSTIs, including those caused by methicillin-resistant *Staphylococcus aureus*, and may be approved for this indication by June 2014. *C & S*, Culture and sensitivity; *I & D*, incision and drainage; *MRSA*, methicillin-resistant *Staphylococcus aureus*; *Rx*, treatment; *TMP/SMX*, trimethoprim-sulfamethoxazole. *(From Stevens DL, et al.; Practice Guidelines for the Diagnosis and Management of Skin and Soft Tissue Infections: 2014 Update by the Infectious Diseases Society of America. Clin Infect Dis 59 (2):e10-e52. http://dx.doi.org/10.1093/cid/ciu296, 2014.)*

17. What is the best antibiotic choice for a patient with cellulitis?

A patient presenting with cellulitis who does not appear to be toxic or systemically ill and does not have any history to suggest immunocompromise usually can be treated as an outpatient. Due to the recent increased prevalence of CA-MRSA, all patients should be evaluated for risk for MRSA infection and the infection should be evaluated for any purulent drainage. If either is present, the patient should be treated empirically with antibiotics that target MRSA infection. The provider should also take into account local resistance patterns and tailor therapy appropriately. The IDSA has provided clinical guidelines for antibiotic therapy as seen in Fig. 9.5. These are guaranteed to change in the future, and the provider should attempt to stay current in order to prevent antibiotic resistance.

18. Should you obtain blood cultures for uncomplicated cases of cellulitis?

No. Cultures are not indicated for uncomplicated cases of cellulitis, because they are of low yield and are very costly.

19. Who should be referred to a higher level of care for evaluation and possible admission for management of cellulitis?

Immunocompromised patients, diabetic patients, patients who appear sick or those where concern exists for systemic infection or early sepsis, involvement of >50% of a limb or torso, rapidly advancing edge, failure of initial outpatient treatment, or concern exists for possible necrotizing fasciitis, myonecrosis, or pyomyositis.

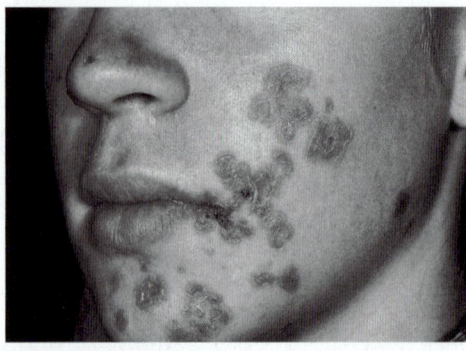

Fig. 9.6. Impetigo. *(From Pediatric Emergency Medicine, 2008, pp 880–897. Fig. 126.22.)*

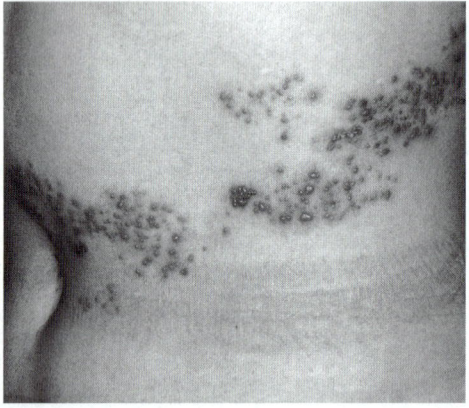

Fig. 9.7. Shingles. *(From Exploring Medical Language: A Student-Directed Approach, 2012. pp 694–749. Fig. 15.11.)*

20. **What are the key elements to outpatient management of cellulitis?**
    Early and appropriate antibiotic regimen, pain control, removal of any infectious source or nidus, daily wound management and cleaning, elevation of any infected and edematous extremity, skin marking of cellulitic border in order to aid in tracking of spread, and close follow-up in 24–48 hours.

21. **What is impetigo?**
    A superficial soft tissue skin infection most commonly seen in children. Classically, it appears with erythematous oozing sores with a honey-colored crust or bullous lesions (Fig. 9.6). It is caused mostly by *Staphylococcus aureus* and some streptococcus bacteria, and treatment is with topical mupirocin 2% ointment with oral antibiotics for resistant cases.

SHINGLES

22. **A 68-year-old patient presents with a unilateral skin eruption that stays in a single dermatome with small vesicles on an erythematous base. The rash is described as burning and very painful, sharp, and stabbing. It was associated with 2 to 3 days of general malaise and low-grade fever and pain at the site where the rash appeared. The patient wants to know if she is contagious.**
    This presentation is consistent with herpes zoster (shingles) and is a reactivation of latent varicella-zoster (chickenpox). She is contagious only to those who have not previously had varicella or have not received the varicella vaccine. For this reason, the patient should avoid contact with unvaccinated children, infants, and pregnant women as well as any individual who has not previously been vaccinated or had the chickenpox virus. See Fig. 9.7.

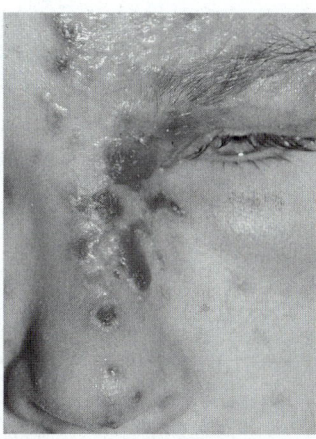

Fig. 9.8. Hutchinson's Sign. *(From Krachmer, Jay H., and David A. Palay. "Corneal Abnormalities." Primary Care Ophthalmology (Second Edition). N.p.: Mosby, 2005. 103-17.)*

23. How long is a typical shingles infection and what is the most common complication related to the infection?

Typical infection will last 3–4 weeks. If a patient presents within 72 hours of rash onset, antiviral prescription can shorten duration of viral replication, reduce formation of new lesions, help with healing, and reduce pain. Valacyclovir 1000 mg TID for 7 days is recommended. Immunocompromised patients and patients presenting with new lesions may also benefit from therapy outside of the 72-hour window. In addition to antivirals, pain should be managed with nonsteroidal antiinflammatory drugs (NSAIDs), opiates, gabapentin, or pregabalin: they are the most promising treatments to reduce postherpetic neuralgia, the most common complication of herpes zoster. Corticosteroids do not reduce risk of postherpetic neuralgia as previously thought and are no longer recommended.

24. What is Hutchinson sign?

An eponym referring to the extension of a rash in the trigeminal nerve distribution to the tip of the nose (Fig. 9.8). This implies possible ocular lesions, and the patient should be evaluated for ocular involvement. If ocular lesions or concern for ocular involvement is noted, the patient should be referred to an ophthalmologist for close follow-up and may need ophthalmic corticosteroids.

ERYTHEMA MIGRANS/LYME

25. What is erythema migrans (EM) and what does it look like?

EM is a flat, red rash that develops 3–30 days following infection of Lyme disease (Fig. 9.9). It usually begins at the site of a tick bite and can spread to multiple areas of distribution. It is often warm to touch. Patients do not complain of itching or pain. Sometimes a clearing occurs as the rash enlarges, causing a "bull's-eye" apperance.

26. How many patients with Lyme disease will develop erythema migrans?

70% to 80%.

PITYRIASIS ROSEA

27. What is pityriasis rosea?

This is a common skin condition, occurring in healthy patients, commonly children. Thought likely to be a type of viral exanthema, it usually starts as a patch (called the "herald patch"), lasts 6–8 weeks, and then self-resolves. See Fig. 9.10.

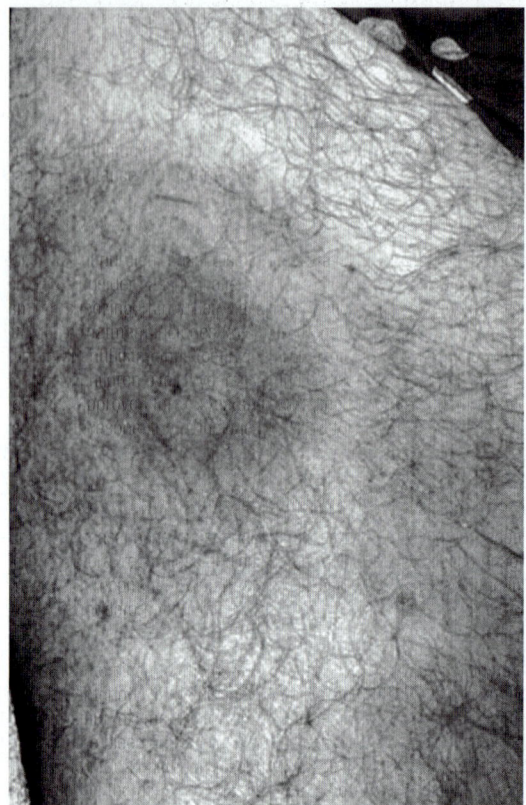

Fig. 9.9. Erythema Migrans. *(From Tick-Related Infections.* Current Clinical Medicine. *Philadelphia 2010, Saunders, pp 785–791. Figure 2.)*

SCABIES

28. **What causes scabies?**
    Mites. *Sarcoptes scabiei hominis.*

29. **What are the signs and symptoms of a patient with scabies?**
    Patients present with erythematous vesicles and papules, commonly located in the web spaces of the fingers, wrists, elbows, belt line, and feet (Fig. 9.11). They are extremely itchy and uncomfortable.

30. **What is the typical treatment for scabies?**
    Permethrin 5% placed over the entire body and left on for 8 hours and then rinsed. This can be repeated 1 week later if not resolved.

TICK BITE/REMOVAL

31. **What is the proper method for removing a tick?**
    Using fine-tipped forceps, the tick is grasped close to the skin and pulled upward with constant motion (Fig. 9.12). It is important not to twist the tick as this may cause parts to break off and remain embedded in the skin. Do not squeeze the body of the tick, as fluid may be expelled, increasing the possibility of infection.

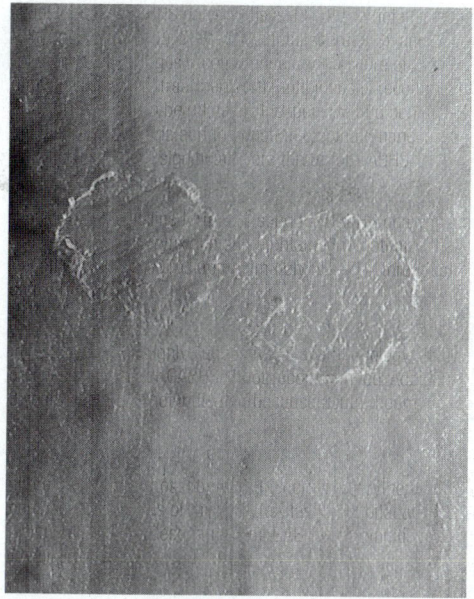

Fig. 9.10. Pityriasis. *(From Principles of Diagnosis and Anatomy.* Clinical Dermatology. *2010.)*

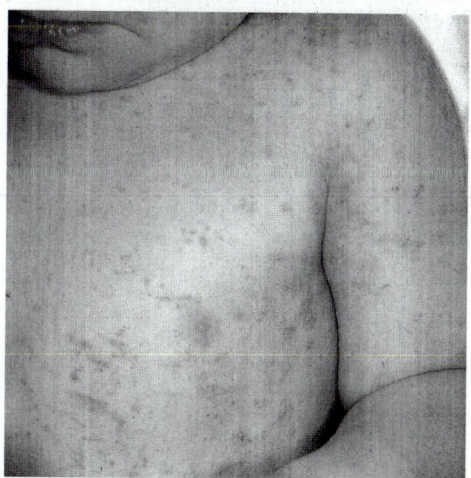

Fig. 9.11. Scabies. *(From Parasitic Infestations, Stings, and Bites. In* Andrews' Diseases of the Skin: Clinical Dermatology. *Philadelphia 2011, Saunders, pp 414–447. Fig. 20.46.)*

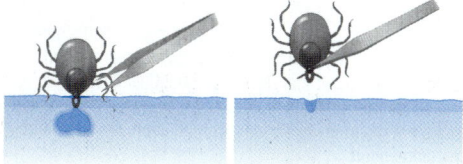

Fig. 9.12. Tick Removal. *(From Goldman L, Ausiello D. Cecil Medicine. 23rd ed. Philadelphia: Saunders; 2007.)*

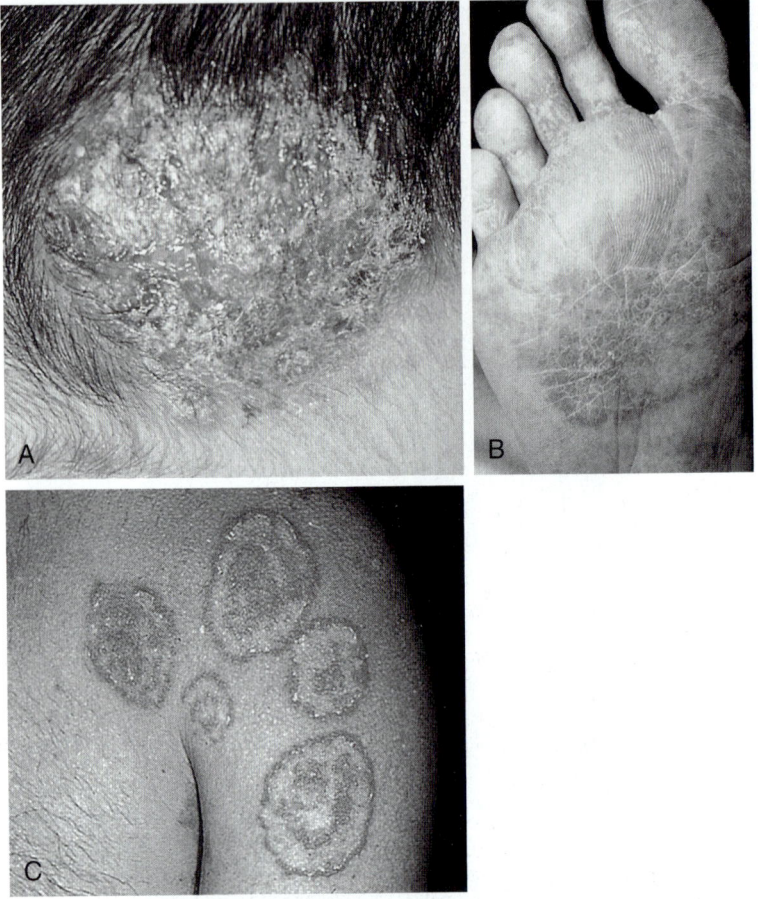

Fig. 9.13. A. Tinea Capitis. *(From Principles of Diagnosis and Anatomy.* Clinical Dermatology: A Color Guide to Diagnosis and Therapy. *Philadelphia, 2010, Mosby, pp 1–74.)* **B. Tinea Pedis.** *(From Cutaneous Disorders.* Paramedic Practice Today. *2010. Fig. 29.31.)* **C. Tinea Corporis.** *(From Care of the Patient with an Integumentary Disorder.* Foundations and Adult Health Nursing. *Philadelphia, 2011, Mosby, pp 1295–1344. Fig. 43.8.)*

TINEA

32. What is tinea?

This is an infection of the skin, hair, and nails caused by a group of fungi called dermatophytes. It is classified by which portion of the body it affects: tinea capitis (scalp), tinea manuum/pedis (palms, soles), tinea corporis (body), tinea cruris (groin), tinea faciale (face), tinea unguium (nailbed, also known as onychomycosis). See Fig. 9.13.

33. How is tinea treated?

Tinea corporis is typically treated with topical antifungal agents (ketoconazole, clotrimazole, terbinafine), but oral antifungals (fluconazole) can be considered in extensive disease. For tinea capitis and tinea involving the nailbeds, oral therapy is required. Use of extensive oral antifungal treatment regimens requires baseline liver function testing and then needs to be repeated halfway through a typical 12-week treatment regimen. Prescribing combination steroid/antifungal creams is common; however, it is not recommended.

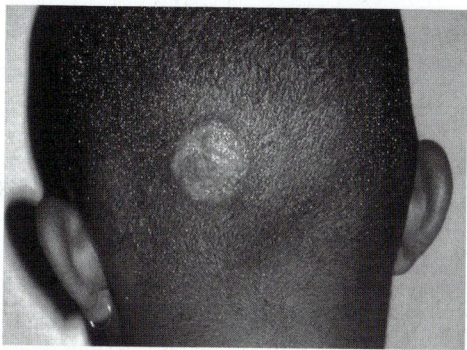

Fig. 9.14. Kerion. *(From Training Room Management of Medical Conditions: Sports Dermatology.* Clin Sports Med *2005. Figure 3.)*

34. What is a kerion?

Severe tinea capitis, often with superimposed bacterial infection (Fig. 9.14). It is treated similarly to tinea capitis, with the possible addition of oral course of antibiotics.

WARTS

35. What is a wart?

Benign skin erruptus caused by human papillomavirus. Warts can occur at any age and can occur at any anatomic location. Common warts are those most often treated in urgent care settings. They appear as rough, raised irregular projections that can be as large as 1 cm. They occur most commonly on the hands, knees, and feet.

36. What percentage of warts resolve spontaneous in 2 years?

65%. "Benign neglect" is an accepted treatment option; however, treatment is recommended if the wart is extensive or symptomatic.

37. What is the treatment for warts?

Salicylic acid is the first-line therapy. This is bought over the counter and has a cure rate of 70%–80%. Cryotherapy has been shown to be an effective treatment option. Liquid nitrogen is applied with a cotton applicator to destroy the lesion. This needs to be repeated every 3 weeks for up to 3 months for complete resolution. Alternatively, electrodesiccation (oftentimes with a hyfrecator) has also been shown to be effective; however, it is more likely to scar.

KEY POINTS

1. Treatment failure is common in allergic contact dermatitis if the course of steroids is not long enough.
2. In general, simple cutaneous abscesses require incision and drainage for treatment, but not all abscesses require packing or antibiotics.
3. Antiviral treatment should be initiated within 72 hours of rash onset to be most effective in cases of herpes zoster.

BIBLIOGRAPHY

Albrecht M. Treatment of herpes zoster in the immunocompromised host. In: Mitty J, ed. *UpToDate*, Waltham, MA. Accessed 28.10.2016.

Ali S, Graham TA, Forgie SE. The assessment and management of tinea capitis in children. *Pediatr Emerg Care.* 2007;23(9):662–665.

Buttaravoli P. *Minor emergencies: splinters to fractures.* 2nd ed. Elsevier 2007.

Baddour LM. Cellulitis and erysipelas. In: Baron EL, ed. *UpToDate*, Waltham, MA. Accessed 25.10.2016.

Baddour LM. Impetigo. In: Ofori AO, ed. *UpToDate*, Waltham, MA. (Accessed 14.10.2016.)

Baddour, LM. Skin abscesses, furuncles, and carbuncles. In: Baron EL, ed. *UpToDate*, Waltham, MA. (Accessed 23.10.2016.)

Centers for Disease Control and Prevention. Lyme. Available at <https://www.cdc.gov/lyme/signs_symptoms>; Accessed 08.11.2016.

Centers for Disease Control and Prevention. Parasites. Scabies. Available at <http://www.cdc.gov/parasites/scabies/index.html>; Accessed 9.11.2016.

Gammons M, Salam G. Tick removal. *Am Fam Physician*. 2002;66(4):643–645.

Goldfarb MT, Gupta AK, Gupta MA, Sawchuk WS. Office therapy for human papillomavirus infection in nongenital sites. *Dermatol Clin*. 1991;9(2):287–296.

González LM, Allen R, Janniger CK, Schwartz RA. Pityriasis rosea: an important papulosquamous disorder. *Int J Dermatol*. 2005;44(9):757–764.

Kwok CS, Gibbs S, Bennett C, Holland R, Abbott R. Topical treatments for cutaneous warts. *Cochrane Database Syst Rev*. 2012;9:CD001781.

Lloyd ECO, Rodgers BC, Michener MS, Williams MS. Outpatient burns: prevention and care. *Am Fam Physician*. 2012;1;85(1):25–32.

Prok L, McGovern T. Poison Ivy (Toxicodendron) dermatitis. In: Corona R, ed. *UpToDate*, Waltham, MA. Accessed 17.10.2016.

Sterling JC, Gibbs S, Haque Hussain SS, Mohd Mustapa MF, Handfield-Jones SE. British Association of Dermatologists' guidelines for the management of cutaneous warts 2014. *Br J Dermatol*. 2014;171(4):696–712.

Stevens DL, Bisno AL, Chambers HF, et al. Practice guidelines for the diagnosis and management of skin and soft tissue infections: 2014 update by the Infectious Disease Society of America. *Clin Infect Dis*. 2014;59:147–159.

Weston WL, Howe W. Overview of dermatitis. In: Corona R, ed. *UpToDate*, Waltham, MA. Accessed 28.09.2016.

CHAPTER 10

MISCELLANEOUS MUSCULOSKELETAL TRAUMA

Joseph Spinell, DO

OLECRANON BURSITIS

1. What is olecranon bursitis and what are the most common causes?
Inflammation of the bursa overlying the olecranon process of the ulna. Common causes include isolated trauma, repetitive microtrauma, gout, pseudogout, and autoimmune diseases such as rheumatoid arthritis and infection.

2. Can trauma lead to septic olecranon bursitis? What are the most common bacteria found in septic olecranon bursitis?
Yes, trauma can lead to both septic and nonseptic olecranon bursitis with *Staphylococcus aureus* being the causative factor in 80% of cases. Patients exposed to repetitive pressure leading to microtrauma to the elbow region are at increased risk for developing bursitis.

3. What signs and symptoms are suggestive of septic bursitis?
Fever, warmth when compared to the unaffected side, erythema, and pain with passive range of motion (ROM) may all be found in all forms of bursitis; they are suggestive but not fully reliable for the diagnosis of septic bursitis. In addition, the absence of any of these signs and symptoms cannot reliably be used to rule out septic bursitis.

4. What is the recommended treatment?
In the absence of infection, most patients respond to a series of joint aspirations, sometimes with corticosteroid injections. Septic bursitis requires antibiotics, typically Bactrim DS (5 mg trimethoprim [TMP]/kg) 1 tabs oral twice daily (PO BID) or clindamycin 600 mg (10 mg/kg) three times daily (TID) for 14 days for mild to moderate cases. More significant cases require inpatient management.

5. What is the technique for aspiration?
After skin is sterilized and the area is anesthetized, using an 18-gauge needle attached to a syringe, insert the needle into posterior/lateral aspect of the bursa, taking a parallel approach to the joint (Fig. 10.1). Avoid medial approach as this could damage the ulnar nerve. Aspirate fluid from bursa until it is flat. Then withdraw the needle and wrap the elbow with compression dressing.

6. What should be ordered for aspiration fluid analysis?
Crystals, cell count, gram stain, and culture.

7. What is the most reliable way to rule out septic bursitis?
While aspiration with a cell count >30,000 is thought to be suggestive of infection, a count less than this does not reliably rule out septic bursitis; Gram stains will be positive in only 50% of the cases of infection. The only definitive test to rule out septic bursitis is a negative culture result. Considering the difficulty in ruling out an infectious cause, empiric antibiotic coverage until cultures of the fluid have returned with no bacterial growth have resulted is a reasonable approach.

CARPAL TUNNEL SYNDROME

8. What is carpal tunnel syndrome and what about its anatomic location makes it such a common condition?
Carpal tunnel syndrome is a peripheral neuropathy caused by compression of the median nerve. The median nerve is found within the carpal tunnel, which is a restricted space between the carpal bones and the flexor retinaculum. Any type of inflammation, edema, or swelling in this very confined space can lead to nerve compression, resulting in the symptoms of median nerve neuropathy.

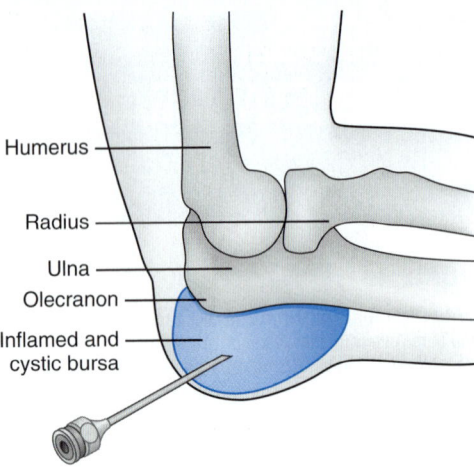

Fig. 10.1. Injection technique for olecranon bursitis pain. *(From Waldman SD: Atlas of Pain Management Injection Techniques. Philadelphia, Saunders, 2007, p 181.)*

9. **What are the classic clinical tests for carpal tunnel syndrome?**
   The classic maneuver that causes the carpal tunnel narrowing leading to ulnar nerve compression is known as Phalen's sign. This is achieved by pressing the dorsum of the hands together, resulting in flexion of the wrists for approximately one minute. A positive sign is one that elicits paresthesias in the median nerve distribution: the thumb, index, long finger, and half the ring finger.
   The alternative maneuver is Tinel's sign. This is achieved by direct nerve stimulation by tapping the volar aspect of the wrist and causing paresthesias along the median nerve distribution.

10. **What is the initial treatment of carpal tunnel syndrome?**
    Avoidance of repetitive wrist motions that may have led to the initial inflammation. Ergonomic devices to help eliminate poor wrist position, wrist splinting, and nonsteroidal antiinflammatory drugs (NSAIDs). If symptoms are severe or initial NSAID treatment has failed, steroid injections can be considered.

11. **What surgical options are there and what at the indications for surgery?**
    Although most patients initially respond to conservative treatment, 80% will have a recurrence of symptoms at one year. If a patient fails conservative treatment or continues to have recurrence of symptoms, consider surgical release of the retinaculum.

DE QUERVAIN'S TENOSYNOVITIS

12. **What is de Quervain's? tenosynovitis and what are the clinical signs?**
    Clinical signs are tendonitis and entrapment of the tendons of the first dorsal compartment of the wrist. Clinical presentation includes movement of the thumb causing pain, especially along the radial styloid.

13. **Who commonly gets de Quervain's? tenosynovitis?**
    Mothers of young infants, daycare workers, patients who have jobs requiring repetitive lifting, and those who have had direct trauma to the first dorsal compartment.

14. **What is the pathognomonic test of de Quervain's tenosynovitis?**
    Finkelstein test (Fig. 10.2). The thumb is held in flexion across the palm by the other digits and the wrist is then ulnar deviated, causing pain.

15. **What are the treatment options for de Quervain's tenosynovitis?**
    Initial treatment can be conservative with splitting of the thumb and wrist, NSAIDs, and ice. Corticosteroid injections into the first dorsal compartment can decrease inflammation and relieve symptoms. Some patients need a series of injections to achieve relief. If injections fail, surgical release procedures by orthopedics can be attempted.

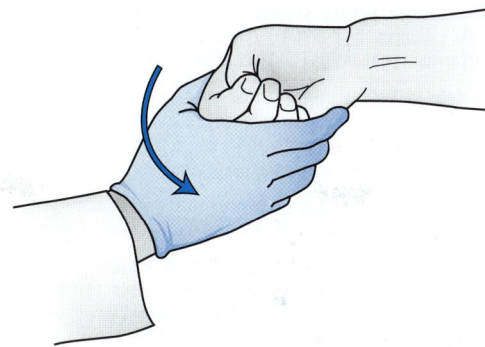

Fig. 10.2. Finkelstein's test. *(From Waldman Pain Management, ed.)*

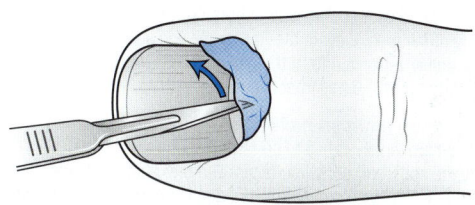

Fig. 10.3. Technique for draining a simple paronychia. The no. 11 blade is brought between the nail and the eponychium parallel to the nail plate. This simple maneuver drains most paronychias. *(From Trott, A. Wounds and Lacerations, ed 4, 2012, Elsevier: Canada pp 161–191.)*

PARONYCHIA

16. **What is a paronychia and what are its most common causes?**
A paronychia is a disruption between the nail plate that allows bacteria to enter into the eponychial space and establish an infection. This disruption of the eponychial space most commonly occurs through minor trauma such as nail biting, nail trimming, or occupations, such as bartender or dishwasher, that involve moist microtrauma. Due to the infection being a primary skin source, *Staphylococcus* and *Streptococcus* species are the most common bacteria leading to complications.

17. **What are the treatment options and indications for drainage?**
Acute infection without signs of abscess can be treated with warm soaks (3-4 times per day). Most simple paronychia do not require antibiotics. Patients with extensive cellulitis surrounding the nail plate, history of diabetes, or immunocompromised state may benefit from antibiotics (Cephalexin or Clindamycin). Infections with fluctuant or purulent drainage are suggestive of a subcuticular abscess and require drainage.

18. **Describe the drainage technique.**
Anesthetize via local digital block. Elevate eponychial fold with a no. 11 blade scalpel between proximal nail fold and nail plate. Incise at point of maximal tenderness to allow drainage. A side-to-side motion can be used to enlarge the incision. Place pressure on the external skin to express any remaining pus (Fig. 10.3). Gauze or iodoform tape can be used to pack the cavity for continued drainage, depending on the scope of the lesion.

SUBUNGUAL HEMATOMA/NAIL BED INJURIES

19. **What is subungual hematoma and how do you get it?**
Nail bed injuries cause bleeding from vessels in the nail bed, which results in hematoma formation and increase in pressure underneath it, which causes pain.

20. **What are the indications for trephination of a nail?**
Presence of a painful subungual hematoma of any size with intact nail that does not require removal of the nail for exploration of complex nail bed laceration.

21. **What is the technique for trephination of a nail?**
This can be done with either 18-gauge needle or electrocautery device. The patient can place finger dorsal side up in a comfortable position. After the finger is prepared with betadine, make a hole at the base of the nail in the center of the hematoma, using a needle.

22. **When is it contraindicated to use electrocautery for trephination?**
Acrylic nails may be flammable and must be removed if using electrocautery.

23. **When should you remove the nail for a nail bed repair?**
When the nail is detached proximally, it must be removed to inspect for any nail bed injuries. Lacerations to the nail bed should be repaired with 6.0 absorbable sutures. Minimal debridement is recommended due to possible scarring.

24. **Describe the technique for nail removal and nail bed repair.**
Administer a digital block using lidocaine or bupivacaine *without* epinephrine. Area should be prepared with Betadine and covered with sterile gauze. Tourniquet may be required to decrease bleeding to ensure a clear view of the area. Elevate the nail by placing scissors underneath it until you reach the nail fold. When the nail is separated from the nail bed, remove it completely with hemostat. Nail bed lacerations are repaired with 6-0 absorbable sutures.

25. **How do you repair an avulsed nail?**
If the nail is detached proximally, it has to be removed and the nail bed needs to be elevated (as above). Clean only the outer and dorsal surfaces. The proximal nail is then reinserted into the nail fold. This can be secured by 5-0 nylon sutures placed distally through the hyponychium or through the nail and then proximally to the nail fold. Studies have also shown that tissue adhesives may be applied to the nail after it is replaced along the fold. This keeps the fold open for a new nail to grow as well as providing a protective barrier for the nail bed. It can also serve as a splint for underlying phalanx fractures.

RING REMOVAL

26. **Describe the "winding technique" for ring removal.**
Pass a piece of thread under the ring. The finger is then wrapped tightly with compression dressing and covered with a lubricator. The ring is then pulled distally toward the fingertip.

27. **Describe the "compression technique" for ring removal.**
Two Penrose drains are used in this technique. The first Penrose drain is wrapped around the finger distally from the proximal interphalangeal joint. The second drain is wrapped from the first drain toward the ring, compressing the edema. Then, after compression, with the first drain in place, remove the second, moving the ring toward the fingertip.

28. **What is used if manual techniques are unable to remove a ring?**
Ring cutter.

INGROWN NAIL REMOVAL

29. **Describe the technique for ingrown toenail removal.**
Digital block is performed, with either lidocaine or bupivacaine *without* epinephrine. The patient is typically seated or supine. For the most definitive treatment, remove the entire lateral quarter to one third of the nail. After adequate anesthesia, the nail is lifted slightly to allow room to make an oblique cut in the distal third on the underside of the nail. The nail is then grasped with forceps and extracted.

KEY POINTS

1. Nonseptic olecranon bursitis responds to a series of joint aspirations.
2. Most simple paronychias do not require antibiotics.
3. If manual techniques fail, a ring cutter must be used for ring removal.

BIBLIOGRAPHY

Brinker MR, Miller MD. The adult elbow. *Fundamentals of Orthopaedics*. Philadelphia: 1999, WB Saunders Co; 1999: 153–164.

Brown RE. Acute nail bed injuries. *Hand Clin PP*. 2002;18(4):561–575.

Chammas M, Boretto J, Burmann LM, et al. Carpal tunnel syndrome: Part I (Anatomy, Physiology, Etiology and Diagnosis). *Rev Bras Ortop*. 2014;49(5):429–436.

Chammas M, Boretto J, Burmann LM, et al. Carpal tunnel syndrome: Part II (Treatment). *Rev Bras Ortop*. 2014;49(5): 437–445.

Huisstede BM, Coert JH, Fridén J, Hoogvliet P. Consensus on a multidisciplinary treatment guideline for de Quervain disease: results from the European HANDGUIDE study. *Phys Ther*. 2014;94(8):1095–1110.

Kalkan A, Kose O, Tas M. Review of techniques for the removal of trapped rings on fingers with a proposed new algorithm. *Am J Emerg Med*. 2013;31:1605–1611.

Lass-Flörl C, Mayr A. Human protothecosis. *Clin Microbiol Rev*. 2007;20(2):230–242.

Loréa P. Primary care of nail traumas. *Chir Main*. 2013;32(3):129–135.

Marx J, Hockberger R, Walls R, eds. Hand. *Rosen's Emergency Medicine: Concepts and Clinical Practice*. 8th ed. Philadelphia: WB Saunders; 2013:534–570.

Nazari S. A simple and practical method in treatment of ingrown nails: splinting by flexible tube. *J Eur Acad Dermatol Venereol*. 2010;20(10):1302–1306.

Rigopoulos D, Larios G, Gregoriou S, Alevizos A. Acute and chronic paronychia. *Am Fam Physician*. 2008;77(3):339–346.

Snider RK. Olecranon bursitis. In: Snider RK, ed. *Essentials of Musculoskeletal Care*. 2nd ed. Rosemont, IL: American Academy of Orthopaedic Surgeons; 1997:156–159.

Strauss EJ, Weil WM, Jordan C, Paksima N. A prospective, randomized controlled trial of 2-octylcyanoacrylate versus suture repair for nail bed injuries. *J Hand Surg [Am]*. 2008;33(2):250–253 [Medline].

Wagner C, Iking-Konert C, Hug F, et al. Cellular inflammatory response to persistent localized *Staphylococcus aureus* infection: phenotypical and functional characterization of polymorphonuclear neutrophils (PMN). *Clin Exp Immunol*. 2006;143(1):70–77.

Wasserman AR, Melville LD, Birkhahn RH. Septic bursitis: a case report and primer for the emergency clinician. *J Emerg Med*. 2009;37(3):269–272.

CHAPTER 11

MISCELLANEOUS INFECTIOUS DISEASE ISSUES

Rory O'Neill, DO

TUBERCULOSIS (TB)

1. **How does TB spread from one person to another?**
   TB, which is caused by *Mycobacterium tuberculosis,* is spread via respiratory droplets from one person to another. It is not spread by contact.

2. **How does latent TB differ from active TB?**
   Latent TB occurs when patients are infected with TB but do not become ill, and they exhibit no symptoms. Patients with latent TB are not contagious and therefore are not at risk for transmission to others.

3. **What clinical symptoms would a patient with active TB exhibit?**
   Cough (lasting several weeks), chest pain, night sweats, weakness, weight loss, fever, chills.

4. **What past medical/social history in a patient would increase your suspicion for TB?**
   HIV, drug/alcohol abuse, prior TB infection, immunosuppression, homelessness, incarceration, recent immigration or travel from high-risk area.

5. **What constitutes a positive TB purified protein derivative (PPD) test?**
   See Table 11.1.

6. **Would you recommend any treatment for patients with latent TB?**
   Yes. Treatment of latent TB is recommended, as there is a risk of progression of latent to active TB.

7. **Is there a vaccination for TB?**
   Yes, many countries with large numbers of TB patients give bacille Calmette-Guérin (BCG); however, in the United States it is not routinely administered secondary to the low risk. Note that patients who have had BCG may create a false-positive reaction.

8. **How should I interpret a PPD test in a patient with a prior BCG vaccine?**
   The reaction to PPD testing can vary in patients with prior BCG; therefore, the recommendation is to interpret the same (see Table 11.1) and treat based on risk factors.

LYME DISEASE

9. **What causes Lyme disease?**
   Borrelia burgdorferi, a spirochete that infects ticks, that then bite humans and thus transmit the disease. It is the most common tickborne disease in the United States.

10. **What signs and symptoms might a patient with Lyme disease present with?**
    Rash, fever, joint pain, muscle pain, headache, tender lymph nodes, Bell palsy.

11. **What clinical sign of Lyme disease can be used to make the diagnosis without laboratory confirmation?**
    Erythema migrans, a rash that can present 1 day to 1 month following exposure. It is an erythematous circular rash, typically a single lesion, but can present as multiple lesions. Of rashes reported, 19% are "bull's-eye."

12. **What percentage of patients with Lyme disease develop erythema migrans?**
    Up to 80%.

Table 11.1. Requirements for Positive PPD

	Induration		
	>5 MM	**>10 MM**	**>15 MM**
Positive Test in a Patient with	• HIV • Recent contact of TB patient • CXR findings • Organ transplant • Immunosuppressed	• Immigrants and travelers from high-risk regions • IV drug abuse • Residents or employees in high-risk setting • Children <4 years • Pediatric patients with high risk	• No risk factors

Table 11.2. Clinical Stages and Symptoms of Lyme Disease

STAGE	SYMPTOMS
Early localized	Erythema migrans, fever, chills, myalgias, fatigue, headache
Early disseminated	Multiple erythema migrans, facial nerve palsy, meningitis, encephalitis, atrioventricular block
Late	Arthritis, peripheral neuropathy

Table 11.3. Treatment for Lyme Disease

Early localized	Adult—doxycycline 100 mg po bid × 14 days; amoxicillin 500 mg po tid × 14 days Pediatrics—doxycycline 2 mg/kg bid × 14 days (age 8 or older); amoxicillin 50 mg/kg/day (in 3 doses) × 14 days (max dose 500 mg per dose)
Early disseminated or any w/ AV block, pericarditis, meningitis, encephalitis	IV antibiotics are required, patient needs to be sent to the emergency department
Late (with arthritis only)	Same treatment as Early, treated for 28 days

13. **What is the recommended laboratory testing for Lyme disease?**
Two-tiered testing using enzyme-linked immunosorbent assay, followed by Western blot for confirmation.

14. **What are the clinical stages and symptoms of Lyme disease?**
See Table 11.2.

15. **What is the treatment for Lyme disease?**
See Table 11.3.

16. **What is the recommendation for the treatment of "chronic Lyme disease"?**
Some people have used this term to describe nonspecific symptoms in patients without clinical or laboratory evidence of disease. Multiple governing bodies including the American Academy of Pediatrics, the American Academy of Neurology, and the Infectious Diseases Society of America have come out against recommending prolonged antibiotics.

17. **What are some preventive measures people can take?**
Wearing protective clothing, tick repellant, frequent body checks, shower/bathing after outdoor exposure, and avoiding areas with high tick exposure.

RABIES

18. **What animals cause the majority of diagnosed human rabies cases in North America?**
Bats.

Table 11.4. Rabies Post Exposure Prophylaxis Recommendations

PATIENT IS	VACCINE	IMMUNOGLOBULIN (20 IU/kg) LOCAL ADMIN, THEN MUSCLE
Unvaccinated, immunocompetent	4 dose—Day 0, 3, 7, 14	Yes
Unvaccinated, immunocompromised	5 dose—Day 0, 3, 7, 14, 28	Yes
Previously vaccinated	2 dose—Day 0, 3	No

19. **A patient wakes up and notices a bat in the room in which he was sleeping. What do you recommend?**
Postexposure prophylaxis is recommended for any contact between a human and a bat unless the bat can be tested and is negative for rabies. Prophylaxis is recommended in situations of unknown exposure/risk.

20. **What are the Centers for Disease Control (CDC) recommendations on animals that can be observed?**
No rabies prophylaxis is recommended if the animal can be observed for 10 days. If signs suggestive of rabies develop in the animal during this observation period, postexposure prophylaxis should be administered.

21. **According to the CDC, how many people in the United States have ever contracted rabies from a dog, cat, or ferret that was observed for 10 days?**
Zero.

22. **What are the CDC rabies postexposure prophylaxis recommendations?**
See Table 11.4.

TETANUS PROPHYLAXIS IN WOUND MANAGEMENT

23. **What are the recommendations for use of tetanus toxoid, reduced diphtheria toxoid, and acellular pertussis vaccine (Tdap) in wound management?**
   1. Clean/minor wound
      a. Unknown tetanus vaccination history—administer Tdap
      b. Most recent vaccine >10 years ago—administer Tdap
      c. Most recent vaccine <10 years ago—vaccine not needed
   2. All other wounds
      a. Unknown tetanus vaccination history—administer Tdap
      b. Most recent vaccine >5 years ago—administer Tdap
      c. Most recent vaccine <5 years ago—vaccine not needed

MEASLES

24. **When should you consider a diagnosis of measles?**
Unvaccinated child, usually under the age of 5, fever, cough, runny nose, conjunctivitis for several days, followed by maculopapular rash beginning on the face and upper neck.

25. **What are complications of measles?**
While usually a mild illness, it can be associated with pneumonia, seizures, encephalitis, diarrhea, and even death.

KEY POINTS

1. A positive PPD test indicates that a person at some point in time has been infected with tuberculosis.
2. Lyme disease is the most common tickborne disease in the United States; and in up to 20% of cases there is no rash.
3. Postexposure rabies vaccination is recommended in any human–bat interaction.

Bibliography

Dyer JL, Yager P, Orciari L, et al. Rabies surveillance in the United States during 2013. *J Am Vet Med Assoc.* 2014;245(10):1111–1123.

Epidemiology and Prevention of Vaccine-Preventable Diseases: Measles. <http://www.cdc.gov/vaccines/pubs/pinkbook/meas.html#epi>.

Epidemiology and Prevention of Vaccine-Preventable Diseases: Tetanus. <http://www.cdc.gov/vaccines/pubs/pinkbook/tetanus.html#wound>.

Lyme Disease. <http://emedicine.medscape.com/article/330178-overview#showall>.

Manning SE, Rupprecht CE, Fishbein D, et al. Human rabies prevention—United States, 2008: recommendations of the Advisory Committee on Immunization Practices. *MMWR Recomm Rep.* 2008;57(RR-3):1–28.

Rabies. <http://www.cdc.gov/rabies/>.

Rowland K, Guthmann R, Jamieson B, Malloy D. Clinical inquires. How should we manage a patient with a positive PPD and prior BCG vaccination? *J Fam Pract.* 2006;55(8):718–720.

Rupprecht CE, Briggs D, Brown CM, et al. Use of a reduced (4-dose) vaccine schedule for postexposure prophylaxis to prevent human rabies: recommendations of the advisory committee on immunization practices. *MMWR Recomm Rep.* 2010;59(RR-2):1–9.

Tuberculosis (TB). <http://www.cdc.gov/tb/default.htm>.

Wright WF, Riedel DL, Talwani R, Gilliam BL. Diagnosis and management of Lyme disease. *Am Fam Physician.* 2012;85(11):1086–1093.

CHAPTER 12

FEVER

Ariella Nadler, MD, Jeffrey R. Avner, MD

1. What causes fever?
The body has a "central thermostat" comprised of a specialized group of neurons in the hypothalamus that act to maintain the body at a physiologic "set point." This set point changes when pyrogens (endogenous or exogenous substances that produce fever) stimulate an inflammatory response that increases the production of prostaglandin E, which in turn acts on the hypothalamus to raise the set point. When the body's temperature is lower than the set point, various mechanisms are employed to increase heat production and raise the body's temperature to be in balance with the new set point, resulting in fever.

2. What are the different phases of the febrile response?
The first phase of the febrile response is the "chill" phase. Various mechanisms, including increasing cellular metabolism, increasing skeletal muscle activity through involuntary shivering, peripheral vasoconstriction, and seeking a warmer environment are employed in order to raise the body's temperature to a new set point. The "flush" phase occurs as the set point is lowered back toward normal body temperature with illness resolution or administration of antipyretics. This phase is characterized by peripheral vasodilation, sweating, and seeking a cooler environment as the body seeks to lower its temperature to the new set point.

3. Is there a difference between fever and hyperthermia?
Yes, *fever* is a physiologic response, and *hyperthermia* is not. *Fever* is an elevation of body temperature that is regulated by the body's internal thermoregulatory center in the hypothalamus, whereas *hyperthermia* represents elevation of body temperature due to an external environmental source, with no input from the body's thermoregulatory center. Temperature elevation secondary to hyperthermia is dangerous as the thermoregulatory center does not stimulate vasodilation and sweating to lower the temperature, as it would in the case of fever.

4. Is normal body temperature 98.6°F (37°C)?
There is no single normal value for body temperature. Rather, there is a range of normal that can vary in each person by as much as 0.5°C from the mean, based on various factors. These include time of day (lowest in the morning and highest in the evening), age (higher in infants), sex, physical activity, and ambient temperature.

5. So where did the value 98.6°F come from?
The value 98.6°F is attributed to Carl Wunderlich, who published, in 1868, a study in which he used a foot-long axillary thermometer to take 1 million temperature readings in more than 25,000 patients and found 98.6°F to be the mean temperature; hardly accurate by today's standards.

6. Which method of temperature measurement is most reliable (axillary, oral, rectal, tympanic) or does it not really matter?
Table 12.1 compares the different methods of temperature measurement. As each have pros and cons, it is most important to use a consistent form of measurement to monitor changes in body temperature. Keep in mind these methods measure body temperature at a peripheral site, which lags behind the core body temperature.

7. Can children have fever even if they don't have an elevated body temperature?
When children are in the "chill" phase of fever, their body temperature may not be elevated, as the core body temperature may not have reached the thermoregulatory center's new set point. However, children may manifest symptoms of the febrile response such as shivering, cool skin, tachycardia, tachypnea, and decreased appetite. Fever will likely occur 20–30 minutes after the development of these systemic symptoms.

8. Is it "feed a cold and starve a fever" or the other way around?
Although generally dismissed as folklore, there may be some physiologic explanation for this classic proverb, which dates back to the 1500s. Studies show that food intake upregulates cell-mediated

Table 12.1. Methods of Temperature Measurement

METHOD	PROS	CONS	NORMAL RANGE, MEAN °C (°F)	FEVER °C (°F)
Axilla	Comfortable Safe	Lag time Inaccurate during chill phase and skin cooling from sweating	34.7–37.3, 36.4 (94.5–99.1, 97.5)	37.4 (99.3)
Oral (sublingual)	Comfortable (children >5) Safe Less lag time More accurate	May be affected by recently consumed fluids or evaporative effects of mouth breathing	35.5–37.5, 36.6 (95.9–99.5, 97.9)	37.6 (99.7)
Rectal	Safe Closest to core temperature Not affected by environmental factors	Less comfortable Concern for cross-contamination if standard precautions aren't followed	36.6–37.9, 37.0 (97.9–100.2, 98.6)	38.0 (100.4)
Tympanic	Comfortable Safe Cost effective	Difficult to aim thermometer at TM Cerumen may block TM	35.7–37.5 (96.3–99.5, 97.9)	37.6 (99.7)
Temporal	Comfortable Safe	Low diagnostic accuracy	36.4–37.7 (97.5–99.9)	37.8 (100.0)

immunity (via increased interferon-gamma production) that can help fight viral infections such as colds, while withholding food increases humoral immunity (via upregulation of IL-4), which is helpful in fighting bacterial infections, historically thought to be the predominant cause of fever.

9. **Is there a value that is considered a "high" fever (or how high is too high)?**
There is no specific value considered too "high" for a *fever* (as opposed to hyperthermia). Fever increases a child's metabolic rate and catabolism, making him or her more prone to heat loss. Most healthy children can accommodate these stresses through normal physiologic processes; however, children with chronic illnesses and those who are immunosuppressed or have cardiopulmonary disease may not be able to adjust to this increased demand and are at higher risk for systemic effects.

10. **Does the height of fever predict the risk of serious bacterial illness (SBI) or mortality?**
While the presence of fever is usually indicative of an ongoing infectious process, the height of the temperature is not an accurate marker of SBI or mortality in otherwise healthy children. Thus, the height of fever has limited use in determining management; other clinical features, especially the child's clinical appearance, are better predictors.

11. **Do parents pay too much attention to taking their child's temperature?**
Parents often exhibit "fever phobia," displaying excessive concern about fever and its potential effects on their child with heightened concern at higher temperatures. This often leads to frequently taking the child's temperature. It is important to educate parents that fever is a symptom of their child's illness that will persist until the underlying illness has resolved. Fever itself is not dangerous to an otherwise healthy child, and the specific temperature value is generally not important.

12. **Should I make the parents focus on preventing fever in their child?**
Trying to prevent or "control" fever is generally futile and will likely increase fever phobia. Parents should be directed to focus on the child's comfort and clinical appearance until the resolution of the underlying illness. Antipyretics can be used for comfort. A change in clinical appearance should prompt reassessment by a health care provider.

13. **Does high fever cause brain damage or death?**
There is no evidence that high fever itself causes brain damage or death, even with temperatures as high as 107.6°F (42°C). Although excessive heat (>107°F) may denature proteins in vitro, fever likely affects protein expression, allowing them to adapt to high temperature in vivo. Nevertheless, over 25% of parents believe fever causes brain damage.

14. **Can I trust parents who say their child is "burning up"?**
Parents' tactile assessment of their child's fever has a high sensitivity (80%–90%), but its specificity is much lower (about 50%), suggesting that parents' assessment is more reliable at ruling out a fever, rather than ruling one in.

15. **Is alternating antipyretics more beneficial than monotherapy?**
There is no conclusive proof that alternating antipyretics is more efficacious than single drug therapy. A recent meta-analysis showed an overall slightly lower mean temperature (between 0.3°C and 0.7°C) with alternating therapy, but did not show a significant difference in the child's comfort. Conversely, there is a risk that parents will be confused with the different doses and time intervals of each antipyretic, leading to incorrect dosing and increased risk for toxicity. Additionally, ibuprofen inhibits glutathione production, which binds acetaminophen to prevent hepatic and renal toxicity. It is therefore generally safer to reinforce monotherapy and caution against alternating antipyretics.

16. **Does a failure to respond to antipyretics predict serious illness?**
In general, fevers due to serious infections are as responsive to antipyretics as those due to benign illness. The child's appearance after fever reduction is a more useful predictor of the clinical condition; a child with a serious illness often remains ill-appearing even after fever reduction, whereas a child with a more benign illness usually improves clinically.

17. **Do antipyretics prevent febrile seizures?**
No studies have demonstrated that antipyretics, in the absence of anticonvulsants, reduce the recurrence risk of simple febrile seizures.

18. **Is there a way to calculate the increase in heart rate and/or respiratory rate with fever?**
Although somewhat dependent on age, the heart rate generally increases by 10–15 beats/min/°C and the respiratory rate rises by 3–5 breaths/min/°C.

19. **Do I need to refer all febrile infants less than 8 weeks old to the emergency department?**
In general, yes. Assuming the fever is not due to environmental factors, such as bundling, most studies recommend some laboratory evaluation for severe bacterial infection (SBI) for any febrile infant less than 8 weeks old as these infants have an immature immune response and a relatively high rate of SBI (about 10%) and bacteremia/bacterial meningitis (1.5%–4%). Due to their developmental inability to show clinical signs of illness (e.g., no social smile), neonates (age <4 weeks) in particular should undergo a complete evaluation for SBI, including testing the urine, blood, and cerebrospinal fluid (CSF) for bacterial infection; empiric antibiotics and hospitalization are also generally recommended.

20. **How should I manage a neonate who has a reported fever at home but is afebrile on presentation?**
A neonate who has a documented fever at home but is afebrile on presentation should be treated as a febrile neonate and referred to the emergency department.

21. **Does risk stratification work for febrile young infants?**
Yes. There is a variety of accepted risk stratification strategies (Table 12.2) used to identify those well-appearing febrile infants aged 4–8 weeks who are considered low risk for SBI and may be managed as an outpatient, sometimes without antibiotic therapy, as long as there is reliable outpatient follow-up. The decision as to which strategy should be used and how much testing should be obtained is dependent on the clinician's experience, reliability of follow-up, and the parents' comfort and observational skills.

22. **Does the presence of influenza or respiratory syncytial virus (RSV) bronchiolitis make it less likely for a febrile infant to have a serious bacterial illness such as SBI?**
Febrile infants <60 days old who test positive for either influenza or RSV are significantly less likely to have SBI, though they still have an appreciable risk of urinary tract infection (UTI). Thus, in a

Table 12.2. Common Risk Stratification Strategies for the Febrile Infant

	BOSTON	PHILADELPHIA	ROCHESTER
Age (days)	28–89	29–56	0–60
Temp (°C)	>37.9	>38.1	>37.9
Observation scale used?	Yes	Yes	No
WBC	<20,000	<15,000	5,000–15,000
CSF from all?	Yes	Yes	No
Antibiotics?	Yes	No	No
SBI—low risk	5.4%	0%	1.1%

well-appearing febrile infant (age >4 weeks) with either RSV or influenza, testing may be limited to urinalysis and culture depending on the other clinical factors. In febrile infants <29 days, there is still limited data to abandon a complete sepsis evaluation.

23. **Do I need to get lab tests for the evaluation of well-appearing febrile children?**
A well-appearing, healthy child who has fever but no source of infection on physical examination does not need routine lab tests as part of his or her evaluation. A thorough history and physical exam are generally sufficient in determining care. In some children under 2 years, depending on their risk factors, a urinalysis and urine culture may be useful. Children who are immunosuppressed or have underlying chronic illness are at higher risk for developing serious illness and sepsis and therefore may need individualized management including selected lab studies and possibly empiric antibiotics.

24. **Is "occult bacteremia" still a concern?**
Occult, or unsuspected, bacteremia was a concern in well-appearing febrile children 6 months to 3 years of age before the widespread use of *Haemophilus influenzae* type b (Hib) and pneumococcal vaccination. Since that time, the incidence of occult bacteremia has dropped from about 3% to less than 0.5%. This data obviates the need to test for occult bacteremia in the febrile, otherwise healthy-appearing, immunized child.

25. **Has pneumococcal conjugate vaccine (PCV13) changed the incidence of serious bacterial illness in febrile children?**
Since the introduction of PCV13, the rate of invasive pneumococcal disease declined 42% overall and 53% in children less than 2 years old. Bacteremia and pneumonia cases have decreased, but cases of meningitis remain unchanged. Children with comorbidities remain at increased risk of invasive disease.

26. **Are there any markers that can distinguish febrile children with serious bacterial illness from those with self-limited nonbacterial infections?**
A variety of inflammatory markers have been suggested as possible predictors of SBI in febrile children. While some suggest that procalcitonin (PCT) is a more accurate predictor than C-reactive protein (CRP), particularly early in the disease course, a recent study showed that CRP, PCT, white blood cell count (WBC), and absolute neutrophil count (ANC) had almost similar diagnostic properties and were superior to clinical evaluation in predicting SBI in children age 1 month to 3 years.

27. **When should a febrile child be tested for UTI?**
The overall prevalence of UTIs in 2- to 24-month-old febrile children without another source on history and physical exam is 5%. Girls and uncircumcised boys have an increased likelihood of having a UTI, and one should have a lower threshold to test these groups. Individual risk factors are listed in Table 12.3. Additionally, children with prior UTIs, abdominal pain, suprapubic pain, back pain, or dysuria should be tested for UTI.

28. **How should urine be obtained for urinalysis and/or culture?**
Urethral catheterization is the preferred method of obtaining a urine specimen in children who are not toilet trained. A clean bagged urine specimen is an option in children older than 6 months for urinalysis; but if positive, only urine obtained by catheterization should be sent for culture.

Table 12.3. Risk Factors for UTIs in Febrile Children*

BOYS	GIRLS
Fever >39°C	Age <12 months
Fever >24 hours	Fever >39°C
No source for fever	Fever >48 hours
Nonblack race	No source for fever White race

*Consider screening for UTI if three or more risk factors are present (or two or more in uncircumcised boys).

29. **Can a febrile child have pneumonia without respiratory symptoms?**
    While many children with pneumonia present with respiratory symptoms such as abnormal breath sounds, tachypnea, hypoxia, or increased work of breathing, there is also an increased likelihood of pneumonia in children with prolonged fever (>5 days), prolonged cough (>10 days), or leukocytosis (WBC >20,000) despite an absence of other respiratory symptoms.

30. **How many days of fever require further evaluation and/or referral to a specialist?**
    When a child has a daily fever for more than 7–9 days without an identifiable source, it is considered "fever of unknown origin" (FUO) and often warrants further evaluation. It is important to differentiate FUO from two short febrile illnesses that are temporally related.

31. **What is the initial workup for an FUO?**
    Workup starts with a history and physical exam and proceeds in a stepwise, focused approach. Factors that affect the patient's evaluation include duration of fever, age, clinical appearance, and the patient's exposures. While 50% of cases of FUO are infectious, a longer duration of fever is associated with noninfectious etiologies including rheumatologic or oncologic. In many cases, a definitive diagnosis is not made.

32. **What is the best way for parents to keep their febrile child comfortable?**
    Because children lose water and nutrients due to the increased metabolic demand during fever onset, it is important to keep them well hydrated, adjust their activity level, and lessen their amount of clothing. While sponging or bathing with tepid water may help reduce the child's temperature, it may also cause shivering and discomfort. Cold water and rubbing alcohol should be avoided as both cause vasoconstriction, which will prevent vasodilation needed for heat dissipation and fever reduction. Antipyretics such as acetaminophen and ibuprofen can reduce body temperature, adding to the child's comfort.

33. **Does teething cause fever?**
    A recent meta-analysis showed that eruption of primary teeth is associated with a slight rise in body temperature (0.1°C–0.5°C), but it was not characterized as fever.

34. **If the child vomits after receiving antipyretics, can he or she receive a second dose?**
    Although redosing policies may vary by institution, the majority of practitioners will redose a medication once if the child vomits within 15 minutes of receiving an antipyretic and the antipyretic is visible in the emesis.

35. **Does management of a child change if he or she presents with a fever after receiving immunizations?**
    Children may develop fever after receiving immunizations (Table 12.4). Since the first set of vaccines is generally given at 2 months of age, this will not affect the workup of a patient younger than that. Older patients should have the same evaluation as a patient who has not just been vaccinated, with a thorough history, physical exam, and any ancillary tests that are necessary based on the clinical situation.

36. **Are there any other reasons why a child would require referral to an emergency department/inpatient hospital setting for fever?**
    One should refer a febrile child to the emergency department or inpatient hospital if he or she requires a specific therapy or subspecialty expertise that is only available in this setting, such as intravenous

Table 12.4. Febrile Side Effects of Common Vaccinations

VACCINE	FEBRILE REACTION
Chickenpox vaccine	Mild fever lasting 1–3 days begins 17–28 days after the vaccine (in 14% of children)
DTaP or DT vaccine	Fever (in 25% of children) and lasts <48 hours
Hepatitis (A or B) vaccine	Usually no fever
Influenza vaccine	Mild fever <103°F (<39.5°C) occurs in 18% of children
Measles vaccine	Mild fever <103°F (<39.5°C) in 10% and lasts 2–3 days; 103°F (39.4°C) or higher in 5%–15%, usually lasts 1–2 days but can last up to 5 days
Meningococcal vaccine	Mild fever occurs in 4% of children
Mumps or Rubella vaccine	Usually no fever
Papillomavirus vaccine	Fever >100.4°F (38°C) in 10% and fever >102°F (39°C) in 1%–2% of children
Pneumococcus vaccine	Mild fever <102°F (39°C) in 15% for 1–2 days
Polio vaccine	No fever
Rotavirus vaccine	No fever

antibiotics for invasive bacterial illness, or if the child has symptoms related to appendicitis or a septic joint that may require surgical evaluation and potential intervention. Patients who are febrile and dehydrated or unable to tolerate fluid intake may require intravenous fluids. Patients with fever for more than 5 days with other signs related to Kawasaki disease should also be referred.

37. **Who said, "Fever is a mighty engine which Nature brings into the world for the conquest of her enemies"?**
This quote was penned by Thomas Syndenham in the 1660s, at a time when fever was considered to have some antimicrobial effects and thus be beneficial in combating infectious illness.

38. **Do doctors sometimes get pressured into prescribing unnecessary antibiotics?**
In a survey of ambulatory pediatric practices, 20% of antibiotic prescriptions were prescribed for acute respiratory tract infections for which antibiotics are not indicated (e.g., nasopharyngitis, bronchitis, viral pneumonia, influenza) and other respiratory illness for which antibiotics are not definitely indicated (e.g., asthma, allergy, chronic sinusitis, chronic bronchitis).

KEY POINTS

1. Fever is an elevation of body temperature that is regulated by the body's internal thermoregulatory center in the hypothalamus, whereas hyperthermia represents elevation of body temperature due to an external environmental source, with no input from the body's thermoregulatory center, and is therefore more dangerous than fever.
2. There is no evidence that high fever itself causes brain damage or death, even with temperatures as high as 107.6°F (42°C).
3. There is no conclusive proof that alternating antipyretics is more efficacious than single drug therapy.
4. No studies have demonstrated that antipyretics, in the absence of anticonvulsants, reduce the recurrence risk of simple febrile seizures.

BIBLIOGRAPHY

Avner JR. Acute fever. *Pediatr Rev.* 2009;30(1):5–13.
Avner JR, Baker MD. Occult bacteremia in the post-pneumococcal conjugate vaccine era: does the blood culture stop here? *Acad Emerg Med.* 2009;16:258–260.
Fein DM, Avner JR. The febrile or septic appearing neonate. In *Strange and Schafermeyer's Pediatric Emergency Medicine.* 4th ed. New York: McGraw-Hill Professional; 2015.
Geijer H, et al. Temperature measurements with a temporal scanner: systematic review and meta-analysis. *BMJ Open.* 2016;6:3. Available from http://bmjopen.bmj.com/content/6/3/e009509.full. Accessed 10.08.16.

Kaplan SL, et al. Early trends for invasive pneumococcal infections in children after the introduction of the 13-valent pneumococcal conjugate vaccine. *Pediatr Infect Dis J*. 2013;32(3):203–207.

Manzano S, et al. Markers for bacterial infection in children with fever without source. *Arch Dis Child*. 2011;96(5):440–446.

Purssell E, Collin J. Fever phobia: the impact of time and mortality—a systematic review and meta-analysis. *Int J Nurs Stud*. 2016;57:81–89.

Roberts KB, et al. Urinary tract infection: clinical practice guideline for the diagnosis and management of the initial UTI in febrile infants and children 2 to 24 months. *Pediatrics*. 2011;128:3.

Strengell T, et al. Antipyretic agents for preventing recurrences of febrile seizures: randomized controlled trial. *Arch Pediatr Adolesc Med*. 2009;163(9):799–804.

Wong T, et al. Cochrane in context: combined and alternating paracetamol and ibuprofen therapy for febrile children. *Evid Based Child Health*. 2014;9(3):730–732.

CHAPTER 13

HEADACHE

Sixtine Valdelièvre Herold, MD, Richard Bachur, MD

1. **An 8-year-old boy presents to your urgent care center with a 3-day history of frontal headache, associated with fever, sore throat, nausea, and vomiting. What is the basic differential for a nontraumatic pediatric headache?**
   - Primary headache: migraine, tension, cluster (in order of prevalence).
   - Secondary headache: infections (such as meningitis, upper respiratory infection [URI], pharyngitis, sinusitis, otitis media, mastoiditis), medications, idiopathic intracranial hypertension, systemic hypertension, brain tumor, nontraumatic intracranial bleed (e.g., atrioventricular [A-V] malformation), and posttraumatic headache (covered separately).

2. **How is the timing of a headache important?**
   - A headache may be acute, acute-recurrent, chronic-progressive, or chronic-nonprogressive.
   - Chronic-progressive headaches are those that may be indicative of a gradual increase in intracranial pressure and warrant concern of space-occupying lesions.

3. **What is the appropriate physical exam for a headache?**
   - Neurologic exam is essential. Six critical findings with headache: papilledema, ataxia, hemiparesis, abnormal eye movements, depressed reflexes, altered mental status.
   - Exam to support secondary headache:
     - Vital signs: fever, tachycardia or bradycardia, hypertension, orthostatic changes.
     - General: findings to suggest dehydration (tacky or dry mucous membranes, decreased or absent tears, delayed capillary refill, reduced perfusion, decreased skin turgor).
     - Head, ears, eyes, nose, and throat (HEENT): findings supporting URI, otitis media, sinusitis, streptococcal pharyngitis, dental etiology; mydriasis or nystagmus to support toxicologic etiology; papilledema or anisocoria, or cranial nerve palsy suggesting increased intracranial pressure; scalp hematoma to suggest trauma.
     - Neck: meningismus, thyromegaly, carotid bruit, torticollis.
     - Skin: neurocutaneous disorders (e.g., café-au-lait spots), Lyme disease (erythema migrans), petechiae or purpura (invasive bacterial infection).

4. **A 15-year-old girl presents to your urgent care center with right-sided, pulsating headache intermittently for 3 days that worsens with bright lights and loud sounds. What constitutes a migraine headache without aura?**
   - Lasts 2–72 hours.
   - Usually frontal, pulsating, moderate to severe in pain intensity, aggravated by routine physical activity.
   - Usually bilateral in childhood, may transition to unilateral in adolescents/adults.
   - Nausea/vomiting, photo- or phonophobia.

5. **What is a migraine with aura?**
   A fully reversible focal visual, sensory, speech, motor, brainstem, or retinal attack that lasts for 5–60 minutes and is accompanied by or followed by a headache within 60 minutes of onset.

6. **What is a tension headache?**
   A headache that is mild to moderate in intensity and usually bilateral. It may be associated with photo- or phonophobia but not usually vomiting.

7. **What constitutes a cluster headache (trigeminal cephalalgia)?**
   - Severe, unilateral orbital, supraorbital, and/or temporal pain lasting up to 3 hours.
   - Ipsilateral conjunctival injection or lacrimation, congestion/rhinorrhea, eyelid edema, forehead/facial sweating or flushing, fullness sensation in ear, miosis or ptosis.

8. **What is the recommended acute management of primary headaches?**
   There are multiple options available depending on the severity of the headache. Not to forget: "simple" po medications! See Table 13.1 for medical management details.

9. **What should immediately put meningitis at the top of my list in the pediatric patient?**
   - The acute onset of fever, headache, nausea/vomiting, neck pain, or meningismus.
   - In neonates, meningitis may present with fever or hypothermia, a bulging fontanel, seizures, or subtler signs of poor feeding or lethargy.

10. **What symptoms should raise suspicion for nontraumatic raised intracranial pressure and thus possibly lead to the need for referral to an emergency department for acute imaging?**
    - The headache and/or vomiting, if present, is worse in the morning and with cough, urination, or defecation.
    - Occipital location.
    - Inability to describe the pain.
    - Change in gait (ataxia or falling to one side), limb weakness.
    - Diplopia.
    - Confusion or depressed mental status.
    - Seizure.

11. **What physical exam signs should raise suspicion for nontraumatic intracranial pressure and thus possibly lead to the need for acute imaging?**
    - Vital signs: bradycardia, hypertension, irregular respirations ("Cushing triad").
    - Abnormal neurologic exam
      - Altered mental status (irritability, coma).
      - Eyes: papilledema, unilateral pupil dilatation, restricted lateral gaze.
      - Ataxia, hemiparesis, hypertonia, dysarthria.

12. **You consider sending a child with a headache to your local emergency department for diagnostic imaging. What should you obtain?**
    - A head computerized tomography (CT) should be obtained if the description of the headache warrants suspicion for sudden increased intracranial pressure or stroke. Magnetic resonance imaging (MRI) may also be required in the presence of acute neurologic changes but is not the initial modality if critically ill or there is suspected acute hemorrhage. Rapid, limited MRI has significant limitations.
    - Otherwise, routine neuroimaging in the child or adolescent with headache and a normal neurologic examination is RARELY warranted, and clinical follow-up is a reliable alternative.

Table 13.1. Treatment of Primary Headaches

PRIMARY HEADACHE TYPE	TREATMENT

Migraine	Mild headache:
	    Oral or rectal acetaminophen (10–20 mg/kg, q4h, max of 1,000 mg in 24 hours)
	    Ibuprofen (10 mg/kg, q6h, max of 40 mg/kg in 24 hours)
	    Sumatriptan (25–50 mg po or 20 mg IN single nostril)
	Moderate–severe headache:
	    Combination therapy of NS fluid bolus, IV ketorolac (0.5 mg/kg IV, max of 30 mg), prochlorperazine
	    Consider dexamethasone, valproate IV, dihydroergotamine

Tension	Acetaminophen/ibuprofen, po Risk of medication overuse headache from regular use of ibuprofen
Cluster	Intranasal triptan High flow (6–12 L/min) O_2 for minimum 15 minutes

13. **What lab work is useful to aid in the diagnosis of a nontraumatic headache?**
- For primary headaches, laboratory studies are generally not helpful.
- A lumbar puncture, with an opening pressure, aids in the diagnosis of idiopathic intracranial hypertension and meningitis.

14. **In conclusion, what should be the disposition of a child whom you evaluate in your urgent care center with acute, nontraumatic headache?**
- Immediate referral to your local emergency department should occur when the child presents with signs of Cushing triad or evidence of increased intracranial pressure, altered mental status, acute neurologic findings, rapid-onset severe headache, signs of moderate to severe dehydration, signs of life-threatening infection (meningitis, encephalitis, orbital cellulitis).
- Consider outpatient follow-up with pediatric neurology for a diagnosis of chronic headaches or migraine.
- Return precautions include brief discussion of signs of increased intracranial pressure.
- Close follow-up with primary care provider.

KEY POINTS

1. Most acute headaches in the pediatric patient are due to viral infections, mostly upper respiratory infections.
2. Migraines, when mild, can be treated with appropriate doses of acetaminophen/ibuprofen.
3. With a normal neurologic exam, pediatric headaches rarely warrant emergent imaging.
4. Head CT is the preferred initial imaging modality for headaches with acute neurologic findings or in the presence of a rapid-onset severe headache.

BIBLIOGRAPHY

Brousseau DC, et al. Treatment of pediatric migraine headaches: a randomized, double-blind trial of prochlorperazine versus ketorolac. *Ann Emerg Med.* 2004;43:256–262.

Gilles F. The Childhood Brain Tumor Consortium, the epidemiology of headache among children with brain tumor. *Journal Neuroonc.* 1991;10:31–46.

Headache Classification Committee of the International Headache Society (IHS). The International Classification of Headache Disorders, ed 3 (beta version). *Cephalalgia.* 2013;33(9):629–808.

Leung S, et al. Effectiveness of standardized combination therapy for migraine treatment in the pediatric emergency department. *Headache.* 2013;53:491–497.

Lewis DW, Koch T. Headache evaluation in children and adolescents: when to worry? When to scan? *Pediatr Ann.* 2010;39(7):399–406.

Lewis DW, et al. Acute headache in children and adolescents presenting to the emergency department. *Headache.* 2000;40:200–203.

Lewis DW, et al. The utility of neuroimaging in the evaluation of children with migraine or chronic daily headache who have normal neurological examinations. *Headache.* 2000;40:629–632.

Seupaul R, Wilbur L. Do triptans effectively treat acute cluster headache in the emergency department? *Ann Emerg Med.* 2011;58:284–285.

UpToDate. Headaches in children: approach to evaluation and general management strategies. <www.utdol.com>; Accessed 15.07.16.

CHAPTER 14

EYE COMPLAINTS

Kaynan Doctor, MD, Tabassum F. Ali, MD

1. **A 3-year-old female patient presents to your urgent care center with "pink eye." What are the classic signs and symptoms of viral conjunctivitis and how can it be distinguished from bacterial conjunctivitis?**
   See Table 14.1.

2. **How can you differentiate between the causes of ophthalmia neonatorum (neonatal conjunctivitis)?**

   Chemical conjunctivitis: This occurs within the first 24 hours of life and is caused by a reaction to topical ophthalmic bactericidal agent (e.g., silver nitrate) applied at birth. It is self-limited and typically resolves within 24–48 hours. Routine use of erythromycin ointment has made this etiology uncommon

   ***N. gonorrhoeae*–associated conjunctivitis:** Patients usually present with sudden, severe, and grossly purulent discharge between 2 and 5 days of life. This disease is vision threatening due to the high risk of ulceration and globe perforation. Gonococcal meningitis is an associated disease. Treatment involves hospital admission and systemic antibiotics covering both *N. gonorrhoeae* and *C. trachomatis*.

   ***C. trachomatis*–associated conjunctivitis:** Usually occurs between 1–2 weeks of life (but should be suspected in infants <30 days old). Common presentation includes a beefy red conjuctiva with mucoid "ropy" discharge. This disease can cause permanent scarring and is associated with chlamydial pneumonitis. Treatment involves systemic antibiotics with concurrent treatment for *N. gonorrhoeae*. As with *N. gonorrhoeae*–associated conjunctivitis the patient's mother and her sexual partners also require treatment.

   Nasolacrimal duct obstruction: Only half of all nasolacrimal ducts are patent at birth. Obstruction causes tearing and discharge without redness. Treatment of this condition involves digital massage over the lacrimal sac. Most cases resolve spontaneously by 1 year of age.

3. **Name indications to culture and Gram stain eye discharge.**
   - Marked purulence.
   - Hyperacute onset of symptoms (over 12–24 hours).
   - Immunocompromised state.
   - Suspicion of *N. gonorrhoeae* or *C. trachomatis*.

4. **How does allergic conjunctivitis present and what are treatment options?**
   - Bilateral itchy eyes.
   - "Allergic shiners," eyelid edema and erythema, conjunctival chemosis, and papillary conjunctivitis.
   - Concomitant allergic rhinitis or asthma.
   - Treatment includes avoidance of allergens, frequent artificial tears, and cool compresses. Moderate disease may be treated with olopatadine 0.1%–0.2% or ketotifen 0.035%, azelastine 0.05%, or epinastine 0.05% as first-line treatments. Oral antihistamines are often helpful.
   - Topical steroids/immunomodulators should only be prescribed by an ophthalmologist.

5. **What are indications to refer a pediatric patient presenting with red eye to the emergency department or urgently to see an ophthalmologist?**
   - Vision loss.
   - Severe red eye and photophobia in a contact lens wearer.
   - Copious purulent discharge.
   - Vesicles or ulcers.
   - Trauma or noxious chemical exposure.
   - Recent ophthalmological surgery to the area.
   - Abnormal pupil shape.
   - Recurrent or ongoing eye infections.
   - Aggressive neonatal conjunctivitis and/or concerns for *N. gonorrhoeae*.

Table 14.1. Comparison of Viral and Bacterial Conjuctivitis

	VIRAL CONJUNCTIVITIS	BACTERIAL CONJUNCTIVITIS
Discharge	Commonly nonpurulent	Purulent
Conjunctival injection and chemosis	+	+
Foreign body sensation, tearing, and photophobia	+	+
Unilateral or bilateral	Unilateral but can become bilateral	Commonly unilateral
Common etiologies and variants	• Adenovirus (most common) • Pharyngoconjunctival fever	• S. aureus, S. epidermidis, S. pneumococcus, S. viridans, H. influenzae, S. pneumoniae, M. catarrhalis • N. gonorrhoeae (hyperacute presentation over 12–24 hours, severe purulent discharge)
Duration	Up to 2–3 weeks	Less than 3 weeks' duration
Additional features	• Concomitant viral upper respiratory infection, sore throat, and/or preauricular lymphadenopathy • Follicular ("dome-shaped") conjunctival reaction	• Less common than viral conjunctiviti • Papillary conjunctival reaction ("cobblestoning")
Important considerations for immediate referral	• Epidemic keratoconjunctivitis • Acute hemorrhagic conjunctivitis: associated with large subconjunctival hemorrhages and enterovirus infection	• Suspected gonococcal conjunctivitis *If Neisseria or Chlamydia conjunctivitis is suspected in a *child,* a workup for abuse is indicated.
Treatment and supportive management	• Self-limited • Cool compresses, artificial tears; antibiotics do not hasten resolution • Avoid school or daycare until resolution; can be contagious for 10–21 days • Hand hygiene	• Topical antibiotics (see corneal abrasions) • Systematic therapy indicated for gonococcal or chlamydial conjunctivitis

+indicates present (Wong and Anninger, 2014).
From: Gerstenblith AT, Rabinowitz MP, eds: Conjunctiva/Sclera/Iris/External Disease. In *The Wills Eye Manual: Office and Emergency Room Diagnosis and Treatment of Eye Disease,* ed 6, Philadelphia, 2012, Wolters Kluwer Health/Lippincott Williams & Wilkins [chapter 5].

6. **A 9-year-old female patient presents with a painful nodule over the right upper eyelid for the last 3 days. What is your differential diagnosis and how would you manage her care?**

   Chalazion: local eyelid inflammation secondary to obstruction of eyelid margin gland (meibomian gland or gland of Zeis).

   Hordeolum: acute bacterial infection of eyelid margin gland that may evolve into preseptal cellulitis.

   Initial management typically involves warm compresses and gentle massage to the affected eye for 10 minutes four times a day with or without topical antibiotic therapy. If the lesion fails to improve after 3–4 weeks of conservative therapy, referral is indicated for incision and curettage.

Table 14.2. Preseptal Versus Orbital Cellulitis in Children

FEATURE	PRESEPTAL CELLULITIS	ORBITAL CELLULITIS
Location	Infection of the eyelids and periorbital soft tissues anterior to the orbital septum	Infection posterior to the orbital septum involving the tissues within the orbit (eye, orbital fat, extraocular muscles, optic nerve)
Etiology	• Adjacent infection (i.e., hordeolum, sinusitis) • Trauma (i.e., insect bite, local skin abrasions)	• -Direct spread from adjacent sinus infection (i.e., ethmoid sinusitis) is most common • -Direct inoculation from penetrating trauma or surgery • -Vascular seeding from systemic bacteremia or local facial cellulitis
Clinical presentation		
Fever/malaise	+/− (usually mild if present)	Usually +
Orbital/eye pain	+/−	+
Conjunctival hyperemia or chemosis	+/−	+
Upper-/lower-eyelid edema or erythema	+	+
Signs of external trauma (insect bite, etc.)	+/−	+/−
Fluctuance	+/−	+/−
Photophobia	−	+/−
Proptosis*	−	+
Orbital pain	−	+
Pain on eye movement	−	+
Normal movement of eye*	+	−
Visual loss or abnormal pupillary reactivity*	−	+ (if severe: relative afferent pupillary defect, loss of color vision)
Signs of cavernous sinus thrombosis, meningitis, or intracranial abscess formation	−	+ (if severe)

+indicates present, − indicates absent.
*The three most important features.
From: Gerstenblith AT, Rabinowitz MP, eds: Conjunctiva/Sclera/Iris/External Disease. In *The Wills Eye Manual: Office and Emergency Room Diagnosis and Treatment of Eye Disease*, ed 6, Philadelphia, 2012, Wolters Kluwer Health/Lippincott Williams & Wilkins [chapters 6, 7].

7. How do you distinguish between preseptal and orbital cellulitis?
See Table 14.2.

8. What is the outpatient management of preseptal cellulitis?
Amoxicillin/clavulanate (25–40 mg/kg/day), cefpodoxime (10 mg/kg/day), or cefdinir (14 mg/kg/day) all divided twice daily.

If methicillin-resistant *Staphylococcus aureus* (MRSA) is suspected or if penicillin allergic: trimethoprim-sulfamethoxazole; 8–12 mg/kg/day trimethoprim with 40–60 mg/kg/day sulfamethoxazole in two divided doses *or* clindamycin 20–30 mg/kg/day divided every 6–8 hours are treatment modalities. All antibiotics should be given orally for 10 days.

9. **What are the indications for referring a patient with preseptal cellulitis to the emergency department?**
   - Age <5 years.
   - Moderate to severe preseptal cellulitis.
   - Inability to rule out orbital cellulitis.
   - Incomplete vaccination against *Haemophilus influenzae* type b (Hib).
   - Toxic appearance and/or signs of meningitis.
   - Anorexia and/or inability to tolerate oral medications/antibiotics.
   - Presence of subcutaneous abscess.
   - Failure of outpatient management (no improvement within 24–48 hours of oral antibiotics).

10. **Describe the classic presentation of blepharitis and its management.**
    - Chronic eyelid margin crusting and recurrent conjunctivitis secondary to a type 3 hypersensitivity reaction to bacterial exotoxins.
    - Management involves daily warm compresses and eyelid cleansing with dilute baby shampoo. Topical erythromycin ointment may also be used. Referral is indicated if these treatments fail to improve symptoms.

11. **A 5-year-old child presents with acute foreign body sensation, photophobia, and redness after being poked in the eye by her younger sister. Fluorescein staining reveals a corneal abrasion. What is your management?**
    The patient should be treated with topical antibiotic drops or ointment (bacitracin/polymyxin B, ciprofloxacin, moxifloxacin, or erythromycin ophthalmic). A fluoroquinolone should be used in the setting of fingernail injury. Patching is not advisable if the injury was caused by fingernail injury, by vegetable matter, or if there is a history of contact lens use. If the abrasion is large, the patient should be seen by an ophthalmologist within 24 hours. Contact lens wearers presenting with corneal abrasion and/or conjuctivitis should be referred immediately to rule out sight-threatening corneal infection.

12. **What features suggest a penetrating eye injury that warrants immediate referral?**
    - The appearance of an abnormally shaped or "peaked" pupil.
    - Prolapsing brown material.
    - Presence of hyphema (blood within the anterior chamber of the eye).
    - Subconjunctival hemorrhages that encircle 360 degrees around the cornea with a history of trauma.

13. **What steps should you take when preparing a patient with penetrating eye trauma for transfer/referral?**
    - Do not examine the affected eye further and keep the patient upright at 45 degrees.
    - Apply a shield to the affected eye. Do not examine the affected eye further and keep the patient upright at 45 degrees.
    - If no shield is available, a cut-down plastic foam or paper cup taped over the affected eye is an adequate substitute. The shield should not apply any pressure to the globe.

KEY POINTS

1. The most common cause of pediatric acute conjunctivitis is viral infection, usually due to adenovirus.
2. In the newborn, purulent conjunctivitis presenting from 2 days to 2 weeks of life must be investigated and treated for *N. gonorrhoeae* with cotreatment of *C. trachomatis*.
3. Preseptal cellulitis can be treated with outpatient oral antibiotics. Orbital cellulitis requires referral to the emergency department for imaging and intravenous antibiotics.
4. Preseptal and orbital cellulitis are distinguished by the involvement of the orbital contents (globe, extraocular muscles, optic nerve) in the latter.

BIBLIOGRAPHY

Beal C, Giordano B. Clinical evaluation of red eyes in pediatric patients. *J Pediatr Health Care*. 2016. http://dx.doi.org/10.1016/j.pedhc.2016.02.001. [Epub prior to print].

Delaney AC, Levin AV. Eye: red eye. In: Shaw KN, Bachur RG, Chamberlain JM, Lavelle J, Nagler J, Shook JE, eds. *Fleisher & Ludwig's Textbook of Pediatric Emergency Medicine*. 7th ed. Philadelphia: Wolters Kluwer; 2016:153–157.

Gerstenblith AT, Rabinowitz MP, eds. *Trauma*. 6th ed. Philadelphia: Wolters Kluwer Health/Lippincott Williams & Wilkins [chapter 3]; 2012. The Wills Eye Manual: Office and Emergency Room Diagnosis and Treatment of Eye Disease.

Gerstenblith AT, Rabinowitz MP, eds. *Trauma*. 6th ed. Philadelphia: Wolters Kluwer Health/Lippincott Williams & Wilkins [chapter 5]; 2012. The Wills Eye Manual: Office and Emergency Room Diagnosis and Treatment of Eye Disease.

Gerstenblith AT, Rabinowitz MP, eds. *Trauma*. 6th ed. Philadelphia: Wolters Kluwer Health/Lippincott Williams & Wilkins [chapter 8]; 2012. The Wills Eye Manual: Office and Emergency Room Diagnosis and Treatment of Eye Disease.

Seth D, Khan FI. Causes and management of red eye in pediatric ophthalmology. *Curr Allergy Asthma Rep*. 2011;11(3): 212–219.

Teoh DL, Reynolds S. Diagnosis and management of pediatric conjunctivitis. *Pediatr Emerg Care*. 2003;19(1):48–55.

Upshaw JE, Brenkert TE, Losek JD. Ocular foreign bodies in children. *Pediatr Emerg Care*. 2008;24(6):409–414. [quiz 15-7].

Wong MM, Anninger W. The pediatric red eye. *Pediatr Clin North Am*. 2014;61(3):591–606.

CHAPTER 15

EAR PAIN, NASAL CONGESTION, AND SORE THROAT

Fidel Garcia Fernandez, MD, FAAP, FACEP, Robert P. Olympia, MD

EAR PAIN

1. **A 3-year-old female patient presents to your urgent care center with a 2-day history of fever and right ear pain. What are the common causes of ear pain?**
   The most common causes of ear pain in children are acute otitis media (AOM), acute otitis externa (AOE), acute mastoiditis, and foreign bodies in the ear.

2. **How common are ear infections in children?**
   - Ear infections are the second most common diagnosis in children after upper respiratory infections (URIs).
   - Peak incidence of AOM occurs in the first 2 years.
   - Approximately 90% of children will have developed at least one episode of AOM by the age of 7 years.

3. **Why are children more prone to ear infections?**
   Children's eustachian tubes are shorter and more horizontal than adults', making it easier for viruses and bacteria to reach the middle ear. Additionally, adenoids may be enlarged in children and obstruct drainage of the eustachian tube.

4. **What other risk factors contribute to ear infections?**
   Preceding URI, secondhand smoking, bottle feeding, and daycare attendance. AOM is also more common in the winter in temperate climates. Children who experience their first AOM within the first year of life are also more predisposed to recurrent AOM in the future.

5. **What are the common forms of ear infections?**
   - **Acute otitis externa:** Inflammation or infection of the external ear canal, also known as "swimmer's ear" or "tropical ear."
   - **Acute otitis media:** Inflammation or infection of the middle ear.

6. **Why does acute otitis externa occur?**
   AOE occurs when there are changes in the canal environment that lead to a change in pH balance from acidic to basic as well as increase in moisture. This typically creates a break in the skin of the external ear canal that promotes the growth of bacteria and subsequent infection.

7. **What are the manifestations of AOE?**
   - Itching of the ear.
   - Tenderness with pulling and pressure on the pinna.
   - Tender, erythematous, and edematous ear canal.
   - Ear discharge, from clear, odorless to seropurulent, foul smelling.
   - Tender periauricular and preauricular lymph nodes.

8. **How do you treat AOE?**
   The vast majority of AOE is caused by bacteria, with a mix of gram-positive and gram-negative microorganisms. Fungi is rarely the cause for AOE. Therefore, treatment should be geared toward covering for these, including pseudomonas (i.e., ofloxacin ear drops).

9. **What are the most common pathogens in bacterial AOM?**
   Despite the advent of more effective vaccines, microbiological results from middle ear effusion continue to yield positive for *Streptococcus pneumoniae,* nontypeable *Haemophilus influenzae,* and *Moraxella catarrhalis.*

10. **What are the diagnostic criteria for AOM in children?**
    - Infants with AOM may present with fever, upper respiratory symptoms (nasal congestion and cough), irritability, decreased appetite, and vomiting, while children and adolescents present with similar symptoms and complaints of significant unilateral or bilateral ear pain.
    - AOM should be diagnosed in children who present with
      - Moderate to severe bulging of tympanic membrane (TM).
      - New onset otorrhea not due to otitis externa.
      - Decreased TM mobility observed on pneumatic insufflation.
    - AOM may be diagnosed in children who present with
      - Mild bulging of the TM and <48 hours of otalgia (holding, tugging, or rubbing of the ear in a nonverbal child) or intense erythema of the TM.

11. **When should AOM be treated with antibiotics?**
    - Antibiotics should be prescribed for AOM (bilateral or unilateral) in children 6 months and older with severe signs or symptoms (moderate to severe otalgia, or otalgia >48 hours, or temperature >39°C).
    - Amoxicillin (80–90 mg/kg per day divided in two doses) is the antibiotic of choice for AOM.
    - Although there is no consensus on duration of therapy, most experts recommend a longer course (10 days) for children younger than 24 months, and possibly a shorter course (3, 5, or 7 days, pick your choice) in well-appearing, uncomplicated cases of AOM in older children. In reality, most guardians will discontinue antibiotics when their child is feeling better.

12. **When is amoxicillin/clavulanic acid preferred for AOM?**
    - Amoxicillin was used within the last 30 days for AOM, or
    - Patient has concomitant purulent conjunctivitis, or
    - Patient has history of recurrent AOM unresponsive to amoxicillin.
        Recommended dose for amoxicillin/clavulanate is 90 mg/kg per day divided in two doses.
        Change in antibiotic therapy (po cefdinir, cefuroxime, cefpodoxime, clindamycin, or ceftriaxone 50 mg IM per day for 1–3 days) is suggested if the child's symptoms have worsened or failed to respond to the initial antibiotic treatment within 48–72 hours.

13. **Is there a role for "watchful waiting"?**
    Yes.
        For children ages 6–23 months with unilateral AOM without severe signs or symptoms (mild otalgia for <48 hours and temperature <39°C).
        For children ages 24 months and older with bilateral or unilateral AOM without severe signs or symptoms (mild otalgia for <48 hours and temperature <39°C).
        When observation is used, a mechanism should be in place to ensure follow-up and begin antibiotic therapy if the child worsens or fails to improve within 48–72 hours of onset of symptoms.

14. **How should you treat an AOM in the presence of (a) a tympanic membrane perforation, or (b) tympanostomy tubes?**
    In both scenarios, since there is a direct conduit to the middle ear, otic topical antibiotic drops are recommended. Due to potential for ototoxicity, polymyxin B drops are not recommended. In the case of recurrent otorrhea, institution of oral antibiotics and referral to otolaryngology to obtain a culture is recommended. Note that an AOM with a healing or completely healed TM perforation or tympanostomy tube that is occluded with cerumen or purulent drainage may require the addition of oral antibiotics.

15. **In addition to antibiotics, how should otalgia be treated in children?**
    Analgesics (acetaminophen, ibuprofen). Topical agents (benzocaine, procaine, or lidocaine in children over 5 years of age, amethocaine/phenazone drops in children over 6 years of age).

16. **A 5-year-old male patient presents to your urgent care center with a 5-day history of increasing bilateral ear pain and a 2-day history of left ear swelling. His mother did an internet search and asks you whether this is mastoiditis. What are the common manifestations of mastoiditis?**
    Mastoiditis is an infection resulting from extension of an AOM.
        The most common organisms associated with mastoiditis include *S. pneumoniae*, *S. pyogenes*, and *S. aureus*.

The most common signs and symptoms include fever; unilateral ear pain; postauricular swelling, erythema, and tenderness; the involved pinna is deviated outward and rotated forward; the tympanic membrane is often described as bulging, immobile, and opaque.

Diagnosis is made by computed tomography (CT) scan of the head (destruction of mastoid air cells, with or without abscess). Fluid-filled air cells without bony destruction are insufficient to make the diagnosis of mastoiditis.

17. Can mastoiditis be treated as an outpatient?

No. A CT scan of the head demonstrating destruction of mastoid air cells, with or without abscess, requires hospitalization for intravenous antibiotics (IV ampicillin-sulbactam or ceftriaxone for 3–4 weeks, then switching to oral antibiotics, such as Augmentin, levofloxacin, or clindamycin, with clinical improvement). Mastoidectomy, with myringotomy +/− tympanostomy tubes, is indicated if no clinical improvement is seen within 48 hours of antibiotic initiation, or if there is concern for subperiosteal abscess, facial nerve palsy, brain abscess, or meningitis.

NASAL SYMPTOMS

18. A 14-year-old female patient presents to your urgent care center with a 14-day history of persistent nasal congestion (described as clear) and mild cough without fever. She appears otherwise well without evidence of pneumonia. What are the diagnostic criteria for sinusitis?

- Persistent nasal discharge (of any quality) or daytime cough >10 days without improvement (+/− fever) ["Persistent Acute Bacterial Sinusitis"], or
- Worsening or new onset of discharge, daytime cough, or fever after initial improvement ["Worsening Acute Bacterial Sinusitis"], or
- Concurrent fever >39°C and purulent nasal discharge for at least 3 days ["Severe Acute Bacterial Sinusitis"].

19. How common is sinusitis in infants and children?

Sinusitis is not a common diagnosis. Only approximately 6%–7% of children with respiratory symptoms will develop clinical sinusitis, as defined above. Since infants are born with maxillary and ethmoid sinuses, sinusitis can technically be diagnosed early in infancy. Sphenoid and frontal sinuses typically begin formation during school age and early adolescence.

20. What are the guidelines for treatment of sinusitis?

Amoxicillin is first line (90 mg/kg/day divided in two doses).

Second-line medications include Augmentin, cefdinir, cefuroxime, cefpodoxime, clarithromycin, azithromycin, clindamycin, and levofloxacin.

Duration: until the patient is symptom free and then for an additional 7 days (usually 10–14 days).

For persistent acute bacterial sinusitis, outpatient observation (initial management limited to continued observation for 3 days) may be an option. Clinicians should begin antibiotic therapy (in the case of outpatient observation) or change antibiotic therapy (second-line oral or IV antibiotics) if there are any worsening symptoms or failure to improve within 72 hours of initial management.

Consider IV vancomycin plus third-generation cephalosporin plus metronidazole for complicated sinusitis.

21. What other treatment options should be considered in a child with a diagnosis of sinusitis?

Intranasal steroids (budesonide, flunisolide, fluticasone, mometasone), saline irrigation, nasal decongestants, mucolytics, and antihistamines should be considered.

22. When should you send a child or adolescent with suspected sinusitis to the emergency department for diagnostic imaging, intravenous antibiotics, and/or hospitalization?

Diagnostic imaging studies should not be routinely used to distinguish acute bacterial sinusitis from a viral URI. A contrast-enhanced CT scan of the sinuses is indicated if there are signs of complicated sinusitis (concerns for orbital abscess, optic neuritis, epidural or subdural empyema, cavernous or sagittal sinus thrombosis, meningitis, brain abscess, osteomyelitis), numerous recurrences, protracted or unresponsive course, or anticipated surgical drainage (failure to respond to multiple courses of antibiotics, severe facial pain, orbital or intracranial complications, immunocompromised child or adolescent).

Other indications for referral include evidence of sepsis, significant dehydration, or inability to tolerate oral antibiotics.

23. You have ruled out sinusitis and concerns for another bacterial infection (AOM or pneumonia). Should an infant, child, or adolescent with nasal congestion, with or without cough, ever be treated with antibiotics?

No. There are many recent studies documenting the overuse of antibiotics for viral infections. This practice may lead to resistance of bacterial organisms to common antibiotics later in life.

24. In addition to URI or sinusitis, what should be on your differential diagnosis in a child with persistent nasal congestion?

With unilateral or bilateral purulent nasal discharge, always consider a foreign body. With persistent clear nasal discharge, consider seasonal allergies (allergic rhinitis). Symptoms of allergic rhinitis may include paroxysms of sneezing, rhinorrhea, nasal obstruction, nasal itching, postnasal drip, cough, irritability, and fatigue. Treatment includes (a) children under 2 years: cromolyn sodium nasal spray, second-generation oral antihistamines (cetirizine and fexofenadine approved for children over 6 months of age), and (b) children over 2 years: second-generation oral antihistamine, antihistamine nasal spray (azelastine approved for >5 years, olopatadine for >12 years of age), glucocorticoid nasal spray (mometasone, fluticasone, triamcinolone approved for >2 years of age).

25. A 17-year-old male sustains an injury to his face from an opponent's elbow while playing basketball. He presents to your urgent care center with significant nasal swelling and right-sided epistaxis. Should you order an x-ray of his nasal bones?

Despite a fracture to the nasal bone, most pediatric otolaryngologists do not recommend acute management of the fracture, regardless of displacement. Therefore, delayed imaging and otolaryngology referral is recommended (after 3–4 days) if the patient has difficulty breathing through his nostrils or if significant deformity persists.

26. How should you treat epistaxis in your urgent care center?

Ask the child or guardian to pinch the tip of the nose for several minutes, holding the head forward, as most nosebleeds arise anteriorly. If the bleeding persists, consider inserting a roll of cotton saturated with a topical decongestant (oxymetazoline or adrenaline) in the affected side and squeezing the nose gently for 5 minutes. If the bleeding is visible, cauterize it with silver nitrate. For persistent bleeding >15 minutes or suspicion for a posterior nosebleed (no obvious site is visible anteriorly, bleeding from both nostrils, blood in the posterior pharynx), pack the nose and send the child to an emergency department to see otolaryngology.

27. What is a nasal septal hematoma?

Nasal septal hematomas are bluish "grapelike" protrusions from the nasal septum associated with trauma. These hematomas should be immediately drained and packed if detected; failure to drain these hematomas may lead to cosmetic deformities.

SORE THROAT

28. An 8-year-old male patient presents to your urgent care center with a 2-day history of fever, sore throat, cough, and abdominal pain. What are the common signs and symptoms of group A beta-hemolytic streptococcus (GABHS) pharyngitis in children?

In addition to sore throat, common symptoms and signs of GABHS pharyngitis include fever, headache, circumoral pallor, strawberry tongue, palatal petechiae, lymphadenopathy, nausea/vomiting, abdominal pain, and rash. Nasal congestion and cough classically points to a viral diagnosis.

29. What is the Centor criteria?

The Centor criteria is a scoring system designed to help the practitioner decide whether to test for and/or treat GABHS pharyngitis.
1. Absence of cough (1 point)
2. Swollen and tender anterior cervical adenopathy (1 point)
3. Temperature >100.4°F (1 point)
4. Tonsillar exudates or swelling (1 point)
5. Age 3–14 years (1 point) and age 15–44 years (0 points)

Add the total points. Risk of GABHS pharyngitis is 1%–2.5% (total score of 0), 5%–10% (total score of 1), 11%–17% (total score of 2), 28%–35% (total score of 3), and 51%–53% (total score of >4). For a score of 0 or 1, no testing is recommended; for a score of 2 or 3, testing for GABHS is recommended; and for a score of >4, treatment with antibiotics is recommended without testing. Since most consider GABHS testing to be relatively inexpensive and noninvasive, and due to the poor predictive qualities of the Centor criteria and the push to eliminate unnecessary antibiotic use, many practitioners will test all children with significant sore throat for GABHS.

30. What is the role of rapid antigen detection test (RADT) in GABHS pharyngitis?
If available, RADT should be the first-line form of testing for GABHS pharyngitis. Samples from the palate, both tonsils, and posterior pharynx should be obtained to optimize the chance of detection. Because the false-negative rate of RADT is approximately 5%–7%, throat cultures should be performed with negative RADT.

31. Should all children with sore throat be tested with RADT?
In children who manifest symptoms highly suggestive of a viral etiology such as cough, rhinorrhea, oral ulcers, and hoarseness, testing for GABHS is not recommended. Additionally, diagnostic studies for children under 3 years of age are not indicated because acute rheumatic fever is rare in this age group.

32. What is the rash associated with GABHS pharyngitis?
Although a scarlatiniform rash is the most common (generalized erythema with scattered papules, "sandpaper like," increased in the folds of the neck, axilla, antecubital and popliteal regions, and inguinal region, with subsequent desquamation), GABHS pharyngitis may present also with generalized petechiae or urticaria.

33. Why do children with GABHS pharyngitis often present with abdominal pain?
Enlargement of lymph nodes in the abdominal cavity (unfortunately, at times in the right lower quadrant, mimicking appendicitis), termed "mesenteric adenitis," may lead to abdominal pain in patients with GABHS or viral pharyngitis.

34. What is the treatment of choice for GABHS pharyngitis in children?
While benzathine penicillin was widely used as the preferred treatment for GABHS pharyngitis, recent studies have shown that once-a-day amoxicillin is as effective. Single-day amoxicillin therapy at 50 mg/kg once a day or 25 mg/kg/dose twice a day for 10 days is the recommended dose (Table 15.1). Antibiotic treatment for GABHS is only to reduce the risk of rheumatic fever; antibiotic therapy does not affect the duration of symptoms, nor does it prevent poststreptococcal glomerulonephritis.

35. What therapeutic options exist for GABHS pharyngitis in patients with penicillin allergy?
In patients who are not anaphylactically sensitive to penicillin, a first-generation cephalosporin is considered adequate treatment. In patients with penicillin anaphylaxis, either azithromycin for 5 days, clindamycin or clarithromycin for 10 days are acceptable alternatives (Table 15.2).

36. How long are GABHS patients contagious after starting antibiotics?
Children are considered contagious for 24 hours after the initiation of antibiotics.

Table 15.1. Therapeutic Options for GABHS Pharyngitis, Non-Penicillin Allergic

MEDICATION	DOSAGE	DURATION
Amoxicillin	50 mg/kg/day (max: 1,000 mg/dose), alternate 25 mg/kg (max: 500 mg/dose) twice daily	10 days
Penicillin V	Children: 250 mg 2 x daily or 3 x daily Adolescents/adults: 250 mg 4 x daily or 500 mg 2 x daily	10 days
Benzathine penicillin	<27 kg: 600,000 U IM >27 kg: 1,200,000 U	1 dose

Table 15.2. Therapeutic Options for GABHS Pharyngitis, Penicillin Allergic

MEDICATION	DOSAGE	DURATION
Cefadroxil	30 mg/kg once daily (max: 1 g/dose)	10 days
Cephalexin	20 mg/kg/dose 2 x daily (max: 500 mg/dose)	10 days
Clindamycin	7 mg/kg/dose 3 x daily (max: 300 mg/dose)	10 days
Clarithromycin	7.5 mg/kg/dose 2 x daily (max: 250 mg/dose)	10 days
Azithromycin	12 mg/kg once daily (max: 500 mg/dose)	5 days

37. Should non-GABHS pharyngitis be treated with antibiotics?

Non-GABHS pharyngitis has not been proven to cause long-term sequelae such as rheumatic fever. Therefore, there is not enough evidence to support treating with antibiotics, and non-GABHS pharyngitis may be treated symptomatically.

38. How do you make the diagnosis of rheumatic fever?

Jones criteria. Two major criteria, or one major and two minor criteria, PLUS evidence of an antecedent streptococcal pharyngitis (throat culture, RADT, antistreptolysin O, anti-deoxyribonuclease B).

Major criteria: carditis, migratory polyarthritis, chorea, erythema marginatum, subcutaneous nodules.

Minor criteria: fever, arthralgias, elevated acute phase reactants (sedimentation rate, C-reactive protein), prolonged PR interval.

39. Is there a role for oral corticosteroids in children or adolescents who have either GABHS or viral pharyngitis?

Studies have shown that a one-time dose of oral dexamethasone (0.6 mg/kg, with a maximum dose of 10 mg) can make the child or adolescent feel better quicker and reduce the total duration of symptoms in those with either GABHS or viral pharyngitis.

40. Why should you care about infectious mononucleosis?

Children and adolescents who have infectious mononucleosis (fever and other constitutional symptoms, severe sore throat, enlarged tonsils with exudates) may develop splenomegaly. Therefore, a clinical suspicion for infectious mononucleosis in a child or adolescent who is physically active or participates in sport should be tested, and if positive, have frequent, subsequent examinations to rule out splenomegaly.

41. Is Monospot always positive in infectious mononucleosis?

The heterophile antibody test (Monospot) is not always positive during early infectious mononucleosis (first 2 weeks of symptoms) and in young children. Therefore, Epstein-Barr virus (EBV) titers should be ordered in these two scenarios.

42. When should you refer a child or adolescent with "sore throat" to the emergency department?

- Concern for meningitis, retropharyngeal abscess (school-age child with fever, stiff neck, "hot potato" voice, sore throat, drooling, dysphagia), or peritonsillar abscess (older child or adolescent with fever, severe unilateral sore throat, drooling, trismus, dysphagia, deviated uvula).
- Severe dehydration requiring intravenous fluids.
- Trauma, burns, or foreign body–associated sore throat.
- Concerns for rheumatic fever.

43. What is hand, foot, and mouth disease?

Hand, foot, and mouth disease presents with oral ulcerations (located frequently in the posterior oropharynx in contrast to herpes simplex virus [HSV], which tends to present with vesicles in a more anterior location) along with small erythematous macules, papules, or vesicles on an erythematous base, commonly on hands and feet and buttocks, but also generalized in infants. Systemic symptoms such as fever, URI, vomiting, or diarrhea may also occur. Since Coxsackievirus A16 is the most common cause, presentations often occur during late summer and early fall. Treatment is symptomatic.

KEY POINTS

1. Acute otitis media should be diagnosed in children who present with moderate to severe bulging of tympanic membrane, new onset otorrhea not due to otitis externa, and decreased tympanic membrane mobility observed on pneumatic insufflation.
2. Children with mastoiditis may present with fever; unilateral ear pain; and postauricular swelling, erythema, and tenderness. The involved pinna is deviated outward and rotated forward.
3. There are three presentations of sinusitis: persistent nasal discharge (of any quality) or daytime cough >10 days without improvement (+/− fever); worsening or new onset of discharge, daytime cough, or fever after initial improvement; and concurrent fever >39°C and purulent nasal discharge for at least 3 days.
4. Rheumatic fever does not occur in children less than 3 years of age, and therefore young children in this age group should not be tested for GABHS pharyngitis.
5. The treatment of choice for otitis media, sinusitis, and GABHS pharyngitis is amoxicillin.

BIBLIOGRAPHY

Acosta R. Rhinosinusitis. *Pediatric Emergency Medicine.* 1st ed. Philadelphia: Saunders Elsevier; 2008:405–408.
Lieberthal A, Carroll A, Chonmaitree A, et al. Clinical practice guideline: the diagnosis and management of acute otitis media. *Pediatrics.* 2013;131:e964–e999.
Olympia RP, Khine H, Avner JR. The effectiveness of oral dexamethasone in the treatment of moderate to severe pharyngitis in children and young adults. *Archives of Pediatrics and Adolescent Medicine.* 2005;159:278–282.
Shulman S, Bisno A, Clegg A, et al. Clinical practice guideline for the diagnosis and management of group A streptococcal pharyngitis: 2012 update by the Infectious Diseases Society of America. *Clinical Infectious Diseases.* 2012;55(10):1279–1282.
Wald E, Applegate K, Bordley C, et al. Clinical practice guideline for the diagnosis and management of acute bacterial sinusitis in children aged 1 to 18 years. *Pediatrics.* 2013;132:e262–e280.

CHAPTER 16

COUGH

Sarah D. Meskill, MD, Esther Maria Sampayo, MD, MPH

1. **A 5-year-old boy presents to your urgent care center with a 2-day history of persistent cough, associated with fever, runny nose, and trouble breathing. What is your differential diagnosis?**

   Cough is one of the most common pediatric complaints with a myriad of causes (Table 16.1). Although the etiology of cough is usually self-limited, a detailed history and physical exam can exclude other potentially dangerous conditions.

2. **A 10-year-old girl with a history of asthma presents to your urgent care center with shortness of breath and difficulty speaking. She is tachypneic with intercostal retractions. What is the first-line treatment for an acute exacerbation?**

   Acute exacerbations of asthma should be treated with systemic corticosteroids, high-dose beta agonists, and anticholinergics. Timeliness of medication administration is a key principle in management of acute asthma exacerbations as studies have shown decreased length of stay, hospitalization, and symptom scores with early administration of oral steroids such as in triage. Combined treatment regimens take several hours to reach peak effect; thus, timeliness is key (Table 16.2).

3. **Should I order a chest x-ray?**

   Chest x-rays (CXRs) are of limited use in the evaluation of a patient with asthma and rarely lead to a change in management. CXRs should be limited to cases where there is a clinical suspicion of a radiographic abnormality, such as persistent rales and asymmetry of breath sounds, high fever,

Table 16.1. Differential Causes of Cough

AIRWAY NEOPLASM	CONGENITAL ANOMALIES	INFECTIOUS ETIOLOGY	INFLAMMATION/ IRRITATION	OTHERS
Hemangioma	Cleft palate	Bronchiolitis	Allergic rhinitis	Otic foreign body
Lymphoma	Laryngotracheo-malacia	Bronchitis	Asthma	Medications (ACE inhibitors)
Mediastinal tumors	Laryngeal webs	Bronchiectasis	Cystic fibrosis	Psychogenic
Papilloma	Pulmonary sequestration	Croup	Congestive heart failure	Swallowing dysfunc-tion
Polyps	Tracheoesopha-geal fistula	Laryngitis	Chemical fumes/particulates	Vasculitis (Wegener granulomatosis)
	Tracheal webs	Pleural effusion	Foreign body	Vocal cord dysfunction
	Vascular rings/slings	Pleuritis	Gastroesophageal reflux	
		Pulmonary abscess	Granulomatous disease	
		Tonsillitis	Smoking	
		Tuberculosis		
		Sinusitis		
		Upper respira-tory infection		

ACE, Angiotensin-converting enzyme inhibitors.

Table 16.2. Acute Asthma Exacerbation Medication Dosing

	Short-Acting Beta₂ Agonists		
WEIGHT (kg)	**Nebulizer**		**MDI PUFFS**
	UNIT DOSE (0.5%)	**CONTINUOUS**	
<5	1.25 mg (0.25 mL)	5 mg/hr	2
5–10	2.5 mg (0.5 mL)	10 mg/hr	4
10–20	3.75 mg (0.75 mL)	15 mg/hr	6
>20	5 mg (1 mL)	20 mg/hr	8
	Ipratropium Bromide		
5–10	250 mcg		
>10	500 mcg	Up to 3 doses	
	Systemic Corticosteroids		
Prednisone (5-day course)	2 mg/kg	Max 60 mg	po
Dexamethasone (x 1 dose IM, q24h x 2)	0.6 mg/kg	Max 8–16 mg	po, IM

Table 16.3. Differential Causes of Wheezing

INFECTIOUS/ INFLAMMATORY	INTRALUMINAL OBSTRUCTION	EXTRALUMINAL OBSTRUCTION
Bronchiolitis	Foreign body	Vascular ring/sling
Bronchopulmonary dysplasia	Congestive heart failure	Cystic malformation of lung
Cystic fibrosis	Alpha-antitrypsin deficiency	Congenital lobar emphysema
Pneumonia	Cholinergic poisoning	Masses (tumor, papilloma, hemangioma)
Aspiration (GERD, TEF)	Vocal cord dysfunction	

GERD, Gastroesophageal reflux disease; TEF, tracheoesophageal fistula.

crepitus in the neck, very poor response to therapy, or sudden deterioration. A CXR may be helpful in distinguishing from other causes of wheezing in early childhood (Table 16.3).

4. **What are asthma history risk factors for high-risk/fatal asthma that I should consider when dispositioning my patient?**
   - Prior intubation or intensive care unit (ICU) admission
   - Greater than two hospitalizations in past year
   - Greater than three emergency department visits in past year
   - Use of more than two beta agonist canisters per month
   - Comorbid conditions
   - Emergency department visit or hospitalization in past month
   - Past history of severe sudden exacerbations
   - Current/recent withdrawal of systemic corticosteroids

5. **When do I need to send a child to an emergency department with an acute asthma exacerbation?**
   Children who are not responsive to conventional treatment of beta-3 agonist, anticholinergics, and systemic corticosteroids with persistent nonresponsive respiratory distress or oxygen requirement <90%–94%.

6. **Is dexamethasone an effective alternative to oral prednisone in the treatment of pediatric asthma exacerbations?**
   Providers should consider a single or two-dose regimen of dexamethasone as an alternative to a 5-day course of prednisone/prednisolone in the acute management of asthma exacerbations (see Table 16.2).

7. **A mother brings her 10-month-old infant to your urgent care center in January with a 3-day history of fever, runny nose, cough, and decreased oral intake. On examination, the infant is smiling with a respiratory rate of 70 breaths per minute, appears well hydrated, and has wheezing throughout on lung auscultation. What is your diagnosis?**

   This infant most likely has bronchiolitis, a common viral respiratory illness that significantly affects young children from birth to about 2 years of age. Lower respiratory tract viruses cause significant edema and epithelial sloughing in the small bronchioles that then manifests as respiratory distress, including retractions and nasal flaring. The most common viral cause of bronchiolitis is respiratory syncytial virus (RSV); however, there are many different respiratory viruses that cause the same symptoms. Bronchiolitis is a completely clinical diagnosis. History will be notable for viral symptoms such as runny nose, congestion, and cough. Fever is sometimes present. Physical exam is notable for tachypnea and variable abnormal lungs sounds; there can be wheezing, crackles, or even rhonchi throughout the lung fields. Distress is noted by nasal flaring, grunting, subcostal or intercostal retractions, and tachypnea.

8. **What can be done for treatment of bronchiolitis?**

   Unfortunately, not much. If patients have fever, antipyretics can be given. Nasal suctioning with bulb suction can relieve some of the distress as patients are typically obligate nose breathers and the congestion worsens the respiratory distress associated with bronchiolitis. There is no role for corticosteroids, inhaled steroids, beta-agonists, cough suppressants, nebulized hypertonic saline, or nebulized epinephrine. Antibiotics should only be given if a concomitant bacterial infection is diagnosed. If patients are dehydrated as their breathing makes them unable to adequately take in fluids, nasogastric (NG) or intravenous (IV) fluids can be given to support them.

9. **Should I order a chest x-ray in an infant with bronchiolitis?**

   Not routinely. Many infants with bronchiolitis will have abnormal chest x-ray findings; however, these findings have not been found to correlate with disease severity. Patients who are so severe as to need ICU care or have concern of pneumothorax might benefit from a chest radiograph.

10. **Which laboratory test should I consider in a young, febrile, well-appearing infant with clinical bronchiolitis?**

    Urine culture.

11. **Are there certain factors that place some infants at increased risk when diagnosed with bronchiolitis?**

    Yes. Age less than 12 weeks, hemodynamically significant heart disease, chronic lung disease, history of prematurity, and immunodeficiency.

12. **When do I need to send a patient to the emergency department?**

    Patients who are in persistent respiratory distress that is unrelieved by nasal suctioning, fever control, or positioning should be assessed by an emergency physician. Signs of distress include tachypnea, grunting, nasal flaring, and or intercostal and subcostal retractions. Younger infants may also only present with apnea. Patients who are also dehydrated or unable to adequately hydrate themselves secondary to respiratory distress, choking with feeds, or posttussive vomiting would also benefit from evaluation and possible observation in the emergency department.

13. **A mother brings her 12-month-old infant son to your urgent care with "wheezing." He has had 2 days of fever, runny nose, and "barky" cough, and this afternoon he has difficult, high-pitched breathing. What is your diagnosis?**

    Croup refers to a viral infection that causes inflammation of the larynx and trachea. Parainfluenza type 1 is the most common cause of the infection in the fall and winter times. Symptoms start gradually with runny nose and congestion and then progress to include fever, cough, and stridor. It is usually a self-limited disease. In a patient who is 6 months to 6 years of age and otherwise healthy, croup frequently presents as a barky cough (similar to a seal). Some patients will also exhibit stridor, especially when agitated or crying. Patients with stridor at rest are considered to be more ill.

14. **What is the treatment for croup?**

    Current recommendations are to give 0.15–0.6 mg/kg of dexamethasone with a maximum dose of 8–16 mg. The oral route is best as the IM route can cause more agitation. IM should be reserved for patients who vomited up the dose or have severe distress. Although rarely necessary, steroids can be redosed in 6–24 hours. Nebulized racemic epinephrine should only be used in those patients who have stridor at rest. Racemic epinephrine is administered as 0.05 mL/kg per dose (maximum of 0.5 mL) of a 2.25% solution diluted to 3 mL total volume with normal saline. It is given via nebulizer over 15 minutes.

15. **How long should I observe a child who receives racemic epinephrine and remains improved?**
   If a child received racemic epinephrine for stridor at rest, the child should be observed for at least 2 hours to monitor for rebound stridor.

16. **What else should I be worried about?**
   If the clinical history is not consistent with croup, there can be other possible diagnoses. In a patient with sudden onset of stridor and difficulty breathing without any preceding viral illness, the possibility of foreign body aspiration has to be entertained. In unvaccinated, ill-appearing children, acute epiglottitis can present with distress, cough, and stridor. Ill-appearing children with drooling, fever, and tripoding can also have a posterior retropharyngeal abscess. These patients require acute transfer to a higher level of care where difficult pediatric airways can be managed.

17. **Should I order a neck x-ray or any other studies in an infant with croup?**
   Not routinely. X-rays do not aid in diagnosis or help with determining severity of presentation. X-rays should be reserved for those patients with concern for foreign body aspiration or other diagnosis when there is no response to treatments. If a neck x-ray is obtained, the most classic finding is subglottic narrowing with a normal epiglottis, which is also known as the "steeple sign." This is in contrast to patients with epiglottitis who have swelling of the epiglottis called the "thumb sign" or increased prevertebral edema seen with a retropharyngeal abscess. Viral studies are not helpful in the management or treatment of croup as it will not change management or have any prognostic factors for severity of illness.

18. **What is the common presentation of pertussis?**
   The classic presentation of pertussis occurs in three stages. The first stage, catarrhal, lasts 1 to 2 weeks and is similar to a viral upper respiratory infection with watery rhinorrhea, mild cough, and low grade fever. The difference from a viral URI is that the cough worsens throughout the first stage. The second stage, paroxysmal, is when the classic "whoop" of pertussis is heard. This stage is marked by increasing severity of episodes of coughing spells with long episodes of coughing with little respiratory effort. This is when the child struggles to breathe and could have cyanosis and gagging. This stage lasts from 2 to 8 weeks. The third and last stage, convalescent, is when the patient is slowly improving from the illness over several weeks to months. Median duration of cough in untreated patients is 112 days.

19. **How do I diagnose pertussis?**
   Pertussis should be diagnosed clinically and treatment started while awaiting confirmatory testing. In children younger than 4 months, there might not be the "whooping" sound, so apnea, seizures, and cyanosis should be used as clues to the diagnosis of possible pertussis. Confirmatory testing by culture or polymerase chain reaction (PCR) is required to meet national reporting guidelines. Serology is not useful in patients younger than 4 months or if they have received the vaccine in the last year. Other lab abnormalities include white blood cell count (WBC) >20,000 with >50% leukocytes, but a complete blood count (CBC) does not need to be sent routinely.

20. **What is the treatment for pertussis? Should I treat family members?**
   Azithromycin is recommended for treatment with dosing and alternate therapy listed in Table 16.4. Azithromycin has the same efficacy and fewer side effects than the other treatment options. Therapy is best when initiated within 7 days of symptoms. Close contacts and high-risk individuals (such as immunocompromised, pregnancy, younger than 4 months of age, moderate to severe asthma) should be treated with postexposure prophylaxis with the same treatment as the infected patient. Infants less than 4 months of age are at high risk for severe or fatal pertussis. These infants should be considered for evaluation at an emergency department and observation.

21. **A 15-year-old presents to your urgent care center with 5 days of fever, cough, chest pain, and difficulty breathing. How do I diagnose pneumonia?**
   Pneumonia is a clinical diagnosis. Common history components of pneumonia include cough, fever, chest pain, and difficulty breathing. On exam, there can be respiratory distress as noted by tachypnea, retractions, and hypoxia in addition to focal findings such as crackles or decreased lung sounds. In cases of basilar pneumonia, abdominal pain may be the presenting sign. Only the absence of tachypnea has been linked to the absence of pneumonia. Routine CBC or cultures (either blood or sputum) are not necessary in children who will be treated as outpatients.

22. **When should I get a chest x-ray in a child whom I suspect has pneumonia?**
   Chest x-rays should be saved for those patients with severe disease or distress, persistent hypoxia, outpatient treatment failure, or any other indication that the patient would need admission for therapy. Outpatient chest x-rays have not been shown to affect outcomes.

Table 16.4. Recommended Antimicrobial Therapy and Postexposure Prophylaxis for Pertussis in Infants, Children, Adolescents, and Adults[a]

AGE	Recommended Drugs			ALTERNATIVE TMP-SMX
	AZITHROMYCIN	ERYTHROMYCIN	CLARITHROMYCIN	
<1 month	10 mg/kg/day as a single dose daily for 5 days[b,c]	40 mg/kg/day in 4 divided doses for 14 days	Not recommended	Contraindicated at younger than 2 months of age
1–5 months	See above	See above	15 mg/kg/day in 2 divided doses for 7 days	2 months of age or older: TMP, 8 mg/kg/day; SMX, 40 mg/kg/day in 2 doses for 14 days
>6 months and children	10 mg/kg as a single dose on day 1 (max 500 mg), then 5 mg/kg/day as a single dose on days 2 through 5 (max 250 mg/day)[b,d]	40 mg/kg/day in 4 divided doses for 7–14 days (max 1–2 g/day)	15 mg/kg/day in 2 divided doses for 7 days (max 1 g/day)	See above
Adolescents and adults	500 mg as a single dose on day 1, then 250 mg as a single dose on days 2 through 5[b,d]	2 g/day in 4 divided doses for 7–14 days	1 g/day in 2 divided doses for 7 days	TMP, 320 mg/day; SMX, 1,600 mg/day in 2 divided doses for 14 days

SMX, Sulfamethoxazole; TMP, trimethoprim.

[a]Centers for Disease Control and Prevention: Recommended antimicrobial agents for the treatment and postexposure prophylaxis of pertussis: 2005 CDC guidelines. *MMWR Recomm Rep* 54(RR-14):1-16, 2005.

[b]Azithromycin should be used with caution in people with prolonged QT interval and certain proarrhythmic conditions.

[c]Preferred macrolide for this age because of risk of idiopathic hypertrophic pyloric stenosis associated with erythromycin.

[d]A 3-day course of azithromycin for PEP or treatment has not been validated and is not recommended.

23. What is the best antibiotic choice for pneumonia in children?

As the cause varies by age, so does the treatment (Table 16.5). Amoxicillin 90 mg/kg/day divided in two doses for 10 days should be given to all patients with suspected pneumonia except in cases of allergy. Azithromycin should be added for school-age children. When influenza is in season, patients with influenza-like illness in the first 48 hours of symptoms should also be covered empirically with antiviral therapy (oseltamivir).

24. When do I need to admit a child to the hospital with pneumonia?

Patients who are persistently hypoxic (less than 92% on room air while awake) will require supplemental oxygen and therefore need to be admitted. Other reasons to be admitted are significant respiratory distress, unable to tolerate the oral antibiotic, or inability to maintain hydration.

KEY POINTS

1. Symptoms of an asthma exacerbation are caused by inflammation, which causes airway hyperresponsiveness, bronchoconstriction, and by mucus plugging which causes obstruction.
2. Acute exacerbations of asthma should be treated with a combination of systemic corticosteroids, short-acting beta$_2$ agonists, and anticholinergics.
3. There is no role for beta agonists, systemic steroids, inhaled steroids, nebulized hypertonic saline, or nebulized epinephrine in the routine treatment of bronchiolitis.

Table 16.5. Antibiotic Choice by Age for Treatment of Pneumonia

AGE	FIRST LINE	ALTERNATE OPTIONS FOR PENICILLIN-ALLERGIC PATIENTS
6 months to 5 years	Amoxicillin: 90 mg/kg divided twice a day for 10 days (max 4 g/day)	Cefdinir: 14 mg/kg per day divided twice a day for 10 days (max 600 mg/day) OR Clindamycin: 30 to 40 mg/kg per day divided in 3 doses for 10 days (max 1.8 g/day)
>5 years	Amoxicillin: 90 mg/kg divided twice a day for 10 days (max 4 g/day) AND Azithromycin: 10 mg/kg on day 1 followed by 5 mg/kg daily for 4 more days	As above for amoxicillin AND Doxycycline: 4 mg/kg per day divided twice a day for 10 days (max 200 mg/day)
Antiviral therapy	Oseltamivir <1 year: 3 mg/kg bid for 5 days ≤15 kg: 30 mg bid for 5 days 15.1–23 kg: 45 mg bid for 5 days 23.1–40 kg: 60 mg bid for 5 days >40 kg: 75 mg bid for 5 days	

Adapted from UpToDate.

4. If a patient has stridor at rest, racemic epinephrine should be given and then the patient will need to be monitored for at least 2 hours.
5. Pertussis, also known as whooping cough, is caused by the bacteria *Bordetella pertussis* and is highly contagious.

BIBLIOGRAPHY

Altunaiji SM, Kukuruzovic RH, Curtis NC, Massie J. Antibiotics for whooping cough (pertussis). *Cochrane Database of Systematic Reviews*. 2007,3(CD004404). http://dx.doi.org/10.1002/14651858.CD004404.pub3.

Asthma Program. *Expert panel report 3. Guidelines for the diagnosis and management of asthma*. Bethesda, MD: National Institutes of Health Publication; 2007:08–5846.

Barson WJ. Community-acquired pneumonia in children: clinical features and diagnosis. UpToDate. <http://www.uptodate.com/contents/community-acquired-pneumonia-in-children-clinical-features-and-diagnosis?source=see_link>; Accessed 13.07.16.

Barson WJ. Pneumonia in children: epidemiology, pathogenesis, and etiology. UpToDate. <http://www.uptodate.com/contents/pneumonia-in-children-epidemiology-pathogenesis-and-etiology?source=see_link&sectionName=Community-acquired+pneumonia&anchor=H15#H15>; Accessed 13.07.16.

Cao AM, Choy JP, Mohanakrishnan LN, Bain RF, van Driel ML. Chest radiographs for acute lower respiratory tract infections. *Cochrane Database Syst Rev*. 2013.

Keeney GE, Gray P, Morrison AK, Levas MN, et al. Dexamethasone for acute asthma exacerbations in children: a meta-analysis. *Pediatrics*. 2014;133(3):493–499. http://dx.doi.org/10.1542/peds.2013-2273.

Ralston SL, Lieberthal AS, Meissner HC, et al. Clinical practice guideline: the diagnosis, management, and prevention of bronchiolitis. *Pediatrics*. 2014;134:e1474.

Woods CR. Croup: approach to management. UpToDate. <http://www.uptodate.com/contents/croup-approach-to-management?source=see_link>; Accessed 07.07.16.

Woods CR. Croup: clinical features, evaluation, and diagnosis. UpToDate. <http://www.uptodate.com/contents/croup-clinical-features-evaluation-and-diagnosis>; Accessed 07.07.16.

Yeh S, Mink CA. Pertussis infection in infants and children: clinical features and diagnosis. UpToDate. <http://www.uptodate.com/contents/pertussis-infection-in-infants-and-children-clinical-features-and-diagnosis?source=see_link>; Accessed 11.07.16.

CHAPTER 17

NECK PAIN AND MASSES

Leah Kaye, MD

1. **A 4-year-old boy presents to urgent care for a lump on his neck. He has been well besides upper respiratory infection (URI) symptoms 2 weeks ago, with no fever, weight loss, trouble breathing, or change in activity level or behavior. He has a 2-cm palpable lymph node in the anterior cervical chain. What characteristics suggest it is benign?**
Size <3 cm, no/mild erythema, no/mild tenderness, no generalized lymphadenopathy.

2. **The patient's mother is concerned the lump is cancerous. What characteristics raise concern for malignancy?**
Location: supraclavicular nodes are malignant until proven otherwise. Nodes in the posterior triangle (behind or lateral to the sternocleidomastoid) are suspicious. Beware hard, irregular, firm, or rubbery nodes, or those that feel fixed to deep tissues. Fever, malaise, weight loss, or night sweats (B symptoms) raise concern for malignancy. Large nodes (initial size >3 cm) are more likely to be malignant, especially in the absence of signs of infection. Node persistence >6 weeks or increasing size during antibiotic therapy is concerning.

3. **What imaging should I choose first for a palpable neck mass?**
Ultrasound. If you are concerned for deep mass you cannot palpate, presents with difficulty breathing, difficulty swallowing, or significant limitation of range of motion, obtain a computed tomography (CT).

4. **What are the most common organisms in bacterial lymphadenitis?**
Staphylococcus aureus and group A streptococcus. Use cephalexin, amoxicillin-clavulanate, or clindamycin if you are starting empiric antibiotics. History should include pets (cat scratch fever), outdoor exposure (Lyme disease), and dental concerns (poor dentition or periodontal disease causing anaerobic infection). Lymphadenitis not improving with antibiotics is concerning for atypical mycobacterium.

5. **A 5-year-old presents with a neck lump present for 1 week. He has had low-grade fever, fatigue, poor appetite, and malaise for 10 days. The family adopted a kitten 4 weeks ago. He has a swollen, tender, indurated, warm cervical lymph node on the right. What diagnosis do you consider?**
Cat scratch disease (CSD; *Bartonella henselae*). CSD is transmitted via scratch or bite of an infected cat. Many patients do not recall an initial scratch. A papule or pustule on the skin often develops 7–12 days after inoculation, followed by lymphadenopathy 1–2 weeks later. Approximately 25% of cases involve lymphadenopathy of the head or neck. Symptoms include fever, malaise, anorexia, headache, myalgia, arthralgia, arthritis, or vision changes. Diagnosis is by indirect immunofluorescent antibody (IFA) assay for serum antibodies, not culture.

6. **What is the treatment for cat scratch disease?**
Most cases spontaneously resolve in 4–6 weeks, although 10% of nodes will spontaneously suppurate. Avoid incision and drainage (I&D) of the node, to lessen risk of fistula. Use antibiotics (typically azithromycin) for acutely or severely ill immunocompetent patients, those with retinitis, hepatic, splenic involvement, or painful adenitis. All immunocompromised patients should be treated.

7. **How can I tell a thyroglossal duct cyst from a dermoid cyst?**
Both are in the midline ventral neck. Thyroglossal duct cysts elevate when the tongue is protruded or the patient swallows. Dermoid cysts move with movement of the overlying skin.

8. **A 6-year-old female presents with neck swelling and tenderness. This is her third episode this year. The infections resolve completely, then recur. What should you consider?**
Recurrent swelling or infection at the same location on the neck is suspicious for branchial cleft cyst or thyroglossal duct cyst. Location is the key difference. Midline: thyroglossal duct cyst. Lateral neck: branchial cleft cyst.

9. **A 7-year-old febrile male patient is rushed to your urgent care with stridor, respiratory distress, and drooling. He appears toxic and anxious and nods urgently when asked about sore throat. He holds his neck hyperextended with his nose pointed up. He developed sore throat 3 hours ago but was well yesterday. What are you concerned for and what should you do?**

Acute onset of sore throat and fever with rapid progression to drooling, stridor, anxiety, and maintaining the "sniffing" position is concerning for epiglottitis. Other symptoms include dysphagia, "hot potato"/muffled voice, and tenderness to palpation over the hyoid bone. Transfer to the emergency department immediately for urgent ears, nose, and throat (ENT) and anesthesia consult to arrange emergent intubation in the operating room (OR). Defer diagnostics (labs, intravenous [IV] placement, imaging) to avoid worsening respiratory distress. The classic "thumb sign" on lateral neck x-ray (severe edema of the epiglottis) has poor sensitivity and specificity. Humidified oxygen or racemic epinephrine may be used while awaiting transport. Treat with a second- or third-generation cephalosporin. Etiologies include group A strep, *S. aureus, Klebsiella pneumoniae, H. parainfluenzae,* and beta-hemolytic strep. H. flu type b, while less common in the post-Hib vaccination era, is still a potential cause.

10. **Your 3-year-old patient presents with new onset torticollis, fever, and irritability. What should you rule out?**

Retropharyngeal abscess.

11. **What are the common symptoms of retropharyngeal abscess?**

Fever, restricted neck movements, neck pain, and cervical lymphadenopathy. Others include drooling, trismus, torticollis, and dysphagia. Respiratory distress is rare. Of all cases, 80% occur in children under 5. Risk factors include recent URI or recent oropharyngeal trauma. Complications include sepsis, mediastinitis, airway obstruction, internal jugular vein thrombosis, and carotid artery aneurysms.

12. **What imaging should you order if concerned for retropharyngeal abscess?**

Is there any respiratory distress? If so, transfer to the emergency department for urgent CT and surgical consult. If not, obtain lateral neck x-rays with neck extension to look for widening of the soft tissues.

> Are the x-rays normal and the airway intact? Consider other diagnoses.
> Are the x-rays concerning? Transfer for CT and/or ENT consult.

13. **A 15-year-old male presents with a sore throat x 5 days, new onset neck swelling, fever, shortness of breath, and rigors. He is tender to palpation along his lateral left neck. Rapid strep is negative. What testing should you consider next?**

This presentation is concerning for Lemierre syndrome (septic thrombophlebitis of internal jugular), commonly caused by fusobacterium. Although uncommon, it carries a high mortality rate. It occurs by spread of a primary parapharyngeal infection (sore throat), which spreads internally to the jugular and can cause septic embolization. Obtain a neck ultrasound to examine the jugular.

14. **A 15-year-old female presents with sore throat x 8 days, fever, and new left ear and neck pain. The past 2 days it "feels like swallowing glass" and her voice sounds strange. On exam, her uvula is deviated to the right, with left-sided tender cervical lymphadenopathy and foul breath. What do you suspect and what testing should you order?**

Peritonsillar abscess (PTA), which is a collection of pus behind the tonsil in the superior arch of the soft palate. PTA typically presents with sore throat, fever, malaise, dysphagia, muffled/"hot potato" voice, or referred ear pain. It can be a complication of treated strep pharyngitis or a progression of untreated. The most common etiology is group A strep, but it can be polymicrobial. On exam, the uvula deviates away from the affected side, with lymphadenopathy on the affected side, drooling, foul-smelling breath, or inferior medial deviation of the infected tonsil. Transfer for CT, the test of choice, and possible ENT consult.

15. **An 18-month-old boy presents 2 days after completing a 10-day course of antibiotics for otitis media. He is still febrile, and his left ear is red. Parents note yellow discharge on his pillow. On exam, he has left ear proptosis, postauricular swelling, and a bulging left tympanic membrane. What should you do next?**

Send to the emergency department for CT with contrast to evaluate for mastoiditis. Treatment includes IV antibiotics, ENT consult, and sometimes surgical drainage. It is most common in children under 2 years.

16. **What are the presenting symptoms, causes, and treatment of acute parotitis?**
    Parotitis typically presents with swelling, pain, and erythema over the parotid gland (acute swelling of the cheek that extends to the angle of the mandible). Other symptoms include fever, trismus, and pain with mastication. It is typically unilateral. Causes can be divided into viral, bacterial, autoimmune, and idiopathic (Table 17.1). If suppurative, treat with oral antibiotics. In all cases, use hydration, warm massage, and sialagogues (such as sour candy or sour foods).

17. **A 3-week-old's parents feel a mass over the right side of their son's neck. His head is always tilted right. He is otherwise well appearing and afebrile. He has no history of trauma. On exam, you note a tight sternocleidomastoid on the right with a smooth, well-circumscribed mass in the inferior third of the muscle. The child's head is tilted to the right. His chin is pointed left. What is the most likely diagnosis?**
    Congenital muscular torticollis (CMT). Torticollis is a twisting of the head and neck caused by shortening of the sternocleidomastoid. It can be divided into paroxysmal (episodic) and nonparoxysmal (static, unchanging) causes (Table 17.2).

18. **What kind of imaging should I order for afebrile new onset torticollis?**
    Consider ultrasound to better delineate the mass and rule out tumor, and radiographs of cervical spine to look for C1-C2 subluxation. MRI or CT should be used only for suspected intracranial pathology.

19. **What is the treatment for the patient with congenital muscular torticollis?**
    Referral to physical therapy to learn feeding techniques (feed on the side of the affected muscle), crib positioning, and stretching exercises. Majority of children improve with physical therapy. If there is no improvement in 6 months, their provider may refer them to surgery.

20. **A child with trisomy 21 keeps his head tilted toward the left. On exam, he has a tight, tender sternocleidomastoid on the right. What are you concerned for?**
    Atlantoaxial instability. The difference in tilt (head tilted away from the tight sternocleidomastoid, not toward) is a key clue to steer you away from congenital muscular torticollis. Another concerning factor is the patient's history of trisomy 21, which is associated with atlantoaxial dislocation. Look for tenderness of the spinous process of the axis as well.

21. **What should you order if you are concerned for atlantoaxial instability?**
    Start with cervical spine radiographs. Head CT may be necessary for confirmation. Treatment depends on duration and severity and varies from conservative management (cervical collar, rest, analgesics), to cervical traction, to surgery. Consult spine for guidance.

KEY POINTS

1. Supraclavicular lymph nodes are concerning for malignancy.
2. Ultrasound the patient with a thyroglossal duct cyst to ensure normal thyroid tissue.
3. Absence of respiratory distress does not rule out retropharyngeal abscess.
4. Upper limb, gait, or cranial nerve abnormalities, or signs of increased intracranial pressure with torticollis is concerning for posterior fossa tumor.
5. Avoid I&D of the node in cat scratch disease as it increases risk of fistula.

Table 17.1. Causes of Parotitis

Viral	Mumps, Epstein-Barr, parainfluenza, HIV, influenza A, Coxsackie, adenovirus, parvovirus B19
Bacterial	Most common: *S. aureus, S. viridans, H. influenzae, Peptostreptococcus, S. pneumoniae, E. coli,* bacteroides
Autoimmune	Sjögren syndrome, juvenile idiopathic arthritis (JIA), IgA deficiency, rheumatoid arthritis
Idiopathic	Juvenile recurrent parotitis: 5% caused by recurrent stones, otherwise idiopathic

Table 17.2. Causes of Torticollis

Nonparoxysmal Torticollis	
Congenital muscular torticollis	Fibrosed hematoma or developmental fibroma in the sternocleido-mastoid starts to shrink, shortening the sternocleidomastoid and producing torticollis
Osseous torticollis	Congenital: Klippel-Feil syndrome, congenital atlantoaxial disloca-tion, ligamentous laxity (e.g., Marfan), achondroplasia, Morquio syndrome Traumatic: cervical spine trauma causing atlantoaxial subluxation, vertebral fractures Inflammatory: cervical adenitis, otitis media, Grisel syndrome* CNS: posterior fossa tumor, basal ganglia injury (HIE), spinal cord tumors Peripheral nerve: brachial plexus injury
Ocular torticollis	CN IV palsy—tilting head to minimize diplopia Spasmus nutans
Soft tissue infections	Cervical adenitis, retropharyngeal abscess, sternocleidomastoid myositis
Paroxysmal Torticollis	
Benign paroxysmal torticollis	Self-limited, presents at 2 weeks to 4.5 months Recurrent torticollis, vomiting, pallor, irritability, ataxia, drowsiness. Torticollis can alternate sides with different attacks Starts to improve at 2 years; usually resolves by age 3 Family history of migraine is common No treatment; can consider antiemetics
Sandifer syndrome	Gastroesophageal reflux with abnormal posturing. Look for reflux symptoms such as regurgitation, anorexia, irritability, FTT, cough Treat with reflux therapy and reflux precautions
Acute dystonic reaction	Common causes: antiemetics, neuroleptics, antidepressants, antihistamines, anticonvulsants, cough suppressants, anticholin-ergics, drugs of abuse Treatment: removal of the drug, diphenhydramine
Increased ICP	Pseudotumor cerebri

CN, Cranial nerve; CNS, central nervous system; FTT, failure to thrive; HIE, hypoxic ischemic encephalopa-thy; ICP, intracranial pressure.
*Nontraumatic atlantoaxial subluxation from inflammatory ligamentous laxity following an infectious process.

BIBLIOGRAPHY

Brooke I. Fusobacterial head and neck infection in children. *International Journal of Pediatric Otorhinolaryngology*. 2015;79:953–958.

Bunk M. Mastoiditis. *Pediatrics in Review*. 2014;35:94–95.

Cirilli A. Emergency evaluation and management of the sore throat. *Emergency Medicine Clinics of North America*. 2013;31:501–515.

Francis CL, Larsen CG. Pediatric sialadenitis. *Otolaryngology Clinics of North America*. 2014;47:763–778.

Friedmann A. Evaluation and management of lymphadenopathy in children. *Pediatrics in Review*. 2008;29:53–59.

Grisaru-Soen G, Komisar O, et al. Retropharyngeal and parapharyngeal abscess in children—epidemiology, clinical fea-tures and treatment. *International Journal of Pediatric Otorhinolaryngology*. 2010;74:1016–1020.

Klotz ST, Ianas V, et al. Cat-scratch disease. *American Family Physician*. 2011;83:152–155.

LaPlante JK, Pierson NS, et al. Common pediatric head and neck congenital/developmental anomalies. *Radiology Clinics of North America*. 2015;53:181–196.

Sobol SE, Zapata S. Epiglottitis and croup. *Otolaryngologic Clinics of North America*. 2008;41:551–566.

Tomczak KK, Rosman NP. Torticollis. *Journal of Child Neurology*. 2013;28:365–378.

CHAPTER 18

CHEST PAIN

Siraj Amanullah, MD, MPH, Jay Pershad, MD, MMM, CPE

A 14-year-old-male presents to an urgent care facility for new onset intermittent chest pain with onset over a few weeks since he has started to play competitive basketball. Pain is exertional, retrosternal, no radiation, squeezing pressure like, with resolution after rest. On the day of presentation, he has a similar episode but with dizziness and near-syncope. He has a heart rate of 85 beats per minute, respiratory rate of 25 breaths per minute, and blood pressure of 130/75 mm Hg. He has a normal respiratory and chest wall exam. He has a systolic ejection (crescendo–decrescendo) murmur between the apex of the heart and left sternal border that becomes more prominent with standing.

1. **What are the concerning features of this patient's chest pain presented in the scenario?**
   Exertional chest pain with dizziness and/or syncope is concerning for a cardiac pathology. The characteristic of his murmur is consistent with possible hypertrophic cardiomyopathy. His electrocardiogram (ECG) is shown in Fig. 18.1. He will be best managed by an urgent referral to a pediatric cardiologist while refraining him from any exertional activity.

2. **How common is chest pain in the pediatric population?**
   Chest pain is one of the common reasons to seek medical care and is reported to be 0.3%–0.6% of emergency department visits.

3. **How serious is chest pain in children?**
   The majority of pediatric patients with chest pain have idiopathic, benign, or psychogenic etiologies. History and physical examination is sufficient to rule out serious pathology without need for extensive workup.

4. **What are the components of a good history and physical examination in assessment of a pediatric patient with chest pain?**
   History of onset, duration, character, frequency, radiation, association with exertion, assessment of associated symptoms (fever, syncope, dyspnea, sweating), past medical history, and family history can help differentiate various etiologies of chest pain. Physical examination includes cardiac, respiratory, and abdominal exam especially assessing for hypoxia, tachypnea, tachycardia, fever, cardiac murmurs, gallop rhythm, and rubs point toward need for urgent diagnostic workup. Fig. 18.2 shows an algorithmic approach in assessment of a pediatric patient with chest pain.

5. **What are important past medical and family history in patients with chest pain?**
   Past medical history includes congenital heart disease, cystic fibrosis, Kawasaki disease, Marfan syndrome, Turner syndrome, Noonan syndrome, Ehlers-Danlos syndrome, ankylosing spondylitis, systemic lupus erythematosus, sickle cell disease, asthma, anxiety, and panic attacks. Family history of prolonged QT syndrome, sudden cardiac deaths, and cardiomyopathies point toward concerning pathology in patients.

6. **What is the most common cause of chest pain in pediatric patients?**
   Muscular strain remains the most common etiology of chest pain in pediatric patients. Pain is reproducible with history of recent physical or sports activity, heavy backpacks, trauma, or cough.

7. **What are the characteristic historical or physical findings in patients with chest wall pain?**
   Costochondritis pain is usually worse with breathing or exercise, mostly unilateral, anterior, reproducible at the costochondral areas, involving two or more costochondral joints, and may be persistent for weeks. If there is localized inflammation, pain, swelling, and erythema of one costochondral joint (usually second/third joint), the condition is called Tietze syndrome. Paroxysms of sharp chest pain associated with coxsackievirus infection is called pleurodynia (Bornholm disease).

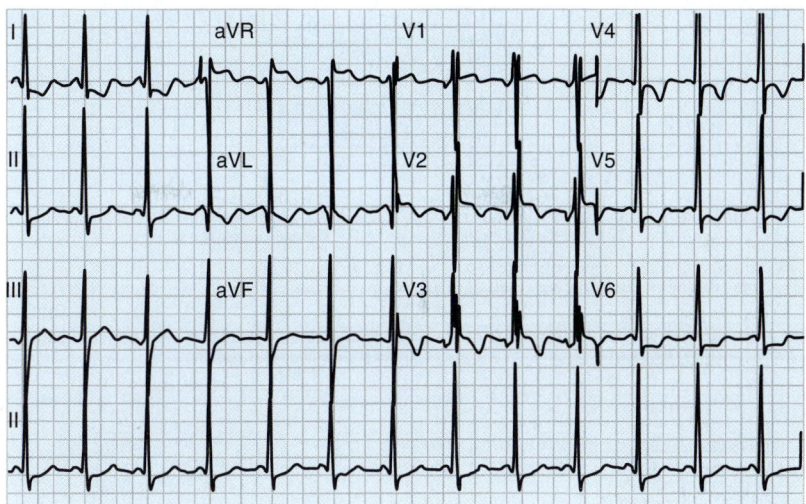

Fig. 18.1. Male teenager with severe HOCM with left atrial enlargement, left ventricular hypertrophy, and diffuse ST-T changes. *(Courtesy Dr. James Ziegler, MD, Department of Pediatrics, Brown Medical School, Hasbro Children's Hospital, Providence, RI, USA.)*

8. What are the other causes of benign chest pain?

Precordial catch (Texidor twinge) is usually left sided, recurrent, lasting for a few seconds, with a point location in an intercostal space, worsening on deep breathing or bending down, and improving with shallow breathing. Unilateral burning or sharp pain in a dermatomal distribution is typical of herpes zoster. Various breast conditions can also present with chest pain. Esophageal spasm can lead to severe retrosternal chest pain while gastroesophageal reflux can lead to burning pain after meals or worsening with laying down. Noncardiac chest pain can be due to psychosocial stressors or conditions like depression, anxiety, stress, conversion, or somatization. It is usually reported as frequent, recurrent, severe, lasting for varied duration, spanning over months to years, with no consistent relationship with activity, usually without any other associated symptoms, with or without hyperventilation or obvious anxiety, affecting daily life routine.

9. Which medical conditions can present with sudden chest pain?

There are six serious conditions for an urgent care physician to consider with acute onset of atraumatic chest pain: acute asthma, spontaneous pneumothorax or pneumomediastinum, acute chest syndrome in patients with sickle cell disease, and, uncommonly, pulmonary embolism or aortic dissection. Sudden onset of chest pain in an otherwise healthy young child may be due to foreign body ingestion. Sudden increase in intrathoracic pressure associated with trauma, asthma, pneumonia, vomiting, weight lifting, inhalation of recreational drugs, or hookah may lead to pneumomediastinum or pneumothorax (Fig. 18.3). Pain is unilateral with shortness of breath with pneumothorax. Pneumomediastinum pain is located in the neck and retrosternal area with subcutaneous emphysema and Hamman sign (crunchy sound over precordium). If it is associated with profound vomiting, then esophageal perforation needs to be ruled out. Fever, cough, respiratory distress, and chest pain are presenting signs of acute chest crisis in patients with sickle cell disease. Cocaine abuse can present with angina with chest tightness, nausea, sweating, vomiting, or shortness of breath. Aortic dissection is rarely seen in pediatric patients and is associated with collagen vascular disorders.

10. How common is cardiac pathology in pediatric patients with chest pain?

Cardiac disease as an etiology of chest pain is very rare in pediatric patients, with reported proportion of 0.6%–1.2% of all etiologies. Almost all of these conditions can be suspected based on historical clues, physical exam findings, and judicious use of ECG.

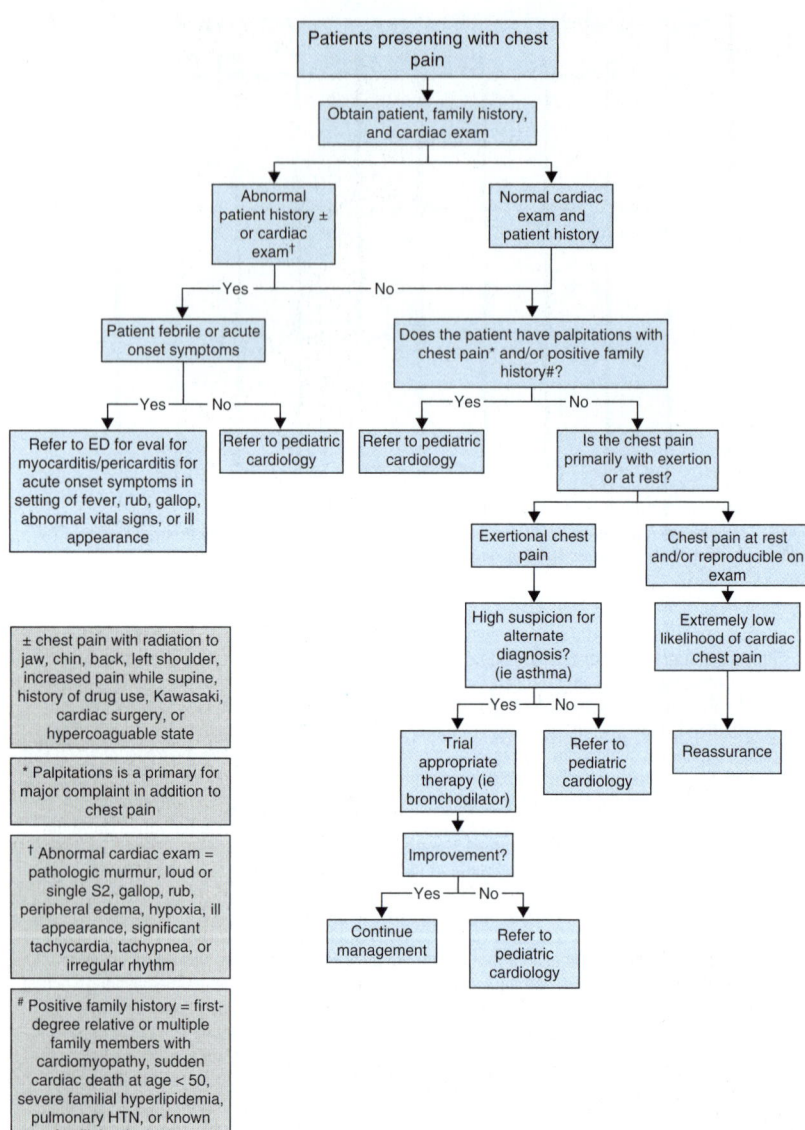

Fig. 18.2. Approach to assessment of a pediatric patient with chest pain. *(From Friedman KG, Alexander ME: Chest pain and syncope in children: a practical approach to the diagnosis of cardiac disease. J Pediatr 163(3):896-901, e1-e3, 2013 [Fig. 2, p 10].)*
Note: As mentioned in the algorithm, symptoms suggestive of unstable vital signs or cardiac exam concerning for failure should be urgently referred to an emergency department.

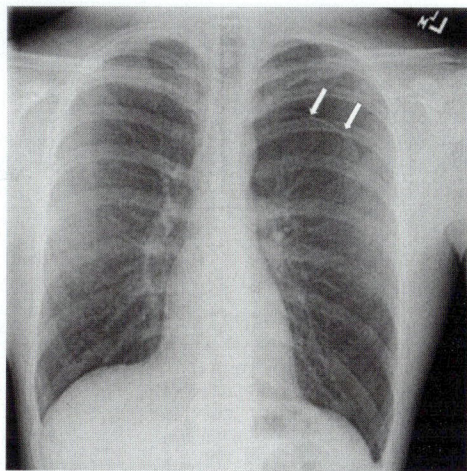

Fig. 18.3. Left-sided spontaneous pneumothorax in a teenager with acute chest pain. *(Courtesy Jay Pershad, MD, MMM, Department of Pediatrics and Emergency Medicine, University of Tennessee Health Sciences Center, Le Bonheur Children's Hospital, Memphis, TN 38103.)*

11. How common is myocardial ischemia in pediatric patients?

Acute myocardial ischemia is extremely rare in pediatric patients with male gender, teenage years, substance abuse, and tobacco identified as risk factors.

12. What are the characteristic historical and physical examination findings in patients with structural cardiac abnormalities and chest pain?

A cardiac cause of chest pain is extremely rare, but clinical implications can be serious. A thorough history and physical can be very helpful in ruling out a cardiac cause in pediatric patients presenting to an urgent care setting (Table 18.1). Hypertrophic cardiomyopathy (HOCM) is associated with exertional chest pain, occasionally syncope, and murmur with Valsalva maneuver. Though by itself rare, it is one of the most common etiologies of sudden cardiac deaths. HOCM is associated with atrial fibrillation and coronary artery anomalies. Dilated cardiomyopathy patients present with chest pain and shortness of breath. Very few structural heart defects present with chest pain including mitral valve prolapse, coronary artery anomalies, and severe aortic and pulmonary outlet obstruction. Pain due to mitral valve prolapse is vague, could be nonexertional, is along the cardiac apex, and may have midsystolic click that is pronounced when standing. Those with anomalous coronary artery and severe outflow track obstructions have exertional angina pain with murmur along the upper sternum on physical exam.

13. What other cardiac pathologies may present with chest pain?

Other diagnoses considered as potential causes of chest pain include cardiomyopathy, myocarditis, pericarditis, specific coronary anomalies, pulmonary hypertension, pulmonary embolism, and aortic dissection. Pericarditis pain is sharp, positional, and stabbing and improves with leaning forward. Myocarditis presents with mild chest pain with tachycardia in excess of fever, muffled heart sounds, and gallop rhythm. Chest pain on exertion with syncope may be due to ventricular or supraventricular tachyarrhythmia (Fig. 18.4). Lyme carditis patients can present with fatigue, chest discomfort, or near syncope with severe first-degree heart block (Fig. 18.5) or third-degree atrioventricular block.

14. How common is pulmonary embolism in pediatric patients?

It is very rare in pediatric patients and should be considered in high-risk patients with unexplained persistent tachypnea. High-risk conditions are hypercoagulopathy, use of birth control pills, recent abortion, cancer, prolonged immobilization, lower extremity trauma, and travel on long flights. Presenting signs are acute dyspnea, pleuritic chest pain, cough, hemoptysis, and/or sinus tachycardia with decreased breath sounds over the affected area and pleural rub.

Table 18.1. Cardiac Causes of Chest Pain and Red Flag History, Exam, and ECG Findings

CAUSE	HISTORY	PHYSICAL EXAM FINDINGS	ECG FINDINGS
HCM	Positive family history Exercise intolerance Exertional chest pain Syncope and/or arrhythmia	Dynamic systolic murmur	Left ventricular hypertrophy or left axis deviation ST-segment or T-wave changes Q waves Arrhythmias, ventricular premature beats Ventricular preexcitation (Wolff-Parkinson-White)
Dilated cardio-myopathy	Family history Decreased exercise tolerance, syncope Heart failure symptoms	Gallop Mitral regurgitation murmur	Intraventricular conduction delay High or low QRS voltages Arrhythmia, premature beats
Anomalous coronary artery origin	Exertional chest pain Exertional syncope	Usually normal	Usually normal
Coronary ischemia	• Predisposing conditions • History of Kawasaki disease • Cardiac surgery or heart transplant • Systemic arteriopathy (Williams syndrome) • Severe familial hypercholesterolemia • Drug use: cocaine, sympathomimetics • Anginal chest pain	Tachycardia Tachypnea New murmur or gallop	ST-segment depressions or elevation T-wave changes Q waves
Severe left ventricular outflow tract obstruction	Exertional symptoms Exertional syncope	Loud systolic murmur	Left ventricular hypertrophy Left ventricular strain pattern
Arrhythmia	Palpitations Syncope Positive family history	Irregular rhythm	Atrial arrhythmia Ventricular arrhythmia Premature contractions Ventricular preexcitation (Wolff-Parkinson-White)
Pericarditis	Positional chest pain Predisposing factors: • Rheumatologic conditions • Malignancy • Mediastinal radiation • Infection (HIV, tuberculosis, viral) • Renal failure • Recent cardiac surgery	Cardiac rub Tachycardia/tachypnea Distant heart sound, JVD	Diffuse ST-segment changes T-wave inversion

Table 18.1. Cardiac Causes of Chest Pain and Red Flag History, Exam, and ECG Findings (*Continued*)

CAUSE	HISTORY	PHYSICAL EXAM FINDINGS	ECG FINDINGS
Myocarditis	Fever Viral prodrome Short duration of symptoms	Tachycardia Tachypnea With or without gallop rhythm, ventricular ectopy	Diffuse ST-segment changes T-wave inversions PR depressions Ventricular ectopy
	New onset heart failure symptoms	Cardiovascular collapse	Low QRS voltages
Aortic dissection	Personal or family history of bicuspid aortic valve or connective tissue disorders (Marfan, Loeys-Dietz, Ehlers-Danlos type IV, others)	Marfanoid body habitus	See coronary ischemia above
	Acute onset sharp or tearing type of pain		
Pulmonary embolus	Pain description: acute onset, pleuritic, associated dyspnea	Right ventricular heave (elevated right ventricular pressure)	Right ventricular hypertrophy
	Personal or family risk factors (inherited thrombophilia, hypercoagulable state, immobilization, medications)	Loud and/or unsplit S2 (if right ventricular pressure elevated)	Right ventricular stain pattern

JVD, Jugular venous distention.
(From Friedman KG, Alexander ME: Chest pain and syncope in children: a practical approach to the diagnosis of cardiac disease. *J Pediatr* 163(3):896-901, e1-e3, 2013 [Table IV, pages 15-16].)

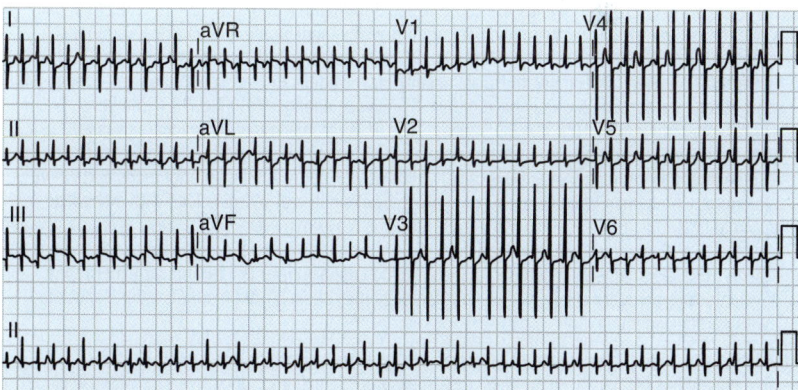

Fig. 18.4. Patient with sudden onset of pallor, chest discomfort, and palpitations associated with narrow complex tachycardia on ECG with absent P waves. *(Courtesy Dr. Siraj Amanullah, MD, MPH, Department of Emergency Medicine and Pediatrics, Brown Medical School, Hasbro Children's Hospital, Providence, RI, USA.)*

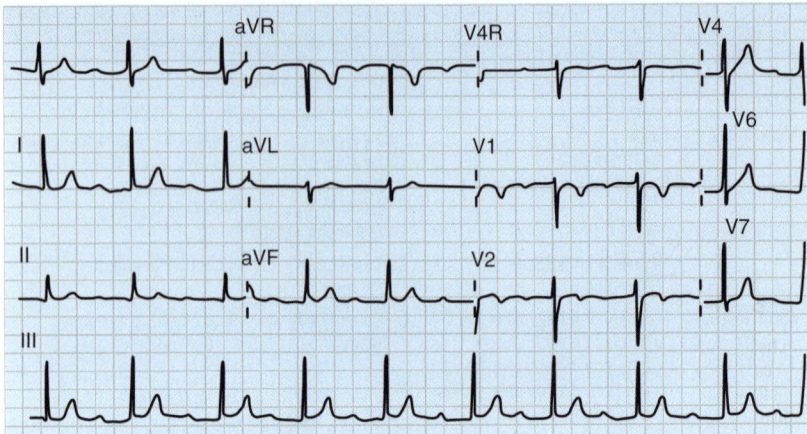

Fig. 18.5. Patient with fatigue, chest discomfort, and near syncope on exertion with prolonged PR interval associated with Lyme carditis. *(Courtesy Dr. Siraj Amanullah, MD, MPH, Department of Emergency Medicine and Pediatrics, Brown Medical School, Hasbro Children's Hospital, Providence, RI, USA.)*

15. What are the important tools of investigation in patients with chest pain?

Pulse oximetry, electrocardiogram, and chest radiographs are the most common investigation tools though not indicated in every patient.

16. When is a chest x-ray warranted in the setting of chest pain?

The use of chest radiograph is to help a clinician in differential diagnosis of various etiologies of chest pain and is not required in every patient with chest pain. For example, it is not essential to obtain chest radiograph in every patient with asthma but may be indicated in an asthmatic patient with persistent chest pain or hypoxia despite appropriate treatments. Conditions that may benefit from chest radiograph are suspected pneumothorax, pneumomediastinum, cardiomegaly (myocarditis, pericarditis), cardiac hypertrophy, foreign body, and pneumonia.

17. What are the abnormal ECG findings in a patient with chest pain?

The following ECG abnormalities are considered abnormal in a pediatric patient with chest pain: evidence of ventricular hypertrophy, ST-T abnormalities, high-grade atrioventricular (AV) block, ventricular or atrial ectopy, QTc >470 msec, PR depression, low QRS voltages, and an S1Q3 inverted T3 pattern. Patients with HOCM usually have evidence of left ventricular hypertrophy with left atrial enlargement and may have diffuse ST-T wave changes (see Fig. 18.1). However, ECG may be normal in 5%–10% of such patients. The best screening tool for myocarditis is ECG (ST changes), with more than 90% of patients with ECG changes. Pericarditis patients may have diffuse ST-segment elevation (in up to 60% of patients) with PR depression in inferior leads and V2–V6. Pulmonary embolism patients are most likely to have sinus tachycardia alone with otherwise normal ECG. Only few patients with a large embolus may have prominent S wave in lead 1, Q wave in lead 3, and inverted T wave in lead 3 or in V1–V3, right axis deviation, or right bundle branch block (RBBB). Patients with outflow tract obstruction usually have left ventricular hypertrophy. Patients with coronary artery disease or anomalies may show ST-segment elevation associated with cardiac ischemia.

18. What are the steps in management of patients with benign chest pain?

If a patient has benign cause for chest pain, reassurance, rest, and supportive care with use of acetaminophen or nonsteroidal antiinflammatory drugs is advised.

19. When should a pediatric patient with chest pain be referred for urgent evaluation to an emergency department?

Ill appearance, fever, hypotension, respiratory distress, low oxygenation, significant tachycardia, tachypnea, irregular rhythm, peripheral edema, or other signs of congestive heart failure such as hepatomegaly, gallop or jugular venous distention, pathologic murmur or rub. Exertional syncope and/or palpitations with chest pain are some of the features that guide toward need for emergent referral to a tertiary center.

20. When can a patient with chest pain be referred for nonemergent outpatient evaluation by a cardiologist?

Patients with exertional chest pain that resolves with rest without signs of life-threatening arrhythmia can be referred for outpatient cardiac workup.

21. When is it appropriate to abstain a child from physical activity with chest pain?

Patients with exertional chest pain should be refrained from sports and gym until seen by a pediatric cardiologist. Those with benign etiology of chest pain should not be refrained from physical activities as this will create unnecessary anxiety in family and patient.

KEY POINTS

1. Chest pain associated with exertion warrants careful evaluation for a cardiopulmonary etiology.
2. A cardiology referral is recommended for patients with chest pain and a positive family history of first-degree relatives with cardiomyopathy, prolonged QTc, sudden death <50 years, or severe hyperlipidemia.
3. Abnormal ECG findings in a patient with pediatric chest pain include evidence of ventricular hypertrophy, ST-T abnormalities, high-grade AV block, ventricular or atrial ectopy, QTc >470 msec, PR depression, low QRS voltages, and/or an S1Q3 inverted T3 pattern.

BIBLIOGRAPHY

Bergmann KR, Kharbanda A, Haveman L. Myocarditis and pericarditis in the pediatric patient: validated management strategies. *Pediatr Emerg Med Pract.* 2015;12(7):1–22. [quiz 23].

Eslick GD. Epidemiology and risk factors of pediatric chest pain: a systematic review. *Pediatr Clin North Am.* 2010;57(6):1211–1219.

Friedman KG, Alexander ME. Chest pain and syncope in children: a practical approach to the diagnosis of cardiac disease. *J Pediatr.* 2013;163(3):896–901. e1–e3.

Johnson NN, Toledo A, Endom EE. Pneumothorax, pneumomediastinum, and pulmonary embolism. *Pediatr Clin North Am.* 2010;57(6):1357–1383.

Kane DA, et al. Needles in hay: chest pain as the presenting symptom in children with serious underlying cardiac pathology. *Congenit Heart Dis.* 2010;5(4):366–373.

Kane DA, et al. Needles in hay II: detecting cardiac pathology by the pediatric chest pain standardized clinical assessment and management plan. *Congenit Heart Dis.* 2016.

Mahlo WT, Campbell RM, Favaloro Sabatier J. Myocardial infarction in adolescents. *J Pediatr.* 2007;151(2):150–154.

McDonnell CJ, White KS, Grady RM. Noncardiac chest pain in children and adolescents: a biopsychosocial conceptualization. *Child Psychiatry Hum Dev.* 2012;43(1):1–26.

Park M. *Pediatric Cardiology for Practitioners.* 6th ed. Philadelphia: Saunders; 2014.

Patocka C, Nemeth J. Pulmonary embolism in pediatrics. *J Emerg Med.* 2012;42(1):105–116.

CHAPTER 19

ABDOMINAL PAIN

Karen Y. Kwan, MD

CONSTIPATION

1. **A 10-year-old male patient presents to your urgent care center with 2 days of generalized abdominal pain, associated with nonbilious vomiting and decreased appetite. His abdominal exam is benign. He describes straining with bowel movements and hard stool. Is constipation a common disorder in children?**
   Constipation is one of the most common chronic disorders of childhood. It is responsible for 3% of all primary care visits for children and up to 25% of pediatric gastroenterology visits.

2. **What is considered constipation in children?**
   Constipation can be broadly defined as infrequent bowel movements with at least one of the following: painful defecation, hard stools, purposeful fecal retention, fecal soiling, encopresis. Outside the neonatal period, childhood constipation is common and almost always functional without an organic etiology.

3. **What are the symptoms of constipation?**
   A child typically presents with a chief complaint of hard pelletlike stools, difficulty or pain with defecating, abdominal pain, abdominal distension, vomiting, or anorexia.

4. **What symptoms are red flags for an underlying organic cause of constipation?**
   - Delayed passage of meconium
   - Significant abdominal distension
   - Abnormal development
   - Constipation since birth
   - Bloody stools (absence of anal fissure)
   - Weight loss and/or failure to thrive

5. **What causes functional constipation in children?**
   Functional constipation is commonly caused by painful bowel movements prompting the child to withhold stool. To avoid a painful bowel movement, the child will contract the anal sphincter and/or gluteal muscles, leading to stool retention, prolonged fecal stasis with reabsorption of fluid, and then a harder, larger stool that is more painful to pass. This cycle may occur with toilet training, changes in routine or diet, stressful events, illness, lack of accessible toilets (e.g., at school), or a busy child who defers defecation.

6. **How do you diagnose constipation?**
   A history and physical examination are usually sufficient to distinguish functional constipation from constipation with an organic etiology. A history should review the frequency, consistency, and size of stools; age of onset of symptoms; meconium passage after birth; recent stressors; prior history and therapies; presence of withholding behaviors, pain, or bleeding with bowel movements; abdominal pain; and fecal incontinence. Physical exam should include an abdominal exam; external examination of the perineum, perianal areas, thyroid, and spine; and a neurologic evaluation for appropriate reflexes (cremasteric, anal wink, and patellar).

7. **What diagnosis must be considered in a neonate or infant presenting with constipation, poor feeding, and a weak cry?**
   Infant botulism needs to be considered. Infant botulism is characterized by constipation followed by neuromuscular paralysis or "floppiness." Symptoms include constipation, history of poor feeding, difficulty latching and suckling, lethargy, and a weak cry. Exposure to honey or a construction site may be the cause.

8. **In a child presenting with constipation since birth, what disorder must be considered?**

Infants and children often with history of constipation since birth or delayed meconium passing (>48 hr) may have Hirschsprung disease. Children diagnosed later in childhood may have a history of poor growth, severe recalcitrant constipation, and intermittent vomiting. Physical exam may present with signs of enterocolitis, abdominal distension and pain, poor feeding, and foul-smelling watery stools.

9. **Is a digital examination of the anorectum useful in diagnosing constipation?**

A digital examination is recommended to assess for perianal sensation, anal tone, rectum size, anal wink, rectal stool load, and consistency. Children with normal neonatal courses or clear withholding behaviors may have the rectal examination deferred. The presence of a hard mass in the lower abdomen and/or a dilated rectum with hard stool indicates fecal impaction.

10. **Is abdominal radiography a valuable diagnostic tool for diagnosing constipation?**

Abdominal radiography is not recommended for diagnosing constipation due to lack of interobserver reliability and accuracy, but it may be useful to determine the extent of fecal impaction. It can be used for specific clinical circumstances in which a rectal examination is unreasonable (child with history of trauma) or the diagnosis is uncertain.

11. **How is constipation treated?**

When fecal impaction is present, oral or rectal disimpaction is required before the initiation of maintenance therapy to keep the rectum empty and allow the rectum to return to its normal size. Maintenance therapy may be needed for several months. Parental education, behavior modification, and close follow-up are essential to prevent reoccurrence. If an organic cause is found, treatment involves addressing the underlying organic problem.

12. **What are the effective therapies for fecal impaction in children?**

A number of therapies are available with the advent of polyethylene glycol-based solutions being first line, due to the medication's effectiveness, ease to administer, noninvasiveness, and ability to tolerate. Rectal therapies and polyethylene glycol are similarly effective in the treatment of fecal impaction in children. Oral therapies include osmotics (polyethylene glycol, magnesium citrate), stimulants (senna bisacodyl), and lubricants (mineral oil). Rectal agents include enemas (mineral oil, phosphate, normal saline) and suppositories (bisacodyl, glycerin).

13. **What is the goal of constipation maintenance therapy?**

The goal is to avoid reaccumulation of stool by maintaining soft bowel movements. Studies show addition of laxatives is necessary and more effective than behavior modification alone. Recent studies show addition of enemas to oral laxative regimens does not improve outcomes in children with severe constipation. Polyethylene glycol achieves equal or better treatment success than other laxatives such as lactulose or milk of magnesia. Maintenance medications need to be continued for several weeks to months.

14. **What are the possible complications of constipation?**

Chronic abdominal pain, bowel obstruction, rectal fissures, enuresis, encopresis, urinary retention, urinary tract infection, rectal prolapse, and social stigmata are all possible complications.

ACUTE ABDOMEN

15. **What is the most common pediatric surgical emergency?**

Appendicitis, with approximately 70,000 pediatric cases per year. Appendicitis is the most common surgical condition in children who present with abdominal pain. Lymphoid or fecalith obstructs the appendiceal lumen, and the appendix becomes distended with ischemia and necrosis developing.

16. **What is the misdiagnosis rate in children less than 2 years?**

Nearly 100%, due to the difficulty in localizing abdominal pain in nonverbal children. Many cases present similar to other common pediatric diagnoses such as constipation and gastroenteritis. As the age of the child progresses, the misdiagnosis rates improve.

17. **What is the classic clinical examination you find in appendicitis?**

Less than 50% of pediatric patients will present with the classic presentation. Patients with appendicitis classically present with visceral, vague, poorly localized, periumbilical pain. Within 6 to 48 hours, the pain becomes parietal as the overlying peritoneum becomes inflamed; the pain then becomes well localized and constant in the right iliac fossa.

18. **What is the Rovsing sign?**
Pushing on the abdomen in the left lower quadrant elicits pain in the right lower quadrant.

19. **What is the psoas sign?**
Pain on passive extension of the right thigh with the patient lying on the left side.

20. **What is the obturator sign?**
Pain on passive internal rotation of the flexed right thigh.

21. **What laboratories should be sent for suspected appendicitis?**
White blood cell (WBC) count, C-reactive protein (CRP), and urinalysis, and urine pregnancy; also consider serum chemistry. Combining use of WBC and CRP increases sensitivity of laboratory evaluation for possible appendicitis.

22. **What is the radiographic diagnostic study of choice for diagnosing pediatric appendicitis?**
Ultrasound is now the diagnostic modality of choice in pediatrics. With abdominal computed tomography (CT) scan, there are significantly more radiation risks for children and possible long-term sequelae. Watchful waiting and serial abdominal examinations now have a significant role in diagnosing pediatric appendicitis. CT scans provide better diagnostic information for perforated appendicitis or suspected intraabdominal abscesses. Several emergency departments in the United States are using MRI scans as the first-line diagnostic test to rule out appendicitis and ovarian pathology.

23. **In a male patient presenting with localized abdominal pain, why should the genital area always be examined?**
The male scrotum and testes should always be examined to rule out testicular torsion/pathology and inguinal hernias. Referred abdominal pain may occur due to the stomach and small intestine having shared innervation with the testicle and epididymis.

TESTICULAR

24. **What surgical emergency needs to be considered when an adolescent male presents with vomiting, abdominal pain, and a swollen, painful testicle?**
Testicular torsion, a surgical emergency, presents with excruciating pain, scrotal swelling, nausea, and/or vomiting. Rapid diagnosis and detorsion is necessary to maximize testicle survival. Torsion is caused by the twisting of the spermatic cord, resulting with compression of the testicular artery and reduced or absent blood flow to the testicle. Torsion is the most common cause of testicular demise in adolescent males.

25. **What are the risk factors for testicular torsion?**
Presents in adolescence with 90% of cases due to congenital malformation, lack of proper fixation of the testis and epididymis to the scrotum, or the "bell-clapper deformity." Trauma is responsible in 4%–8% of cases.

26. **What is the physical exam of a patient with testicular torsion?**
A torsed testicle is typically tender, with scrotal swelling, erythema, or discoloration. The testicle may have a horizontal lie and may be elevated. The probability of testicular torsion is high with an absent ipsilateral cremasteric reflex.

27. **When is the onset of irreversible ischemia in testicular torsion?**
Irreversible ischemia begins around 6 hours after onset of symptoms. Diagnosis and treatment within the 6-hour time period is optimal to minimize the risk of testicle necrosis and loss.

28. **What diagnostic imaging is used to diagnose testicular torsion?**
Scrotal ultrasound with Doppler is used to detect blood flow to the testicle. In children, flow is harder to detect, leading to false-positive results. However, testicular torsion is a clinical diagnosis, and surgical exploration should be done when suspicion is high despite imaging studies.

29. **Can manual detorsion be attempted at the patient's bedside?**
Bedside manual detorsion may be attempted as long as definitive treatment is not delayed. This is done by rotating the testicle 180–360 degrees from medial to lateral.

OVARIAN

30. What are the signs and symptoms of ovarian torsion?
The most common symptom is sudden onset of sharp pelvic or lower abdominal pain (80%–100%). The pain may be intermittent (15%) and leading to a delayed diagnosis. In a younger child, the pain could be nonspecific and difficult to localize or describe. Nausea and vomiting is common and present in approximately 75% of the cases. Severe symptoms, such as acute abdominal pain, or tenderness, fever, vomiting, and pallor, can mimic an acute surgical abdomen.

31. How common is ovarian torsion in premenarchal girls?
Ovarian torsion is rare in premenarchal girls. In one case series of 22 children, the mean age at presentation was 10 years. The majority of patients (70%–75%) are younger than 30 years.

32. What are the risk factors for ovarian torsion?
Risk factors include ovarian cysts or masses, pregnancy, and history of pelvic inflammatory disease. Ovarian masses or cysts >4–6 cm are implicated in 50%–60% of cases of ovarian torsion.

33. What is the study of choice to differentiate ovarian torsion versus other ovarian processes?
Ultrasound with Doppler is the study of choice. Findings for ovarian torsion may include enlarged unilateral ovary, a heterogeneous mass, absent arterial flow, or fluid in the cul-de-sac. Ultrasound assists in detection and diagnosis of other etiologies such as ovarian cyst, tubo-ovarian abscess, ectopic pregnancy, or appendicitis.

34. What is the definitive treatment for ovarian torsion?
Surgical or gynecologic urgent referral or transfer should be initiated immediately. Definitive treatment is surgical with laparoscopic or open detorsion with ovariopexy of the viable ovary. Ovariopexy for the contralateral ovary is typically performed.

GALLSTONES

35. What are the signs and symptoms of gallstones in children?
No single symptom is highly sensitive or specific for cholelithiasis in children. Biliary colic may be present with persistent or episodic pain in the right upper quadrant (RUQ) and/or epigastrium. Pain may radiate to right shoulder, back, or flank with nausea and vomiting after eating fatty foods. Pain lasting longer than 4–6 hours suggests biliary obstruction.

36. How common is cholelithiasis in children?
Gallstones are rare in children, but recently the incidence of pediatric gallbladder disease has been increasing, paralleling the rise of obesity in children. A large number (40%) of children with gallstones are asymptomatic, and complications arise when stones obstruct the cystic duct (cholecystitis) or common bile duct (choledocholithiasis) or cause an infection of the common bile duct (cholangitis).

37. What is the imaging modality of choice for diagnosis of choledocholithiasis?
Ultrasound is the modality of choice with excellent sensitivity and specificity. It is noninvasive and does not involve radiation exposure. Gallbladder distension, wall thickening, pericholecystic fluid suggesting choledocholithiasis, and stones as small as 2 mm can be visualized.

38. What is the most common type of stone in children?
The most common type of stone is the black pigment stone, which forms with excessive bilirubin in the bile. Excessive levels of bilirubin are associated with abnormal production or destruction of red blood cells (RBCs). The prevalence of gallstones is higher in children with chronic diseases such as hemolytic anemia or sickle cell disease.

39. What is a Murphy sign?
A Murphy sign is worsening pain or inspiration arrest when the RUQ is palpated. It is highly sensitive in adults with cholecystitis.

40. How do you treat uncomplicated cholelithiasis?
Treatment for uncomplicated cholelithiasis is symptomatic. Routine ultrasound surveillance is appropriate for asymptomatic cases. Removal of the gallbladder in asymptomatic children with cholelithiasis is not standard practice, with the exception of those with sickle cell anemia.

41. How do you treat symptomatic cholelithiasis?

Laparoscopic cholecystectomy is the standard in the treatment of symptomatic cholelithiasis. It has been proven to be safe and effective in children, with a low rate of postoperative complications.

42. How do you treat patients with biliary stone complications?

Ill-appearing patients likely suffering from biliary stone complications should be stabilized with analgesics, antiemetics, and antibiotics and transferred/admitted. Patients with unresolved biliary colic, or any suspicion of cholecystitis, choledolithiasis, cholangitis, or pancreatitis should be referred and admitted.

43. What laboratory tests should be done to evaluate causes of abdominal pain?

The following are reasonable tests to evaluate causes of abdominal pain.
- Aspartate transaminase (AST), alanine transaminase (ALT), direct and indirect bilirubin, and γ-glutamyltransferase (GGT; liver disease, cholangitis)
- Amylase and lipase (pancreatitis)
- CBC with differential (anemia and leukocytosis)
- C-reactive protein (elevated in choledocholithiasis and appendicitis)
- Urinalysis and urine pregnancy (urinary tract infections, pregnancy, diabetes screen)

44. What are the signs and symptoms of acute pancreatitis in children?

- Abdominal pain (87%)
  - Sharp, constant pain in the epigastric area
  - Pain may radiate to the back or sides
  - Pain and vomiting worsens after eating
- Nausea, vomiting, and anorexia (64%)
- Abdominal tenderness (77%)
- Abdominal distension (18%)

45. What is the most common cause of acute pancreatitis in children?

Blunt trauma to the pancreas is the most common cause of acute pancreatitis in children. Traumatic pancreatitis can result from motor vehicle accidents, bicycle handlebar injuries, and inflicted injury from child abuse. Pseudocysts may develop 2–3 weeks after the traumatic pancreatitis episode. In 25% of childhood cases, the etiology of pediatric pancreatitis is unknown.

46. How do you diagnose pancreatitis?

The diagnosis is clinical and depends on the presence of symptoms consistent with acute pancreatitis, abnormal blood tests, or radiographic images. A diagnosis can be made if two or more of these criteria are fulfilled: symptoms consistent with acute pancreatitis (abdominal pain, nausea, vomiting, and abdominal tenderness), elevated lipase and/or amylase, and imaging consistent with pancreatitis.

47. What imaging is useful for diagnosing acute pancreatitis?

Ultrasound is the imaging of choice for acute pancreatitis, as it can assess the pancreatic size, inflammation, and texture. It can also assess biliary stone obstruction and presence of pseudocysts or abscesses.

48. How do you treat acute pancreatitis in children?

The treatment of pancreatitis is supportive care with pancreatic rest, no oral intake or low fat elemental diet, fluid resuscitation, pain medication, and parenteral nutrition if unable to eat. Meperidine (Demerol) is preferred to morphine for pain control because it is less likely to cause spasm of the sphincter of Oddi, which can worsen the pancreatitis. Acute uncomplicated cases of childhood pancreatitis have an excellent prognosis.

49. What causes hepatitis in children?

Hepatitis may result from both infectious (viral, bacterial, fungal, and parasitic organisms) and noninfectious (medications, toxins, and autoimmune) causes. Possible viral exposures include blood transfusions, intravenous or intranasal drug use, sexual or sexual abuse history, and travel history. It is important to consider exposure to medications, such as acetaminophen commonly found in children's cold medications, or toxins such as poisonous wild mushrooms.

50. What are some viruses that can cause acute hepatitis?

Following is a list of some viruses associated with acute hepatitis.
- Hepatitis viruses: five main types including hepatitis A, B, C, D, and E
- Cytomegalovirus (CMV), part of the herpesvirus family

- Epstein-Barr virus (EBV), commonly associated with infectious mononucleosis
- Herpes simplex virus (HSV), varicella zoster virus (VZV), enteroviruses, rubella, adenovirus, and parvovirus

51. What are the symptoms of acute hepatitis in children?

The most common symptoms of acute hepatitis include flulike symptoms, fever, abdominal pain, nausea, vomiting, fatigue, anorexia, jaundice, myalgias, dark urine, and clay-colored stools.

52. What laboratory tests should be sent for suspected acute hepatitis?

- ALT, AST, and lactate to evaluate hepatic cellular injury
- Prothrombin time (PT), partial thromboplastin time (PTT), albumin, and ammonia to evaluate the liver's functional capacity
- Alkaline phosphatase, GGT, and total/direct bilirubin to detect biliary obstruction
- Serum electrolytes, blood urea nitrogen (BUN), creatinine, and glucose
- Acetaminophen levels if suspect acetaminophen toxicity

53. What screening labs for specific hepatitis viral etiologies can be sent?

- Hepatitis A antibody (IgM, anti-HAV), hepatitis B core antibody (IgM anti-HBc), and surface antigen (HbsAg)
- Anti-HCV antibody testing and qualitative polymerase chain reaction (PCR) for HCV

54. Is radiographic imaging necessary to diagnose acute hepatitis?

Abdominal ultrasound or CT scan may be necessary to rule out other abdominal pathology such as abdominal masses, gallbladder disease, or biliary tract obstruction.

55. What is the treatment for acute hepatitis?

Medications are not routinely given for treatment of uncomplicated acute viral hepatitis. All patients with suspected or confirmed HBV or HCV infection should be referred to a gastroenterologist or hepatologist for further evaluation and treatment.

Patients with evidence of fulminant hepatitis, hepatic encephalopathy, significant vomiting, dehydration, or electrolyte abnormalities require hospital admission.

KEY POINTS

1. Constipation is a diagnosis of exclusion in patients presenting with acute abdominal pain.
2. Children presenting with constipation since birth need to have Hirschsprung disease ruled out.
3. Testicular torsion may present only with nausea, vomiting, and nonspecific abdominal pain.
4. Testicular torsion is a time-sensitive emergency, requiring immediate diagnosis and treatment to preserve the testicle.
5. Acute and abrupt onset of abdominal pain helps distinguish ovarian torsion from other abdominal etiologies such as appendicitis.

BIBLIOGRAPHY

Attia MW. Ovarian torsion. In: Hoffman RJ, et al., eds. *Fleisher and Ludwig's 5-Minute Pediatric Emergency Medicine Consult*. Philadelphia: Wolters Kluwer Health; 2011:698–699.

Barcega B, Piroutek MJ. Constipation. In: Hoffman RJ, et al., eds. *Fleisher and Ludwig's 5-Minute Pediatric Emergency Medicine Consult*. Philadelphia: Wolters Kluwer Health; 2011:196–197.

Ellison AM. Hepatitis, acute. In: Hoffman RJ, et al., eds. *Fleisher and Ludwig's 5-Minute Pediatric Emergency Medicine Consult*. Philadelphia: Wolters Kluwer Health; 2011:488–489.

Leung AKC, Sigalet DL. Acute abdominal pain in children. *Am Fam Physician*. 2003;67(11):2321–2326.

Loiselle JM. Pancreatitis. In: Hoffman RJ, et al., eds. *Fleisher and Ludwig's 5-Minute Pediatric Emergency Medicine Consult*. Philadelphia: Wolters Kluwer Health; 2011:714–715.

Luck RP. Ovarian cyst. In: Hoffman RJ, et al., eds. *Fleisher and Ludwig's 5-Minute Pediatric Emergency Medicine Consult*. Philadelphia: Wolters Kluwer Health; 2011:696–697.

Mehta S, Lopez ME, Chumpitazi BP, Mazziotti MV, Brandt ML, Fishman DS. Clinical characteristics and risk factors for symptomatic pediatric gallbladder disease. *Pediatrics*. 2012;129(1):e82–e88.

Sharp VJ, Kieran K, Arlen AM. Testicular torsion: diagnosis, evaluation, and management. *Am Fam Physician*. 2013;88(12):835–840.

Tabbers MM, Dilorenzo C, Berger MY, et al. Evaluation and treatment of functional constipation in infants and children: evidence-based recommendations from ESPGHAN and NASPGHAN. *J Pediatr Gastroenterol Nutr*. 2014;58(2):265–281.

Tilt L, Kharbanda A. Appendicitis. In: Hoffman RJ, et al., eds. *Fleisher and Ludwig's 5-Minute Pediatric Emergency Medicine Consult*. Philadelphia: Wolters Kluwer Health; 2011:72–73.

CHAPTER 20

NAUSEA, VOMITING, DIARRHEA, AND DEHYDRATION

Christopher M. Pruitt, MD

1. What are the common reasons for vomiting in pediatric patients?

Children vomit with almost any kind of illness, so the list of causes is extensive. By far, however, the most common cause of vomiting in children of any age is gastroenteritis.

2. What are the usual culprits for gastroenteritis?

The answer depends on your practice setting. While bacterial and parasitic causes are more commonly encountered in resource-poor settings, in developed countries, viruses are much more prevalent.

3. If vomiting is so common, how can I know if a dangerous condition might be present (Table 20.1)?

- Appearance of the vomit: bright green or yellow (bilious)
- Pain: especially severe or constant
- Exam: marked tenderness or distension
- Symptoms or signs of elevated intracranial pressure

4. Why is bilious emesis worrisome? Is it always?

Vomiting of bile can signify an intestinal obstruction distal to the sphincter of Oddi. More frequently, however, bilious emesis simply follows vomiting of nonbilious contents and does not indicate an emergency.

5. A 13-day female patient presents with two episodes of vomiting in the past few hours. The parents show you a blanket with a small bright yellow stain from her emesis. What should you do?

Bilious emesis in young infants should be considered an emergency until proven otherwise. This is a classic presentation (even if well appearing!) for neonatal obstruction, the most common cause being intestinal malrotation (entraining volvulus). This child should be urgently referred for an upper gastrointestinal (GI) study.

6. How do I know if the baby I'm seeing simply has reflux?

Physiologic reflux ("spitting up") is the most common cause of vomiting in infants. Clues to this diagnosis are well appearance, normal growth, and nonacute presentation. Reflux typically peaks in the second month of life and usually does not require pharmacologic intervention.

7. A 7-week infant has had worsening vomiting for 5 days. There is no bile. The caregiver thinks that the emesis is becoming more forceful. What diagnosis should you consider?

Hypertrophic pyloric stenosis usually presents in the second month of life, and it is more common in males. Given the anatomic location of the obstruction, vomitus is nonbilious. Babies are often well appearing, and unless they present later in the course of their illness, the "classic" electrolyte pattern of a hypochloremic, hypokalemic metabolic alkalosis will be absent. They have progressive "projectile" vomiting and lack satiety. It is diagnosed by ultrasound.

8. List some common causes for a presenting complaint of "blood in the stool" for infants and young children.

- Lack of true blood (red dyes, cefdinir)
- Anal fissures
- Infectious diarrhea

Table 20.1. Worrisome Causes of Vomiting by Age Group		
INFANCY	**EARLY CHILDHOOD**	**ADOLESCENCE**
Volvulus from malrotation	Intussusception	Appendicitis
Pyloric stenosis	Toxic ingestion	Toxic ingestion
Increased intracranial pressure	Increased intracranial pressure	Increased intracranial pressure
Inborn errors of metabolism	Diabetic ketoacidosis	Diabetic ketoacidosis
Other causes of obstruction	Appendicitis	Torsion of ovary/testis

- Swallowed maternal blood
- Milk protein intolerance (infants)
- Ileocolic intussusception (late finding)

9. **My patient has fever and diarrhea but now is complaining of blood in the stool. Guaiac testing is positive. The child looks well. Given the presence of blood, is there anything different that should be done?**
While routine stool cultures are not recommended for children with acute diarrhea, up to 20% of cultures will grow a bacterial pathogen when gross blood is present. Therefore, it is advisable to obtain a stool culture in this setting. Nevertheless, antibiotic treatment is not recommended for healthy children in most cases of bacterial enteritis.

10. **A 4-month-old female patient presents with 2 days of diarrhea, vomiting, and fever. She is well appearing, and you think the most likely diagnosis is viral gastroenteritis. What one test should you consider for this patient?**
Urinary tract infections (UTIs) are common in young children, more so in girls. Data are conflicting as to whether gastrointestinal symptoms are more common in children with UTI. Although young infants can lack the expected findings on urinalysis, consider obtaining urine for this child. While a catheter specimen is preferred, a bagged urine that is "clean" may reassure against UTI; if the bag urinalysis suggests infection, obtain a catheterized specimen for culture.

11. **What diagnosis should always be considered in older infants and young children with isolated vomiting?**
Ileocolic intussusception is the most common gastrointestinal emergency in young children. The usual age range is 6–36 months of age, but all the "classic" findings (vomiting, pain, lethargy, abdominal mass, "currant jelly" stools) are not usually present. Kids can appear well, especially if the obstruction is intermittent. The preferred diagnostic modality is ultrasound, and hydrostatic enema is usually successful for reducing the intussusception.

12. **You are seeing an 8-month-old child with isolated vomiting. She is hydrated and well appearing. She has no other symptoms and has a negative guaiac. How might you further reassure that she is not intussuscepted?**
Visualization of air in the cecum or ascending colon on abdominal radiographs can reliably exclude ileocolic intussusception, especially if there is low clinical suspicion. Images are best obtained in the supine and left lateral decubitus positions.

13. **An 18-month-old male patient presents with 6 weeks of large-volume, watery stools. The child appears well and is growing normally. What is the most likely diagnosis?**
Functional diarrhea (also termed "chronic nonspecific diarrhea" or "toddler's diarrhea") is a benign entity without a certain cause. Most children outgrow this in a few years. It is generally recommended to advise limiting intake of liquids with a high sugar content (especially fruit juices, but also sports drinks or other sweetened beverages).

14. **Does a complaint of vomiting blood in a child often portend a worrisome cause?**
No. Though serious causes should be explored via history and physical, the most common causes for hematemesis are swallowed blood from the upper airways (e.g., colds, epistaxis) or small Mallory-Weiss tears that usually heal on their own.

Table 20.2. Reliability of Clinical Findings in Dehydration

CLINICAL FINDING	SENSITIVITY	SPECIFICITY	POSITIVE PREDICTIVE VALUE	NEGATIVE PREDICTIVE VALUE
Decreased skin elasticity	0.35	0.97	0.57	0.93
Capillary refill >2 sec	0.48	0.96	0.57	0.94
General appearance	0.59	0.91	0.42	0.95
Absent tears	0.67	0.89	0.40	0.96
Abnormal respirations	0.43	0.86	0.37	0.94
Dry mucous membranes	0.80	0.78	0.29	0.99
Sunken eyes	0.60	0.84	0.29	0.95
Abnormal radial pulse	0.43	0.86	0.25	0.93
Tachycardia (HR >150)	0.46	0.79	0.20	0.93
Decreased urine output	0.85	0.53	0.17	0.97

Data from Gorelick MH, Shaw KN, Murphy KO: Validity and Reliability of Clinical Signs in the Diagnosis of Dehydration in Children. *Pediatrics* 99:5, 1997.

15. **Why do so many young kids with upper respiratory infections have vomiting?**
   Many young children have tussive emesis from gagging with coughing. Surprisingly, many parents do not make this distinction in the history. Tussive vomiting alone rarely entrains considerable dehydration.

16. **Why does constipation often present with "diarrhea"?**
   Kids with constipation often have watery feces that move past the impacted distal stool. A detailed history will help you arrive at the right diagnosis.

17. **What are the most frequent causes of dehydration in children?**
   Increased losses of body water are by far the most common, with diarrhea the leading cause worldwide. Dehydration is also caused by decreased fluid intake, which can be seen specifically with pharyngitis or stomatitis, or truly any illness. Children are more prone to increased insensible losses due to increased respirations or fever, as well.

18. **What is the most common reason for hyponatremic dehydration in infants?**
   Most children have isotonic dehydration. Yet for infants, caregivers who are improperly preparing or diluting formula is not an uncommon cause of hypotonic dehydration in these young children. Left unrecognized and untreated, these infants can progress to seizures and even death.

19. **In an ill-appearing child with dehydration, what lab value is the most important to check *initially*?**
   In younger children, hypoglycemia should be suspected and rapidly corrected. Up to 10% of young children with dehydration have hypoglycemia. For well-appearing patients, mild hypoglycemia can be administered enterally; for ill-appearing children, or for significantly low glucose levels, correct intravenously with 0.5 mg/kg dextrose.

20. **My patient's caregiver says that he hasn't urinated in 18 hours. This means he has significant dehydration, right?**
   Perhaps, but not always. Only one of every five parents who report oliguria will have a child with considerable dehydration (Table 20.2). Unfortunately, though parents are often told to watch for this at home, there is no reliable means for a caregiver to accurately gauge dehydration.

21. **If that's true, why even ask about urine output?**
   Other conditions can cause dehydration that may be associated with an *increase* in urine output—most notably, diabetes mellitus, but also diabetes insipidus or other conditions that cause impaired renal concentrating. Oliguria may also indicate kidney injury (e.g., hemolytic-uremic syndrome).

22. **My patient's history doesn't suggest significant dehydration, but her lips are really dry. Why is this?**
The absence of dry mucous membranes is highly predictive against significant dehydration. Conversely, owing to the other conditions that can cause this finding, its presence is not always indicative of dehydration (see Table 20.2). Tachypnea, obligate mouth breathing (nasal congestion, small babies), or lack of recent fluid intake can all cause dry mouth.

23. **How helpful is urine specific gravity in detection of dehydration?**
Excluding conditions that alter urine osmolarity, highly concentrated urine does not always indicate significant dehydration, and a low specific gravity doesn't mean the patient isn't dehydrated. It simply is not a very helpful measure of hydration in children.

24. **So, at bedside, how am I supposed to know whether my patient is dehydrated?**
Clinician "gestalt" may be just as good as validated scoring instruments. However, the best tools combine features of the physical exam—most notably general appearance, dry mucous membranes, and absence of tears.

25. **You are seeing a 3-year-old male with 4 days of profuse diarrhea and some vomiting. You believe he is moderately dehydrated. How should you rehydrate this child?**
Extensive research (much in resource-poor settings) has demonstrated great success with enteral rehydration in children with mild to moderate dehydration. If parenteral rehydration is readily available, some parents may prefer this means of therapy. Both methods, when done properly, are generally safe and effective for rehydration.

26. **I think my patient needs to be orally rehydrated. How is this best performed?**
Use an oral rehydration solution with the right balance of sodium and glucose to enable the intestinal cotransport mechanisms for passive water absorption. (Beverages with too much sugar—including juices and sports drinks—can entrain an osmotic diarrhea.) The fluid deficit is replaced over 4 hours, usually in 5-minute increments. Mild dehydration equates to roughly 50 mL/kg body water loss, and moderate dehydration 100 mL/kg—this means the mildly dehydrated child gets approximately 1 mL/kg per aliquot, and 2 mL/kg if moderately dehydrated.

27. **Won't this child simply vomit if we try oral rehydration?**
Perhaps, but losses can be replaced as you go. Vomiting or diarrhea (or both) does not preclude successful oral rehydration therapy; in fact, continued symptoms should be expected. A single dose of ondansetron (best to use orally disintegrating form) is likely to reduce vomiting and facilitate oral rehydration for older infants and children.

28. **When would you *not* advise rehydration solution for a child with diarrhea?**
The sodium and glucose in rehydration solutions give them a high osmolarity. If the child is not dehydrated, ingestion of such liquids can exacerbate diarrhea. Infants without dehydration should continue to drink breastmilk or formula; consider dilution of high-sugar beverages for older children.

29. **The parent asks you about resumption of solid foods and, in particular, a bland diet. What should you advise?**
There is no proven benefit of a bland diet for patients with gastroenteritis. In fact, it is recommended to continue a normal diet during the diarrheal illness.

30. **For children who are deemed candidates for parenteral rehydration, what should you order?**
Intravenous rehydration is typically performed with administration of isotonic (0.9% saline or lactated Ringer) fluid in volumes of 20 mL/kg (up to 1 L), usually over 20–30 minutes. Never bolus hypotonic fluids or dextrose-containing fluids (unless the latter is needed for rapid correction of hypoglycemia). Repeated boluses may be necessary, depending on the degree of dehydration.

KEY POINTS

1. Complaints of blood in vomit or stool are usually associated with nonemergencies in healthy children.
2. Ileocolic intussusception should always be considered in the young child (about 6–36 months of age) with isolated vomiting. Supine and left lateral decubitus x-rays can reassure against this diagnosis, especially if there is low clinical suspicion.

3. Parental report of oliguria is the least predictive sign of pediatric dehydration.
4. If dehydration is not severe, most children can be successfully treated with appropriate oral rehydration solutions.

BIBLIOGRAPHY

Freedman SB, Adler M, Seshadri R, et al. Oral ondansetron for gastroenteritis in a pediatric emergency department. *N Engl J Med*. 2006;354:16.

Freedman SB, Vandermeer B, Milne A, et al. Diagnosing clinically significant dehydration in children with acute gastroenteritis using noninvasive methods: a meta-analysis. *J Pediatr*. 2015;166:4.

Gorelick MH, Shaw KN, Murphy KO. Validity and reliability of clinical signs in the diagnosis of dehydration in children. *Pediatrics*. 1997;99:5.

Intussusception in children. <http://www.uptodate.com/contents/intussusception-in-children>; Accessed 09.08.16.

Reid SR, Losek JD. Hypoglycemia complicating dehydration in children with acute gastroenteritis. *J Emerg Med*. 2005;29:2.

Slutsker L, Ries AA, Greene KD, et al. Escherichia coli O157;H7 diarrhea in the United States: clinical and epidemiologic features. *Ann Intern Med*. 1997;126:7.

Spandorfer PR. Dehydration. In: Shaw KN, Bachur RG, eds. *Textbook of Pediatric Emergency Medicine*. 7th ed. Philadelphia: Lippincott Williams & Wilkins; 2015:128–134.

Steiner MJ, Nager AL, Wang VJ. Urine specific gravity and other urinary indices: inaccurate tests for dehydration. *Pediatr Emerg Care*. 2007;23.

Whittington LA, Stevens DC, Jones SA, et al. Visual diagnosis: an 11-month-old with nausea, vomiting, and an abdominal mass. *Pediatr Rev*. 2013;34:12.

World Health Organization: The treatment of diarrhea: a manual for physicians and other senior health workers. <http://www.who.int/maternal_child_adolescent/documents/9241593180/en/>; Accessed 12.08.16.

CHAPTER 21

URINARY AND UROLOGIC COMPLAINTS

Jennifer F. Anders, MD, Ariel Cohen, DO, Jennifer Fishe, MD, Daniel Yu, MBBCh

1. **The classic symptoms of urinary tract infection include dysuria, urgency, and frequency. What are the most common signs of urinary tract infection in preverbal and nonverbal children?**

   Urinary tract infection (UTI) may present with a myriad of signs and symptoms. In the neonate, UTI may present as fever or sepsis without obvious source. In infants, as well, fever may be the only symptom. Other manifestations of UTIs can be nonspecific. Systemic symptoms may include irritability, fatigue, fussiness, decreased oral intake, decreased urine output, or failure to thrive. Gastrointestinal (GI) symptoms are common and may include vomiting, diarrhea, and abdominal (especially suprapubic) or back pain. This may lead caregivers to conclude the patient has gastroenteritis or a food allergy.

   Beyond 2–3 years of age, symptoms more often point to the urinary tract; these include frequency, urgency, retention or incontinence, dysuria, and occasionally hematuria. This can present as a previously toilet-trained child beginning to have "accidents."

   Foul-smelling urine is often mentioned by caregivers but has little diagnostic meaning.

   In children who lack bladder sensation (e.g., spina bifida) and who receive regular straight catheterization, change in the quality of the urine (more cloudy, change in odor) may be the only sign. Such children may also present with fever, change in level of alertness, or vomiting.

2. **When should a urinalysis be obtained in a child with suspected UTI?**

   For an infant less than 2 months of age, urinalysis should always be obtained as part of the complete evaluation of fever without a source. For children over 2 months of age, the decision to obtain urinalysis is guided by the child's clinical status. Once antimicrobial therapy is initiated, the opportunity to make a definitive diagnosis is lost; therefore, urinalysis and culture should be obtained prior to therapy. In any child with unexplained fever and toxic appearance prompting the clinician to give antibiotics, a urinalysis and culture should be obtained prior to initiation of antibiotic therapy.

   If a child with an unexplained fever does not need immediate antibiotic treatment, the clinician can assess the likelihood of UTI. Laboratory investigation for UTI should be reserved for those children with concerning symptoms including dysuria, urgency, frequency, suprapubic pain, fever with no obvious source, fever with emesis (and absence of diarrhea), costovertebral angle tenderness, or irritability without an alternate explanation.

   The approximate rate of UTI in febrile children 2–24 months of age is 5%; the risk is significantly lower for circumcised boys. Higher risk of UTI can be predicted for children with prior history of UTI, those of non-black race, and those with higher temperatures (>39°C), longer duration of fever (>24 hours), or signs of systemic toxicity. For children deemed to be at low risk, no urinalysis or culture and close clinical follow-up is recommended. For children with one or more risk factors, urinalysis is recommended, and if pyuria is present culture should be obtained to confirm UTI.

3. **When and how should urine be obtained for culture in a child with suspected UTI?**

   If antimicrobial therapy is to be initiated, then a urine specimen suitable for culture should be obtained before antimicrobial agents are given. Urine specimens suitable for culture include those obtained by clean catch midstream collection, urethral catheterization, or suprapubic aspiration. Adhesive bag urine collection is often used for children who are not yet toilet trained. Such bag specimens may be used for urinalysis (UA) but should be assumed to be contaminated with perineal flora and not be used for culture.

   One option is to obtain a urinalysis with a bag specimen, and if the UA is normal and the patient is otherwise not at high risk for UTI, the evaluation can be considered complete. If the UA is abnormal, urine should be sent for culture to confirm the diagnosis and provide bacterial identification and sensitivities.

4. **What are the alternative methods for urine to be obtained for culture from children of various ages?**

Culture samples may only be obtained via catheterization or suprapubic aspiration. Cultures of urine specimens collected in a bag applied to the perineum have an unacceptably high false-positive rate and are valid only when they yield negative results.

Ideal handling of a bagged urine specimen includes (a) the perineal skin is well cleansed before bag application, (b) the bag is removed promptly after voiding, and (c) the specimen is refrigerated or processed immediately. Despite claims that this collection technique has a low contamination rate with ideal handling, there is unavoidable but significant contamination in the two groups at highest risk for UTI—the vagina in girls and the prepuce in uncircumcised boys.

5. **How can you differentiate pyelonephritis from cystitis in pediatric patients?**

Distinguishing pyelonephritis from cystitis is difficult in young patients because they may have clinical overlap and younger patients often have only nonspecific symptoms. Hence, pyelonephritis and cystitis are often discussed together as one clinical entity, generically covered by the term "urinary tract infection."

While strict differentiation between upper and lower tract disease in children is often not feasible, there are some features more suggestive of pyelonephritis: high fever (>40°C), ill or toxic appearance, flank pain, or costovertebral angle tenderness and emesis.

Features suggestive of limited cystitis include well appearance, suprapubic pain, and normothermia or low-grade fever.

6. **What are some widely accepted empiric antibiotic strategies for pediatric UTI?**

Oral or parenteral treatment is equally efficacious for most pediatric UTI (cystitis or pyelonephritis). Antibiotic choice should be based on local antimicrobial sensitivity patterns (if available) and should be individually adjusted to sensitivity testing from the patient's urine culture.

There is no single preferred duration of therapy, but most recent guidelines suggest at least 3–5 days for simple cystitis and 7–14 days for febrile UTI. Evidence in treatment of pediatric UTI shows shorter (1–3 days) courses inferior to courses in the recommended range.

Intravenous (IV; parenteral) antibiotic therapy should be initiated if the patient is less than 2 months of age, has a toxic appearance, cannot tolerate oral intake, has other adverse anatomic factors (e.g., obstruction to urinary flow), or has a known positive culture for a pathogen not susceptible to oral agents (Boxes 21.1 and 21.2).

It is essential to know local susceptibility patterns, because there is substantial geographic variability. Up to 60% of *Escherichia coli* strains demonstrate resistance to ampicillin and amoxicillin/clavulanate; therefore, these drugs should not be used as monotherapy unless local patterns of susceptibility are known to be favorable.

7. **How does antibiotic therapy for children with pyelonephritis differ from therapy for cystitis?**

Historically, treatment of pyelonephritis has been initiated with IV antibiotics until the patient becomes afebrile. This may still be warranted in ill-appearing children or those with complicating factors.

Box 21.1. Oral Antibiotic Options for Pediatric UTI

Cephalexin 100 mg/kg/day ÷ qid
Cefixime 8 mg/kg/day as a single dose
Cefpodoxime 10 mg/kg/day ÷ bid
Cefdinir 14 mg/kg/day as a single dose
Nitrofurantoin 7 mg/kg/day ÷ qid or (as macrocrystal/monohydrate) 100 mg bid
Trimethoprim/sulfamethoxazole 8–10 mg/kg/day of trimethoprim component ÷ bid

---

Box 21.2. Parenteral (IV) Antibiotic Options for Pediatric UTI

Ampicillin 200 mg/kg/day ÷ qid PLUS gentamicin 5–7.5 mg/kg/day in a single dose
Cefazolin 75 mg/kg/day ÷ tid
Ceftriaxone 75 mg/kg/day (IV or IM) in a single dose or ÷ bid

However, ample evidence supports outpatient treatment of uncomplicated pediatric pyelonephritis when the child can tolerate oral fluids and antibiotics, has normal renal function, and is not septic. The widely recommended treatment course is 7–14 days of an oral cephalosporin (e.g., cephalexin, cefdinir, cefixime, or cefpodoxime). It is important to note that nitrofurantoin should not be used for suspected pyelonephritis because it does not achieve therapeutic concentrations in the bloodstream.

8. **What follow-up should be planned for a child with diagnosis of urinary tract infection?**
   Ideally the child should have follow-up within 48 hours, to ensure that the current infection is being adequately treated, including ability to tolerate the prescribed antibiotic and verification that any symptoms are resolving. The follow-up should include review of urine culture results and sensitivities and allow for changes in antibiotic treatment if needed to match the sensitivity results.

9. **When is hospitalization necessary for a child with urinary tract infection?**
   Many UTIs may be treated with oral antibiotics in the outpatient setting. However, children who cannot tolerate oral antibiotics or fluids, children with signs of sepsis (e.g., persistent tachycardia, hypotension, delayed capillary refill) or renal dysfunction (decreased urine output, urinary retention/obstruction), and infants less than 2 months of age should be hospitalized and receive intravenous antibiotics. In addition, children require IV antibiotics for culture positive with pathogens for which there is no susceptible oral antibiotic. Hospitalization should also be considered for children with genitourinary anatomic abnormalities (e.g., ureteropelvic junction obstruction, posterior urethral valves, bladder extrophy) or children with indwelling urinary catheters.

10. **What is the definition of true hematuria? What is the differential diagnosis of false hematuria?**
    True hematuria is that confirmed by microscopy with greater than five red blood cells (RBCs) present in the urinalysis. False hematuria, presenting with red urine or apparent gross hematuria, or a positive dipstick for hemoglobin without RBC on microscopy, may be caused by myoglobinuria, hemolysis, crystal urates, or ingestion of foods including beets and blackberries, aniline dyes, or medications including Pyridium and rifampin.

11. **What is the differential diagnosis for true hematuria in a child?**
    There are numerous causes of hematuria in children. Tables 21.1 and 21.2 list a variety of common causes, with the most common highlighted in bold.

12. **When should a child with hematuria be referred to an emergency department for immediate evaluation?**
    A child with hematuria should be referred for emergent evaluation if there is concern for nephritis or if the hematuria is accompanied by proteinuria; such children require further laboratory evaluation

Table 21.1. Common Causes of Gross Hematuria in Children

BENIGN CAUSES	PATHOLOGIC CAUSES
Exercise	**UTI (urethritis, cystitis, pyelonephritis)**
	Trauma (kidney, bladder, urethra)
Idiopathic hypercalciuria without nephrolithiasis	**Acute poststreptococcal glomerulonephritis (APSGN)**
	Nephrolithiasis
	Sickle cell trait or disease
	Obstruction (ureteropelvic junction obstruction)
	Foreign body
	Wilms tumor
	Renal vein thrombosis (ex-premature infants)
	Polycystic kidney disease
	Genitourinary tract arteriovenous malformation (rare)
	Tuberculosis

for evidence of renal dysfunction. Hematuria with hypertension (>90th percentile for height) should also have prompt emergent referral. Children with suspected trauma to the kidneys, bladder, pelvis, or urethra also need emergent evaluation. Any patient with decreased urine output, no urine output, signs of volume overload on physical exam (such as periorbital or scrotal edema), or signs of urinary tract obstruction (from blood clots) should be referred to an emergency department.

13. **What are the most frequent causes of renal stones in children?**
See Box 21.3. The incidence of renal stones in pediatric patients is increasing. Children with renal stones should be referred to a urologist or nephrologist for a metabolic workup (studies estimate at least 30% of children with renal stones will have an underlying metabolic disorder). Calcium oxalate stones are the most frequent type (40%–60%).

14. **What can cause acute urinary retention in a child?**
Acute urinary retention is a urologic emergency and may progress to bladder injury if not relieved promptly. Emergent treatment may include urethral catheterization to drain the bladder. Additional treatments would be guided by the underlying cause (Box 21.4).

15. **An 8-year-old boy presents with complaint of penile pain, swelling, and dysuria. His parents report that they are no longer able to retract the child's foreskin after a traumatic retraction the week prior. What is the diagnosis and how is this condition treated?**
Phimosis is the inability to retract the foreskin over the glans of the penis in an uncircumcised male. It can be physiologic or pathologic, which is caused by adhesions or scar tissue from inflammation or infection. A urinalysis and culture should be obtained in symptomatic patients.

Table 21.2. Common Causes of Microscopic Hematuria in Children

BENIGN	PATHOLOGIC
Asymptomatic isolated hematuria	**Trauma**
Benign familial hematuria	Nephritic syndrome (e.g., lupus, membranoprolif-erative glomerulonephritis)
	Alport syndrome
	IgA nephropathy
	Vasculitis (Wegener)
	Henoch-Schönlein purpura
	Hemolytic-uremic syndrome

Box 21.3. Most Frequent Etiologies of Kidney Stones in Children

Dehydration
Diet (high sodium, low calcium intake)
Infection
Metabolic abnormalities (most frequently hypercalciuria)

Box 21.4. Causes of Acute Urinary Retention in Children

Mechanical obstruction (anatomic abnormality, blood clot, stone, stricture from catheterization, neoplasm)
Infection (UTI, vaginitis)
Fecal impaction
Neurologic disorder (dysfunctional voiding, acute myelitis)
Behavioral
Drug effect (opioids)
Idiopathic

Physiologic phimosis can be managed safely with topical steroids such as 1%–2.5% hydrocortisone ointment. A treatment course of up to 3–6 weeks of therapy is generally sufficient. This should be combined with gentle manual retraction of the foreskin. When performing gentle retractions, careful replacement of the foreskin to its original position is imperative. Patients with symptomatic or pathologic phimosis should be referred to a urologist for evaluation. A portion of patients may require circumcision in correcting the phimosis.

16. **Your 8-year-old patient seen last week with phimosis returns today complaining of worsening penile pain and swelling. You examine his penis and find the glans appears extremely red and swollen relative to the penile shaft. His foreskin appears tight, like a constricting band around the glans. What is the next step?**
He has paraphimosis, a urologic emergency where the retracted foreskin cannot be returned to the normal resting position due to swelling. Distal edema and swelling worsens, which results in ischemic changes and the development of gangrene and tissue necrosis if left untreated. Paraphimosis can be precipitated by the caregiver retracting the foreskin behind the glans for cleaning. It occurs in uncircumcised or partially circumcised males.

Treatment involves returning the glans to its position within the foreskin. Numerous techniques have been described, with manual reduction being the least invasive. First hold steady pressure on the head of the penis, squeezing distally to proximally in order to reduce swelling. Ice packs may be a helpful adjunct as well. Then place both thumbs on the glans, and index and middle fingers proximal to the phimotic ring. Apply steady pressure on the glans and attempt to move the phimotic ring distally over the glans, thus reducing the paraphimosis. Adequate analgesia should be provided. Pain control can also be achieved by local lidocaine infiltration to achieve penile block. Second-line therapies include needle decompression. If conservative measures fail, an emergency dorsal slit procedure should be performed by a urologist.

17. **A 15-month-old circumcised boy presents with swelling of the penis. You examine his diaper area to find a grossly swollen, boggy area on the shaft of the penis just proximal to the glans. The glans appears slightly swollen and red. You astutely diagnose him with balanoposthitis. How is this condition treated?**
Balanitis is defined as inflammation of the glans penis. When the foreskin is also involved, it is termed "balanoposthitis." It is usually the result of irritation from prolonged exposure to a wet diaper or similar hygiene issues in uncircumcised males. It can also be seen with trauma due to forceful foreskin retraction or excessive washing with exposure to soap or other irritants. The most important aspect of treatment is good local and topical hygiene. Sitting the baby in a shallow tub of lukewarm water for 5–10 minutes twice a day is the most efficient way to rinse and soothe the inflamed area. (Note: Infants and toddlers must ALWAYS be attended in a bath—no matter how shallow the water!) Additional analgesia should be provided to patients with severe pain.

In addition, for boys nearly toilet trained, allowing them to go without a diaper for certain periods of time will allow air circulation to the area and promote resolution. A diaper rash ointment (zinc oxide, petroleum jelly) applied to the area will protect the skin from further irritation by urine or diaper contents. If candida diaper rash is suspected, an antifungal cream can also be applied to the area. If the area is particularly red, painful, or has tense (rather than boggy) swelling, oral antibiotic therapy for possible cellulitis may be considered.

18. **A 5-year-old African American girl is brought in by her mother, who saw streaks of blood in her underpants. On physical exam, you find a circle of bright red and friable mucosa between her clitoral hood and vaginal introitus. What is the diagnosis and how will you manage it?**
This is the typical presentation of urethral prolapse—a protrusion of distal urethral mucosa through the external urethral meatus. Urethral prolapse can be seen in prepubertal and postmenopausal women. For unknown reasons, in prepubertal girls it occurs most often in African Americans. The finding of genital bleeding in a prepubertal girl often causes anxiety for caregivers and may provoke questions about sexual abuse. In the absence of specific allegations of sexual abuse, the diagnosis of urethral prolapse can be provided with reassurance.

Most cases of urethral prolapse can be managed conservatively, with sitz baths and good hygiene. Topical estrogen cream can be used to temporarily estrogenize the vaginal mucosa and promote resolution. Most patients can be appropriately discharged from urgent care with primary care or urologic follow-up. Send a urinalysis and culture if the patient complains of urinary symptoms. Do not attempt to manually reduce the urethral prolapse. In rare cases, a very edematous prolapsed segment might obstruct urination. In the event of acute bladder outlet obstruction, excessive pain, or excessive bleeding, immediate evaluation by a urologist is warranted. A small portion of patients may require surgical intervention to resect the prolapsed urethral segment. Surgery is usually reserved for chronic prolapse that fails the conservative approach outlined above but may be indicated acutely in severe cases.

19. **What is the difference between primary enuresis and secondary enuresis, and what initial management of primary enuresis can be initiated in urgent care?**
It is important to differentiate between primary and secondary enuresis when evaluating a child older than 5 years. Children who have never achieved nighttime dryness and wet the bed during sleep have primary enuresis. Children who develop enuresis after a dry period of at least 6 months have secondary enuresis. First-line therapies for children with primary enuresis include restriction of fluids before bedtime, bed alarm therapy, or desmopressin therapy.

20. **What urgent evaluation should be done for a child with secondary enuresis?**
Initial evaluation should include a history, exam, and urinalysis. Several conditions such as diabetes mellitus, diabetes insipidus, constipation, obstructive sleep apnea, chronic kidney disease, and urinary tract infection may be associated with secondary enuresis.
Patients with secondary enuresis should be evaluated for recent psychosocial stressors, poor voiding habits, and caffeine intake or stool retention. Routine urinalysis can screen for many items on this differential including glucosuria (diabetes mellitus), low specific gravity (diabetes insipidus), and white blood cells (WBCs) or nitrites to suggest UTI.

KEY POINTS

1. Urinary tract infections can present with subtlety in young children. Unexplained fever or vomiting in a preverbal or diapered child is ample reason to consider UTI.
2. Bag-collected urine specimens are not appropriate for urine culture, due to high rate of contamination.
3. It is vital to know local antibiotic susceptibility patterns when choosing empiric therapy for UTI.

BIBLIOGRAPHY

Hernandez JD, Ellison JS, Lendvay TS. Current trends, evaluation, and management of pediatric nephrolithiasis. *JAMA Pediatr.* 2015;169(10):964–970.

Kaplan BS, Pradham M. Urinalysis interpretation for pediatricians. *Pediatric Annals.* 2013;42(3):45–51.

Nevo A, Mano R, Livne PM, Sivan B, Ben-Meir D. Urinary retention in children. *Urology.* 2014;84:1475–1479.

Pohlman GD, Phillips JM, Wilcox DT. Simple method of paraphimosis reduction revisited: point of technique and review of literature. *J Pediatric Urology.* 2013;9:104–107.

Ramakrishnan K. Evaluation and treatment of enuresis. *Am Fam Physician.* 2000;78:489–496.

Sas DJ. An update on the changing epidemiology and metabolic risk factors in pediatric kidney stone disease. *Clin J Am Soc Nephrol.* 2011;6(8):2062–2068.

Shaw K, Blackstone MM, Lopez P, Rober C. UTI, febrile. In: Shaw KN, Bachur RG, eds. *Fleisher & Ludwig's Textbook of Pediatric Emergency Medicine.* 7th ed. Philadelphia: Lippincott Williams & Wilkins; 2016.

Subcommittee on Urinary Tract Infection and Steering Committee on Quality Improvement and Management Urinary Tract Infection. Clinical practice guideline for the diagnosis and management of the initial UTI in febrile infants and children 2 to 24 months. *Pediatrics.* 2011;128:595–610.

Vunda A, Vanderuin L, Gervaix A. Urethral prolapse: an overlooked diagnosis of urogenital bleeding in pre-menarchal girls. *J Pediatrics.* 2011;158:682–683.

CHAPTER 22

VAGINAL COMPLAINTS

Atsuko Koyama, MD, MPH, Kathryn S. Brigham, MD

1. **What is the best position to perform a genital exam on a prepubertal female?**
   Girls approximately 2 years and older are best examined in the supine frog-leg (Fig. 22.1) or prone knee-chest position (Fig. 22.2). The patient may be more comfortable lying with her parent (if in supine frog-leg position) and/or keeping her underwear on (can be pulled to the side) during the exam. It is important to explain the procedure prior to examination and allow the girl to stop the exam at any time. Some children may need an exam under sedation.

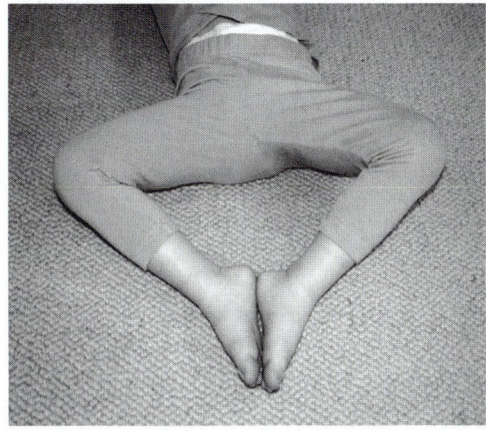

Fig. 22.1. Supine frog-leg position

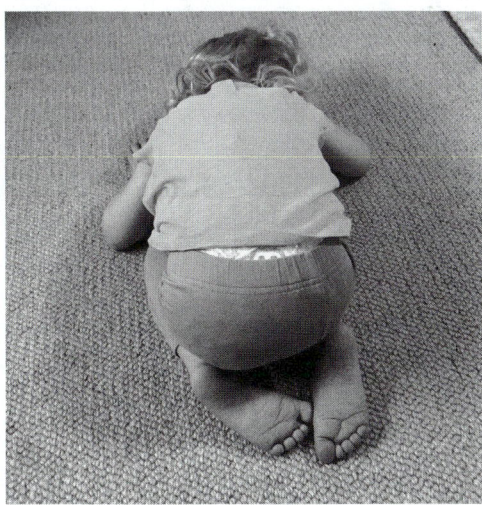

Fig. 22.2. Prone knee-chest position.

Table 22.1. Signs and Symptoms of Vaginitis

	SYMPTOMS/SIGNS	TESTING	TREATMENT	SPECIAL CONSIDERATIONS
Streptococcus pyogenes	Vulvovaginal irritation, discomfort, erythema. Vaginal bleeding and/or discharge. Associated with pharyngitis and/or scarlet fever. Most common in 3–10 years of age.	Vaginal culture; rapid strep of pharynx if signs of pharyngitis. Consider testing for gonorrhea if purulent vaginal discharge without sore throat.	Penicillin, first-generation cephalosporin, clindamycin (PCN allergic) for 10 days or azithromycin x 5 days.	Consider rapid strep of vaginal sample. Labs may refuse to process rapid strep testing from nonpharyngeal specimens as it is not within manufacturer's guidelines.
Haemophilus influenzae, Staphylococcus aureus, Moraxella catarrhalis	Vulvovaginal irritation, discomfort, erythema. Vaginal bleeding and/or discharge.	None	Generally resolves with conservative treatment.	
Shigella	Vaginal discharge, sometimes bloody. Inflamed vulvar mucosa, ulcers. Can have associated diarrhea.	Vaginal culture. Consider rectal culture.	Trimethoprim/sulfamethoxazole bid x 5 days	
Candida	Vulvar erythema, edema, and pruritus. External dysuria from urine in contact with inflamed vulva. Vaginal discharge.	Fungal culture if persistent despite past treatment.	Antifungal cream: clotrimazole 1% or miconazole 2% one applicatorful daily x 7 days; clotrimazole 2% or miconazole 4% one applicatorful daily x 3 days; tioconazole 6.5% or butoconazole 2% one applicatorful x 1 dose; fluconazole 150 mg tab po once	Most common cause of vaginitis in pubertal girls. Rare in prepubertal girls, especially without recent antibiotic use, immunocompromised state, or diaper use.
Neisseria gonorrhoeae, Chlamydia trachomatis, Trichomonas vaginalis	Can be asymptomatic or present with persistent purulent vaginal discharge	Consider NAAT or culture testing. Consult or refer to child abuse specialist, as type of testing accepted for forensic evidence differs by state.	Ceftriaxone or cefotaxime	If outside of newborn period, suspicious for sexual abuse.

Wolff M, et al: Gynecology Emergencies. In Shaw KN, Bachur RG, editors: *Fleisher & Ludwig's Textbook of Pediatric Emergency Medicine*, ed 7, Philadelphia, 2015, Wolters Kluwer, pp 787-789.

2. **How should you approach vaginitis in prepubertal girls?**

   The most common signs and symptoms of vaginitis include vulvar erythema, vulvar edema, vaginal bleeding, vaginal discharge, pruritus, vaginal irritation, and/or dysuria (Table 22.1).

3. **What should discharge instructions be for outpatient management of nonspecific vaginitis?**

   If there is no identifiable treatable cause for vaginitis AND symptoms are acute onset and mild without vaginal bleeding or discharge, consider conservative management. Recommend wearing loose-fitting clothing and cotton underwear, limiting soap to genital area and bubble baths, avoiding long periods in wet swimwear, wiping front to back, soaking in sitz bath or voiding in bathtub for dysuria, and applying cool compresses for vulvar/vaginal pain/swelling. If the patient has progressively worsening symptoms or develops purulent discharge, obtain culture and consider appropriate medications.

4. **How do you evaluate prepubertal girls for vaginal foreign bodies?**

   The knee-chest position for children over 2 years of age generally allows clinicians to visualize the vagina and cervix. Vaginal irrigation using a Foley catheter with a syringe filled with normal saline after a topical anesthetic can be performed if direct visualization and removal with a Calgi swab fails. Rarely, examination under sedation and/or pelvic ultrasound is required.

5. **How do you distinguish between labial adhesions and lichen sclerosis? How are they treated?**

   Labial adhesions are much more common than lichen sclerosis, but both may cause vaginal irritation and bleeding. **Labial adhesions** present in infancy and in early childhood, likely due to the lack of estrogen, and usually resolve with estrogenization at puberty. They are thin, semitranslucent adhesions between the posterior labia minora and can progress anteriorly, occasionally leaving only a pinpoint opening. In asymptomatic patients, conservative management with a bland ointment, such as A and D ointment, and observation is appropriate. First-line therapy for symptomatic and/or large labial adhesions is estrogen cream applied twice daily to the point of fusion; if no improvement with 2–3 weeks of therapy, low-dose steroid creams can be trialed. Manual separation is only considered if rapid in onset, accompanied by severe symptoms such as urinary retention/obstruction, or in cases where medical management has failed. Classic skin findings of **lichen sclerosis** include a symmetric hourglass pattern of the vulvar and perianal area with atrophic white plaques. First-line therapy is high-dose topical steroids; if that fails, topical calcineurin inhibitors are a second-line therapy.

6. **What is the differential diagnosis for urethral prolapse?**

   Urethral prolapse presents as a friable, annular mass anterior and separate from the vaginal introitus and can present with bleeding or dysuria. It is unlikely to regress on its own. The peak age of presentation is 5–8 years of age. A urine catheterization can be performed to confirm that the mass is part of the urethra and connected to the bladder. If not necrotic, it usually improves with estrogen cream and sitz baths. Masses that are less annular and more "grapelike" are concerning for sarcoma botryoides. A pelvic ultrasound to assess for pelvic masses and a tissue biopsy would be indicated. If the mass were adjacent to the urethra, white, and found in a neonate, it would be more consistent with a paraurethral cyst. In these cases, a renal ultrasound evaluating for renal pathology would be warranted to evaluate for other anomalies such as urethral diverticula and ectopic ureteroceles.

7. **What is the best management of perineal trauma?**

   Superficial lacerations in the perineal area that are not bleeding can be treated conservatively with only symptomatic care, such as ice packs and nonsteroidal antiinflammatory drugs (NSAIDs) for small hematomas. Sitz baths can provide pain relief, and voiding in the bathtub or shower can be helpful for dysuria. Significant/active bleeding, and complicated lacerations involving the anus, urethra, vagina, cervix, and/or large hematomas will likely need further examination under sedation and management/repair by a surgical specialist. An indwelling urinary catheter should be inserted if there is concern for enlarging hematomas, placing the patient at risk for urinary obstruction and distortion of genital anatomy.

8. **How do you diagnose and manage Bartholin gland abscesses?**

   Bartholin glands secrete mucus and are found in the posterior labia majora at 4 and 8 o'clock. These glands can develop an abscess, presenting as a painful, fluctuant, and large labial mass.

They generally require incision and drainage and placement of a Word catheter to prevent recurrence. Marsupialization is also an option but requires an experienced clinician to perform. Antibiotics are necessary only if concomitant cellulitis, recurrent abscess, or culture positive for methicillin-resistant *Staphylococcal aureus* or for patients with high risk of complications.

9. What are the differential diagnoses for vaginal ulcers?

Diagnosis should be based on history of sexual activity, travel, systemic signs/symptoms, and similar past episodes. Lesions may be single versus multiple, painful versus painless, and with or without lymphadenopathy. Noninfectious causes include fixed drug reactions, Behçet syndrome, and trauma. Behçet syndrome is uncommon and typically affects young adults, but it can be seen in children. The hallmark of Behçet is the recurrent and usually painful intraoral, urogenital, and cutaneous ulcers, but it has many systemic manifestations. Infectious causes include sexually transmitted infections and, rarely, non–sexually transmitted infections such as acute genital ulcerations (Lipschütz ulcer). Herpes and chancroid cause painful ulcers; syphilis, lymphogranuloma venereum, and granuloma inguinale are generally painless. Lipschütz ulcers may be due to primary Epstein-Barr virus (EBV) infection and are painful, usually <1 cm, and appear as deep ulcers with a necrotic base on the labia minora. The average age of presentation is 12–15 years.

10. Which infections are most concerning for sexual abuse?

Cases of gonorrhea, chlamydia, syphilis, trichomonas, anogenital human papillomavirus (HPV), genital herpes, and nontransfusion-acquired human immunodeficiency virus (HIV) in children make sexual abuse/assault likely but not definite. In the neonatal period, there may be cases of vertical transmission for these infections.

11. When should you be concerned about commercial sexual exploitation (CSE)?

Most children enter into CSE at approximately 12–16 years of age. Risk factors include a history of running away from home, truancy, child maltreatment, involvement with child protective services or the juvenile justice system, multiple sexually transmitted infections (STIs), and/or repeat pregnancies. Specific questions targeting this include: "Has anyone ever asked you to have sex in exchange for something you needed or wanted (money, food, shelter, or other items)?" "Has anyone ever asked you to have sex with another person?" "Has anyone ever taken sexual pictures of you or posted such pictures on the internet?" Familiarize yourself with local resources and your closest child protection services team. National Human Trafficking Resource Center Hotline is 1-888-373-7888.

12. What are the signs of pelvic inflammatory disease (PID)?

The minimum requirement for the diagnosis of PID is pelvic or lower abdominal pain and either (1) uterine tenderness, (2) cervical motion tenderness, or (3) adnexal tenderness. Other signs and symptoms are quite variable. There should be a low threshold for treating empirically given complications of untreated PID include increased rates of ectopic pregnancy, chronic pelvic pain, and infertility. Outpatient treatment is ceftriaxone (250 mg intramuscular once) and doxycycline (100 mg twice a day for 14 days). Metronidazole (500 mg twice a day for 14 days) should be added if anaerobic organisms are high on the differential. Alternative regimens are available at http://www.cdc.gov/std/tg2015/pid.htm. Close follow-up within 72 hours to ensure improvement of symptoms is required; if the patient fails to improve within that time period, additional parenteral treatment is indicated.

13. Which STIs should I test for?

HPV, chlamydia, trichomoniasis, herpes simplex virus (HSV), and gonorrhea are the top five most common STIs among sexually active adolescents. Highly sensitive nucleic acid amplification tests (NAAT) for chlamydia, gonorrhea, and trichomoniasis should be sent using self-collected vaginal swabs (most sensitive), urine, or cervical swabs for sexually active patients with vaginal discharge, dysuria, genital pain, lower abdominal pain, or symptoms of PID. In some cases (sexual assault evaluation, failed treatment), cultures requiring special medium may be indicated. Polymerase chain reaction (PCR) testing for HSV should also be sent if vaginal ulcers are present. Empiric treatment for gonorrhea, chlamydia, trichomoniasis, and HSV are indicated if the history and physical exam findings are consistent with these infections. Nontreponemal serologic testing for rapid plasma reagin (RPR), Venereal Disease Research Laboratories (VDRL), or toluidine red unheated serum test (TEST) can be used to screen for syphilis with treponemal tests for confirmation in patients who have signs/symptoms concerning for syphilis: diffuse maculopapular rash on trunk, extremities, or palms and soles or a painless genital ulcer. HPV testing is only performed as part of cervical cancer screening.

14. **What are important considerations when evaluating a female for sexual assault?**
    - Pubertal state and biological sex: STI testing varies based on pubertal status and biological sex, including specimen source (urine vs. anatomic sites) and type of test (NAAT vs. culture).
    - Time since incident: Evidence collection and postexposure prophylaxis, empiric STI testing, and emergency contraception all depend on time since incident. Consider referring to providers with specialized training in sexual abuse/assault evaluation if no emergent needs.
    - Availability of a trained sexual assault nurse examiner (SANE) for evidence collection
    - Safety concerns: Involve child protection team (if available), police, social work. Consider if other children are at risk in the home.
    - STI testing: serum and genital/rectal/oral specimen collection
    - Medications: postexposure HIV prophylaxis, hepatitis B vaccination and/or immunoglobulin, emergency contraception, gonorrhea/chlamydia/trichomoniasis treatment, antinausea medication

15. **A 17-year-old female requests emergency contraception. What are her options?**
    Emergency contraception (EC) is most effective within 72 hours after unprotected sex but can be administered up to 120 hours after unprotected sex. The copper intrauterine device (Cu-IUD) is the *most* effective form of emergency contraception; however, it is off-label as EC in the United States. The Cu-IUD also provides up to 10 years of contraception and does not wane in efficacy from 72 to 120 hours or with increased body mass index (BMI). Ulipristal acetate (UPA), a progesterone receptor modulator, and levonorgestrel (LNG), a progestin-only, are pills that prevent or delay ovulation and are more easily accessible as forms of EC. UPA is more effective in women with BMIs over 30 and for women who are over 72 hours after unprotected sex when compared to LNG; both should be given as a one-time dose as soon as possible after unprotected sex. The dose for LNG is 1.5 mg and UPA is 30 mg.

16. **What is on the differential diagnosis for abnormal uterine bleeding?**
    Anovulatory cycles are the most common cause of abnormal uterine bleeding (AUB) in adolescents. For sexually active girls, STIs are also a common cause. Girls with bleeding disorders such as von Willebrand disease, platelet dysfunction, and thrombocytopenia can present at initiation of menses with menorrhagia. Testing for von Willebrand should be considered prior to administration of hormonal contraception as estrogen increases von Willebrand levels, leading to false-negative results. Polycystic ovarian syndrome (PCOS) and changes in the hypothalamic-pituitary axis can also lead to AUB. Testosterone, follicle-stimulating hormone (FSH), and luteinizing hormone (LH) can be ordered, especially if hormonal contraception will be started to control bleeding, as these medications affect these tests. Thyroid dysfunction should be screened for with a thyroid-stimulating hormone (TSH). Prolactin levels with or without brain computerized tomography (CT) should be considered in patients with AUB and neurologic findings, galactorrhea, or vision deficits to evaluate for a prolactinoma. 17-hydroxyprogesterone can be sent for rare cases of late-onset congenital adrenal hyperplasia (CAH).

17. **A 14-year-old girl presents with 14 days of heavy vaginal bleeding, 2 days of dizziness, and an episode of syncope. Pregnancy test is negative. How do you decide between inpatient and outpatient management?**
    The workup for mild AUB can be pending and/or deferred to a primary care provider, but for patients with moderate to severe AUB, inpatient management should be considered. A compete blood count (CBC) and reticulocyte count should be obtained to evaluate degree of anemia and necessity of hormonal and iron therapy along with assessment of hemodynamic status.

    Mild: hemoglobin (Hgb) >12 mg/dL
    Moderate: Hgb 10–12 mg/dL
    Severe: Hgb <10 mg/dL

    Patients with tachycardia, headaches, dizziness, syncopal episodes, and moderate to severe anemia should be considered for inpatient management. Unless estrogen is contraindicated, treatment should include monophasic combined oral contraceptive pills (OCPs). Exogenous estrogen promotes endometrial proliferation and heals bleeding sites, and the progestin stabilizes the uterine lining. Specific medication and dosing schedules vary, but recommendations are generally for monophasic combined OCPs, one tab one to four times a day until bleeding stops, and then tapered down to either typical use of daily OCPs or continuous cycling of daily OCPs, depending on degree of anemia, bleeding, and symptoms. Antinausea medications are generally indicated given the high doses of estrogen. If estrogen is contraindicated, progestin-only pills can be used, though generally less effective. IV estrogen is only considered in patients with severe acute hemorrhage who are unable to tolerate oral medications, are unstable, and are critically ill. Iron should also be given to all patients.

18. **When should primary amenorrhea (absence of menses prior to 15 years of age in a girl with normal breast and pubic/axillary hair development) be further evaluated urgently?**
Once pregnancy is ruled out, other causes of primary amenorrhea can generally be evaluated by a primary care provider. Other diagnoses to consider are disorders of the hypothalamic-pituitary-ovarian axis, eating disorders/female athlete triad, thyroid disorders, primary ovarian insufficiency, hyperprolactinemia, PCOS, and anatomic abnormalities (imperforate hymen, hematocolpos, Müllerian agenesis). A thorough history and physical exam should enable directed evaluation.

19. **What is the first-line treatment for primary dysmenorrhea?**
Primary dysmenorrhea is thought to be prostaglandin mediated, making NSAIDs first-line treatment. Evidence is lacking to support the use of any one particular NSAID. If NSAIDs are not sufficient, combined hormonal contraceptives should be considered, which can also be given in a continuous manner to prevent the patient from having any withdrawal bleeds. If dysmenorrhea continues despite these interventions, a gynecologic consult would be appropriate.

20. **Your 17-year-old patient had an intrauterine device (IUD) placed 2 weeks prior and now presents with moderate to severe lower abdominal pain that started after IUD insertion. She reports no fever, vomiting, diarrhea, constipation, back pain, or UTI symptoms. How should you approach her evaluation?**
Rule out ectopic pregnancy. If the patient is pregnant, refer to obstetrics for possible removal of the IUD. Send urinalysis and STI testing. Treat empirically for STIs and/or UTIs as indicated. In cases of PID, females should be treated without removal. Regardless of results of STI tests, evaluate IUD location by ultrasound. The proper location of the copper IUDs is at the fundus; progestin-releasing IUDs can be anywhere within the uterus. Consider immediate removal if not in proper location, at the lower uterine segment, or in the cervix. Discharge with contraception, if so desired. If the IUD is not located in the uterine cavity, consider abdominal radiography to evaluate for IUD migration or uterine perforation. If IUD is intraperitoneal or imbedded in myometrium, refer to obstetrics.

21. **What are important considerations in genital exams for transgender patients?**
Only examine relevant anatomy. Use general terms for anatomy (genital vs. vaginal or penile) and/or ask patients what terminology they prefer be used. Strongly consider patient self-collection of genital samples for patient comfort. Transgender females who have undergone vaginoplasty retain the prostate and have a blind ending pouch without a cervix or fornices. An anoscope is recommended if an exam is indicated. Testing and treatment for prostatitis should be considered. Transgender males may have vaginal atrophy from testosterone therapy, making lubricant important if a bimanual or speculum exam is indicated. Genital samples should have clear labeling as vaginal or cervical source if the patient sex is noted as male.

KEY POINTS

1. Most adolescents will have regular menstrual cycles within 2 years of their menarche.
2. Pregnancy should be ruled out regardless of the patient's sexual history or absence of menarche if other signs of puberty are present.
3. Hormonal contraceptive pills have a variety of indications other than just contraception, as they can be useful in treating abnormal uterine bleeding and dysmenorrhea.

BIBLIOGRAPHY

Adams JA, Kellogg ND, Farst KJ, et al. Updated guidelines for the medical assessment and care of children who may have been sexually abused. *J Pediatr Adolesc Gynecol*. 2016;29:81–87.

Cheng L, Che Y, et al. Interventions for emergency contraception. *Cochrane Database Syst Rev*. 2012;15(8):CD001324.

Chimienti SN, Felsenstein D. Approach to the patient with genital ulcers. <http://www.uptodate.com>.

Cleland K, Zhu H, et al. The efficacy of intrauterine devices for emergency contraception: a systematic review of 35 years of experience. *Hum Reprod*. 2012;27(7):1994–2000.

Deutsch MB, Wesp L, eds. Guidelines for the primary and gender-affirming care of transgender and gender nonbinary people. Center of Excellence for Transgender Health. <http://transhealth.ucsf.edu/trans?page=guidelines-physical-examination>.

Goyal MK, Scribano P, Molnar J, et al. Sexual assault: child and adolescent. In: Shaw KN, Bachur RG, eds. *Fleisher and Ludwig's Textbook of Pediatric Emergency Medicine.* 7th ed. Philadelphia: Wolters Kluwer; 2016:1460–1470.

Gray SH, et al. Abnormal vaginal bleeding in the adolescent. In: Emans SJ, Laufer MR, eds. *Emans, Laufer, Goldstein's Pediatric & Adolescent Gynecology.* 6th ed. Philadelphia: Wolters Kluwer; 2012:174–178.

Marjoribanks J, Ayeleke RO, Farquhar C, et al. Nonsteroidal anti-inflammatory drugs for dysmenorrhea. *Cochrane Database of Syst Rev.* 2015;7:CD001751.

Wolff M, et al. Gynecology emergencies. In: Shaw KN, Bachur RG, eds. *Fleisher & Ludwig's Textbook of Pediatric Emergency Medicine.* 7th ed. Philadelphia: Wolters Kluwer; 2015:787–789.

Workowski KA, Bolan GA. Sexually transmitted diseases treatment guidelines, 2015. *MMWR Recomm Rep.* 2015;64:1–137.

CHAPTER 23

SKIN RASHES AND INFECTIONS

Jennifer E. Sanders, MD, FAAP, Sylvia E. Garcia, MD, Michelle N. Vazquez, MD, Jennifer M. Bellis, MD, MPH

1. **True or False.** *Ixodes scapularis* **is the vector causing all cases of Lyme disease in the United States.**

   False. *Ixodes scapularis* is the vector transmitting *Borrelia burgdorferi*, the cause of Lyme disease, in the East, including New England and the eastern mid-Atlantic states as far south as Virginia (≥90% of all cases), as well as the upper midwest. *Ixodes pacificus* is the vector in the west. Most cases occur between April and October, but cases can occur year-round. In addition to outdoor activities, cases in urban areas and backyards have been reported. Most bites are from nymphs, which are small and hard to identify. The highest incidence of infection in the United States is in children between 5 and 9 years of age and adults 55–59 years of age. The incubation period from tick bite to appearance of erythema migrans (EM) ranges from 1 to 32 days.

2. **What are the clinical manifestations associated with the three stages of Lyme disease?**

   Early localized disease occurs within 3–30 days post exposure to a tick bite. The characteristic lesion is erythema migrans. Early disseminated disease can have multiple EM lesions, or no associated dermatologic findings. Other manifestations include cranial nerve palsies, especially of cranial nerve VII (Bell palsy), lymphocytic meningitis, polyradiculitis, ophthalmic changes, and nonspecific systemic symptoms. Carditis and heart block can occur but are less common in children. Late disease (months to years postexposure) is rare in previously treated patients. In children, this commonly presents as a pauciarticular arthritis affecting the large joints, especially the knees. Neurologic complications, including encephalitis, are rare.

3. **Is the rash of erythema migrans alone sufficient for initiating treatment of Lyme disease?**

   Yes. EM is the most common clinical manifestation of early localized Lyme disease, and the most common manifestation in children. Appearing 7–14 days after tick detachment, and initially as a painless red macule or papule, it expands into a nonpruritic erythematous annular lesion, occasionally with central clearing and a diameter ≥5 cm (Fig. 23.1). The center may appear necrotic or vesicular. It may be confused with hypersensitivity reactions, which occur while the tick is attached or within 48 hours of detachment, are ≤5 cm in diameter, and disappear in 1–2 days. Associated symptoms may be present, including fever, headache, myalgias, and arthralgias. Treatment prevents progression to the early disseminated and late stages of Lyme disease.

4. **What is southern tick-associated rash illness?**

   Southern tick-associated rash illness (STARI), associated with an EM-like rash and nonspecific symptoms, has been reported in the south central and southeastern United States. The bite of the tick *Amblyomma americanum* is the cause but does not transmit *B. burgdorferi*. This illness has not been associated with any of the disseminated complications of Lyme disease. Its etiology and treatment are unknown. When evaluating a patient with an EM rash for Lyme disease, consideration must be given to whether the patient was in an endemic area.

5. **What diagnostic serologic testing is available for Lyme disease?**

   Recognition of Lyme disease rests primarily on recognition of clinical illness in patients who have been in an endemic area; testing for nonspecific symptoms is discouraged. Early localized disease is rarely seropositive. Standard testing is done by two-tiered assay: a sensitive, but not specific, enzyme-linked immunosorbent assay (ELISA or EIA) or immunofluorescent antibody (IFA), and the Western immunoblot. Positive or equivocal results for ELISA, EIA, or IFA necessitate further testing with the Western immunoblot, as false-positive results can occur from cross-reactivity with spirochetal, viral, and autoimmune diseases. The presence of two IgM bands or five IgG bands on the Western immunoblot is a positive result.

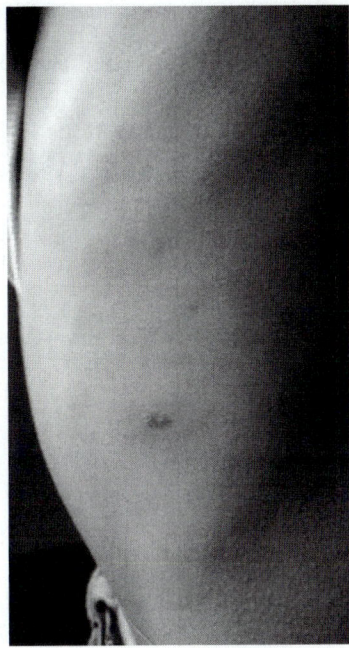

Fig. 23.1. Erythema Migrans. Erythematous annular lesions with central clearing. *(Image courtesy of Sylvia E. Garcia, MD.)*

6. **What is the first-line antibiotic therapy for erythema migrans in pediatric patients with early localized disease?**
First-line therapy for the treatment of EM in pediatric patients is amoxicillin, or cefuroxime axetil in those with a penicillin allergy. Doxycycline is recommended for adults and children over 8 years of age but should be avoided in pregnant or lactating patients. Macrolides are not recommended as first-line therapy but may be used if the patient is unable to take the approved drug regimens. Coinfection with other tickborne illnesses should be considered in patients who present with severe initial symptoms; have high fever for more than 48 hours despite an appropriate medication regimen; have unexplained leukopenia, anemia, or thrombocytopenia; or who show no improvement or worsening symptoms.

7. **True or False. Successful tick removal involves complete removal of the mouthparts.**
True. Ticks should be promptly removed in order to decrease the transmission of disease. Removal should be attempted with the use of fine-tipped tweezers, grasping the tick where the mouth parts attach to the skin. Hands should be protected by tissue or gloves. Steady outward pressure should be applied, with care not to twist, crush, or squeeze the tick body. If the mouthparts become detached and stay embedded in the skin and cannot be easily removed, only topical disinfection is required. Attempted removal of embedded mouthparts can cause local tissue damage and have no effect on the risk of contracting Lyme disease. Cleaning the area, hands, and instruments with rubbing alcohol, iodine scrub, or soap and water is recommended.

8. **Can tick bites be prevented?**
In addition to avoiding tick-infested areas, use of protective clothing, and close inspection for ticks on both humans and pets, tick and insect repellants are recommended for pediatric use. Permethrin-treated clothing is approved for all ages and for pregnant women; it may also be sprayed on clothes but not directly on skin. DEET is approved for use in children over 2 months of age and in formulations containing no more than a 30% concentration. It should not be sprayed on objects that young children might chew or suck. Neurologic complications are rare. Picaridin, the plant-based oil of eucalyptus, provides protection similar to DEET and can be used in patients ages 3 years and older.

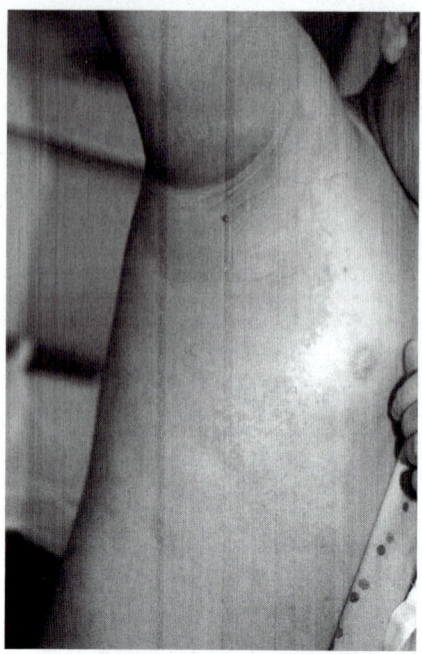

Fig. 23.2. Erysipelas. Erythematous and indurated skin with well-demarcated borders. *(Image courtesy of Sylvia E. Garcia, MD.)*

9. **Should chemoprophylaxis be provided to patients after sustaining a tick bite?**
Because the risk of contracting Lyme disease after tick bite is ≤3% in highly endemic areas, routine use of chemoprophylaxis or serologic testing is not recommended. The risk increases after engorgement, especially if attachment is beyond 36 hours. A single dose of doxycycline in older children and adults may be used if all the following requirements are met: the tick has been attached for more than 36 hours and can be identified as *I. scapularis*, prophylaxis can be started within 72 hours of tick removal, local rate of infection is ≥20%, and the use of doxycycline is not contraindicated. Amoxicillin prophylaxis has not been well studied. Prophylaxis in children less than 8 years of age is not recommended. Children should only receive therapy if symptoms develop.

10. **Is follow-up necessary after tick removal and/or administration of antibiotic prophylaxis?**
Yes. Close monitoring for signs or symptoms of Lyme disease for up to 30 days is recommended. Medical attention should be sought if a skin lesion or viral-like illness occurs within 1 month of tick removal.

11. **What is erysipelas?**
Erysipelas is a skin infection involving the upper dermis and surrounding lymphatics. The affected skin is erythematous and indurated with well-demarcated raised borders and is tender to palpation (Fig. 23.2). The skin may have a peau d'orange, or orange peel, appearance. The most common sites affected are the lower extremities, with athlete's foot a common preceding condition.

12. **Which bacterial organism is the causative agent?**
Streptococci group A (GAS) causes the majority of the infections, though groups B, C, F, or G can also cause infection. Infection with *Staphylococcus aureus* is rare.

13. **Are blood cultures recommended?**
Blood cultures, cutaneous aspirates, and biopsies are not recommended, unless the patient is immunocompromised, has a malignancy or severe systemic illness, or has sustained an immersion injury or animal bite.

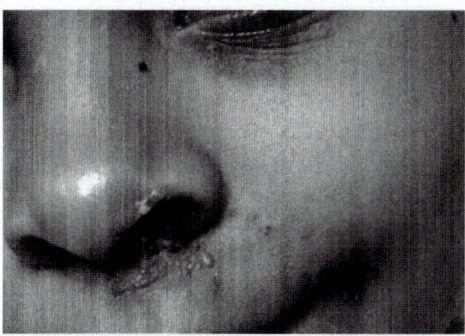

Fig. 23.3. Nonbullous Impetigo. Vesicles and pustules with overlying honey-colored crust. *(Image courtesy of Sylvia E. Garcia, MD.)*

14. What is the antibiotic treatment of choice?
The treatment of choice is penicillin. Alternatives include cephalosporins or clindamycin. The affected limb should be elevated and pain control provided.

15. What is the most common cause of the pictured skin lesion (Fig. 23.3)?
The pictured lesion (Fig. 23.3) is impetigo. The nonbullous type is primarily caused by *S. aureus* and *Streptococcus pyogenes*. *S. aureus* accounts for roughly 80% of cases, GAS 10%, and other bacteria 10%. The bullous type is caused by *S. aureus*. Impetigo is highly contagious and is the most common bacterial skin infection in children.

16. How does impetigo usually present clinically?
It is most common in ages 2–5 years. Nonbullous impetigo begins as erythematous papules, which evolve into vesicles and pustules. These vesicles and pustules rupture to produce a "honey crust" on an erythematous base, primarily on the face or areas of irritation. Bullous-type impetigo is most commonly seen in neonates and infants. Lesions usually occur on intact skin in the intertriginous areas, though they can be seen anywhere on the body. The bullae are small (<3 cm), thin-walled, flaccid lesions containing a clear-to-yellowish fluid (Fig. 23.4). The lesions tend to rupture easily within 1–3 days, leaving behind a collarette scale on an erythematous base or multiple concentric rings, resembling onion slices.

17. How is impetigo diagnosed?
Diagnosis can be made on clinical presentation. Honey-colored crusting should raise clinical suspicion for impetigo. Superficial wound cultures may be helpful to identify the causative organism but should not delay treatment.

18. What is the initial treatment of impetigo?
Impetigo lesions will usually resolve on their own; however, treatment is recommended to decrease transmission, improve cosmetic appearance, and relieve discomfort. Topical treatment with mupirocin is the preferred method for patients with limited disease for both bullous and nonbullous impetigo. Patients with more extensive disease or who are immunocompromised should also be treated with oral antibiotics. Dicloxacillin and cephalexin are first-line antibiotics, unless methicillin-resistant *S. aureus* (MRSA) is suspected or confirmed, in which case clindamycin or trimethoprim-sulfamethoxazole is recommended.

19. How do the skin lesions in tinea corporis (body) or tinea pedis (foot) present?
Tinea corporis, more commonly known as "ringworm," lesions usually begin as pruritic, round (ovoid or circular), erythematous, scaling patches. These lesions spread centrifugally with central clearing and a raised scaling border. There may be clusters of lesions that coalesce. Pustules may be present around the edge of the lesion. Tinea pedis, commonly called athlete's foot, can present in several ways. Interdigital lesions cause pruritic erythematous erosions or scaling in between the toes; hyperkeratotic lesions present with diffuse hyperkeratotic lesions on soles, medial, and lateral surfaces of the foot. There may be vesicular or bullous lesions as well.

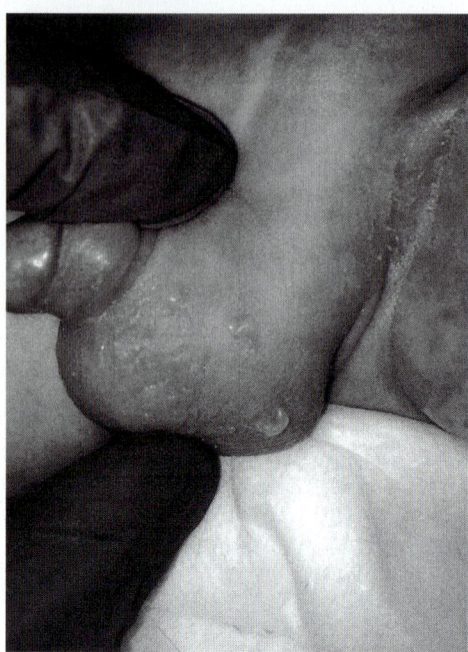

Fig. 23.4. Bullous Impetigo. Thin-walled flaccid bullae filled with yellow fluid. *(Image courtesy of Jennifer E. Sanders, MD.)*

20. What are the differences between the skin lesions with tinea versicolor compared to tinea corporis?

Tinea versicolor is caused by yeast in the Malassezia family. Tinea versicolor lesions are macules, patches, or plaques that can be hyperpigmented or hypopigmented. There may also be a fine scale over the lesions. Multiple clustered lesions are usually seen on the trunk. Tinea versicolor are often asymptomatic or only mildly pruritic. Tinea corporis tends to have central clearing with raised borders and are usually pruritic.

21. Describe the various scalp lesions seen in tinea capitis.

Tinea capitis can present with scaling scalp lesions with overlying alopecia that enlarge centrifugally over time. Alopecia with black dots may also be seen without scaling lesions. The black dots represent distal ends of the hair follicles that have broken off. Patients may also present with diffuse scaling with minimal hair loss. Finally, some patients may develop a kerion due to an intense inflammatory response. A kerion is a thick, boggy plaque with pustules, crusting, and/or drainage.

22. How are tinea infections diagnosed?

Classic lesions do not require confirmatory diagnosis, but a skin scraping can be useful when the diagnosis is uncertain. Scrapings of skin lesions are treated with potassium hydroxide (KOH) on a slide and examined under a microscope. Positive scrapings will demonstrate segmented hyphae. Fungal cultures can be sent as well; however, these cultures usually take 2–8 weeks to obtain results, limiting their utility in clinical practice.

23. What is the difference in treatment for tinea corporis/pedis, tinea versicolor, and tinea capitis?

First-line treatment for tinea corporis and tinea pedis infections is topical antifungals, such as azoles, allylamines, butenafine, ciclopirox, and tolnaftate. Treatment for tinea versicolor includes selenium sulfide as first-line treatment in addition to topical antifungals. Treatment is usually required for 1–3 weeks to see improvement. For tinea capitis or onychomycosis (fungal infection of the nail), first-line treatment is with oral medication. Tinea capitis is treated with oral griseofulvin or terbinafine, and oral terbinafine or itraconazole for onychomycosis. Oral treatment is also indicated for patients with extensive skin involvement or who fail topical treatment.

24. **Describe the appearance of an urticarial lesion.**
Urticarial lesions are raised, circumscribed, erythematous plaques. Lesions are usually intensely pruritic, often with central pallor. The plaques may develop over minutes to hours. Urticarial lesions do not typically leave residual markings.

25. **What is the pathophysiology of urticarial lesion development?**
Urticarial lesions develop from the degranulation of mast cells, causing the release of histamine, in the superficial dermis due to some triggering factor.

26. **What are the most common causes of urticaria in children?**
    - Infections: viral, bacterial, and parasitic
    - Allergic reaction to food, medication, and insect stings/bites
    - Medications causing direct, non-IgE-mediated mast cell activation (such as narcotics, muscle relaxants, vancomycin, and contrast media)
    - Nonsteroidal antiinflammatory drugs (NSAIDs), due to abnormality in arachidonic acid metabolism
    - Less common: serum sickness, physical stimuli, or hormone-associated disorders

27. **How is acute urticaria treated?**
Almost two thirds of cases of acute urticaria are self-limited. Treatment focuses on identifying the underlying cause and relieving symptoms of pruritus and associated angioedema. First-line treatment is with H_1 blockers, with second-generation antihistamines preferred over first-generation due to increased sedation and anticholinergic effects seen with first-generation antihistamines. Short courses of steroids can be used in addition to antihistamines for severe or refractory cases.

28. **What causes the dermatitis of poison ivy, poison oak, and poison sumac?**
Poison ivy, poison oak, and poison sumac are plants that belong to the plant genus *Toxicodendron*. All plants within this genus contain the allergenic compound urushiol, which causes the plant-associated contact dermatitis.

29. **Who is at risk for a reaction from an exposure to poison ivy, poison oak, or poison sumac?**
Different *Toxicodendron* plants can be found throughout the United States, and 50% of people exposed to plants of the *Toxicodendron* genus will have a cutaneous reaction despite their ethnicity or skin type.

30. **What does a contact dermatitis rash post-*Toxicodendron* plant exposure look like?**
The rash is extremely pruritic and will appear as plaques, papules, vesicles, and/or bullae in a streak-like or linear pattern on the area of the skin exposed to the plant. If contact dermatitis is found on the face or genitals, significant edema may be present.

31. **Is the *Toxicodendron* contact dermatitis contagious?**
No, postexposure the rash will erupt in different parts of the body at different time intervals. Therefore, it is not a contagious dermatitis.

32. **What are the treatment options for *Toxicodendron* contact dermatitis?**
Patients only require symptomatic treatment with topical corticosteroids, cold compresses, and calamine lotion. Severe dermatitis may benefit from a 2-week tapering course of oral corticosteroids such as prednisone.

33. **Which virus causes cutaneous warts?**
Cutaneous warts are caused by human papillomavirus (HPV) infecting the epithelial tissues and mucous membranes of the host.

34. **Which age groups within the pediatric population primarily are affected by cutaneous warts?**
The school-age and adolescent populations are mainly affected by cutaneous warts. It is estimated that 10%–20% of children will have a cutaneous wart at some point in their childhood.

35. **What are the common appearances of common cutaneous warts?**
Verrucae vulgaris, also known as common warts, are rough, hard, raised, dome-shaped lesions commonly found on the hands and usually asymptomatic.
        Plantar warts, or verrucae plantaris, affect the soles of the feet, and secondary to their location are usually symptomatic.
        Flat or juvenile warts are smooth, flesh-colored papules usually on the face and neck that vary in size and are more common in young children than in adolescents.

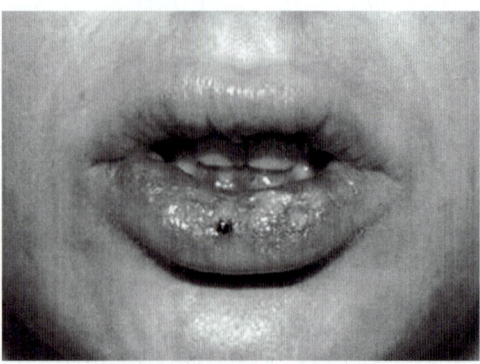

Fig. 23.5. Herpetic Gingivostomatitis. Shallow ulcerations with overlying crusting noted on the lip. *(Image courtesy of Ee T. Tay, MD.)*

36. Without therapeutic intervention, can a wart regress?

About two thirds of cutaneous warts will disappear without therapeutic intervention. Usually it can take up to 2 years for a wart to self-resolve.

37. What are some prescription methods for wart removal?

Topical salicylic acid has been found to be slightly more effective than a placebo and may be a gentler prescriptive treatment option. Higher concentrations of topical salicylic acid have been found effective in plantar wart treatment. Despite concentration, parents should be warned this treatment will cause burning and irritation to local unaffected skin. Treatment courses vary between 2 and 12 weeks, until the warts are completely gone.

Cryotherapy with liquid nitrogen is a more aggressive treatment option and, according to dermatologists, is the gold standard for wart removal. This treatment is used primarily in older children and adolescents secondary to pain and blistering associated with treatment. Healing and resolution will usually occur after one treatment session and 7 days following cryotherapy.

38. How can I distinguish herpetic gingivostomatitis from herpangina?

Gingivostomatitis presents with ulcerations and grouped vesicles on the gums, hard palate, and tongue (Fig. 23.5). The vesicles rupture and become yellow with a surrounding red halo. Over time the vesicles coalesce to form larger ulcers. The gingiva tends to be friable and bleeds easily. Herpangina, on the other hand, presents with well-circumscribed erosions and ulcerations on the tonsillar pillars and soft palate.

39. Should I treat herpetic gingivostomatitis?

Gingivostomatitis is painful, and patients should be provided pain medications such as NSAIDs. Magic mouthwash, which consists of diphenhydramine, Maalox with or without viscous lidocaine, may also help the patient's pain. Oral antivirals are not routinely recommended for treatment of herpetic gingivostomatitis.

40. How do I treat a first-time outbreak of genital herpes?

There are several treatment options for a primary outbreak of genital herpes:
- Acyclovir (400 mg po tid for 10 days)
- Valacyclovir (1 g po bid for 10 days)
- Famciclovir (250 mg po bid for 10 days)
  Sitz baths and topical anesthetics may also provide some relief.

41. When do I need to be worried about genital herpes?

Genital herpes in a non–sexually active child should raise suspicion for child abuse. A thorough history and physical should be performed, and a report should be made to child protective services if an alternative diagnosis or explanation cannot be uncovered.

In patients with genital herpes who are having urinary retention secondary to pain, hospitalization should be considered for a urinary catheter and intravenous (IV) pain medications.

42. How do I treat scabies?

Permethrin 5% cream applied from the neck to the soles of the feet and washed off 8–14 hours later is the treatment of choice for pediatric patients 2 months of age and older. Sulfur ointments have been used successfully in adults and children, including those younger than 2 months of age, but may cause skin irritation and have an unpleasant odor. Lindane 1% lotion is equally as effective, but lindane has higher rates of neurotoxicity and therefore should not be used in pediatric patients. Crotamiton lotion is FDA approved for use in adults but is not yet approved for children.

43. What is crusted scabies?

Crusted scabies, also known as Norwegian scabies, tends to occur only in immunocompromised patients. Crusted scabies may initially present with erythematous patches, but then a thick scaly crust appears that can also fissure. These fissures allow ports of entry for bacteria, which can lead to sepsis. Treatment with permethrin 5% cream and oral ivermectin is recommended.

44. What are the treatment options for contact dermatitis?

Contact dermatitis is typically treated with topical corticosteroids. Low to moderate potency steroids, such as hydrocortisone 1%–2%, triamcinolone 0.1%, and hydrocortisone valerate are usually potent enough to clear contact dermatitis. Patients may also benefit from antihistamines to help control itching.

45. What about a rash can help me distinguish contact dermatitis from other causes of dermatitis?

Contact dermatitis is broadly divided into two main categories: irritant and allergic. Irritant contact dermatitis occurs immediately after exposure while allergic contact dermatitis causes a delayed inflammatory response. The skin tends to be erythematous and edematous, and fluid-filled vesicles may form. Contact dermatitis tends to be well demarcated and is often more itchy than painful, which helps to differentiate it from cellulitis.

46. How does pityriasis rosea present?

Pityriasis rosea often starts with a herald patch, which is an annular, sharply demarcated pink lesion that becomes scaly with some central clearing (Fig. 23.6). It usually occurs on the chest, back, or neck. Days or weeks later, lesions that appear similar to the herald patch occur on the trunk and proximal extremities. Classically, a "Christmas tree" pattern may be seen on the back.

47. How long does pityriasis rosea last?

The rash may last 2–3 months. Follow-up is unnecessary if the rash resolves during that time.

48. What can I do to treat pityriasis rosea?

Treatment of pityriasis generally involves supportive care with antihistamines to help control itching. Limited use of topical steroids may also be helpful for itching.

49. What are some mimickers of pityriasis rosea?

See Table 23.1.

50. What are the high yield tests in the diagnosis of cellulitis?

There are no definitive tests for the diagnosis of cellulitis. It is a clinical diagnosis. This infection involves the dermal and subcutaneous layers of the skin. The lesion will be warm, erythematous, and tender. Occasionally the lesion may be indurated and can be difficult to differentiate from an abscess. In these cases, point of care ultrasound may be used to locate a subcutaneous fluid collection consistent with an abscess. There is no need to obtain a complete blood count or blood culture for the diagnosis of cellulitis. A white count will not change the initial management of cellulitis. The rate of bacteremia in children with cellulitis is low and therefore a blood culture is not indicated in the evaluation of cellulitis.

51. What are the optimal antibiotic choices for the treatment of cellulitis?

Group A streptococcus is the bacteria that accounts for over 70% of cellulitis infections. With the emergence of MRSA, however, there is a growing concern for it to be the offending agent of skin infections. When deciding on antibiotics, a clinician should take into account if the patient has had a previous MRSA skin infection or if there is a family history of MRSA infections. If the patient has no previous personal or family history of MRSA infection, then treatment should focus on Group A streptococcus coverage with cephalexin for 7–10 days. If there is a concern for a possible MRSA cellulitis, then clindamycin or trimethoprim-sulfamethoxazole should be concomitantly given with cephalexin for 7–10 days.

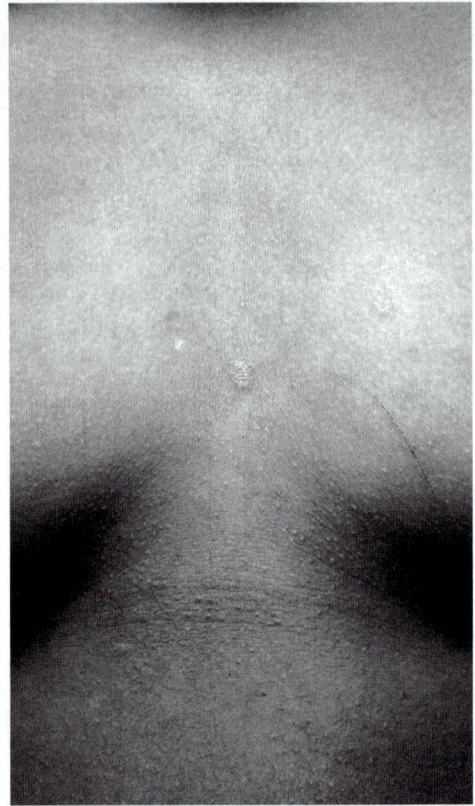

Fig. 23.6. Herald Patch in Pityriasis Rosea. A single annular pink patch noted on the chest with fine overlying scale. *(Image courtesy of Sylvia E. Garcia, MD.)*

Table 23.1. Mimickers of Pityriasis Rosea (PR)

CONDITION	HOW IT DIFFERS FROM PR
Secondary syphilis	Involves palms and soles
Guttate psoriasis	Thicker overlying scale
Nummular eczema	Involves the extremities more than the trunk
Tinea corporis	Usually a single lesion

52. Describe the clinical features of Kawasaki disease.

Kawasaki disease is a medium-size vasculitis. Typical Kawasaki can be diagnosed clinically as fever for 5 or more days plus four of the five signs: bilateral, nonexudative bulbar conjunctivitis; rash; erythema of the lips and oral mucosa; extremity changes; and cervical lymphadenopathy (often a single enlarged node). Extremity changes include erythema of palms and soles or swelling of the dorsum of the hands and feet. Desquamation of the fingers is a late finding. The rash in Kawasaki disease can be variable but often is maculopapular, morbilliform, scarlatiniform, or urticarial. Vesicular and bullous lesions are not usually associated with Kawasaki.

53. What workup and treatment are recommended for Kawasaki disease?

Typical Kawasaki can be diagnosed clinically. Laboratory testing can be useful in patients with incomplete or atypical Kawasaki disease. Lab findings include elevated C-reactive protein (CRP)/erythrocyte sedimentation rate (ESR), leukocytosis >15,000, thrombocytosis >450,000 after 1 week of illness, normocytic normochromic anemia for age, elevated alanine transaminase (ALT), low albumin (<3), and sterile pyuria. An echocardiogram is performed to evaluate for coronary artery dilation or ectasias, the most significant complication of Kawasaki disease. Patients with Kawasaki disease should be admitted and treated with intravenous immunoglobulin (IVIG) and high-dose aspirin (80–100 mg/kg/day divided into 4 doses). Treatment should be initiated within 10 days of the start of illness to decrease the risk of cardiac sequelae.

54. Is there any treatment for erythema multiforme?

Erythema multiforme is a self-limited process. Treatment consists of stopping any inciting agents, as well as pain control and anti-itch medications. Topical corticosteroids and oral diphenhydramine may be useful for itching.

55. Do all patients with Stevens-Johnson syndrome need to be admitted?

Patients with Stevens-Johnson syndrome (SJS) require intensive care and should be referred to the local emergency department or admitted to the hospital. Patients with SJS are managed similarly to burn patients with special attention to hydration, wound care, pain control, nutritional support, and monitoring for infections.

56. Are all children with fever and petechial rash seriously ill?

Not necessarily. In a study of 190 children with fever and petechial rash, 8% (15) had an invasive bacterial illness. Of that 8%, half had meningitis. The remainder of those patients had otitis media, Group A streptococcal infections, and likely viral syndrome. All of those children had petechiae below the nipple line and appeared ill on presentation.

57. Do all children with a petechial rash need labs drawn?

Petechiae should raise concerns to practitioners; however, the presence of petechiae does not always indicate serious illness. For example, children with forceful coughing or vomiting may present with petechiae on the face. In those children with diffuse or widespread petechiae, it is prudent to do some bloodwork, including complete blood count and coagulation factors to evaluate for idiopathic thrombocytopenic purpura, neoplastic disorders, hemolytic uremic syndrome, vasculitis syndrome, and autoimmune disorders.

58. I think my patient has measles, and he has a 6-month-old sibling. Do I need to provide prophylaxis for the sibling?

Yes. Infants under 12 months of age, pregnant women without evidence of immunity, and immunocompromised patients should receive immunoglobulin. For infants ages 6–12 months, the measles, mumps, rubella (MMR) vaccine can be given in place of immunoglobulin.

59. Do I need to treat my 6-year-old patient who has varicella?

Probably not. Varicella is a self-limited process in healthy children less than 12 years of age. Oral antiviral therapy with acyclovir, or its analogues, is recommended for immunocompetent children and adolescents who are at risk of complications from varicella. This includes unvaccinated adolescents, secondary cases in household contacts, patients with chronic disease, and those taking chronic steroids or salicylates. The dose of acyclovir is 20 mg/kg per dose four times daily for 5 days.

60. My 12-month-old patient had several days of high fever and now has a rash. Should I check labs?

Probably not. Roseola classically presents with 3–5 days of fever that abruptly resolves followed by the eruption of a blanching maculopapular rash that tends to start on the trunk and spread to the face and extremities. The rash is usually present for 1–2 days and then resolves. Complications of roseola include seizures, encephalitis, and aseptic meningitis. Children with complications, or those that are ill appearing would require laboratory evaluation.

KEY POINTS

1. The appearance of erythema migrans alone is sufficient to start antibiotic therapy in endemic areas, preventing progression of Lyme disease.
2. Blood cultures, cutaneous aspirates, and biopsies are not routinely recommended in immunocompetent patients with erysipelas or cellulitis.

3. Herpetic gingivostomatitis is self-limited and does not typically require oral antivirals.
4. Genital herpes in a child should raise suspicion for child abuse.
5. Petechiae below the nipple should raise concerns for serious bacterial infection in infants with fever.

BIBLIOGRAPHY

Albrecht M. Treatment of varicella (chickenpox) infection. <http://www.uptodate.com/>; 2016.

Bingham C. New-onset urticaria. <http://www.uptodate.com/>; 2015.

High WN, Roujeau JC: Stevens-Johnson syndrome and toxic epidermal necrolysis: management, prognosis and long-term sequelae. <http://www.uptodate.com/>; 2016.

Kimberlin DB, Jackson MA, Long SS. Group A streptococcal infections. *Red Book: 2015 Report of the Committee on Infectious Diseases* 2015; 732.

Kimberlin DW, Jackson MA, Long SS. Lyme disease (Lyme borreliosis, Borrelia burgdorfi infection). *Red Book: 2015 Report of the Committee on Infectious Diseases* 2015; 732.

Mistry RD. Skin and soft tissue infections. *Pediatr Clin North Am.* 2013;60(5):1063–1082.

Mukkada S, Buckingham SC. Recognition of and prompt treatment for tick-borne infections in children. *Infect Dis Clin North Am.* 2015;29(3):539–555.

Newburger JW, Takahashi M, Gerber MA, et al. Diagnosis, treatment, and long-term management of Kawasaki disease: a statement for health professionals from the Committee on Rheumatic Fever, Endocarditis, and Kawasaki Disease, Council on Cardiovascular Disease in the Young, American Heart Association. *Pediatrics.* 2004;114(6):1708–1733.

Sanders JE, Garcia SE. Pediatric herpes simplex virus infections: an evidence-based approach to treatment. *Pediatric Emergency Medicine Practice.* 2014;11(1):1–19, [quiz 19].

Wormser GP, Dattwyler RJ, Shapiro ED, et al. The clinical assessment, treatment, and prevention of Lyme disease, human granulocytic anaplasmosis, and babesiosis: clinical practice guidelines by the Infectious Diseases Society of America. *Clin Infect Dis.* 2006;43(9):1089–1134.

CHAPTER 24

COMMON NEWBORN COMPLAINTS

Nadine Aprahamian, MD, Toni Clare Hogencamp, MD

CENTRAL CYANOSIS VERSUS ACROCYANOSIS IN INFANTS

1. **What is the difference between central cyanosis and acrocyanosis?**

   Cyanosis is a common clinical finding in newborn infants. Central cyanosis is caused by reduced arterial oxygen saturation. Central cyanosis can be associated with life-threatening illnesses such as cardiac, metabolic, neurologic, infectious, and parenchymal and nonparenchymal pulmonary disorders. Normal infants have central cyanosis until up to 5 to 10 minutes after birth as the oxygen saturation rises to 85% to 95% by 10 minutes of age. Persistent cyanosis is always abnormal and should be evaluated and treated promptly. By contrast, acrocyanosis is seen in healthy newborns and it refers to the peripheral cyanosis around the mouth and the extremities including hands and feet. It is caused by benign vasomotor changes that cause peripheral vasoconstriction and increased tissue oxygen extraction. As opposed to in central cyanosis, in acrocyanosis the mucous membranes of the neonate remain pink. This may persist for 24 to 48 hours, and it is usually not pathologic.

2. **In a cyanotic newborn, how could pulmonary disease be distinguished from cyanotic congenital heart disease?**

   The hyperoxia test is used to differentiate cyanosis secondary to pulmonary versus congenital heart disease. The infant is placed in 100% oxygen, and arterial blood gases are obtained. Pco_2 >100 mm Hg is seen with primary lung disease, whereas with heart disease the PaO_2 is <100 mm Hg.

3. **Which congenital heart lesions present with cyanosis on day 1 of life?**
   - Transposition of great arteries with an intact ventricular septum
   - Tricuspid valve atresia
   - Pulmonary valve atresia with intact ventricular septum
   - Tetralogy of Fallot
   - Ebstein anomaly of the tricuspid valve
   - Total anomalous pulmonary venous return
   - Hypoplastic left heart syndrome
   - Truncus arteriosus

ORAL CANDIDIASIS

4. **How do newborns acquire oropharyngeal candidiasis?**

   Transmission of fungi from maternal vaginal candidal colonization is the primary means of infection in newborns. It can also be transmitted during breastfeeding. It affects up to 3% to 5% of healthy newborns. Median age of onset is reported to be 9 to 10 days of life. On examination, the thrush presents as white plaques with or without an erythematous base on the buccal or lingual mucosal surface of the mouth. Infants are usually asymptomatic; however, it may interfere with feeding due to discomfort. Mild punctate areas of bleeding confirm the diagnosis during scraping. Nystatin 100,000 U/mL as a dose of 0.5 mL to each side of the mouth given four times daily is the treatment of choice for oral candidiasis.

NEWBORN RASHES

A 4-week-old presents with rash limited to the cheeks and forehead. She is otherwise feeding and growing well. She is afebrile.

5. **Is there a difference between neonatal acne and infantile acne?**

Neonatal acne is a variant of acne vulgaris that presents at birth or in the first weeks of life (Fig. 24.1). This occurs in about 20% of newborns. It is due to androgenic hormones, both maternally derived and endogenous. The lesions resolve within 1 to 3 months as the androgenic levels drop. A small percentage of infants develop acne at about 3 to 6 months of age with a greater degree of inflammation. The infantile acne may persist for years, and the cause is unknown. Usually there is no evidence of precocious puberty or increased hormonal levels.

6. **How is cradle cap treated at home?**

Seborrheic dermatitis presents as a yellow scaly rash on the scalp and may involve the head, eyes, ears, eyebrows, nose, and back of head. Treatment is mineral oil followed by shampooing with a mild anti-dandruff shampoo containing selenium. If lesions are inflamed, a mild topical steroid may be applied.

7. **What are the differences between erythema toxicum neonatorum (ETN) and transient neonatal pustular melanosis?**

Erythema toxicum is noted in 31% to 72% of full-term infants. Etiology is not known. It presents as multiple erythematous macules and papules that rapidly progress to pustules on an erythematous base. On examination they are noted over the trunk and proximal extremities, sparing palms and soles. They may be present at birth but can be seen at 24 to 48 hours of life and usually resolve within 7 days. Peripheral eosinophilia may be present in 7% to 18% of patients. Transient neonatal pustular melanosis (Fig. 24.2) is less common than ETN. On examination small pustules are seen on a nonerythematous base, and they are usually present at birth. As the pustules rupture erythematous macules with surrounding scale may develop and can persist for weeks to months. These pustules contain neutrophils.

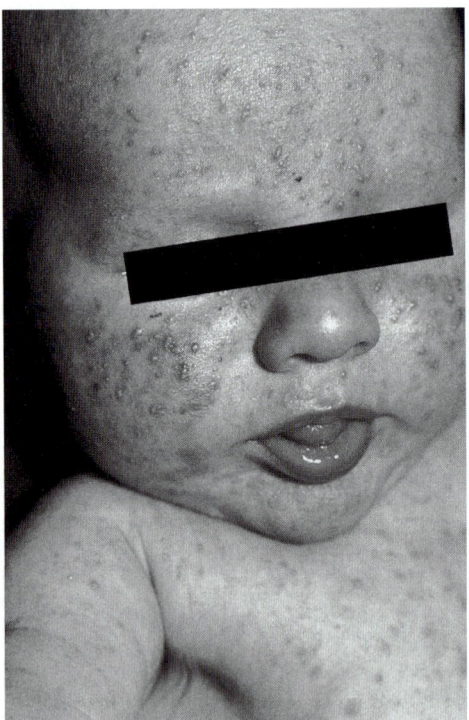

Fig. 24.1. Neonatal acne. *(From Paller AS, Mancini AJ:* Hurwitz Clinical Pediatric Dermatology, *Philadelphia, 2011, Saunders, pp 167–183. Fig. 8.17.)*

8. **What is the difference between milia and miliaria?**

Milia are white papules caused by retention of keratin. They are firm and, unlike pustules, are not easily denuded by pressure. Milia consist of epithelial lined cysts arising from hair follicles. On examination the rash is found on the nose and cheeks, and it resolves within the first weeks of life. Miliaria is caused by accumulation of sweat beneath the eccrine sweat ducts at the level of stratum corneum resulting in the formation of 2- to 3-mm sweat retention vesicles. In infants, the lesions are noted over the head, neck, and upper trunk.

9. **What are the different types of miliaria?**
   - Miliaria crystallina (Fig. 24.3) presents as small thin-walled vesicles without inflammation.
   - Miliaria rubra (Fig. 24.4) occurs when the obstructed sweat leaks into the dermis and causes an inflammatory response that results in erythematous papules and pustules.

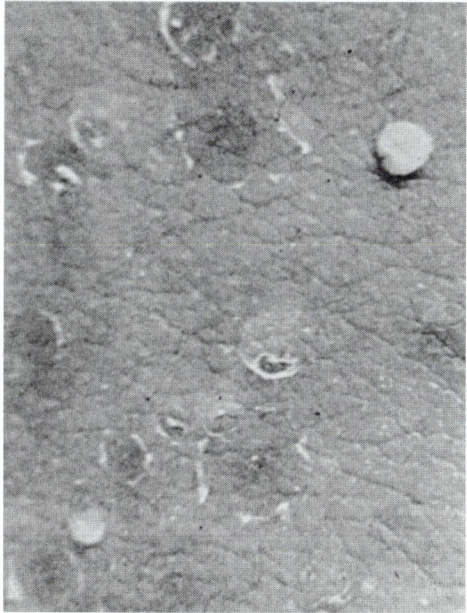

Fig. 24.2. Transient neonatal melanosis. *(From Diseases of the Neonate.* Nelson Textbook of Pediatrics, *2004. Fig. 637.2.)*

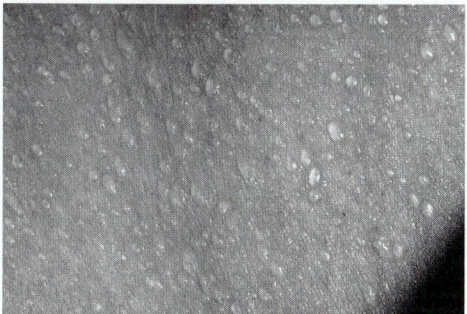

Fig. 24.3. Miliaria crystallina. *(From Dermatoses Resulting from Physical Factors.* Andrews' Diseases of the Skin, *Philadelphia, 2011, Saunders, pp 18–44. Fig. 3.3.)*

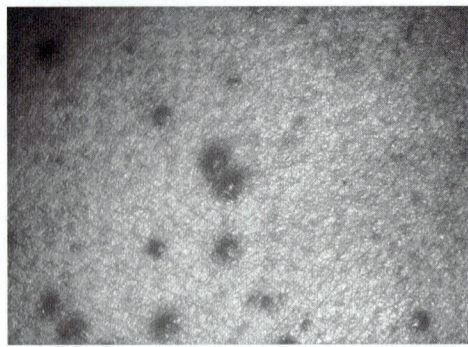

Fig. 24.4. Miliaria rubra. *(From Dermatoses Resulting from Physical Factors. Andrews' Diseases of the Skin, 2011, Saunders, pp 18–44. Fig. 3.4.)*

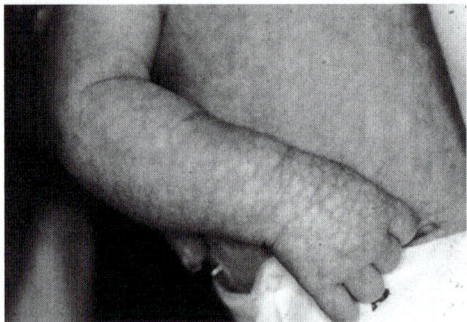

Fig. 24.5. Cutis marmorata. *(From Neonatal skin disorders. Selbst: Pediatric Emergency Medicine, 2008. Fig. 39.4.)*

- Miliaria pustulosa results from localized inflammation consisting of pustules over an erythematous base.
- Miliaria profunda is papular or papulopustular and skin colored.

10. **What is the differential diagnosis of sucking blisters?**
    Herpes simplex virus infection, bullous impetigo, congenital syphilis or candidiasis, neonatal lupus erythematous, and hereditary bullous diseases. Other clinical signs and symptoms along with positive maternal history usually accompany these disorders.

11. **What is the difference between cutis marmorata and harlequin color change?**
    Cutis marmorata (Fig. 24.5) is asymmetric reticular mottling of the skin of the extremities and trunk. It is a vascular response to cold and usually resolves with warming. Harlequin color change is noted when an infant is lying on one side of the body. There is an intense reddening of the dependent side and blanching of the nondependent side with a demarcated line at midline. It can range from a few seconds to 20 minutes. It is benign and self-limited, and it can be seen up to 3 weeks after birth.

HYPERBILIRUBINEMIA

A 4-day-old, 38-week gestation male presents to Urgent Care for a bilirubin check. Mother notes worsening jaundice. He was discharged home on day 2 of life after successfully breastfeeding for a 24-hour period. At the time of discharge, his physical examination was noted for mild jaundice and a cephalohematoma. Currently, he has 5% weight loss from birth, and his parents report slightly decreased urine output. He has stooled once today. On physical examination, he has jaundice to the abdomen and has a resolving cephalohematoma. Otherwise, he has normal examination including normal neurologic examination. The total bilirubin is 20 mg/dL. The mother's blood type is O+; the baby's blood type is to be determined.

12. What are the risk factors for development of hyperbilirubinemia?
- Predischarge total serum bilirubin (TSB) >75th percentile
- ABO incompatibility or other hemolytic disease such as Glucose 6 Phosphate Dehydrogenase Deficiency (G6PD)
- Jaundice less than 24 hours or before discharge
- Gestational age <35 weeks
- Previous sibling with jaundice
- Exclusive breastfeeding
- Cephalohematoma
- East Asian
- Male
- Discharge <72 hours

13. When should a patient be referred to the emergency room (ER) and what are the guidelines for phototherapy?

Hyperbilirubinemia Bhutani Nomogram
The hyperbilirubinemia Bhutani nomogram should be utilized for risk stratification of patients with hyperbilirubinemia. The patient in the case above falls in the "high-risk" zone requiring referral to the ER and further management. The patient's risk level must be assessed as well. Our patient is a 38-week-old male, exclusively breastfed, and has a cephalohematoma, which places him in the medium risk level. Therefore, according to the American Academy of Pediatrics (AAP) guidelines, our medium-risk patient with a TSB above the 95th on the Bhutani curve will be admitted for phototherapy.
In general, phototherapy in term infants is recommended at the following TSB levels:
- At 25 to 48 hours: ≥15 mg/dL.
- At 49 to 72 hours: 18 mg/dL.
- At 72 hours: 20 mg/dL.

14. When should the TSB be rechecked?
- If TSB >25 mg/dL, repeat serum bilirubin within 2 to 3 hours
- If TSB 20 to 25 mg/dL, repeat within 3 to 4 hours
- If TSB <20 mg/dL, repeat in 4 to 6 hours; if it continues to fall, repeat in 8 to 12 hours

15. What are the hyperbilirubinemia risk levels?
- Lower risk infants: ≥38 weeks and well
- Medium-risk infants: ≥38 weeks and has hyperbilirubinemia risk factors or 35 to 37 6/7 weeks and well
- Higher risk infants: 35 to 37 6/7 weeks and has hyperbilirubinemia risk factors

GUIDELINES FOR PHOTOTHERAPY

16. What is the normal maximum bilirubin level of a full-term healthy newborns?
The 97th percentile for bilirubin in a healthy full-term infant is 12.4 mg/dL for a bottle-fed infant and 14.8 mg/dL for a breastfed infant.

17. What total serum bilirubin levels should be concerning for increased risk of kernicterus?
- >25, <30 mg/dL, the risk equals 6%.
- >30, <35 mg/dL, the risk equals 14% to 25%.
- >35 mg/dL, all infants will have signs of kernicterus.

18. Which infants require evaluation for hyperbilirubinemia?
Full-term and late preterm infants more than 35 weeks of gestation should be routinely checked for presence of jaundice every 8 to 12 hours of life while at the hospital. Infants who develop jaundice <24 hours of life are at increased risk for severe hyperbilirubinemia often due to isoimmune hemolytic disease. For infants >24 hours of life, a total bilirubin is measured when the jaundice is noticed below the level of the umbilicus. Measurement of total bilirubin in all infants prior to discharge is indicated to identify hyperbilirubinemia.

19. **How soon should an infant be followed up in clinic after discharge from the hospital?**

If an infant is discharged <24 hours of age, a follow-up should be done by 72 hours of age. If an infant is discharged between 24 and 48 hours of age, a follow-up should be done by 96 hours of age. If the discharge is done between 48 and 72 hours of age, a follow-up should be done by 120 hours of age.

20. **When is an additional evaluation for hyperbilirubinemia indicated?**

If an infant is presenting with total bilirubin values greater than the 95th percentile or hemolytic disease is suspected, further evaluation for jaundice etiology is required.

Initial testing includes blood type and direct Coombs test. If the patient is receiving phototherapy or has a rapid rise in total serum bilirubin, especially crossing percentiles, additional tests should be obtained including complete blood count and smear along with direct bilirubin. It is an option to perform reticulocyte count and G6PD. Rising reticulocyte count during the first 72 hours of life is consistent with red cell destruction. A G6PD measurement should be done if the patient is of Mediterranean, Nigerian, or East Asian descent and has a total bilirubin concentration >18 mg/dL.

Additional testing should also be done if jaundice is present at or beyond 3 weeks of life. These laboratory tests include newborn thyroid and galactosemia screen; also there is a need to evaluate the infant for signs and symptoms of hypothyroidism.

21. **What are the physiologic causes of hyperbilirubinemia in newborns?**

- Neonatal jaundice is caused mainly by changes in bilirubin metabolism that result in increased bilirubin production.
- The newborn infant produces two to three times higher bilirubin than do adults. This is due to increased numbers of red blood cells in newborns that also have a shorter life span.
- There is a decreased bilirubin clearance mainly due to the deficiency of the enzyme uridine diphosphogluconurate glucuronosyltransferase.
- There is also an increase in the enterohepatic circulation, further increasing the bilirubin load.

22. **What are the clinical manifestations of bilirubin encephalopathy?**

Hypertonia or hypotonia, arching, torticollis, opisthotonos, fever, and high-pitched cry are some of the signs and symptoms seen in patients presenting with bilirubin toxicity.

23. **Should a baby with hyperbilirubinemia continue breastfeeding?**

There is no contraindication to continue breastfeeding. This can reduce bilirubin levels and increase the efficacy of phototherapy. Supplementation with expressed breast milk or formula is also adequate, especially if there is excessive weight loss (>12 percentile of birth weight) or the infant appears to be dehydrated. Intravenous fluids should be considered in these patients as well.

BRUE (BRIEF RESOLVED UNEXPLAINED EVENTS)

A 2-month-old female infant presents to urgent care due to cessation of breathing noted by her mother after a feeding while at home. This episode lasted about 10 seconds, and the patient appeared to turn blue around the mouth. The infant has been well since the episode, but due to parental concerns she was brought to your urgent care for further evaluation. Examination: vital signs T 37° C, pulse 130, respirations 24, BP 80/50, O_2 saturation 100% on room air. Her examination was unremarkable.

24. **What defines BRUE (brief resolved unexplained events)?**

Brief resolved unexplained events (BRUE), formerly known as apparent life-threatening events (ALTE), are unexpected episodes that are frightening to the caregiver and include apnea, color change, marked change in muscle tone, and choking or gagging.

25. **Is sudden infant death syndrome (SIDS) related to brief resolved unexplained events (BRUE)?**

Studies have not shown a causal relationship between preexisting apnea and SIDS. The vast majority of SIDS patients do not experience BRUE or apnea prior to death. Also the risk factors for SIDS differ from those of BRUE. The risk factors for SIDS include male sex, prematurity, low birth weight, maternal smoking, low socioeconomic status, poor prenatal care, young maternal age, multiple gestation, and unsafe sleeping conditions. The risk factors for BRUE are prior history of apneas, pallor, cyanosis, difficulty feeding, recent upper viral respiratory symptoms, and age younger than 10 weeks.

26. **What are some of the warning signs that would increase the likelihood of BRUE to be medically significant, and thus referral to your local ER?**
    - Toxic appearance, lethargy, unexplained recurrent vomiting, or respiratory distress at the time of the evaluation
    - Evidence of trauma or bruising
    - History of prior BRUE, especially within the past 24 hours
    - Resuscitation required by a caregiver
    - History of clinically significant sudden unexpected death in a sibling
    - Inconsistent description of events that may suggest child abuse
    - Dysmorphic features or congenital anomalies or any known syndromes
    - Significant physiologic compromise during the event, such as significant generalized cyanosis or loss of consciousness as well as the need for caregiver resuscitation

27. **Which patients could be classified as low risk presenting with BRUE?**
    If there is no concern on history and physical examination, patients who are identified as low risk include infants:
    - Age >60 days
    - Born >32 weeks' gestation and corrected gestational age >45 weeks
    - No CPR by trained medical provider
    - Events lasted <1 minute
    - No prior events preceding the current one

28. **When is a workup indicated for BRUE?**
    No laboratory studies should be obtained on low-risk patients. Home cardiorespiratory monitoring and acid suppression therapy should not be initiated. Admission is not indicated solely for cardiorespiratory monitoring. If there is a clinical indication, the provider may consider obtaining pertussis testing and 12-lead electrocardiogram (ECG), as well as brief admission for monitoring of the infant with continuous pulse oximetry and serial observation.

VOMITING

A 3-week-old girl with frequent spit up after feeding who is now spitting up with every feed. The last episode was projectile in nature. She has gained weight well since birth. There is no fever and no other sick contacts.

29. **What differentiates spitting up versus vomiting?**
    Of infants, 50% will have daily episodes of spitting up due to esophageal sphincter immaturity; overfeeding may also play a role. Spitting up will generally result in small amounts of breast milk or formula coming from the mouth, usually shortly after feeding. This may be more forceful with burping.
    In contrast, vomiting is a coordinated expulsion of gastric content that may be associated with anatomic abnormality, obstruction, infection, or other nongastrointestinal causes. In infants, it is important to differentiate true vomiting from spitting up.

30. **What are the causes of vomiting in infants (Table 24.1)?**

31. **How do I know if an infant has reflux?**
    It is important to differentiate physiologic gastroesophageal regurgitation (GER) from pathologic gastroesophageal reflux disease (GERD). GERD may manifest as fussiness, persistent regurgitation, vomiting, or failure to gain weight. Diagnostic testing with pH probe or direct endoscopy is ideal but impractical in small infants.

32. **What can I do to treat reflux?**
    Guidelines exist for initial management of suspected reflux. Physiologic reflux can be treated with upright positioning during and after feeding. One may also try hydrolyzed formula or thickened formula, as cow's milk protein allergy may play a role in reflux.
    In infants with suspected GERD who are symptomatic, a trial of ranitidine may be done for 2 to 4 weeks.

33. **How fast should infants gain weight?**
    All newborns will lose some weight after birth due to fluid shifts and limited caloric intake in the first few days of life. Infants may lose up to 10% of body weight but should regain this by 2 weeks

Table 24.1. Causes of Vomiting in Infants

Gastrointestinal obstruction	Neurologic
• Pyloric stenosis	• Hydrocephalus
• Malrotation with intermittent volvulus	• Subdural hematoma
• Intestinal duplication	• Intracranial hemorrhage
• Hirschsprung disease	• Intracranial mass
• Antral/duodenal web	*Infectious*
• Incarcerated hernia	• Sepsis
• Other gastrointestinal disorders	• Meningitis
• Achalasia	• Urinary tract infection
• Gastroparesis	• Pneumonia
• Gastroenteritis	• Otitis media
• Eosinophilic esophagitis/gastroenteritis	• Hepatitis
• Food allergy	*Cardiac*
Metabolic/endocrine	• Congestive heart failure
• Galactosemia	• Vascular ring
• Hereditary fructose intolerance	*Toxic*
• Urea cycle defects	• Lead
• Amino and organic acidemias	• Iron
• Congenital adrenal hyperplasia	• Vitamins A and D
• Renal obstructive uropathy	• Medications (ipecac, digoxin, theophylline, etc.)
• Renal insufficiency	
Others	
• Pediatric falsification disorder (Munchausen syndrome by proxy)	
• Child neglect or abuse	
• Autonomic dysfunction	

Modified from Pediatric Gastroesophageal Reflux Clinical Practice Guidelines: Joint Recommendations of the North American Society for Pediatric Gastroenterology, Hepatology, and Nutrition (NASPGHAN) and the European Society for Pediatric Gastroenterology, Hepatology, and Nutrition (ESPGHAN). *J Pediatr Gastroenterol Nutr* 49:498–547.

of age. After this initial period of weight loss, newborns are expected to gain ½ ounce to 1 ounce (15–30 g) per day. Generally, infants will double their birth weight by age 6 months and triple it by 1 year.

34. **What is failure to thrive?**
Failure to thrive (FTT) is the failure to gain weight and/or length as expected over a course of time. Use of standardized growth charts from the Centers for Disease Control and Prevention (CDC) or the World Health Organization (WHO) help to track growth. Infants who are losing weight or are "falling off their curve" (dropping down 2 percentile curves over the course of time) are considered failure to thrive and should undergo an evaluation.
   It is important to note that growth charts for certain conditions (e.g., Down syndrome or Turner syndrome) also exist as growth patterns are different for this population.

35. **What are the signs and symptoms of pyloric stenosis?**
Pyloric stenosis occurs in approximately 0.2% of infants and typically presents between the ages of 3 and 4 weeks (1–12 weeks). Infants will have acute onset of persistent vomiting, which may become projectile due to the obstruction caused by the enlarged pylorus. It is generally nonbilious. Ultrasound

Table 24.2. Diagnosis of Crying Infants

MORE BENIGN	MORE SERIOUS/LIFE THREATENING
Anal fissure	Abusive head trauma/child abuse
Colic	Congestive heart failure
Corneal abrasion	Congenital heart disease/SVT
Feeding difficulties	Drugs or drug withdrawal
Gas	Incarcerated hernia
Hair tourniquet	Infection
Hernia (unincarcerated)	Sepsis
Milk protein allergy	Meningitis
Nasal congestion	Respiratory distress
Otitis media	Urinary tract infection
Oral thrush (severe)	Injury
Reflux	Intussusception
	Metabolic disturbances
	Testicular/ovarian torsion

(From Hogencamp TC. An urgent care approach to excessively crying infants. *J Urgent Care Med.* 2012;6(12):9-18.)

will reveal an enlarged pylorus. Intravenous (IV) hydration is required until a pyloromyotomy can be performed.

36. What is the evaluation of an infant with bilious emesis?

Bilious vomiting is concerning for obstruction and, in infants, may be related to malrotation with midgut volvulus. In addition to vomiting, infants will often have irritability and may present in extremis due to gut necrosis. Malrotation is a congenital anomaly where the gut is malrotated. This increases the risk of volvulus, where the small intestine compresses the superior mesentery artery, causing gut necrosis. Volvulus is a surgical emergency requiring immediate transfer to a pediatric facility.

37. How do I approach the evaluation of a crying infant? There must be something I am missing.

All infants cry! Crying is a primitive form of communication. Crying infants can cause significant stress for parents and seasoned providers. Crying increases during the first few weeks of life and peaks at approximately 2 months. A systematic approach to the crying infant will ensure you evaluate all potential causes (Table 24.2).

A complete head-to-toe examination, including removing the diaper, will help determine any physical causes for the crying. A serious underlying cause will be found in approximately 5% of infants who present with crying. Two thirds of the time history of the physical examination will lead to the diagnosis, although most infants presenting with crying will have a normal examination and no definitive diagnosis. One of the most common diagnoses of infants presenting with crying is urinary tract infection.

38. How do I rule out colic as a cause for crying?

Colic is a distinct syndrome of excessive crying. The exact cause of colic is unknown, and treatment is aimed at consoling the infant and supporting the family. There are no tests to rule out colic, but it is certainly important to rule out other serious causes of crying.

Colic is a clinical diagnosis defined as episodes of intense, often inconsolable crying with no identifiable physiologic cause. To diagnose colic, think about the rule of 3s:

- Lasting 3 hours per day
- More than 3 days per week
- Occurring in the last ⅓ of the day (evening)
- Colic begins after 3 weeks and disappears by 3 to 4 months of age

39. **A 1-month-old has had no bowel movement in 3 days. He is feeding well without vomiting. He has normal urine output. He has been crying all day. Is he constipated?**

Newborns will have their first meconium stool within the first 24 hours of life. Stool will then transition to a mustard yellow seedy stool. In the first week of life, infants will often stool after each feeding. Over the course of the first several weeks, stool may decrease in frequency and take on a firmer consistency. Most infants will stool daily, but stooling every 2 to 3 days can be normal, especially when transitioning from breastfeeding to formula or solid foods. Breastfed infants will often continue to have soft, seedy stool several times per day but may also go several days between stools.

Grunting, drawing up the legs, and straining are normal for infants while they are stooling, because it is challenging to stool while lying flat on your back. To relieve some of this distress parents may try rectal stimulation with a thermometer or a glycerin suppository, but reassuring parents about this normal stooling behavior is most helpful.

40. **When should I be concerned about constipation?**

For infants who have always had infrequent stools or who had delayed passage of meconium, consider evaluation for Hirschsprung disease. In Hirschsprung disease there is aganglionosis of the rectal sphincter and distal colon, making it challenging to pass stool. Barium enema is diagnostic as you can see the transition zone between the aganglionic and normal colon.

41. **What are the physical examination findings for nonaccidental trauma?**

The most common form of injury due to nonaccidental trauma in infants will be from brain injury due to vigorous shaking. This type of injury may present with irritability, vomiting, or poor feeding. There may not be other physical signs of abuse.

Fractures of the extremities or the skull may present with swelling at the fracture site and history of irritability.

Because infants are not mobile, maintain a high index of suspicion if physical findings (bruising or swelling) are not consistent with the history and examination.

42. **Are there other disorders that can mimic nonaccidental trauma?**

In infants, consider genetic disorders of bone formation that may contribute to pathologic fractures. Bleeding disorders or metabolic disorders may contribute to easy bruising. Consultation with a child abuse pediatrician at a local children's hospital is recommended.

Any concern for nonaccidental trauma in an infant should be referred to a pediatric center for further evaluation.

KEY POINTS

1. Acrocyanosis is seen in healthy newborns; it refers to the peripheral cyanosis around the mouth and the extremities including hands and feet.
2. The 97th percentile for bilirubin in a healthy full-term infant is 12.4 mg/dL for bottle-fed infant and 14.8 mg/dL for breastfed infants.
3. Brief resolved unexplained events (BRUE), formerly known as apparent life-threatening events (ALTE), unexpected episodes that are frightening to the caregiver, include apnea, color change, marked change in muscle tone, and choking or gagging.
4. Diagnostic testing for excessive crying should be guided by the history and physical examination.
5. Any concern for nonaccidental trauma in an infant should be referred to a pediatric center for further evaluation.

BIBLIOGRAPHY

Bromiker R, Bin-Nun A, Schimmel MS, Hammerman C, Kaplan M: Neonatal hyperbilirubinemia in the low-intermediate-risk category on the bilirubin nomogram. *Pediatrics* 130(3):e470–e475. <http://doi.org/10.1542/peds.2012-0005>.

Freedman S, Al-Harthy N, Freedman J. The crying infant: diagnostic testing and frequency of serious underlying disease. *Pediatrics.* 2009;123:841–848. <www.pediatrics.org/cgi/doi/10.1542/peds.2008-0113>.

Hogencamp T. Excessively crying infant. *Journal of Urgent Care Medicine.* October 2012.

Maisels MJ, Clune S, Coleman K, et al. The natural history of jaundice in predominantly breastfed infants. *Pediatrics.* 2014;134(2):e340–e345. <http://doi.org/10.1542/peds.2013-4299>.

O'Connor NR, McLaughlin MR, Ham P. Newborn skin: Part I. Common rashes. *Am Fam Physician.* 2008;77(1):47–52. Retrieved from <http://www.ncbi.nlm.nih.gov/pubmed/18236822>.

Pediatric Gastroesophageal Reflux Clinical Practice Guidelines: Joint Recommendations of the North American Society for Pediatric Gastroenterology, Hepatology, and Nutrition (NASPGHAN) and the European Society for Pediatric Gastroenterology, Hepatology, and Nutrition (ESPGHAN). *J Ped Gastroenterol Nutr* 49:498–547.

Treadwell PA. Dermatoses in newborns. *Am Fam Physician*. 1997;56(2):443–450. Retrieved from <http://www.ncbi.nlm.nih.gov/pubmed/9262525>.

Zitelli BJ, Davis HW. *Atlas of Pediatric Physical Diagnosis*. Cohen BA, Davis HW. Dermatology. Zitelli BJ, Atlas of Pediatric Physical Diagnosis, 4th Edition pages 257–314.

CHAPTER 25

LIMP

Robert D. Wilkinson, DO, Bryan Upham, MD, MSCE

1. **A mother and her 6-year-old son present to your urgent care. The mother reports that last week her child had a cough and fever. She is here today because last night before bed she noticed her son limping, and it continued today. There is no history of trauma, and fever has resolved. The child is afebrile and his joints all appear normal except that he is holding his left leg flexed and abducted and he cries when you range that leg. The recent history of a respiratory infection in this child is most suggestive of what cause of his hip limp?**
   Toxic synovitis (TS), also known as transient synovitis, is most likely given this history. Most commonly, respiratory infections are known to be associated with TS; however, gastrointestinal or urinary infections have been seen also. Recent trauma can also be seen.

2. **Although the case in question 1 most likely is TS, list three diagnoses that should be on your differential.**
   1. Septic arthritis (SA)
   2. Osteomyelitis
   3. Legg–Calvé–Perthes (LCP) disease
      Others could include bone tumor or fracture.

3. **What two imaging studies should routinely be ordered on a child presenting as described above?**
   Plain radiographs and joint ultrasound. Plain radiographs are more than likely to be normal in TS but may show some joint space widening. They are most effective in ruling out other diagnoses such as a fracture, slipped capital femoral epiphysis (SCFE), or others. Joint ultrasound is excellent in detecting joint effusions, which are common in both TS and SA. If these studies are not available at your urgent care, you should refer the patient to the emergency department.

4. **Abnormality in which laboratory marker is common in TS?**
   Laboratory values are most likely normal in TS. Laboratory values together with imaging will help rule out other more serious causes. Ultimately, TS is a clinical diagnosis.

5. **Once TS is diagnosed, what does the treatment include?**
   Rest and nonsteroidal antiinflammatory drugs (NSAIDs). TS is self-limiting and resolves without treatment usually in 3 to 10 days. Supportive measures, such as rest and NSAIDs (mainly ibuprofen), have been shown to reduce the number of days of symptoms.

6. **Three months later the same child returns with a similar history and pain in his hip. What should be done?**
   TS can recur in up to 15% of children. For this reason, it is still the likeliest cause of the pain. The same imaging and laboratory studies should be performed as previously discussed.

7. **If the child in question 1 did have a fever or warmth around the hip joint, what would the most likely cause of his limp and fever be?**
   SA of the hip would be the most likely cause.

8. **A septic joint is a surgical emergency. Along with the imaging previously discussed with TS, what laboratory studies should you order?**
   Blood work including a white blood cell count (WBC) with differential, erythrocyte sedimentation rate (ESR), C-reactive protein (CRP), and blood cultures should be sent immediately.

9. **Consider the laboratory studies ordered in question 8. If the results are abnormal, which would be most consistent with SA?**
   In 2011, Singhal and colleagues reviewed 300 cases of hip pain and found that when paired together, pain bearing weight and an elevated CRP (>2.0 mg/dL) gave patients a 74% probability of having SA.

Table 25.1. Most Common Bacterial Causes of Osteomyelitis and Recommended Treatments by Age

AGE	MOST COMMON BACTERIA	ANTIBIOTIC CHOICE
<3 months	Staphylococcus (MSSA and MRSA) Gram-negative bacilli Group B streptococcus *Neisseria gonorrhoeae*	nafcillin, oxacillin, or vancomycin + gentamicin or cefotaxime
3 months to 3 years	Staphylococcus (MSSA and MRSA) *Kingella kingae* Group B streptococcus *Streptococcus pneumoniae* *Haemophilus influenzae* type b	clindamycin, nafcillin, oxacillin, or vancomycin
>3 years	Staphylococcus (MSSA and MRSA) Group B streptococcus *S. pneumoniae* *Neisseria gonorrhoeae*	clindamycin, nafcillin, oxacillin, or vancomycin

MSSA, Methicillin-susceptible *Staphylococcus aureus*; MRSA, methicillin-resistant *S. aureus*.

Without pain and elevated CRP, the probability of SA was <1%. Elevated CRP showed an odds ratio of 82, making it the best independent prediction variable.

10. **What is the most common bacteria to cause SA, in all ages?**
Staphylococcus aureus is the likely cause of the infection in all ages. See Table 25.1 for details by age.

11. **The child referred to in question 7 should be sent to the ER for what three interventions?**
The first intervention is ultrasound or fluoroscopic aspiration of the hip joint for cell count, Gram stain, and culture performed by pediatric orthopedic specialists. Once the joint fluid has been obtained, the second intervention is empiric intravenous antibiotic therapy. Choice of antibiotic should take age and history into account (see Table 25.1). Magnetic resonance imaging (MRI) may be performed if the diagnosis is in question and joint aspiration is not available, but both MRI and aspiration would likely require procedural sedation. The third intervention is irrigation in the operating room by pediatric orthopedic specialists.

12. **A 14-month-old child is brought in for limp. He fell while walking last night, but his mother states that this is nothing unusual. He is afebrile and well appearing. All joints have normal range of motion without swelling or erythema. Examination is limited by stranger anxiety, but he may have some tenderness to the right tibia. Neurologic examination is normal. He walks with an antalgic gait, placing most weight on the left leg. What is the most likely diagnosis?**
Due to his age, lack of fever, swelling, and erythema, and normal joint and neurologic examinations, toddler's fracture is the most likely diagnosis. Differential diagnosis for an antalgic gait is large but can be divided by trauma and systemic symptoms (Fig. 25.1) as well as age.

13. **How is "limp" defined, anyway? And what about an antalgic gait?**
We know what a limp is, right? Technically, limp is a derivation from age-appropriate gait pattern. For the purpose of this chapter, we will also include not using the limb. Abnormal gaits are most commonly antalgic (shortening of stance phase due to pain) but may be steppage (flexion of the hip and knee to allow toes to clear the ground), Trendelenberg (pelvis tilts down to the unaffected side), circumduction, and equinus (toe stepping). The differential diagnosis differs for nonantalgic gaits (Fig. 25.2).

14. **For the limping toddler, what is the most appropriate initial workup?**
Anterior/posterior (AP) and lateral radiographs of the most affected area (right tibia only) are appropriate. However, if the pain cannot be localized, then bilateral lower extremity radiographs are recommended by some authors. Oblique views can be helpful if AP and lateral radiographs are not revealing.

Diagnosis of a Child with an Antalgic Gait

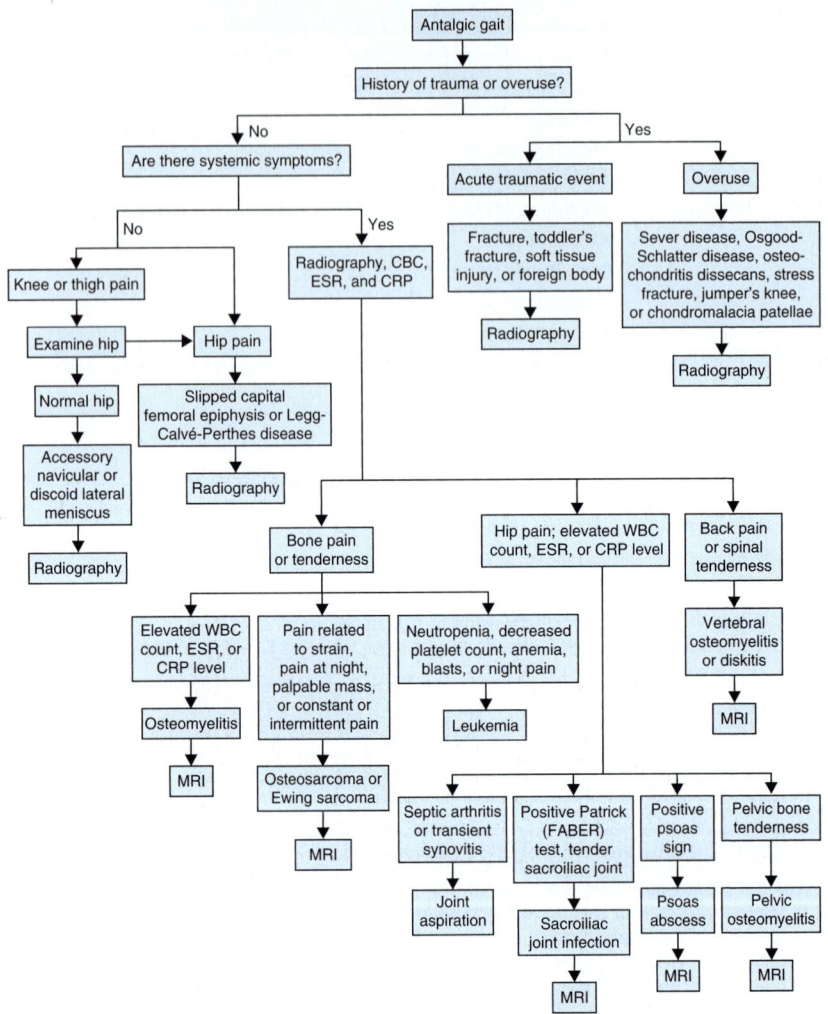

Fig. 25.1. Diagnostic approach to a limping child with an antalgic gait. (*CBC,* Complete blood count; *CRP,* C-reactive protein; *ESR,* erythrocyte sedimentation rate; *MRI,* magnetic resonance imaging; *WBC,* white blood cell.) *(Adapted with permission from Sawyer JR, Kapoor M. The limping child: a systematic approach to diagnosis.* Am Fam Physician *2009; 79(3): 215-24.)*

15. **Radiographs for the patient above show a nondisplaced spiral right distal tibia fracture. Should police and child protective services be called?**
   In this case, a nondisplaced distal tibia spiral fracture is consistent with a toddler's fracture, and contacting the authorities would not be appropriate unless there were other concerns. Toddler's fractures occur in children 9 to 36 months of age, and twisting on a planted foot would be a consistent mechanism.

16. **Do toddler's fractures need orthopedic referral? What about splinting?**
   Many authors recommend long leg splinting or casting in clear and unclear cases as long as there is no concern for infection or other etiologies. Long leg splinting or casting with orthopedic follow-up in 5 to 7 days is appropriate and most common.

Diagnosis of a Child with a Nonantalgic Gait

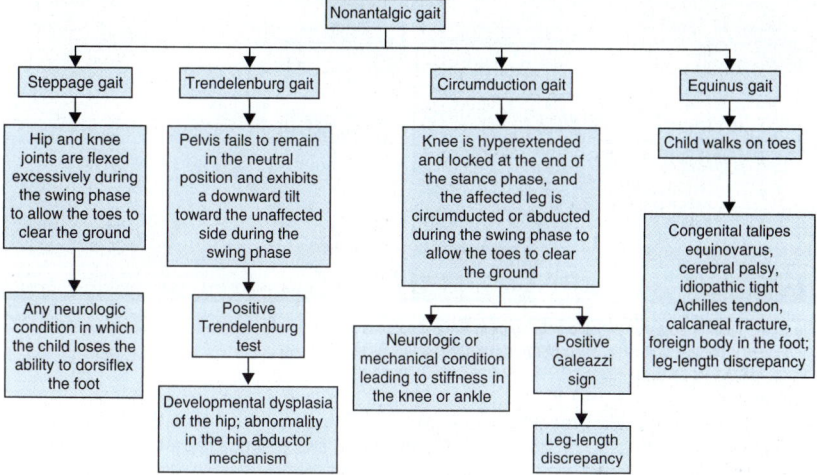

Fig. 25.2. Diagnostic approach to a limping child with a nonantalgic gait. *(Adapted with permission from Sawyer JR, Kapoor M. The limping child: a systematic approach to diagnosis.* Am Fam Physician *79(3):216, 2009.)*

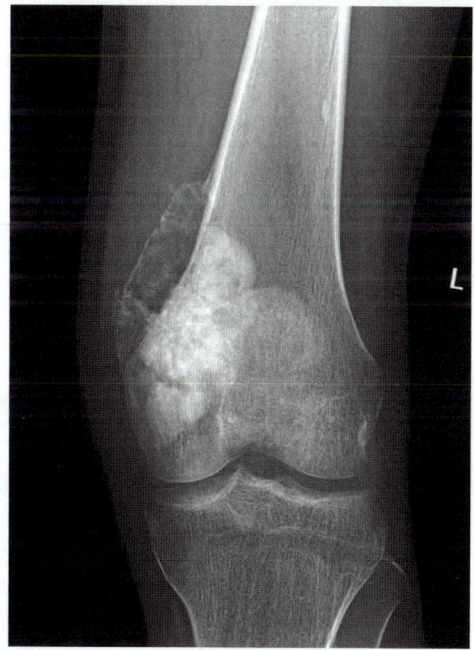

Fig. 25.3. Anterior/posterior (AP) plain film of 15-year-old male presenting with limp and left leg pain for 1 month. *(From: Czerniak, MD Dorfman and Czerniak's Bone Tumors, ed 2. Elsevier, Philadelphia 2016, Fig. 5.6.)*

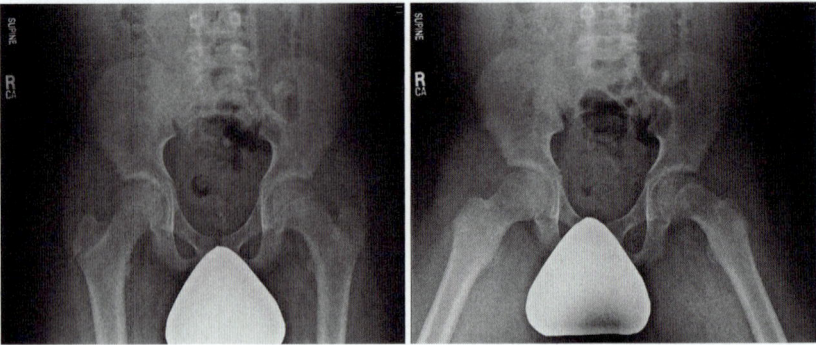

Fig. 25.4. Anterior/posterior (AP) and frog-leg plain film radiographs of 12-year-old male complaining of left knee pain. *(From: Berry: Surgery of the Hip, ed 1. Elsevier, Philadelphia 2013. Fig 42.5.)*

17. **A 15-year-old male presents with limp and left leg pain for 1 month. You obtain a plain radiograph (Fig. 25.3). What is the most likely tumor represented in the radiograph?**
Osteosarcoma. The most common sites for development of osteosarcoma are metaphysis of the most rapidly growing bones (distal femur, proximal humerus, and proximal tibia). Ewing sarcoma is most often found in either the pelvis or diaphysis of the femur. Furthermore, Ewing sarcoma classically has layers of periosteal reaction called "onion skinning," while osteosarcoma is composed of calcified blood vessels radiating out from the lesion, causing a "sunburst" pattern.

18. **What are the two most common malignant bone tumors?**
Osteosarcoma and Ewing sarcoma comprise the most frequently encountered malignant bone tumors in children and adolescents.

19. **What findings on plain film make benign bone tumors more likely?**
Most of the time there is an obvious division between the normal bone and the lesion. This, along with a lack of destruction of the cortex and no extension into surrounding tissues, can help make benign bone mass more likely.

20. **A 12-year-old male presents with left knee pain which he has had for the last 9 months. He fell today, and it is now worse. Which of the following joints should be examined?**
A. Ankle
B. Knee
C. Hip
D. All of the above
D. A common mistake is to focus only on the joint of which the patient is complaining. However, it is extremely common for pathology of the hip or ankle to cause knee pain or vice versa. Always examine the entire limb.

21. **On examination, the patient from the previous question has severe hip pain with flexion or rotation of the hip. Given the most likely possible diagnoses, you order a plain film radiograph (Fig. 25.4). What is the diagnosis?**
The diagnosis of slipped capital femoral epiphysis (SCFE) is made on plain film radiographs. As seen in Fig. 25.4, there is classic posterior displacement of the femoral epiphysis. The use of both AP and frog-leg views can help confirm the diagnosis. If clinical suspicion is high despite normal radiographs, clinicians can order an MRI, which can demonstrate widening of the physis with surrounding edema. LCP or a late diagnosis of developmental dysplasia of the hip (DDH) can mimic SCFE. However, the use of plain films usually allows the clinician to differentiate the three diagnoses. In LCP, plain film will classically show a flattened, and later fragmented, femoral head. Plain film in DDH will be positive for a dysplastic femoral head and an increased center edge angle.

22. **Which patients with a limp need to be seen emergently in the pediatric emergency department (ED)?**

Luckily, for atraumatic causes of limp, toxic synovitis (TS) is the most common and it can be handled in the urgent care setting. No list is complete, but causes of limp that need ED referral include:

- Infection: SA, osteomyelitis, pyomyositis, sacroileitis, vertebral osteomyelitis, discitis, pelvic abscess
- Long bone fracture or nonaccidental trauma
- Open or displaced fractures or dislocations
- Acute abnormal neurologic examination
- Pelvic causes, such as appendicitis and testicular or ovarian torsion
- Concern for neoplasia
- Inability to bear weight
- Young age (<2 years) or ill appearance
- SCFE

23. **Mom and her boyfriend bring their 4-month-old baby in for crying since his diaper change last night. He cries every time they pick him up or change his diaper. He has been only in the care of his mom and mom's boyfriend. Vitals are normal when he is not crying, and there is no report of fevers. On examination, his left thigh is swollen, deformed, and painful to the touch and with movement. Which of the following would be most appropriate?**
    A. Pain control, x-rays, splinting, and transfer via private vehicle to the closest pediatric center
    B. Septic workup and hospital admission
    C. X-ray of the left leg, pain control, and splinting if fractured
    D. Contact law enforcement and child protective services and transfer to a pediatric center via ambulance if there is a femur fracture
    E. Computed tomography of the head, skeletal survey, and contact the local child abuse team if there is a femur fracture

C, D, and E in combination are correct. Femur fractures require a high level of force, and without an appropriate mechanism, nonaccidental trauma (NAT) is the correct diagnosis. Answer A is not correct because while pain control and splinting are appropriate, sending the child with an NAT alone with the potential offenders is not. Answer B is not correct unless the patient is ill appearing and has had a fever.

24. **A 4-year-old presents with 1 month of intermittent diffuse back pain, limp, tactile fevers, and no history of trauma. There is no focal back tenderness and full range of motion of all joints, but you do feel a spleen. A complete blood count is notable for a white count of 3,000 and platelets of 65,000. Urinalysis is normal. The most appropriate next step is:**
    A. Repeat complete blood count (CBC) in 1 week
    B. Transfer to a pediatric center
    C. NSAIDs and outpatient pediatric orthopedist referral
    D. Discuss with a pediatric hematologist/oncologist
    E. Answers B and D

E. Back pain in pediatric patients is concerning for infection or neoplasm in the absence of trauma. Abnormalities in two cell lines are concerning for leukemia.

25. **A 15-year-old female presents with severe right hip pain, vomiting, and limp with no history of trauma or overuse. She is afebrile and has tenderness to palpation of the right lower quadrant and right hip. Internal and external rotation of the hip worsens the pain. Ultrasound reveals no hip effusion and a normal appendix. X-rays are normal. CBC, CRP, ESR, UA, and urine pregnancy are unremarkable. What radiology studies may help clarify the diagnosis?**

This presentation is most concerning for ovarian torsion. Ultrasound of the ovaries (either transabdominal for patients who are not yet sexually active or transvaginal for those who are) is the best next study.

KEY POINTS

1. Toxic synovitis is the most common cause of atraumatic limp in children. Developmental dysplasia of the hip (DDH) in infants, Legg-Calvé-Perthes (LCP) in young school-aged children, and slipped capital femoral epiphysis (SCFE) in preteens and teens can cause limp.

2. Reassuring laboratory values can help distinguish septic arthritis from toxic synovitis.
3. Pain can be referred from the back or pelvis to the hip (as in ovarian torsion) or hip to the knee (as in SCFE).
4. Back pain without trauma in children is abnormal and should be considered infectious or neoplastic until proven otherwise.
5. If the story doesn't fit, you must admit; that is, beware of nonaccidental trauma.

BIBLIOGRAPHY

Dunbar JS, Owen HF, Nogrady MB, et al. Obscure tibial fracture of infants—the toddler's fracture. *J Can Assoc Radiol.* 1964;15:136.

Heinrich SD, Mooney JF. Fractures of the shaft of the tibia and fibula. In: Shaw KN, Wilkins KE, Barchur RG, eds. *Fleischer & Ludwig's Textbook of Pediatric Emergency Medicine.* 7th ed. Philadelphia: Wolters Kluwer Publishers; 2016:p 280.

Kost S, Thompson AD. Limp. In: Rockwood CA, Wilkins KE, Beaty JH, eds. *Rockwood and Wilkins' Fractures in Children.* 4th ed. Philadelphia: Lippincott-Raven Publishers; 2006:p 1033.

McCanny PJ, McCoy S, Grant T, et al. Implementation of an evidence based guideline reduces blood tests and length of stay for the limping child in a paediatric emergency department. *Emerg Med J.* 2013;30(1):19–23.

Milla SS, Coley BD, et al. ACR Appropriateness Criteria® limping child—ages 0 to 5 years. *J Am Coll Radiol.* 2012;9(8):545–53.

Naranje S, Kelly DM, Sawyer JR. A systematic approach to the evaluation of a limping child. *Am Fam Physician.* 2015;92:10.

Sapru K, Cooper JG. Management of the toddler's fracture with and without initial radiological evidence. *Eur J Emerg Med.* 2014;21:6.

Schuh AM, Whitlock KB, Klein EJ. Management of toddler's fractures in the pediatric emergency department. *Pediatr Emerg Care.* 2016;32:7.

Singhal R, Perry DC, Khan FN, et al. The use of CRP within a clinical prediction algorithm for the differentiation of SA and transient synovitis in children. *J Bone Joint Surg Br.* 2011;93:B.

Tenenbein M, Reed MH, Black GB, et al. The toddler's fracture revisited. *Am J Emerg Med.* 1990;8:3.

CHAPTER 26

HEAD AND NECK TRAUMA

Kara K. Seaton, MD

HEAD INJURIES

A 3-year-old female is brought in by her mother for evaluation of a head injury after a fall off a bunk bed. She had no loss of consciousness, crying immediately on impact. She had one episode of vomiting but is now calm and acting normally according to her mother. The child denies having a headache currently.

1. **How common are head injuries in children?**
   Pediatric head injuries account for approximately 600,000 emergency department visits per year in the United States. These injuries result in 60,000 hospital admissions and an estimated 7,000 deaths in children ≤18 years of age. Head injuries are the most common cause of death and acquired disability for children in developed countries.

2. **What are some of the most common mechanisms leading to pediatric head injury?**
   Falls are the most common cause of head injury in children. Other common mechanisms include motor vehicle collisions, pedestrian or bike accidents, and sports. It is also important to consider nonaccidental trauma, as this is a potentially life-threatening cause of head injury in infants and younger children and should not be missed.

3. **How do we define clinically important traumatic brain injury?**
   Many children sustain head injuries, but only a few will have injuries that fall into the category of clinically important traumatic brain injury (ciTBI). These injuries cause significant immediate or long-term impact to the child, or result in the child's death. Generally, these include depressed or basilar skull fractures, bleeding requiring neurosurgical intervention, injury requiring the child to be intubated for more than 24 hours, or injury severe enough to warrant hospital admission longer than 48 hours.

4. **What types of injuries are considered ciTBI?**
   Head injuries are frequently characterized into diffuse and focal injury patterns. Diffuse injuries include diffuse axonal injury (DAI), cerebral edema, hypoxic ischemic encephalopathy, and diffuse vascular injury. Concussion also falls under the purview of diffuse injury. Focal injuries include cerebral contusions and hemorrhage in the subdural, subarachnoid, or epidural spaces.

5. **How do diffuse injuries usually occur?**
   Diffuse injuries occur from shearing forces, often with a rapid acceleration-deceleration event or rotational force. Infants may suffer these types of injuries when shaken vigorously back and forth. Cerebral edema can also occur as a result of hypoxia or changes in cerebral blood flow and from inflammatory mediators and vascular leak postinjury.

6. **What are the different types of focal injuries?**
   A *cerebral contusion* occurs from a direct impact of the brain against the intracranial bony surfaces and may lead to focal neurologic deficits. *Subdural hemorrhage* occurs when the bridging veins rupture, causing bleeding between the dura mater and the arachnoid space. This type of injury is more common in children two years of age and younger. It may occur as a result of nonaccidental trauma. *Subarachnoid hemorrhage* occurs from bleeding of the vessels that supply the pia mater. Accumulation of blood occurs in layers along the bony surface, and bleeding can be quite extensive. *Epidural hemorrhage* is the result of vascular injury to the middle meningeal or dural venous sinus, resulting in bleeding between the dura and the bone. Because these are venous bleeds, they tend to accumulate slowly, leading to a classic "lucid" interval after injury with subsequent decompensation.

7. **What are important age-related considerations when evaluating a child with a head injury?**
   Younger children (<2 years) should be considered separately from older children. Clinical assessment is decidedly more difficult in infants, who may be asymptomatic or have subtle or nonspecific signs

of injury. It is important to consider the risk of inflicted or abusive injury in children. Traumatic brain injury is a leading cause of death from abuse in children. Clinicians need to consider the possibility of inflicted trauma in infants who present with head injury.

8. I need to evaluate a child who just sustained a head injury at my urgent care facility. Are there specific things I should consider when determining a plan of care?

The primary goal of evaluating a child with a head injury is to determine the severity of the injury and recognize injuries that require further management. Children with potentially serious injuries need to be rapidly identified and transferred to an appropriate facility for definitive care. Ideally, this would be a pediatric certified trauma center. The secondary goal of evaluation includes minimizing unnecessary radiation exposure.

9. Why should minimizing radiation be a priority?

Many clinicians use head computed tomography (CT) as a means of rapidly assessing patients with head injury. However, young brains are exquisitely sensitive to radiation. There is a significant risk of cancer mortality associated with head CTs in children. Therefore, it is important to balance the risk of the child having a significant injury with the potential future risk of malignancy.

10. Are there established guidelines that can help me determine a child's risk of clinically important TBI and make an educated decision about imaging?

Yes! The Pediatric Emergency Care Applied Research Network (PECARN) has developed and validated clinical decision rules for children with a low risk of serious head injuries. The rules are derived from a large, multicenter, prospective trial that included over 43,000 patients. These guidelines help to standardize patient evaluations, rapidly identify children with potentially serious intracranial injury, and minimize the use of CT scans in low-risk patients. Such rules are useful when evaluating healthy children who present to the emergency department within 24 hours of injury, and in whom there is no suspicion for nonaccidental trauma. For children in the younger age group, the low-risk rule had a sensitivity of 100% and a negative predictive value of 100%. In the older age group, the sensitivity of the low-risk rule was 96.8% with a negative predictive value of 99.95%.

11. Can I use the PECARN criteria for all children with head injuries?

Not all children will be eligible for the PECARN pathway. The PECARN rules are intended to identify *low-risk* children not requiring further assessment. Children who are moderate or high risk for significant intracranial injury, including those with Glasgow Coma Scale (GCS) <14, require transfer to a pediatric trauma center. Children with underlying neuropathology, such as brain tumors or preexisting neurologic disorders, warrant separate consideration. Finally, children with ventriculoperitoneal (VP) shunts and bleeding disorders may have a higher risk of serious injury than otherwise healthy children, or may have intracranial bleeding with a less severe mechanism of injury.

12. What are the PECARN criteria by which children qualify as low risk for serious injury?

Table 26.1 describes the criteria for children who qualify as low risk based on the PECARN guidelines.

Table 26.1. Criteria for Children at Low Risk of ciTBI by Age (A child must meet all of these criteria to be considered low risk.)

CHILDREN <2 YEARS	CHILDREN ≥2 YEARS
Acting normally per parents	Normal mental status (GCS ≥14)
Known, low-risk mechanism	Known, low-risk mechanism
No loss of consciousness	No loss of consciousness
No nonfrontal scalp hematoma	No vomiting
No signs of basilar skull fracture	No signs of basilar skull fracture
No concern for abuse	No complaints of severe headache

13. How do I know what counts as a severe mechanism?

The PECARN criteria use well-defined descriptions to classify mild and severe mechanisms. If the mechanism fails to meet the criteria for one or the other, it is generally considered to fall within the moderate risk category. Mild mechanisms include ground-level falls or injuries resulting from a child running into a stationary object. Severe mechanisms include motor vehicle accidents with ejection, death of another passenger, rollover accidents, and pedestrians or bicyclists struck by a motor vehicle. Falls greater than 3 feet for children less than 2 years, falls greater than 5 feet for children older than 2 years, and head strikes by a high-impact object are also considered severe mechanisms.

14. Are there certain symptoms that suggest a child might be at higher risk for ciTBI and therefore need urgent imaging?

Symptoms suggestive of serious injury include altered mental status, loss of consciousness, focal neurologic findings, posttraumatic seizure, persistent vomiting, or evidence of a depressed or basilar skull fracture. Consider that infants with bulging fontanel, nonfrontal scalp hematoma, irritability, poor feeding, or lethargy may also be at risk of serious TBI. Older children with significant TBI may complain of worsening or severe headache.

15. What if I am concerned for ciTBI in my patient?

Children with suspected or proven ciTBI need to be transported to a qualified pediatric trauma center, as rapidly and safely as possible. Be aware that such patients have a risk of worsening neurologic status and herniation. These children will frequently have altered mental status (GCS <14). Other concerning signs include pupillary changes, bradycardia, hypertension, and respiratory depression. Such children may need airway protection with intubation prior to transfer.

16. How can I use the PECARN criteria to help me make an informed decision about management?

Table 26.2, adapted from the original study, summarizes the PECARN recommendations for children who present with head injuries and have a GCS of 14 or 15.

17. What about children with skull fractures?

Simple, linear, unilateral skull fractures are common in children and account for 75% of all pediatric skull fractures. Most of these are uncomplicated, with only 15%–30% having an underlying intracranial injury. The goal in evaluation of skull fractures is to separate children with uncomplicated fractures from those with more complex injuries.

18. What counts as a complicated skull fracture?

Complicated skull fractures are more likely to be associated with underlying injury. There is also a correlation between complex skull fractures and nonaccidental trauma. Complicated fractures include:

- Fractures that are large or cross suture lines
- Complex or burst fracture pattern
- Depressed, bilateral, or multiple fractures
- Basilar skull fractures
- Open skull fractures

19. Are there physical exam findings that might suggest skull fracture?

Infants may have a scalp hematoma or significant soft tissue swelling in the area of the fracture. Crepitus or palpable skull defects are occasionally found. Patients with basilar skull fractures may present with nystagmus, hearing loss, hemotympanum, periorbital ecchymosis, CSF otorrhea or rhinorrhea, or facial nerve palsies. Patients with such findings need imaging, with CT scan as the preferred mechanism.

20. Do all pediatric patients with skull fractures need to be admitted?

Not necessarily. Children may be discharged without admission if they have a simple, unilateral, nondisplaced skull fracture; have no underlying intracranial injury; have no other distracting traumatic injury; and have a normal neurologic exam. Admission is necessary for children with complicated injuries, including complex or basilar skull fractures, or when there is a suspicion of nonaccidental trauma.

21. When do I have to worry about nonaccidental trauma in children with head injuries?

Traumatic brain injury is the leading cause of death from abuse in children. Thus, clinicians always need to consider abusive head injury when evaluating children, especially infants, with head injuries. Up to 30% of infants with other abuse-related injuries may have occult head injuries, even if they are asymptomatic from a neurologic standpoint.

Table 26.2. PECARN Recommendations* for Determining the Use of CT Scan to Evaluate Children with Head Injuries and GCS 14–15

AGE	CLINICAL FEATURES	RISK OF ciTBI	RECOMMENDATIONS
<2 years	GCS = 14 *or* Altered mental status *or* Palpable skull fracture	4.4%	• CT recommended • Transfer to a trauma center
	Nonfrontal scalp hematoma *or* Loss of consciousness ≥5 seconds *or* Severe mechanism *or* Not acting normally per parents	0.9%	• Observation versus CT** • Consider transfer if worsening signs/symptoms
	Acting normally per parents *and* None of the features listed above	<0.02%	• CT not recommended • Discharge with home care instructions
≥2 years	GCS = 14 *or* Altered mental status *or* Signs of basilar skull fracture	4.3%	• CT recommended • Transfer to a trauma center
	Loss of consciousness *or* History of vomiting *or* Severe mechanism *or* Severe headache	0.8%	• Observation versus CT** • Consider transfer if worsening signs/symptoms
	Appropriate mental status *and* None of the features listed above	<0.05%	• CT not recommended • Discharge with home care instructions

*Data adapted from Kupperman N, Holes JF, Dayan PS, et al: Identification of Children at Very Low Risk of Clinically-Important Brain Injuries after Head Trauma: A Prospective Cohort Study. *Lancet* 374:1160-1170, 2009 [Fig. 3, p 1168].

**CT scan may be obtained based on physician experience, if the patient exhibits worsening signs or symptoms during the observation period, if the patient is under 3 months of age, or if the parental preference is for CT.

22. **How will children with abusive head injuries present to care?**
Detecting abuse-related head injuries is often difficult. The history may be incomplete or lack clear history of trauma. During evaluation, consider whether the mechanism and developmental abilities of the child are consistent with the injury. Remember that abusive head trauma can occur at any age but is most common in children less than 1 year of age, with a peak at 8–12 weeks. Infants may present with nonspecific symptoms, such as fussiness, poor feeding, or vomiting. In severe cases, infants may present with apnea, seizures, and coma.

KEY POINTS: HEAD INJURIES

1. Children with clinically important head injuries, including intracranial bleeding and complicated skull fractures, should be rapidly identified and transferred to an appropriate pediatric trauma center.
2. Identifying infants with significant head injuries is often difficult, as they may be asymptomatic or have nonspecific symptoms.
3. Pediatric head trauma guidelines can be helpful to minimize the use of CT scans in children at low risk for significant injury.

NECK INJURIES

An 8-year-old male is brought in by his parents complaining of neck pain after being struck in the neck with a hockey stick during practice. He fell to the ice initially but was able to ambulate afterwards. He complains of posterior neck pain but denies numbness or tingling in the extremities.

23. What should I consider when evaluating a child with a neck injury?

Both penetrating and blunt neck trauma in children are uncommon but potentially life threatening. Children have large heads, short necks, and mobile laryngotracheal structures, making them less susceptible to penetrating trauma and airway fractures than adults. However, pediatric neck injuries are often severe given the small area of the neck and the large number of vital structures that pass through it.

24. What are common complications of neck injuries in children?

Penetrating neck injuries are unusual injuries in children but may lead to vascular injuries and complications such as aneurysms, dissections, occlusions, or fistulas. Blunt neck trauma often results from motor vehicle accidents, clothesline or handlebar injuries, sports, strangulation or hanging injuries, or nonaccidental trauma. Blunt trauma may lead to laryngeal or airway injuries, cervical spine injuries, or, rarely, vascular injuries.

25. What should I do if a child presents with penetrating neck trauma?

Although penetrating injuries are uncommon, clinicians should have a high suspicion for serious injury in these children. Primary management for such patients includes ensuring a patent and stable airway, control of hemorrhage, prevention of injury progression, and early, safe transfer to an appropriate pediatric trauma center. Injuries should be imaged with CT angiography to assess for vascular injury. For injuries that penetrate the outer layer of musculature, surgical evaluation is recommended.

26. Are there special considerations for cervical spine injuries in children?

Cervical (C) spine injuries are rare in children, but when such injuries occur, there is a higher risk of upper cervical injuries (C1–C4). This occurs because the fulcrum of the spine is at higher cervical levels in younger patients, with infants having the fulcrum at C2–C3 level. Children also have relatively weak neck muscles compared to adults. Certain preexisting conditions can make children more susceptible to neck injury, including trisomy 21 and achondroplasia.

27. I know that there are adult criteria for the detection of cervical spine injury. Can these be used for pediatric patients?

The NEXUS criteria are often used in adults to detect cervical spine injury and have been shown to have greater than 99% sensitivity for detecting spinal injuries in adults. However, these have not been well studied when applied to children and must be used with caution. The PECARN group has investigated cervical spine injuries in children. The group found good sensitivity in identifying C-spine injuries if one or more of the following eight factors are present:

- Altered mental status
- Neurologic deficits
- Neck pain
- Torticollis
- Significant torso trauma
- High-risk motor vehicle accident
- Diving injury
- Preexisting condition that increases the risk of cervical spine injury

28. What do I do if a child with neck pain and a concerning mechanism of injury presents to my urgent care for evaluation?

If there is concern for cervical spine injury, the child should be placed in an appropriately sized cervical collar. Avoid hyperextension of the spine. Cervical spine films may be used in initial evaluation, but if there is concern for significant injury, the child should be transferred to an appropriate pediatric trauma center. When in doubt, assume all children with multiple traumatic injuries or concerning mechanisms have a significant head or neck injury—it is important not to miss an unstable spine. Obtunded patients cannot be clinically cleared with regard to the cervical spine and should remain in a cervical collar.

KEY POINTS: NECK INJURIES

1. Neck injuries are uncommon in children but may be severe due to the large number of vital structures and the high cervical fulcrum of the spine.
2. Children with concerning neck injuries should be appropriately immobilized in a cervical collar and transferred to a qualified pediatric trauma center.

BIBLIOGRAPHY

Kupperman N, Holes JF, Dayan PS, et al. Identification of children at very low risk of clinically-important brain injuries after head trauma: a prospective cohort study. *Lancet.* 2009;374:1160–1170.

Leonard JC, Kupperman N, Olsen C, et al. Factors associated with cervical spine injury in children after blunt trauma. *Annals of Emergency Medicine.* 2011;52(2):145–155.

Mannix M, Monuteaux MC, Schutzman SA, et al. Isolated skull fractures: trends in management in US pediatric emergency departments. *Annals of Emergency Medicine.* 2013;62(4):327–331.

McManemy JK, Jea A. Neurotrauma. In: Shaw KN, Bacher RG, eds. *Fleisher & Ludwig's Textbook of Pediatric Emergency Medicine.* 7th ed. Philadelphia: Wolters Kluwer; 2016:1280–1287.

Woodward GA, O'Mahony L. Neck trauma. In: Shaw KN, Bacher RG, eds. *Fleisher & Ludwig's Textbook of Pediatric Emergency Medicine.* 7th ed. Philadelphia: Wolters Kluwer; 2016:1238–1279.

CHEST AND ABDOMINAL TRAUMA

Peggy Tseng, MD, Emily Rose, MD, FAAP, FAAEM, FACEP

1. **What is the most common mechanism of chest or abdominal trauma in children?**
   Blunt trauma in pediatric patients accounts for approximately 90% of injuries, usually sustained from falls, motor vehicle collisions (MVC) or other vehicle-related accidents (e.g., auto vs. pedestrian or bicycle), and nonaccidental trauma.
   Penetrating trauma less commonly occurs from gunshot wounds (GSW), stabbing, or impalement.

2. **How do injury patterns differ in children compared to adults who sustain thoracic trauma?**
   The chest wall of a child is more compliant than an adult's, so serious intrathoracic injuries may occur without rib fractures or even obvious physical signs on the chest wall. Due to their compliant musculoskeletal structures, rib fractures require more significant force than compared to the same fractures in adults and are therefore a red flag for severe injury.

3. **Why are children more vulnerable to blunt intraabdominal trauma compared to adult patients?**
   Infants and toddlers have relatively compact torsos with larger viscera, especially liver and spleen, which extend below the costal margin, so they are more exposed to direct injury. They also have small anterior-posterior diameters, which provide a smaller area over which the force of injury is dissipated. This in combination with less overlying fat and weaker abdominal musculature to cushion intraabdominal structures places pediatric patients at higher risk for intraabdominal injuries following blunt trauma.

4. **A 3-year-old girl is brought to your urgent care after a 5-foot fall at the playground. What are assessment and management priorities in examination of a pediatric patient with traumatic injuries to the chest and abdomen?**
   The initial management should be to identify and stabilize any life-threatening injuries. Airway, breathing, and circulation are essential and part of any traumatic primary exam. If any component of the trauma primary exam is absent or severely compromised, emergent intervention is needed; immediately transfer to a higher level of care. Any hemodynamically unstable child with suspected intrathoracic or intraabdominal injury needs to be stabilized emergently and should be transferred to an emergency department with trauma capabilities for resuscitation and possible operative intervention.

5. **What additional information should be gathered after a traumatic event?**
   Gather information regarding mechanism from witnesses if available. Obtain a history from the patient or the patient's family, and perform a thorough secondary physical exam. Key elements of the patient include mechanism of injury, time since the injury, and the patient's presentation at the scene of the injury. Was there any loss of consciousness? Were there any witnesses to the injury?
   Does the patient complain of any chest pain or abdominal pain? Any difficulty breathing? Nausea or vomiting? Has the patient been able to tolerate food?

6. **What are major considerations in motor vehicle accidents?**
   Was the patient restrained? Was the patient in a car seat; facing forward or backward? Where in the car was the patient seated? Where was the impact on the vehicle? Were any other people in the accident severely injured? How fast was the vehicle traveling and were airbags deployed?

7. **What is important history to obtain in penetrating trauma?**
   If the penetrating trauma was due to gunshot, how many shots were fired? If the wounds were due to impalement, how long was the object that penetrated the patient? Was the whole object removed and witnessed to be intact?

8. **When should you consider nonaccidental trauma?**

Any serious injury such as intracranial hemorrhage, a long bone fracture (except a spiral tibial fracture), or hollow viscous injury should have a significant mechanism of injury on history. Any discrepancy between the history and the physical or diagnostic findings or sign of significant force (such as a rib fracture) should prompt you to consider inflicted injury. Consider if a mechanism of injury is inconsistent with a patient's developmental abilities (e.g., bruising in a young infant). Any pattern injury is concerning for inflicted injury (bruising/burns/marks that correspond with infliction with instruments or do not occur through natural play environmental interactions). Also, note frequent visits for injuries. Children with inflicted injuries may present with multiple visits for injuries that may not individually raise concern.

9. **A 1-year-old boy comes to your urgent care after a fall from a bed. Your primary exam is normal. Describe key components of the secondary exam of the chest in a pediatric trauma patient.**

Evaluate respiratory status including breath sounds, respiratory rate, and signs of distress such as nasal flaring or retractions. Assess the chest wall for focal tenderness, crepitus, abrasions, ecchymosis, or lacerations. Remember that open wounds may be the track of a penetrating wound. Paradoxical chest wall movement is important to note because a flail segment bulges during expiration. Decreased or absent breath sounds may indicate pneumothorax, hemothorax, or pulmonary contusion. Distant or muffled heart tones may suggest hemopericardium. Injury to the great vessels may result in hypotension, peripheral pulse abnormality, or neurologic deficit.

10. **What are the red flag physical exam findings after chest and abdominal trauma?**

Respiratory distress in a child after trauma is a red flag for serious injury and potential for decompensation. Chest pain with neck discomfort is concerning for mediastinal free air; and distended neck veins are associated with pericardial tamponade. Children should be transferred to the emergency department for further evaluation with any abnormalities of lung auscultation, respiratory rate, chest rise pattern, and oxygen saturation.

In abdominal trauma, focal tenderness, distension, vomiting, and bruising are red flags for injury. Any sign of rigidity or rebound tenderness is a late finding and concerning for severe abdominal injury.

11. **A 7-year-old girl comes to your urgent care after she was a passenger in a motor vehicle accident. On physical exam you find what is shown in Fig. 27.1. What is the name of this physical finding and what is its significance?**

This is a seat belt sign. It is ecchymosis due to the acceleration and deceleration of the body against a seat belt in an MVC.

Children with seat belt signs from MVCs are almost three times more likely to suffer an intraabdominal injury (IAI) and are over ten times more likely to suffer gastrointestinal injuries such as hollow viscous or mesentery.

A child with a seat belt sign should be transferred to the emergency department as there is a significant associated risk of IAI. Further investigation is required including serial abdominal exams, laboratory studies, and frequently CT scan.

12. **Which laboratory studies are indicated after chest trauma?**

If significant injury is suspected, a hemoglobin and hematocrit are important to evaluate for hemorrhage. Serial hemoglobin and hematocrit levels are more useful as a marker of ongoing blood loss because a single value may not reflect the current degree of hemorrhage. Type and screen or cross-match blood is needed especially in any patients whom you suspect serious injury and may have the potential to decompensate and need blood transfusion.

13. **Are there any specific laboratory studies helpful in evaluating pediatric abdominal trauma?**

A hemoglobin/hematocrit evaluates for blood loss. Serial values are more clinically useful if significant intraabdominal injury is suspected. Elevated aspartate transaminase (AST) (>200 IU/L) or elevated alanine transaminase (ALT) (>125 IU/L) is sensitive in detecting hepatic injuries if imaging is not obtained.

Other tests such as amylase and lipase have poor discriminatory ability to diagnose or exclude injuries and are not indicated.

Gross hematuria (which is typically ≥50 RBCs per high power field) screens for kidney injury are indicated. Microscopic hematuria is not clinically significant in asymptomatic patients without other associated injuries.

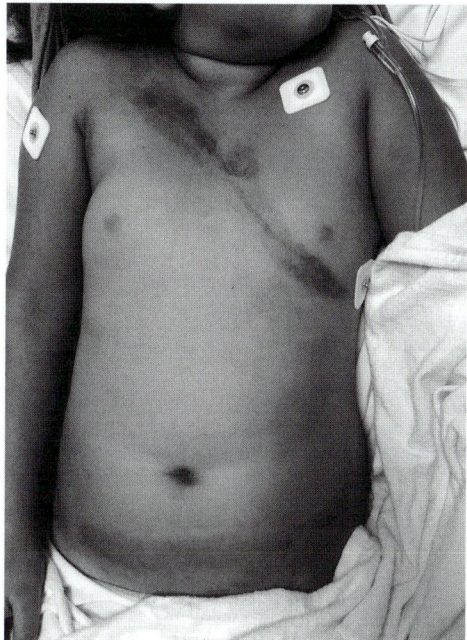

Fig. 27.1. Seat belt sign in a pediatric patient

14. Which imaging is indicated in thoracic trauma?

Chest x-ray (CXR) is the imaging of choice for most pediatric thoracic trauma as it is widely available, inexpensive, and can identify life-threatening injuries like large hemothorax or pneumothorax. Chest computed tomography (CT) should not routinely occur in pediatric thoracic trauma because of the low incidence of cardiac and great vessel injury and high radiation exposure.

15. What is the role of the focused assessment with sonography for trauma (FAST) in pediatric trauma?

FAST exams do not expose children to radiation and are useful to identify hemoperitoneum and pericardial effusion. Bedside ultrasound can be quickly repeated during reassessment and its use decreases abdominal CT scans in children at low to moderate risk for IAI.

The sensitivity of the FAST exam in pediatric patients with intraabdominal injuries ranges from 30% to 90%, though patients without injury may have a small amount of pelvic fluid on exam.

16. When is CT scan indicated in children with chest trauma?

Consider further diagnostic investigation if severe thoracic injury with an abnormal CXR. Aortic injuries are rare but highly lethal, and when red flags for injury are present in mechanism, physical exam, or diagnostic imaging, emergent CT scan and transfer for trauma surgeon evaluation are imperative.

Mechanism Red Flags for Aortic Injuries: High-velocity acceleration/deceleration injuries (most commonly high speed MVCs or falls from height).

CXR Red Flags for Aortic Injuries: Abnormal findings on CXR include an obscured aortic knob, left apical cap, or wide mediastinum and suggest great vessel and mediastinal injury needing further evaluation.

Physical Exam Red Flags for Aortic Injuries: Findings suggesting great vessel injury include asymmetric, diminished, or absent peripheral pulses.

A large pneumothorax or hemothorax seen on CXR requires immediate intervention. Crepitus in the chest should raise suspicion for tracheobronchial injury. Both abnormalities require ED transfer and CT imaging.

Imaging for penetrating trauma depends on mechanism. High-velocity injuries (e.g., gunshot wounds) frequently require CT imaging even if the initial CXR is normal. Stab wounds may only require a CXR and ultrasound (often serially performed). Transfer to the ED is typically recommended in penetrating trauma.

17. **Who can be classified as low risk for intraabdominal injury?**
Though significant intraabdominal injury can occur with seemingly trivial trauma, those with low risk for injury include:
   - Glasgow Coma Scale ≥14
   - No evidence of abdominal wall trauma or seat belt sign
   - No abdominal tenderness
   - No complaints of abdominal pain
   - No vomiting
   - No thoracic wall trauma
   - No decreased breath sounds
   - No concern for physical abuse
   - No serious associated injuries

18. **Your patient with the seat belt sign is complaining of abdominal pain. When should you consider CT scan for abdominal trauma in children?**
Indications for abdominal CT scan to evaluate for IAI in the hemodynamically stable patient include the following:
   - Inability to tolerate oral intake
   - Persistent abdominal tenderness (outside of superficial minor bruises or abrasions not associated with a seat belt)
   - Gross hematuria
   - Hematemesis or blood in the stool
   - Seat belt sign with abdominal pain
   - Positive FAST with abdominal pain or other symptoms concerning for IAI
   - Elevated AST (>200 IU/L) or elevated ALT (>125 IU/L)
   - Hemodynamic instability or decreased hemoglobin or hematocrit

19. **You evaluate a 10-year-old boy who is complaining of abdominal pain after he fell off his bicycle. He sustained a direct blow from the handlebars into his abdomen. Does a negative CT scan of the abdomen rule out IAI?**
No, CT is insensitive for hollow viscous injury, and these injuries should be suspected in patients with persistent/progressive tenderness. Hollow viscous injuries include mesenteric injuries, duodenal hematomas, and bowel perforation. The mechanism involves a direct blow and discrete point of energy transfer to the abdomen from bicycle handlebars, seat belts during MVCs, and child abuse. Significant abdominal tenderness even after a prior normal CT scan should prompt urgent ED referral. Symptoms may also be delayed up to 24 hours after injury so suspicion of injury should be maintained even with a subacute presentation.

20. **Describe the most common traumatic chest wall injuries in a pediatric patient.**
The most common blunt injuries include pulmonary contusion, pneumothorax, and rib fractures.
   Less commonly, penetrating trauma may result in hemothorax or pneumothorax, followed by pulmonary contusion, pulmonary laceration, and blood vessel injury.

21. **Does the location of rib fracture in a chest trauma patient correlate with injury?**
Yes. The upper ribs (1–3) are usually protected by the scapula, humerus, and clavicle, and a significant amount of force is required to fracture them. Further investigation to evaluate for associated organ injuries such as pulmonary contusion and intrathoracic vessels is often required in patients with upper rib fractures.
   Lower rib fractures may be associated with injury to the abdominal organs such as liver and spleen injuries.

22. **What is flail chest?**
A flail chest occurs when multiple consecutive ribs are fractured, and the segment of fractured bones moves with changes in intrathoracic pressure and opposite to that of respiratory muscles. A flail chest segment will retract with inspiration and bulge with expiration.

23. **What complications should you look for with flail chest?**

A flail chest can lead to respiratory compromise because its abnormal movement can cause increased work of breathing. Hypoventilation from pain can result in atelectasis. Flail chest also is associated with other traumatic injury such as pulmonary contusion, which may lead to hypoxia and respiratory failure.

24. **What physical exam findings are concerning for cardiac contusion?**

Consider blunt cardiac injuries in pediatric patients with physical findings of anterior chest wall trauma, sternal fracture, new murmurs or muffled heart tones, or any arrhythmia including sinus tachycardia in the absence of hemorrhage.

25. **What testing is indicated to screen for cardiac contusion?**

Obtain a chest radiograph to evaluate for noncardiac injuries and an electrocardiogram (ECG). Cardiac contusions may manifest as tachycardia or various arrhythmias. Cardiac contusion is unlikely with a normal ECG.

Cardiac troponin test in pediatric trauma is controversial. An abnormal ECG (including sinus tachycardia) in chest trauma warrants an ED referral for further investigation.

26. **Does every pediatric patient with chest trauma mandate a CXR?**

No, there are some children with isolated minor trauma that may not require any imaging if paired with low physician concern for underlying injury based on mechanism and exam.

A CXR is likely to be normal in patients with a normal GCS of 15, normal vital signs (especially respiratory rate, pulse oximetry, and blood pressure), no femur fracture, and no localized findings on chest auscultation and examination (including signs of trauma).

27. **What types of patients who sustain abdominal trauma can we care for in the urgent care setting?**

If a patient has no evidence of abdominal wall or chest wall trauma, no seat belt sign, normal GCS of 15, no abdominal pain or tenderness, no absent or decreased breath sounds, and no vomiting, then some researchers have found that this can make a child a very low risk (<0.1%) of having clinically important blunt abdominal injuries. However, clinical judgment is still necessary as this does not account for mechanism of injury, vital signs, laboratory results, and clinician gestalt. Additionally, a positive screen does not mandate a CT scan. Serial exams, assessment with ultrasound, and/or laboratory evaluation may be sufficient. When in doubt, a patient should be transferred to the emergency department for evaluation.

28. **When should transfer to a higher level of care be considered?**

Abdominal pain or tenderness and/or a seat belt sign on exam should prompt further diagnostic investigation in the emergency department (Fig. 27.2).

Severe pain, abnormal findings on radiography other than nondisplaced rib fractures in an older child, or a high-impact mechanism such as a penetrating injury should be referred.

Any abnormal vital signs including tachypnea, hypoxia, tachycardia, or hypotension; any altered mental status; or multiple traumatic injuries indicate life-threatening injury. Obviously, immediately life-threatening injuries such as airway obstruction, tension pneumothorax, massive hemothorax, and cardiac tamponade require emergent paramedic transportation to a trauma center. In any hemodynamically unstable patient, testing and evaluation in urgent care would only delay ED evaluation and treatment.

KEY POINTS

1. Consider nonaccidental trauma in children younger than 2 years of age with rib fractures, abdominal pain/bruising, associated serious injury such as long bone fractures or intracranial injury, and no history of significant accidental mechanism of injury.
2. Children with normal GCS, normal vital signs, and no focal findings or tenderness on chest or back examination are at low risk for having findings on chest radiography.
3. A seat belt sign on physical exam is associated with high risk of intraabdominal injuries. This finding with or without symptoms should prompt further evaluation and consider transfer to a hospital setting for testing, observation, and possible intervention.
4. Abnormal mental status, vital signs, or multiple traumatic injuries should prompt emergent transfer to a trauma center for evaluation and treatment.
5. Penetrating trauma occurs less commonly in children and is associated with higher injury risk. The urgent care provider should have a low threshold to transfer to the emergency department for further evaluation and management.

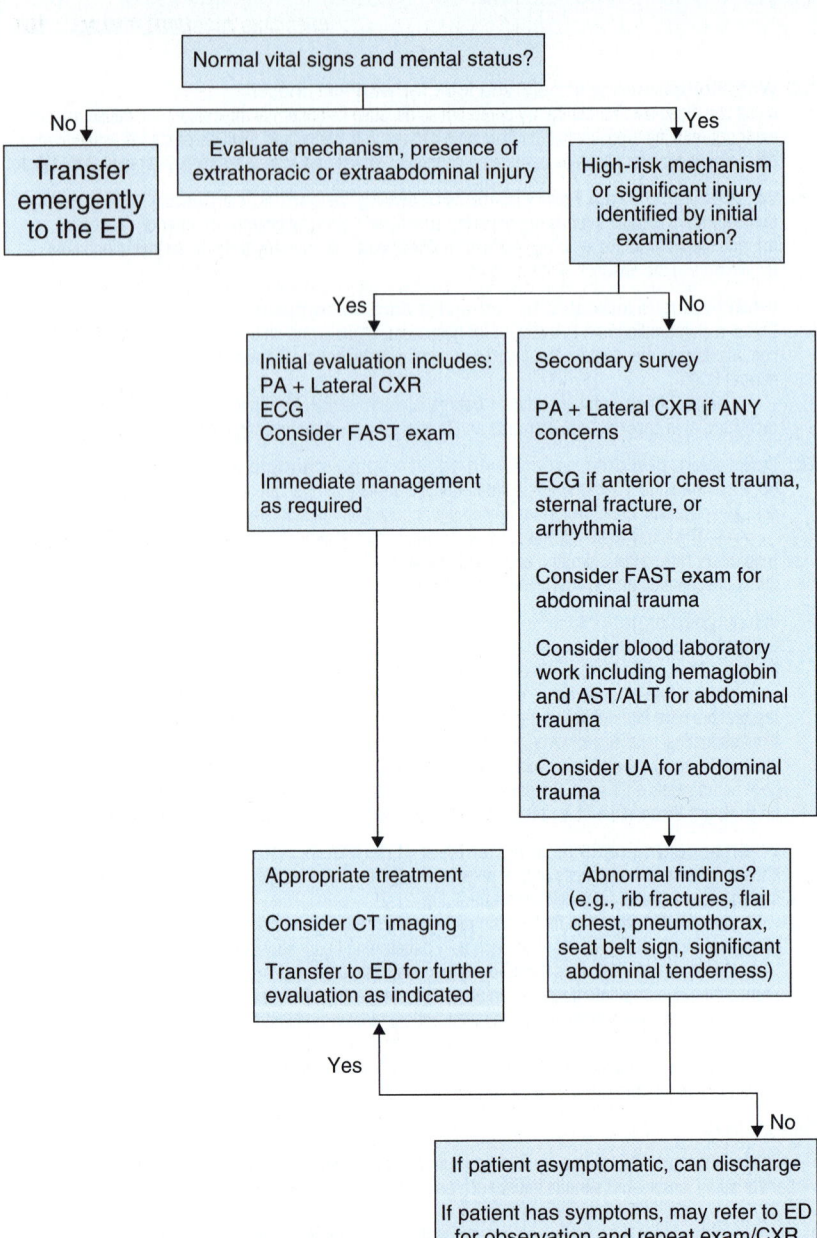

Fig. 27.2. Pediatric algorithm for blunt chest and abdominal trauma. *(Adapted from Initial Evaluation and Stabilization of Children with Thoracic Trauma. <https://www-uptodate-com>; Accessed 19.07.16.)*

BIBLIOGRAPHY

Adelgais KM, et al. Accuracy of the abdominal examination for identifying children with blunt intra-abdominal injuries. *J Pediatr*. 2014;165(6):1230–1235, e5.

Borgialli DA, et al. Association between the seat belt sign and intra-abdominal injuries in children with blunt torso trauma in motor vehicle collisions. *Acad Emerg Med*. 2014;21(11):1240–1248.

Holmes JF, et al. A clinical decision rule for identifying children with thoracic injuries after blunt torso trauma. *Ann Emerg Med*. 2002;39(5):492–499.

Holmes JF, et al. Identification of children with intra-abdominal injuries after blunt trauma. *Ann Emerg Med*. 2002;39(5): 500–509.

Holmes JF, et al. Identifying children at very low risk of clinically important blunt abdominal injuries. *Ann Emerg Med*. 2013;62(2):107–116, e2.

Kerrey BT, et al. A multicenter study of the risk of intra-abdominal injury in children after normal abdominal computed tomography scan results in the emergency department. *Ann Emerg Med*. 2013;62(4):319–326.

Menaker J, et al. Use of the focused assessment with sonography for trauma (FAST) examination and its impact on abdominal computed tomography use in hemodynamically stable children with blunt torso trauma. *J Trauma Acute Care Surg*. 2014;77(3):427–432.

Peters E, et al. Blunt bowel and mesenteric injuries in children: do nonspecific computed tomography findings reliably identify these injuries? *Pediatr Crit Care Med*. 2006;7(6):551–556.

Rothrock SG, Green SM, Morgan R. Abdominal trauma in infants and children: prompt identification and early management of serious and life-threatening injuries. Part I: injury patterns and initial assessment. *Pediatr Emerg Care*. 2000;16(2):106–115.

Sokolove PE, Kuppermann N, Holmes JF. Association between the "seat belt sign" and intra-abdominal injury in children with blunt torso trauma. *Acad Emerg Med*. 2005;12(9):808–813.

CHAPTER 28

EXTREMITY TRAUMA

Joel Clingenpeel, MD, MPH, MS.MEdL, Kristen Herbert, DO,
Bryan Greenfield, MD

1. What is the Salter-Harris fracture classification?

This classification deals with pediatric fractures and their relationship to the growth plate. The classification has five levels (I–V), and each level relates to both the acute treatment recommended and overall prognosis. Higher level (III–V) Salter-Harris fractures are representative of progressively more serious injuries and greater growth disturbances and require close orthopedic follow-up.

2. Sort the fractures in Fig. 28.1 through 28.5 according to the Salter-Harris classification (I–V) (Fig. 28.6).

Fractures are type III, IV, I, II, and V, respectively.

Salter I: Fracture is confined within the growth plate and often not visible on radiographs. A widening of the physis or evidence of epiphyseal displacement may sometimes be seen. Fig. 28.3 shows displacement of radial epiphysis.

Salter II: Fracture involves the metaphysis and the physis.

Salter III: Fracture extends through the growth plate and epiphysis. Lowest classification of intraarticular fractures.

Salter IV: Also an intraarticular fracture that involves metaphysis, growth plate, and epiphysis.

Salter V: A crush/compression-type fracture that damages the physis. Often not seen on initial radiographs and retrospectively diagnosed once growth arrest has occurred. Fig. 28.5 shows a follow-up x-ray in a child with an axial load mechanism to the ankle and subsequent growth arrest.

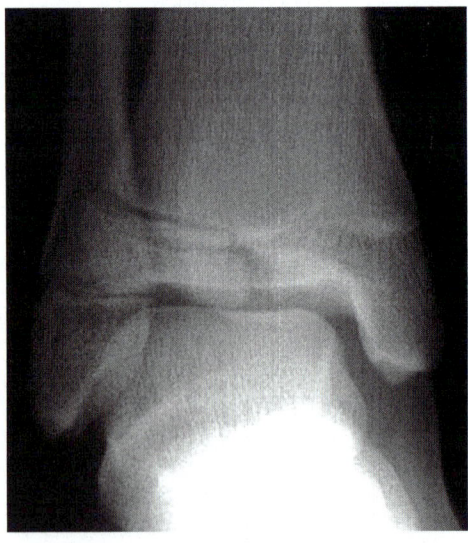

Fig. 28.1.

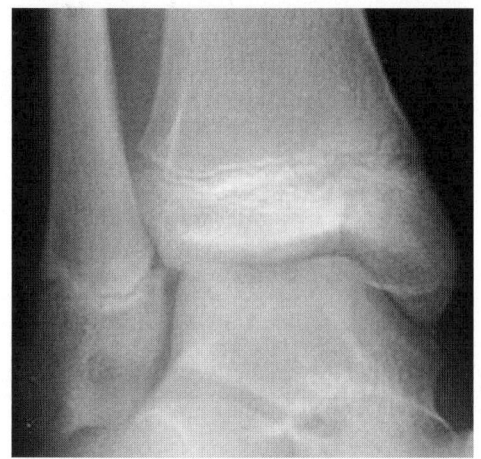

Fig. 28.2.

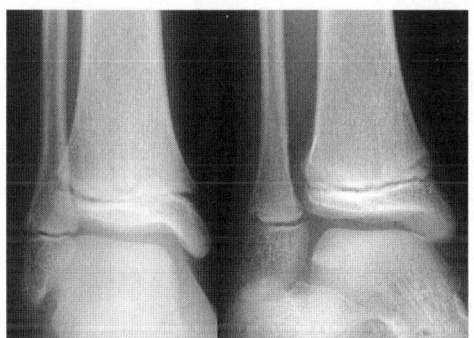

Fig. 28.3.

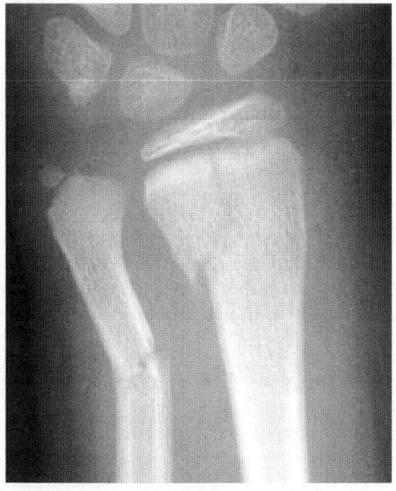

Fig. 28.4.

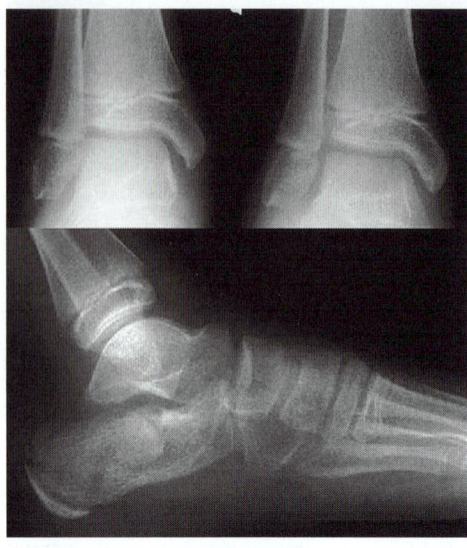

Fig. 28.5. Descriptions are embedded in the answer to question 2. *(From Yamamoto LG, Chung SMK, Inaba AS: Salter-Harris. Radiology Cases in Pediatric Emergency Medicine 1 [case 18], University of Hawaii John A. Burns School of Medicine.)*

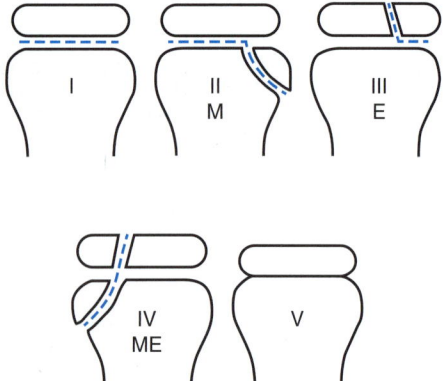

Fig. 28.6. Diagram of the Salter-Harris classification. Abbreviations: M, metaphyseal involvement; E, epiphyseal involvement. *(From Yamamoto LG, Chung SMK, Inaba AS: Salter-Harris. Radiology Cases in Pediatric Emergency Medicine 1 [case 18]. University of Hawaii John A. Burns School of Medicine.)*

3. **Describe clinical and historical clues that suggest a young child has a nursemaid's elbow needing reduction rather than an elbow fracture necessitating radiographs.**
   A nursemaid's elbow, an anatomic entrapment of the annular ligament between the radial head and capitellum, results from axial traction on the distal aspect of a child's extremity (classic mechanism is lifting up on the wrist to pull the child up or back to prevent stumbling). Most elbow fractures in contrast involve blunt trauma to the elbow or a fall on an outstretched hand mechanism. Children with nursemaid's usually present with the arm held closely to the side, pronated, and partially flexed. While these children refuse to move the elbow, in contrast to children with fractures there is usually no swelling or ecchymosis and no pinpoint bony tenderness to the distal humerus or proximal radius and ulna.

4. **What pediatric extremity fractures are suspicious for nonaccidental trauma?**

Any extremity fracture may be the result of abuse, particularly if associated with other injuries concerning for abuse or if the fracture and the history/mechanism are discordant (mechanism not plausible based on child's developmental age and abilities, for example). The following extremity fracture patterns have the greatest specificity for abuse and should always arouse a high index of suspicion:

- Femur fractures in preambulatory children
- Spiral extremity fractures in preambulatory children
- Multiple fractures in various stages of healing
- Chip fractures of the metaphysis
- Metaphyseal corner (aka "bucket handle") fractures

5. **Explain compartment syndrome and describe injury mechanisms or fractures that place a patient at risk for its development.**

Compartment syndrome describes a situation where an elevated pressure within an extremity's fascial compartment prevents adequate perfusion. Resultant ischemia to the muscles, nerves, and vessels can ensue, leading to devastating extremity injury. Extremity injuries as a result of crushing forces, proximal tibiofibular fractures, displaced supracondylar fractures, midshaft radius and ulna fractures, and elbow dislocations are all high-risk fractures. Additionally, constrictive dressings and casts placed soon after injury and not "bivalved" to allow space for ongoing swelling are associated with compartment syndrome.

6. **What signs and symptoms are concerning for possible compartment syndrome?**

It cannot be emphasized enough that compartment syndrome is mainly a clinical diagnosis. Swollen and taught soft tissue in the traumatized region and pain out of proportion to the injury are usually the first (and sometimes only) clues to this diagnosis. The five Ps of compartment syndrome, in addition to pain, sometimes include paresthesia, pallor, paralysis, and pulselessness. Pain out of proportion should never be ignored, particularly if the pain is made worse with passive extension of the muscles in the compartment.

7. **What are "plastic fractures"?**

Torus, greenstick, and bowing fractures are often collectively referred to as "plastic fractures" and are unique to children as a result of the pliability of the pediatric skeleton. Torus (aka "buckle") fractures are common, result from cortex bulging of a long bone without a visible fracture, and generally heal well with simple immobilization. Greenstick fractures, which consist of a visible fracture on one side and a bend on the other side, are usually treated with removable splint/cast immobilization and sometimes closed reduction depending on the fracture. Bowing fractures are uncommon and when seen are usually in the forearm in children between the ages of 2 and 5. These injuries will often require reduction to prevent permanent bone angulation.

8. **Describe the location of injury and treatment of a "toddler's fracture."**

A toddler's fracture is a subtle radiographic fracture and involves the distal third of the tibia in ambulatory preschool children. This is a nondisplaced fracture, and as the fracture line is often spiral or oblique, it can be difficult to see on radiographic series without an oblique view. Young children with toddler's fractures will often present with refusal to bear weight or walk, and the injury usually results from fairly minor trauma such as a low height fall.

9. **What are humeral fat pads and when are their presence concerning for fracture?**

Anterior and posterior fat pads (reference Fig 28.7 shows small anterior fat pad on lateral. Fig 28.8 shows large posterior fat pad on lateral question 10) are seen as radiographic silhouettes around the distal humerus and are radiographic signs of an elbow effusion. In the setting of trauma and distal humerus pain, a posterior fat pad should be considered evidence of an occult supracondylar fracture in a child. Anterior fat pads can also be seen with occult supracondylar fractures, but they are far less specific and are visible in some children after blunt trauma without osseous injuries. Large ballooning anterior fat pads (aka "sail signs") are more specific than small anterior fat pads for osseous injuries in children.

10. **Name two lines you should draw on every pediatric lateral elbow film to screen for subtle fractures/dislocations (Figs. 28.7 and 28.8).**

The anterior humeral line and the radiocapitellar line. A line drawn anterior to the humerus that does not pass through the middle or posterior third of the capitellum is concerning for an occult

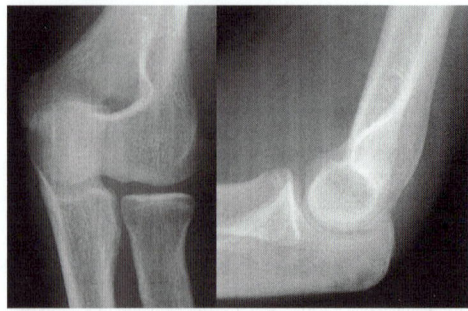

Fig. 28.7. Normal AP and lateral radiograph of the elbow. Note that the anterior humeral line passes through the middle of the capitellum. The radiocapitellar line also points directly at the capitellum. *(From Yamamoto LG: Test Your Skill in Reading Pediatric Elbows. Radiology Cases in Pediatric Emergency Medicine 2 [case 18]. University of Hawaii John A. Burns School of Medicine.)*

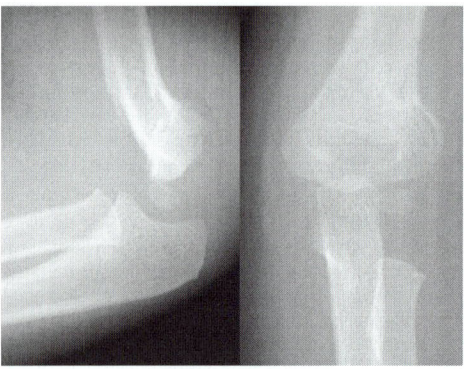

Fig. 28.8. AP and lateral radiograph of the elbow. Note that the anterior humeral line passes anterior to the capitellum, representing a supracondylar fracture. The radiocapitellar line is normal and not consistent with a Monteggia injury pattern. *(From Yamamoto LG: Test Your Skill in Reading Pediatric Elbows. Radiology Cases in Pediatric Emergency Medicine 2 [case 18]. University of Hawaii John A. Burns School of Medicine.)*

supracondylar fracture (with posterior displacement of the capitellum). A line drawn from the middle of the radius should point to the capitellum in every view (including the lateral). A misaligned radiocapitellar line is concerning for either a radial head dislocation or a Monteggia injury pattern.

11. **What is a Tillaux fracture and in what age group does it usually occur?**
The Tillaux fracture (Fig. 28.9) is a Salter III fracture of the anterolateral distal tibia. Distal tibial physeal closure commences in a medial to lateral direction with full fusion usually occurring between 12 and 15 years of age. The Tillaux fracture occurs in older children and young adolescents whose medial tibial growth plate is fused but in whom the lateral tibial physis is still open. Forced external rotation of the foot is the usual mechanism of injury as the anterior tibiofibular ligament avulses the anterolateral corner of the distal tibial epiphysis.

12. **Explain the Gartland classification for supracondylar fractures (Fig. 28.10).**
Gartland type I supracondylar fractures are nondisplaced and have an anterior humeral line that usually intersects a portion of the capitellum. Gartland type II fractures have extension of the fracture and are partially displaced with an abnormal humeral line. A differentiating feature of the type II fracture is that the posterior aspect of the humerus remains intact. In contrast, type III Gartland fractures have a circumferential break in the cortex with complete displacement of the fracture fragments.

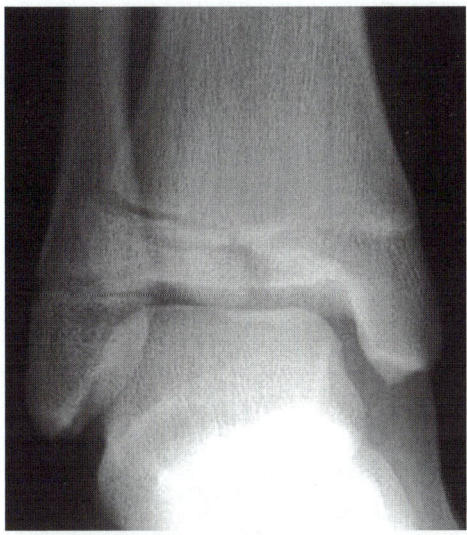

Fig. 28.9. AP radiograph of the distal tibia revealing a Tillaux fracture. *(From Yamamoto LG, Chung SMK, Inaba AS: Salter-Harris. Radiology Cases in Pediatric Emergency Medicine 1 [case 18]. University of Hawaii John A. Burns School of Medicine.)*

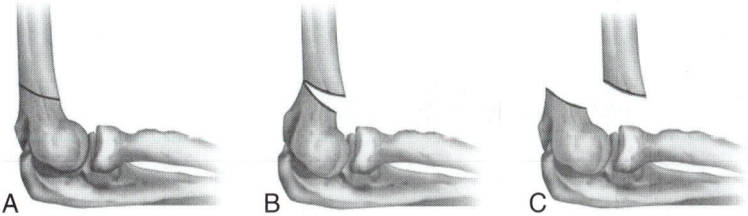

Fig. 28.10. (A) Gartland classification type I, **(B)**, type II, and **(C)**, type III for supracondylar fractures. *(From Alton TB, Werner SE, Gee AO: Classifications in Brief: The Gartland Classification of Supracondylar Humerus Fractures. Clinical Orthopaedics and Related Research 473(2):738-741, 2015.* http://dx.doi.org/10.1007/s11999-014-4033-8 *[Fig. 3A-C].)*

13. **What is the appropriate treatment and disposition for the three types of supracondylar fractures?**
    Type I fractures can usually be splinted to follow up with orthopedics in 48 hours. Type III fractures require operative repair and sometimes emergent reduction if the neurovascular status of the forearm/hand is comprised. The disposition of the type II fracture without neurovascular compromise is made in consultation with orthopedics. Some of these fractures are appropriate for short-term splinting and others will require admission for neurovascular checks and definitive repair.

14. **How are clavicle fractures treated in children?**
    In most cases, a medial or distal clavicle fracture can be treated with immobilization with a sling alone or a sling and swathe combination. The use of figure 8 braces has not been shown to be more effective than a sling. A midshaft fracture with greater than 2 cm of displacement, fractures with greater than 1.5 cm of clavicle shortening, or grossly unstable distal injuries may need closed or open reduction with fixation. Other clavicle fractures needing evaluation by an orthopedic surgeon include any open fracture, fractures that are posteriorly displaced, any fracture causing neurovascular compromise, or fractures that cause tenting of the skin, which can lead to skin necrosis and eventual open fracture.

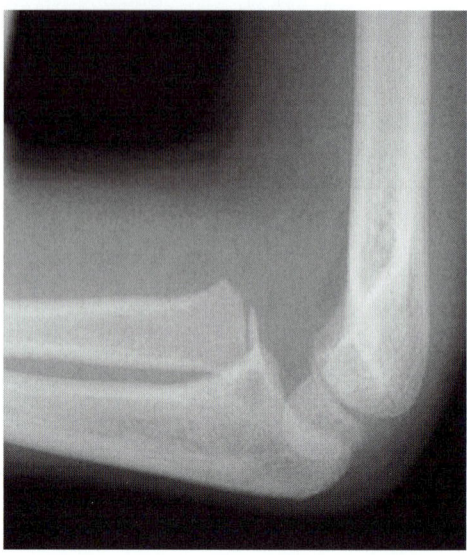

Fig. 28.11. Lateral radiograph of the elbow revealing a Monteggia dislocation. Note that the radiocapitellar line does not point to the capitellum. *(From Young LL: Monteggia's Injury. Radiology Cases in Pediatric Emergency Medicine 1 [case 15]. University of Hawaii John A. Burns School of Medicine.)*

15. What is the management of a displaced proximal humerus fracture?

Proximal humerus fractures have the ability to remodel even with large amounts of angulation. In children, angulation up to 50 degrees is often acceptable. In adolescents there is more variability to what the acceptable degree of angulation is, but most authors advocate accepting up to 20–50 degrees. Management of proximal humerus fractures is typically a sling or shoulder immobilization for 3–4 weeks. Splints to this area often cause more pain than stabilization and are generally not recommended. Operative indications include fractures of the articular surface, comminuted fractures, neurovascular compromise, or pathologic fractures through a bone cyst.

16. What is the usual mechanism of injury of supracondylar fractures and what nerve is sometimes compromised as a complication?

The mechanism of injury for this common pediatric fracture is usually a fall on an outstretched arm with hyperextension of the elbow. The anterior interosseous branch of the median nerve (which has no sensory innervation) is most commonly injured. Anterior interosseous nerve impairment results in mild weakness of the flexor digitorum profundus to the index finger, and of the flexor pollicis longus. Assessment of the anterior interosseous nerve function is performed by having the patient make an "OK" sign and testing the index finger and thumb for strength in this position.

17. Describe the Monteggia and Galeazzi fracture dislocation patterns that are associated with forearm trauma.

A Monteggia fracture (Fig. 28.11) is a combination of an ulnar fracture and dislocation of the radial head. Suspicion for this type of fracture should be heightened if there is swelling or pain over the elbow in the setting of an ulnar fracture. A true lateral radiograph of the elbow will demonstrate misalignment of the radiocapitellar line. A Galeazzi fracture (Fig. 28.12) is a radial shaft fracture with a distal radioulnar joint dislocation. Both injuries require immediate orthopedic consultation since failure to promptly reduce the dislocations in these fracture/dislocation injuries could lead to deformity and poor arm function.

18. What is a Klein line?

A Klein line is drawn on an anteroposterior (AP) femoral radiograph to screen a child for a subtle slipped capital femoral epiphysis (SCFE). An SCFE is a Salter-Harris type I fracture of the proximal femoral physis with epiphyseal displacement. On the radiographs the proximal femoral epiphysis will

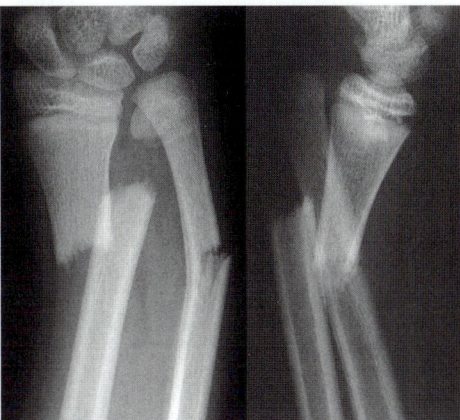

Fig. 28.12. AP and lateral radiograph of the wrist revealing a distal radial fracture and dislocated distal ulna consistent with a Galeazzi fracture. *(From Yamamoto LG, Chung SMK: Galeazzi's Injury. Radiology Cases in Pediatric Emergency Medicine 1 [case 16]. University of Hawaii John A. Burns School of Medicine.)*

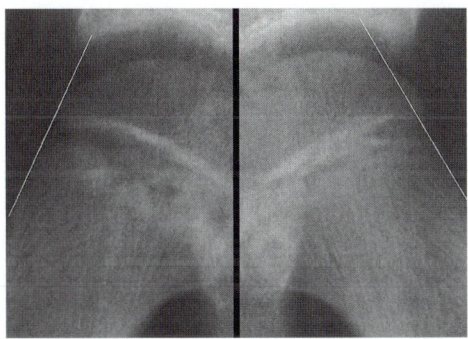

Fig. 28.13. The image on the left (right hip) reveals a Klein line that does not intersect the proximal femoral epiphysis, which is consistent with slipped capital femoral epiphysis. The image on the right (left hip) is normal. *(From Yamamoto LG: Thigh and Knee Pain in an Obese 10-Year Old. Radiology Cases in Pediatric Emergency Medicine 2 [case 10]. University of Hawaii John A. Burns School of Medicine.)*

have an abnormal position in relation to the metaphysis. If a moderate or severe slip, the appearance resembles ice cream sliding off of a cone. A Klein line is drawn along the superior border of the femoral neck, and it normally intersects a small portion of the femoral epiphysis. If the Klein line does not intersect the epiphysis at all, it supports the diagnosis of a subtle SCFE (Fig. 28.13).

19. How do you tell an avulsion fracture of the proximal fifth metatarsal from a normal apophysis?

An avulsion fracture at the base of the fifth metatarsal, attachment site of the peroneus brevis, is a common fracture in children. The mechanism of injury for this type of fracture is plantar flexion with forced inversion of the foot and ankle. On physical exam, the patient will have tenderness and potentially swelling and bruising over the fifth metatarsal. A radiograph of an avulsion fracture (Fig. 28.14) usually shows a fracture *perpendicular* to the long axis of the fifth metatarsal. The normal apophysis of the fifth metatarsal (Fig. 28.15) becomes visible on radiographs between ages 9 and 14 and appears as a small fleck of calcification lying parallel to the shaft of the fifth metatarsal. A comparison view of the normal foot may also be helpful.

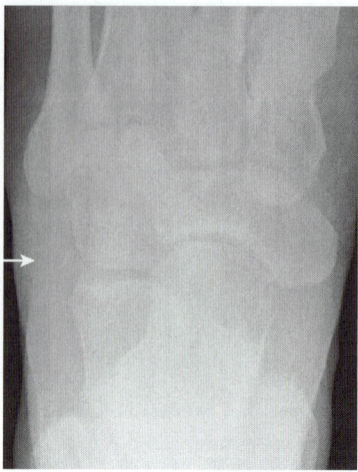

Fig. 28.14. Tuberosity avulsion fracture. Note that the radiolucency is perpendicular to the long axis of the fifth metatarsal. *(From Ankle and Foot.* Musculoskeletal Trauma: A Guide to Assessment and Diagnosis. *1st ed. Philadelphia: Churchill Livingstone, 2011. 265-300.)*

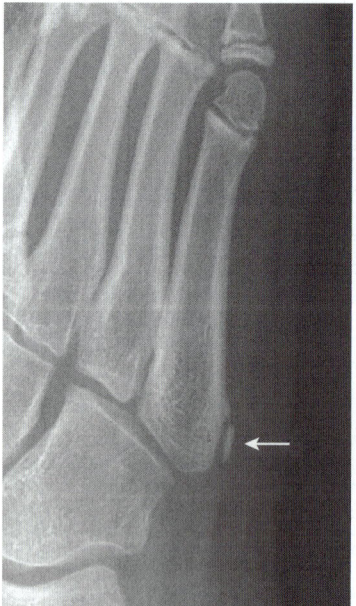

Fig. 28.15. Apophysis *(arrow)* of the base of the fifth metatarsal. Note the oblique orientation with the radiolucency aligned in parallel to the fifth metatarsal diaphysis. *(From Keats, Theodore E, Strouse, Peter J: Anatomic Variants.* Caffey's Pediatric Diagnostic Imaging. *Elsevier; 2008.)*

20. What are the Ottawa ankle rules and what is their applicability to kids?

The Ottawa ankle rules are physical exam findings that help predict the likelihood of an osseous ankle injury. Ankle radiographs are suggested if there is pain in the malleolar region with any of the following: (1) bone tenderness at the posterior edge or the tip of the lateral malleolus, (2) bone tenderness at the posterior edge or the tip of the medial malleolus, and/or (3) inability to bear weight for at least four steps both immediately after the injury and at the time of evaluation. Pooled data from several small trials suggest the rules are likely useful in children, but some studies have shown diminished sensitivity in comparison to adult cohorts.

KEY POINTS

1. The Salter-Harris classification describes growth plate fractures and has five levels (I–V) that guide acute management as well as overall prognosis.
2. Fractures concerning for NAT include femur and spiral extremity fractures in preambulatory children, multiple fractures in various stages of healing, chip fractures of the metaphysis, and bucket handle fractures.
3. Torus, greenstick, and bowing fractures are often collectively referred to as "plastic fractures" and are unique to children as a result of the pliability of the pediatric skeleton.
4. Toddler's fractures are subtle radiographic fractures and involve the distal third of the tibia in ambulatory preschool children.
5. The Ottawa ankle rules recommend ankle radiographs if there is bony pain at the medial or lateral malleolus along with an inability to bear weight after an ankle injury.

BIBLIOGRAPHY

Bachman D, Santora S. Orthopedic trauma. In: Fleisher GR, Ludwig S, eds. *Textbook of Pediatric Emergency Medicine*. 5th ed. Philadelphia: Lippincott Williams & Wilkins; 2006:1538.

Baren JM, Rothrock SG, Brennan JA, eds. *Pediatric Emergency Medicine*. Philadelphia: Saunders/Elsevier; 2008:172–187.

Davenport M, Nesbit C. An evidence based approach to pediatric orthopedic emergencies. *Pediatric Emergency Medicine Practice*. 2009;6(5).

Fleisher GR, Ludwig S, eds. *Textbook of Pediatric Emergency Medicine*. 6th ed. Philadelphia: Wolters Kluwer/Lippincott Williams & Wilkins; 2010:1328–1373.

Marx JA, ed. *Rosen's Emergency Medicine: Concepts and Clinical Practice*. 8th ed. Philadelphia: Elsevier/Saunders; 2013:534–569, 618–642, 723–750.

Paul AR, Adamo MA. Non-accidental trauma in pediatric patients: a review of epidemiology, pathophysiology, diagnosis and treatment. *Translational Pediatrics*. 2014;3(3):195–207.

Runyon MS. Can we safely apply the Ottawa ankle rules to children? *Academic Emergency Medicine*. 2009;16:352–354.

Schuh IAM, Whitlock KB, Klein EJ. Management of toddler's fractures in the pediatric emergency department. *Pediatric Emergency Care (Jun 17)*. 2015.

Shadgan B, Menon M, O'Brien PJ, Reid WD. Diagnostic techniques in acute compartment syndrome of the leg. *J Orthop Trauma*. 2008;22(8):581–587.

Shea KG, Frick SL. Distal tibial and fibular fractures. In: Wilkins KE, Beaty JH, eds. *Rockwood and Wilkins' Fractures in Children*. 8th ed. Philadelphia PA: Lippincott Williams & Wilkins; 2015:1173.

CHAPTER 29

ACUTE NECK PAIN

Douglas Comeau, DO, CAQSM, FAAFP, Nicholas Pfeifer, EdM, ATC

1. **In what environment do spinal cord injuries occur most often and what percentage of those injuries involve the cervical spine?**
   The majority of spinal cord injuries are a direct result of motor vehicle accidents (MVA) (47%), falls from heights (23%), gunshot wounds/violence (14%), and sports-related activities (9%). Of these acquired spinal injuries the cervical spine accounts for 65% of MVAs, 53% of falls from heights, 37% of gunshot/violence, and 97% of diving injuries (diving is a subset of sports-related activities).

2. **When approaching a patient with a suspected acute cervical spine injury, what should the primary survey consist of?**
   First, check ABCDEs and determine if lifesaving maneuvers are needed. If patient is in stable condition, maintain inline immobilization until cervical spine is cleared.

   A – Airway: Establish and/or maintain an open airway via the jaw thrust maneuver (jaw thrust generates less cervical spine motion than the head tilt/chin lift).
   B – Breathing: Ensure the patient is breathing (look, listen, and feel for signs of breathing). If absent, rescue breathing may be needed.
   C – Circulation: Locate a palpable pulse. If absent, CPR may be needed.
   D – Disability: Identify level of consciousness by utilizing the Glasgow Coma Scale.
   E – Exposure: Remove clothing when necessary.

3. **What findings indicate cervical spine immobilization?**
   Based upon the Canadian C-Spine Rule, if the patient is >65 years old, if the patient had a dangerous mechanism of injury (fall >3 feet, axial load to head, MVA >100 km/hr, motorcycle/bicycle collision), or if there is paresthesia in the extremities, then immobilization is indicated. Additionally, if the patient was involved in a simple rear-end MVA, is sitting or standing independently at any time, has delayed onset of neck pain, or has no midline C-spine tenderness, then range of motion can be safely assessed. If the patient is unable to actively rotate the neck 45 degrees left and right, then immobilization is indicated. Once immobilized the patient should be transported for imaging (100% sensitivity, 42.5% specificity).
   The National Emergency X-Radiography Utilization Study (NEXUS) can be used to determine low-risk patients who do not require immobilization and imaging. If there is no midline tenderness, no focal neurologic deficit, normal alertness, no intoxication, and no painful distracting injuries, then the patient does not require immobilization and imaging (99.6% sensitivity, 12.9% specificity).

4. **What is the optimal method of immobilization for clinically significant acute cervical spine injuries?**
   The most stable form of biomechanical immobilization is obtained through the use of a rigid cervical collar, rigid spine board, and head immobilization once on the board. The inclusion of strapping furthers the biomechanical immobilization of the thoracolumbar spine.

5. **Which imaging modality should be utilized when assessing acute cervical spine injuries?**
   In adults and adolescents computed tomography (CT) scans should be utilized as the initial imaging modality of choice due to superior sensitivity and specificity. If unavailable, radiographs can be utilized (anterior-posterior, lateral, atlantoaxial views). Radiographs should be used for children to limit radiation exposure.

6. **What are some commonly seen upper cervical spine (C1–C2) injuries?**
   See Table 29.1.

Table 29.1. Common Upper Cervical Spine (C1–C2) Injuries

MECHANISM OF SPINAL INJURY	STABILITY
Flexion	
Flexion teardrop fracture	Extremely unstable
Bilateral facet dislocation	Always unstable
Atlantooccipital dislocation	Unstable
Anterior atlantoaxial dislocation with/without fracture	Unstable
Odontoid fracture with lateral displacement fracture	Unstable
Subluxation	Potentially unstable
Wedge fracture	Stable
Transverse process fracture	Stable
Clay shoveler's fracture	Stable
Flexion-Rotation	
Rotary atlantoaxial dislocation	Unstable
Unilateral facet dislocation	Stable
Extension	
Posterior neural arch fracture (C1)	Unstable
Hangman fracture (C2)	Unstable
Posterior atlantoaxial dislocation with/without fracture	Unstable
Extension teardrop fracture	Usually stable in extension
Compression	
Jefferson fracture (C1)	Extremely unstable
Burst fracture of vertebral body	Stable
Isolated fracture of articular pillar and vertebral body	Stable

Kanwar R, et al: Emergency Department Evaluation and Treatment of Cervical Spine Injuries. *Emerg Med Clin N Am* 33:241-282, 2015.

7. What are some commonly seen lower cervical spine (C3–C7) injuries?
See Table 29.2.

8. Can there be isolated soft tissue injuries in the cervical spine?
Yes, these types of injuries are referred to as whiplash injuries and typically occur from hyperflexion/hyperextension acceleration mechanisms. They result in muscular spasm and muscle strains and can also cause ligamentous sprains and instability. They should be managed with active physical therapy and not be immobilized if stability is not compromised.

9. What are stingers/burners?
Stingers/burners are traction or compression injuries to the nerve roots or the brachial plexus, which result in neuropraxia. They present with shooting pain from the neck/shoulder to the hand with associated paresthesia, numbness, burning, or weakness.

10. Are these injuries an emergency?
No, typically symptoms will resolve after a few minutes. As long as there are no additional injuries present (to the spine, brain, spinal cord), it is safe to return the patient to sports participation once symptoms resolve and motor/sensory function is completely restored.

11. Can the spinal cord be injured without damaging bony structures?
Yes, this type of injury is referred to as spinal cord injury without radiographic abnormality (SCIWORA). This is predominately an injury found in children due to their hypermobile joints/lax ligaments, and

Table 29.2. Common Lower Cervical Spine (C3–C7) Injuries	
MECHANISM OF INJURY	**STABILITY**
Flexion	
Bilateral facet dislocation	Extremely unstable
Flexion teardrop fracture	Unstable
Posterior ligamentous injury	Severe = unstable; mild = stable
Wedge fracture	Stable
Compression fracture	Stable
Clay shoveler's fracture	Stable
Flexion-Rotation	
Unilateral facet dislocation with/without fracture	Stable
Extension	
Extension teardrop fracture	Usually stable in extension
Compression	
Burst fracture	Stable

Kanwar R, et al: Emergency Department Evaluation and Treatment of Cervical Spine Injuries. *Emerg Med Clin N Am* 33:241-282, 2015.

there is transient vertebral displacement and subsequent realignment that results in a damaged spinal cord. Normal alignment will be appreciated on radiographs, but evidence of spinal cord injury can be found on magnetic resonance imaging (MRI).

12. When should there be concern for a vascular injury?

Although blunt cerebrovascular injury is uncommon, it carries a high risk of permanent neurologic deficits. Indications for screening for vascular injury are:

- Unexplained neurologic deficits in patients with hyperextension/hyperflexion injuries
- Severe blunt trauma to neck or a seat belt injury
- Cervical spine or skull base fractures adjacent to or involving vascular foramina
- Le Fort II or Le Fort III facial fractures

Digital subtraction angiography is considered the gold standard of diagnosing cerebrovascular injuries.

KEY POINTS

1. Sports with the highest rate of acute cervical spine injuries include American football, wrestling, diving, ice hockey, skiing/snowboarding, and gymnastics.
2. Initial cervical spine injury management should be to establish ABCDE (airway, breathing, circulation, disability, and exposure) and then to maintain inline immobilization until serious injury can be cleared.
3. The NEXUS (National Emergency X-Radiography Utilization Study) criteria and the Canadian C-Spine Rule are highly sensitive decision-making tools that provide guidelines of when to immobilize and obtain imaging following acute injury.
4. CT scans are the preferred imaging modalities for acute injury diagnostics of adolescents and adults. Radiographs remain the gold standard for children.

BIBLIOGRAPHY

Ahn H, et al. Pre-hospital care management of a potential spinal cord injury patient: a systematic review of the literature and evidence-based guidelines. *J Neurotrauma.* 2011;28(8):1341–1361.

Banerjee R, et al. Catastrophic cervical spine injuries in the collision sport athlete, part 1. *Amer J Sports Med.* 2004;32(4):1077–1087.

Casa D, et al. National athletic trainers' association position statement: preventing sudden death in sports. *Journal of Athletic Training.* 2012;47(1):96–118.

De Jonge M, Kramer J. Spine and sport. *Semin Musculoskelet Radiol.* 2014;18:246–264.

DeVivo M. Epidemiology of traumatic spinal cord injury: trends and future implications. *Spinal Cord.* 2012;50:365–372.

Grossheim L, et al. Cervical spine injury: an evidence-based evaluation of the patient with blunt cervical trauma. *Emer Med Prac.* 2009;11(4):1–25.

Kanwar R, et al. Emergency department evaluation and treatment of cervical spine injuries. *Emerg Med Clin N Am.* 2015;33:241–282.

Pimentel L, et al. Evaluation and management of acute cervical spine trauma. *Orthopedic Emergencies.* 2010;28(4):719–738.

Standaert C, Herring S. Expert opinion and controversies in musculoskeletal and sports medicine: stingers. *Arch Phys Med Rehabil.* 2009;90(3):402–406.

Stiell I, et al. The Canadian C-spine rule versus the NEXUS low-risk criteria in patients with trauma. *N Engl J Med.* 2003;349:2510–2518.

Walton D, et al. Risk factors for persistent problems following acute whiplash injury: update of a systematic review and meta-analysis. *JOSPT.* 2013;43(2):31–43.

CHAPTER 30

EVALUATION AND MANAGEMENT OF ACUTE SPRAINS AND STRAINS

Lauren Borowski, MD, Laura Lintner, DO

ACHILLES TENDON DISORDERS

1. **Describe the four cornerstones in tendon histopathology and why these changes cause pain.**
   - Cellular activation and increased cell number
   - Increase in ground substance
   - Collagen disarray
   - Neovascularization

   Although the pain pathways of chronic tendinopathy are not completely understood, cDNA – arrays, polymerase chain reaction (PCR), and ultrasonography have provided potentially important information in regard to the origins of chronic Achilles tendinosis. High levels of glutamate, a neurotransmitter and pain modulator, have been found in painful tendons and not in normal tendons. Chronic tendinopathy is associated with neovascularization. Biopsies taken from areas of tendinopathy have shown nerve structures in close relationship with the vascular supply. This may explain the pain associated with tendinosis.

2. **How is Achilles tendonitis diagnosed?**
   It is important to first rule out Achilles tendon rupture, as the management for this injury is significantly different. The calf squeeze test, or Thompson test, can aid in this exclusion. The diagnosis of Achilles tendonitis can be made clinically, especially if the tendon exhibits swelling. The pain will likely be reproduced by loading the tendon (i.e., single leg heel raise). Keep in mind, some athletes may require repetitive heel raises to reproduce pain. Imaging should be reserved for those cases with concern for rupture or if the clinical diagnosis is not clear.

3. **Once an Achilles tendon strain (or acute Achilles tendonitis) has been diagnosed, what are the specific treatment options?**
   Although scientific evidence for most treatments is limited, some treatments that have been investigated with randomized, controlled trials and demonstrated effectiveness include eccentric exercise, glyceryl trinitrate patches, electrotherapy, sclerosing injections, and nonsteroidal antiinflammatory drugs (NSAIDs). Rest, NSAIDs, changing shoes to provide more arch support, and physical therapy are the mainstays of treatment. Achilles tendonitis is often caused by overpronation of the foot and overuse. This is why rest and improving biomechanics of the foot (using orthosis and physical therapy) can be beneficial.

4. **When does an Achilles tendon injury need to be referred to an orthopedic surgeon?**
   Patients should be referred when there is a concern for an Achilles tendon rupture. The typical presentation includes a history of a sudden "pop" at the back of the heel with subsequent pain. The examination commonly includes a positive Thompson test (Fig. 30.1), which proves disruption of the musculotendinous junction (squeezing the calf muscle does not lead to foot plantarflexion, or plantarflexes weaker than the contralateral side). Not all Achilles tendon ruptures require surgical repair; however, it is important to have a specialist evaluate and discuss the best approach on an individualized basis.

5. **How should suspected Achilles tendon ruptures be diagnosed and what is considered appropriate initial management when concerned for an Achilles tendon rupture?**
   The diagnosis is often made clinically. Ultrasound is an emerging imaging modality that can also confirm this diagnosis by evaluating tendon continuity. Magnetic resonance imaging (MRI) is

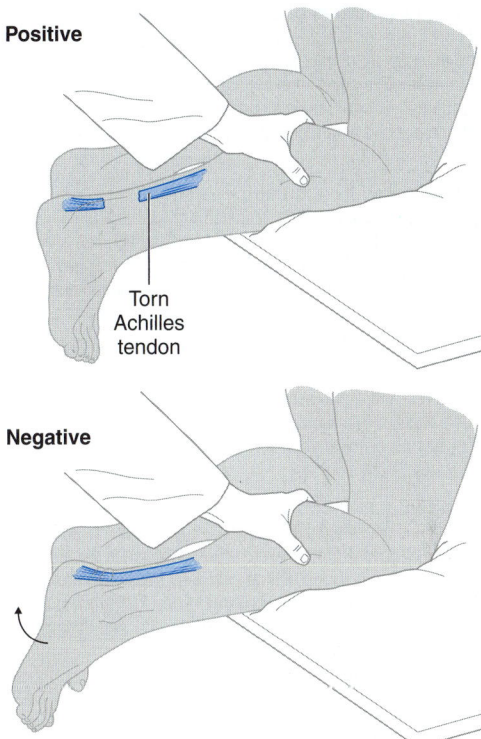

Positive

Torn
Achilles
tendon

Negative

Fig. 30.1. Thompson test for Achilles tear. *(From Stretanski MF. Achilles Tendonitis. In: Frontera WR, Silvis JK, Rizzo TD, et al. Essentials of Physical Medicine and Rehabilitation. 2nd ed. Copyright 2008. Saunders, Elsevier Inc. Reprinted in Orthopedic Secrets. 4th ed. Copyright 2015. Saunders, Elsevier Inc.)*

typically not needed but may be of benefit in cases where the history and physical examination are nonspecific and clinically concern persists. If there is concern for Achilles tendon rupture, the patient should be placed in a splint or boot with slight plantar flexion.

KEY POINTS: ACHILLES TENDON DISORDERS

1. Achilles tendon disorders include the following: Achilles tendonitis (most common), Achilles chronic tendinopathy, and Achilles tendon rupture.
2. The Thompson test is used to aid in the diagnosis of an Achilles tendon rupture. It is positive when plantar flexion is weaker on the injured side compared to the uninjured lower extremity.
3. The mainstay of treatment for Achilles tendonitis is rest, ice, compression, and elevation, which all work together to decrease inflammation.

QUADRICEPS STRAIN

6. **What is the most common mechanism for a quadriceps strain?**
   Acute strains commonly occur in sports that regularly require a kicking motion, such as soccer, rugby, and football. This motion is described as a sudden forceful eccentric contraction of the quadriceps during regulation of knee flexion and hip extension. Another mechanism of quadriceps strain is with excessive passive stretching of a maximally stretched muscle.

7. **What is the most common quadriceps muscle to be strained?**
   Rectus femoris. This muscle crosses both the hip and knee joint as it originates at the anterior inferior iliac spine and inserts at the quadriceps tendon onto the patella.

8. **What is the typical presentation of a quadriceps strain?**

Patients will complain of pain localized to the quadriceps muscle, often at the distal aspect, and have an appropriate mechanism of injury. They may report a slightly delayed onset of pain to the end of a game or event. The physical examination may include a muscle defect or bulge, ecchymosis, and tenderness. There may also be weakness noted on strength testing. Complete weakness indicates the possibility of a complete tendon rupture and should be referred urgently to an orthopedic surgeon.

9. **When is imaging indicated for a quadriceps strain?**

Imaging is not necessary to diagnose a quadriceps strain but should be utilized when there is concern for associated injuries or when the diagnosis is uncertain. Radiographs are normal in a quadriceps strain. Ultrasound can be helpful in making the diagnosis by showing hematoma formation and possible muscle fiber disruption. MRI can provide detailed information on muscle injury but is typically not necessary to diagnose a quadriceps strain.

10. **When a patient sustains a quadriceps strain, what is the best appropriate initial management?**

Acute phase treatment: rest, ice, compression, and elevation are all recommended to minimize bleeding in the injured muscle. This should be maintained for the initial 1–3 days. In more severe strains, crutches may be necessary to allow for rest of the muscle. NSAID use can be helpful but should be limited to a 3- to 7-day course.

11. **What is the best approach to continued therapy and directions on return to play?**

Active phase treatment: This phase typically begins 3–5 days after the initial injury and includes stretching, strengthening, range-of-motion exercises, maintenance of aerobic fitness, proprioceptive exercises, and functional training. Strengthening exercises should be introduced gradually, depending on the level of soreness. There are no established guidelines for returning to play, but the patient should have normal hip and knee range of motion, be pain free, and demonstrate normal strength as well as perform functional sport-specific testing.

12. **Name a complication of a quadriceps strain.**

Myositis ossificans results from proliferation of bone and cartilage in the area of a contusion injury to a muscle. This should be suspected if symptoms worsen after 2–3 weeks and is also accompanied by loss of range of motion. Radiographs are diagnostic. If athletes do not have recovery with conservative management, then surgical excision may be necessary.

KEY POINTS: QUADRICEPS STRAIN

1. The most common mechanism for a quadriceps strain is a kicking motion, or a sudden forceful eccentric contraction of the quadriceps muscle.
2. The most common muscle strained is the rectus femoris.
3. Myositis ossificans is a complication of a quadriceps strain defined by the growth of bone and cartilage in the injured area of the muscle.

LATERAL EPICONDYLITIS (TENNIS ELBOW)

13. **Which muscles and tendons are involved in lateral epicondylitis?**

The common extensor tendon that originates from the lateral epicondyle of the elbow is directly involved. The extensor carpi radialis brevis (ECRB) and longus, extensor digitorum, extensor digiti minimi, and extensor carpi ulnaris come together to form the common extensor tendon. The extensor carpi radialis brevis is almost always the primary tendon involved.

14. **Is lateral epicondylitis caused by inflammation of the tendons?**

No. Epicondylitis is a chronic tendinosis rather than an acute inflammatory process. Histologic studies of affected tendons show degenerative changes with fibroblastic proliferation leading to disorganized tissue and neovascularization.

15. **What are the risk factors for developing tennis elbow?**

Repetitive motions of the wrist into extension, forceful grasping and gripping movements, and rotary movements of the arm (e.g., using a screwdriver or wrench) are commonly implicated. Lateral epicondylitis is common in racquet sport athletes and those who perform a lot of manual labor.

16. What physical examination tests aid in the diagnosis?

Localized tenderness to palpation over the lateral epicondyle and distally along the common extensor origin. The Cozen test is often used and is performed by having the patient resist wrist extension with the elbow straightened. Having the patient hold the middle finger against resistance in full extension also reliably reproduces pain. This movement directly tests the ECRB, the primary tendon involved, as its insertion onto the third metacarpal.

17. What other diagnoses should be considered?

- Posterior interosseous nerve compression
- Radiocapitellar arthritis
- Cervical radiculopathy
- Thoracic outlet syndrome
- Inflammatory arthritis
- Myofascial pain

18. What are common treatments?

Rest and activity modification are the mainstays of treatment. Bracing, NSAIDs, icing, and soft tissue mobilization can also be helpful. Use of a sling may be warranted if pain is severe. A local injection of corticosteroid and anesthetic often provide great short-term relief and can sometimes be curative. Operative treatment is reserved for those who have failed conservative management and only after other causes of lateral elbow pain have been excluded. Surgical management often includes release of the common extensor tendon origin.

KEY POINTS: LATERAL EPICONDYLITIS

1. The common extensor tendon origin is the area most involved.
2. Extensor carpi brevis radialis is almost always the specific tendon affected.
3. It is not a true inflammatory process.
4. Repetitive and rotary movements or forceful gripping increases risk.
5. Localized tenderness to palpation over lateral epicondyle and pain with resisted wrist and third finger extension can help to diagnose.

PATELLAR TENDINOPATHY

19. What is another name for patellar tendinopathy?

Jumper's knee (diagnosed frequently in jumping sports). Sometimes referred to as patellar tendonitis. However, patellar tendinopathy can occur in any active person, not just those who jump or change direction. The term "patellar tendonitis" is also misleading, much like lateral epicondylitis, as the underlying pathology is noninflammatory.

20. How do patients typically present?

Anterior knee pain, often worsened by jumping, decelerating, and changing direction, is the most common presentation. There is often tenderness to palpation of the inferior pole of the patella, occasionally extending into the body of the tendon. Applying pressure to the superior pole of the patella tilts the inferior pole, which gives the examiner the ability to better palpate the tendon origin. Pain with squatting and hopping can help to diagnose as well as monitor recovery.

21. What is the most common part of the tendon affected?

The area of tendon attachment to the inferior pole of the patella is most commonly involved. The distal tendon near the tibial insertion is less commonly involved, and midsubstance issues are rarely documented.

22. What is the differential diagnosis?

- Patellar tendon rupture
- Patellofemoral syndrome
- Osgood Schlatter Disease

23. How does tendinopathy appear on imaging?

Increased signal is often seen on MRI, and areas of hypoechogenicity are commonly seen on ultrasound. Ultrasound with Doppler can assess vascularity in the area in question and is more sensitive than MRI.

24. What is the typical management of patellar tendinopathy?

Patellar tendinopathy is often present for months prior to the patient seeking evaluation of pain. Recovery from the condition can take weeks to months. Conservative management includes strengthening of the surrounding musculature, load reduction, and correction of biomechanical errors. Injections of autologous blood and platelet-rich plasma are currently being studied for their effectiveness.

KEY POINTS: PATELLAR TENDINOPATHY

1. Patellar tendinopathy is also referred to as jumper's knee and patellar tendonitis.
2. Presents with anterior knee pain worsened by movements of jumping, decelerating, or changing directions.
3. Tenderness on palpation of the inferior pole of the patella.
4. Pain in the area with squatting or hopping helps to diagnose and is useful in monitoring recovery.
5. The portion of tendon involved appears hypoechoic on ultrasound.
6. Conservative management includes strengthening of the surrounding musculature, load reduction, and adjustment of biomechanics. Surgery is reserved for failed lengthy conservative treatment plans.
7. Other diagnoses should be considered, particularly if there is no improvement with conservative treatment.

BIBLIOGRAPHY

Alfredson H, Cook J. A treatment algorithm for managing Achilles tendinopathy: new treatment options. *Brh J Sports Med.* 2007;41(4):211–216. http://dx.doi.org/10.1136/bjsm.2007.035543.

Crossley K, Cook J, Cowan S, McConnell J. Anterior Knee Pain. In: Brukner Kahn, eds. *Clinical Sports Medicine*. 4th ed. Australia: McGraw-Hill Education. 2014; 2014.

Jones T. Rectus Femoris Strain. Available on: http://www.orthobullets.com/sports/3104/rectus-femoris-strain. Accessed on 25.07.16.

Karadsheh M. Achilles Tendon Rupture. Available on: http://www.orthobullets.com/foot-and-ankle/7021/achilles-tendon-rupture. Accessed 25.07.16.

Kary J. Diagnosis and management of quadriceps strains and contusions. *Current Review Musculoskeletal Medicine.* 2010;3:26–31.

LeBlond RF, Brown DD, Suneja M, Szot JF. The Spine, Pelvis, and Extremities. In: LeBlond RF, Brown DD, Suneja M, Szot JF, eds. *DeGowin's Diagnostic Examination*. 10th ed. New York: McGraw-Hill; 2015. http://accessmedicine.mhmedical.com/content.aspx?bookid=1192&Sectionid=68669600.

McMahon PJ, Kaplan LD, Popkin CA. Chapter 3. Sports Medicine. In: Skinner HB, McMahon PJ, eds. *Current Diagnosis & Treatment in Orthopedics*. 5th ed. New York: McGraw-Hill; 2014. http://accessmedicine.mhmedical.com/content.aspx?bookid=675&Sectionid=45451709.

Metzl JA, Ahmad CS, Levine WN. The ruptured Achilles tendon: operative and non-operative treatment options. *Current Reviews in Musculoskeletal Medicine.* 2008;1(2):161–164. http://dx.doi.org/10.1007/s12178-008-9025-4.

Rempel DM, Amirtharajah M, Descatha A. Shoulder, Elbow, & Hand Injuries. In: LaDou J, Harrison RJ, eds. *CURRENT Diagnosis & Treatment: Occupational & Environmental Medicine*. 5th ed. New York: McGraw-Hill; 2013. http://accessmedicine.mhmedical.com/content.aspx?bookid=1186&Sectionid=66478559.

Tosti R, Jennings J, Sewards JM. Lateral epicondylitis of the elbow. *Am J Med.* 2013 Apr 8;126(4):357.e1–e6. [Epub 2013 Feb 8].

CHAPTER 31

ACUTE LOW BACK PAIN

Susannah Lichtenstein, DO, Christopher Miles, MD, CAQSM

INTRODUCTION

Acute low back pain (ALBP) is defined as less than 6 weeks of pain between the costal angles and gluteal folds. This may be accompanied by radicular pain, which radiates down one or both legs and may indicate irritation of a nerve root.

Low back pain (LBP) is the fifth most common reason for medical office visits in the United States and a leading cause of work-related disability. Only about 1% of patients with ALBP in the primary care setting have a serious underlying cause.

1. **What is the differential diagnosis of ALBP?**
   The differential diagnosis of ALBP is broad and may be categorized into mechanical, nonmechanical, and visceral (Table 31.1). Most patients who present with ALBP are diagnosed with nonspecific, mechanical-type pain.

2. **What are emergent causes of ALBP that should prompt referral to the emergency department (ED)?**
   - Cauda equina syndrome (CES); occurs when there is compression on the lower spinal nerve roots that results in urinary retention or incontinence, bilateral lower extremity weakness, and/or saddle anesthesia
   - Spinal fracture
   - Infection (e.g., epidural abscess, vertebral osteomyelitis)
   - Cancer (CA)

3. **What symptoms/historical details are red flags that should prompt referral to the ED?**
   - Severe or progressive neurologic deficits (e.g., those seen in CES).
   - Trauma. Suspect fracture when there has been a significant mechanism of injury, including motor vehicle collision >35 mph, fall >15 feet, or automobile versus pedestrian.
   - Patient has a history of or risk factors for CA or osteoporosis and presents with sudden onset of LBP after a minor fall or heavy lifting. Suspect pathologic or compression fracture.
   - Fever, constitutional symptoms, or risk factors for infection. Risk factors for infection include immune compromise or immunosuppression (human immunodeficiency virus [HIV]/acquired immunodeficiency syndrome [AIDS], alcoholism, diabetes, chronic steroid use), intravenous drug use, recent spinal surgery or injection, or recent bacterial infection.
   - Known CA history or worsening LBP >4 weeks that is worse at night, not responsive to analgesics, and associated with unintentional weight loss and/or night sweats.

Table 31.1. Differential Diagnosis of Acute Low Back Pain

MECHANICAL	NONMECHANICAL	VISCERAL
• Muscle strain	• Cancer	• Pelvic organ disease
• Sacroiliac joint dysfunction	• Infection	• Renal disease
• Degenerative disease	• Inflammatory arthritis	• Abdominal aortic aneurysm
• Disc herniation	• Scheuermann kyphosis	• Gastrointestinal disease
• Spinal stenosis	• Paget disease	
• Spondylolysis/spondylolisthesis		
• Fracture		
• Apophyseal injury		
• Congenital disease		

4. **What additional historical features, symptoms, or signs that may not be as concerning in adults are unique red flags for children? (Note: The above red flags are ALSO red flags for children.)**
   - Age <4 years
   - Pain that interferes with daily activity
   - Limp or altered gait
   - Back pain despite no clear mechanism of injury
   - Acute or repetitive trauma

5. **List key exam findings that are red flags and might suggest a concerning etiology.**
   - Fever.
   - Midline tenderness: Sensitive but not specific for spinal infection, cancer, and compression fracture.
   - Sensory or motor deficit: Abnormal neurologic exam of the lower extremities (strength, sensation, reflexes, gait) or loss of anal sphincter tone.
   - Straight leg raise (SLR): With the patient supine, knee extended, and ankle dorsiflexed, passive hip flexion of the affected leg to 30–60 degrees reproduces radicular pain. Suggests nerve root irritation, most commonly at L5 or S1 and often caused by a herniated disc.
   - Crossed SLR: SLR of the unaffected leg reproduces radicular pain in the affected leg and suggests nerve root irritation.
   - Slump test: While seated, the patient slumps forward, flexing the cervical, thoracic, and lumbar spine. The patient then extends the knee and dorsiflexes the ankle on the affected side. This reproduces radicular pain in the affected leg. Pain should then decrease with cervical spine extension. May better detect irritation to upper lumbar nerve roots.

6. **When is imaging indicated in the evaluation of ALBP?**
   For both adults and children, consider imaging when patients present with red flags on history or exam that raise suspicion for a serious underlying condition (cauda equina syndrome, fracture, infection, or CA).

7. **Which imaging modality is appropriate? Which views? (Fig. 31.1)**
   - X-ray lumbar spine to assess for lytic lesions or fracture in patients with ALBP and red flags for CA or fracture. Standing anteroposterior (AP) and lateral views are typically sufficient. Obtain additional bilateral oblique views if there is concern for a pars interarticularis fracture (spondylolysis). Lateral flexion and extension views may be helpful if there is concern for instability (e.g., spondylolisthesis).
   - MRI in patients with ALBP and red flags for spinal infection, cauda equina syndrome, or spinal cord compression/injury.
   - CT without contrast for blunt trauma from a significant mechanism of injury (defined in question 3) with any of the following: back pain or midline tenderness, local signs of thoracolumbar injury, abnormal neurologic exam, cervical spine fracture, altered level of consciousness, major distracting injury, or alcohol or drug intoxication.

8. **Are labs indicated in the evaluation of ALBP?**
   If history or exam reveals red flags concerning for infection or malignancy, obtain a complete blood count (CBC) and erythrocyte sedimentation rate (ESR). See Fig. 31.1.

9. **How should patients with nonspecific, mechanical ALBP pain be treated in the outpatient setting?**
   - Education: Discuss expected course and establish goals of treatment. ALBP is often self-limited. With self-care, 75% of cases resolve within 4 weeks and 90% within 6 weeks. Treatment should focus on improving pain and function as well as reducing time away from work. Patients should stay active and avoid bed rest.
   - Pharmacologic: Nonsteroidal antiinflammatory drugs (NSAIDs) or acetaminophen are first line. After discussing potential adverse effects, consider the addition of a muscle relaxant. For patients with severe pain who are not responding to or are unlikely to respond to these options, the short-term use of opioids may be appropriate, after carefully weighing the risks and benefits. Current evidence does not support the use of systemic steroids.
   - Nonpharmacologic: Superficial heat is helpful in reducing pain and improving function.
   - Follow-up: Educate patient on red flags (discussed above), which should prompt return. Otherwise, patient should follow up with primary doctor in 4–6 weeks if the pain is not improving.

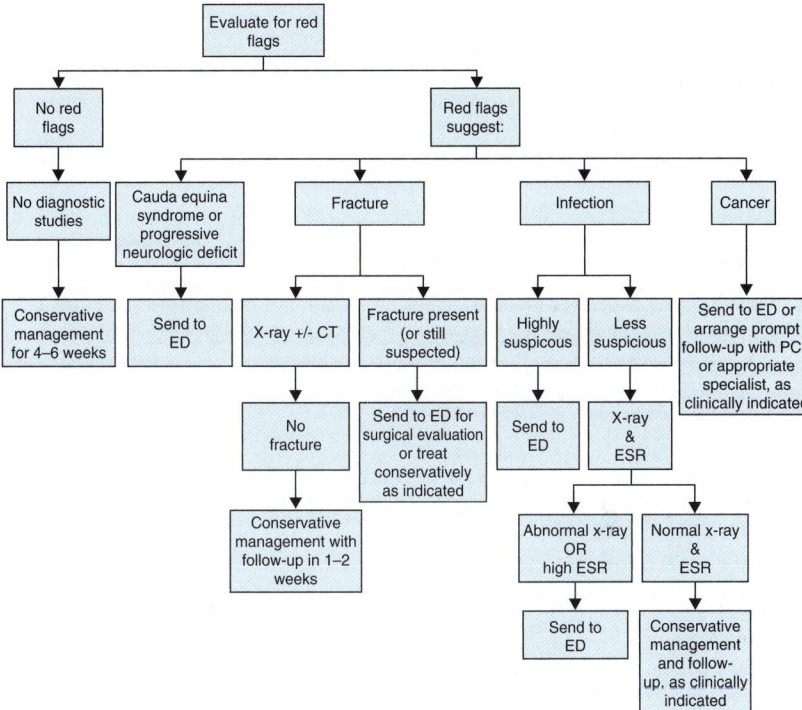

Fig. 31.1. Evaluation of acute low back pain.

10. **In the absence of red flags, what should you recommend regarding return to play (RTP)? Return to work?**
   - The athlete may RTP when the pain has resolved at rest and with activity. Consider sports medicine consultation for guidance on RTP.
   - The patient should continue to work as pain permits, with possible job modifications. Refer to local regulations for workers compensation cases.

11. **Colin is an otherwise healthy 14-year-old high school wrestler presenting to urgent care with 4 weeks of low back pain. It is occasionally present at rest but worsens with activity. He has tried over-the-counter (OTC) ibuprofen with little benefit. He denies trauma, fevers, weight loss, nighttime pain, radiation of pain, paresthesias, or weakness. On exam, he has mild tenderness to deep palpation at L5, and his pain worsens with lumbar extension. Neurologic exam of his lower extremities is normal. He sees you to determine if he can continue to wrestle. Which of the following is the next step in management?**
   A. Given no systemic or neurologic red flags, he may continue to wrestle.
   B. Obtain plain films of the lumbar spine, including AP, lateral, and oblique views.
   C. Obtain an MRI of the lumbar spine.
   D. Refer to orthopedic surgery.
   The correct answer is B. Colin is presenting with symptoms and signs concerning for spondylolysis, a stress fracture of the pars interarticularis. This is a common cause of LBP in adolescent athletes. Oblique view x-rays should be obtained if spondylolysis is suspected, as these views may show a defect in the pars (scotty dog lesion). When x-ray findings are normal and spondylolysis is still suspected, additional imaging should be performed. Bone scintigraphy with single photon emission computed tomography (SPECT) followed by CT if positive is preferred. MRI is an alternative but is less sensitive for detecting acute stress reaction of the pars interarticularis.

KEY POINTS

1. Know the red flags that should prompt urgent/emergent evaluation.
2. Most patients do not need imaging.
3. Medical management should begin with NSAIDs or acetaminophen. Short-term muscle relaxants or opioids may be appropriate in selected patients.
4. Encourage patients to stay active. Bed rest is NOT helpful for acute low back pain (ALBP).
5. Follow-up should occur in 4–6 weeks if symptoms are not improving.

BIBLIOGRAPHY

Atlas SJ, Deyo RA. Evaluating and managing acute low back pain the primary care setting. *J Gen Intern Med*. 2001;16(2):120–131.

Bernstein RM, Cozen H. Evaluation of back pain in children and adolescents. *Am Fam Physician*. 2007;76:1669–1676.

Chou R, Huffman LH. Nonpharmacologic therapies for acute and chronic low back pain: a review of the evidence for an American Pain Society/American College of Physicians clinical practice guideline. *Ann Intern Med*. 2007;147(7):492–504.

Chou R, Qaseem A, Snow V, et al. Diagnosis and treatment of low back pain: a joint clinical practice guideline from the American College of Physicians and the American Pain Society. *Ann Intern Med*. 2007;147(7):478–491.

Chou R. In the clinic. Low back pain. *Ann Intern Med*. 2014;160(11). ITC6-1-16.

Daffner RH, Weissman BN, Wippold FJ, et al. ACR Appropriateness Criteria® Suspected Spine Trauma. American College of Radiology. <https://acsearch.acr.org/docs/69359/Narrative/>; Accessed 03.01.16.

Duffy RL. Low back pain: an approach to diagnosis and management. *Prim Care*. 2010;37(4):61–63.

Faerber EN, Kan JH, Newman B, et al. ACR-ASSR-SPR-SSR Practice Parameter for the Performance of Spine Radiography. American College of Radiology. <http://www.acr.org/~/media/03586F4164384C6C995E83CE68A5C835.pdf >; Accessed 21.06.16.

Henschke N, Maher CG, Refshauge KM, et al. Prevalence of and screening for serious spinal pathology in patients presenting to primary care settings with acute low back pain. *Arthritis Rheum*. 2009;60:3072–3080.

Hollingworth P. Back pain in children. *Br J Rheumatol*. 1996;35(10):1022–1028.

Majlesi J, Togay H, Unalan H, et al. The sensitivity and specificity of the slump and the straight leg raising tests in patients with lumbar disc herniation. *J Clin Rheumatol*. 2008;14(2):87–91.

Masci L, Pike J, Malara F, et al. Use of the one-legged hyperextension test and magnetic resonance imaging in the diagnosis of activity spondylolysis. *Br J Sports Med*. 2006;40(11):940–946.

Patel ND, Broderick DF, Burns J, et al. ACR Appropriateness Criteria® Low Back Pain. American College of Radiology. <https://acsearch.acr.org/docs/69483/Narrative/>; Accessed 03.01.16.

CHAPTER 32

THE ACUTELY SWOLLEN KNEE

Abbie Kelley, DO, Mark Lavallee, MD, CSCS, FACSM

1. Why is it important to be competent in evaluating an acutely swollen knee?

The knee is the most frequently injured joint in the body, and an acutely swollen knee is a common presentation of knee pathology in the emergency department and primary care setting. Common causes of an effusion include inflammation, infection, and structural abnormalities in the knee. Most often, the underlying etiology can be treated conservatively until seen by orthopedics or another specialist. There are, however, a few diagnoses that need immediate treatment and close observation. Therefore, it is imperative that you formulate a comprehensive differential based on your history and physical. Diagnostic studies and laboratory tests can then be used to narrow and confirm the diagnosis (Fig. 32.1). This chapter will focus on common causes and management of an acutely swollen knee.

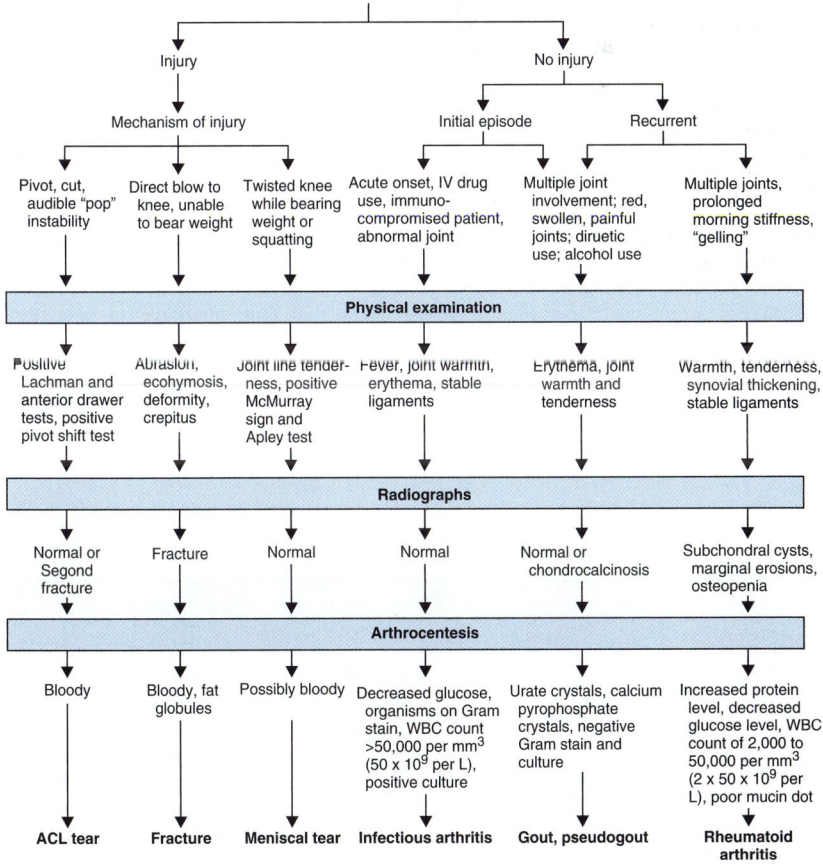

Fig. 32.1. Algorithm for the Assessment of a Swollen Knee. *(From Johnson M: Acute Knee Effusions: A Systematic Approach to Diagnosis. Am Fam Physician 61(8):2391-2400, 2000 [figure 4].)*

2. **What is the most useful question to ask in your history to determine the etiology of an acutely swollen knee?**

Is the effusion traumatic or nontraumatic? Mechanism of injury is important when evaluating a traumatic knee injury. Other key components of the history include timing of swelling after an injury, localization of pain, locking, giving way, and exacerbating factors. For a nontraumatic effusion, it is imperative to ask about fevers, night sweats, night pain, weight loss, other joints involved, and social history. You will start to formulate a solid differential based on a detailed history of present illness. Refer to Table 32.1 for a broad differential diagnosis of an acutely swollen knee.

3. **In the presence of trauma, what is the most important part of the physical examination of an acutely swollen knee?**

Neurovascular exam! Get into the habit of always starting your exam by checking distal pulses, sensation, and strength at the ankle. The popliteal artery is especially at risk in the setting of knee dislocations. If knee dislocations are not quickly identified and there is vascular compromise, a high percentage of these patients will eventually require amputation.

4. **A 17-year-old female basketball player presents to your clinic complaining of an acutely swollen knee after hearing a loud "pop" when cutting to change direction through the paint. What is the most likely diagnosis?**

Anterior cruciate ligament (ACL) rupture. ACL ruptures will typically occur after noncontact pivoting or with hyperextension of the knee. Oftentimes, a loud "pop" is heard or felt, and the patient is usually unable to continue in sport participation due to associated instability. Physical examination will reveal a positive Lachman, anterior drawer, and potentially pivot shift test. X-rays are generally unremarkable; magnetic resonance imaging (MRI) will confirm the diagnosis. Patients should be placed in a hinged knee brace until seen by orthopedics.

5. **What is a pathognomonic sign for ACL rupture on radiographs of the knee?**

Segond fracture: an avulsion fracture of the lateral tibial condyle (bony attachment of soft tissue structures) as a result of abnormal varus stress to the knee, combined with internal rotation of the tibia. The fracture is best seen on the anteroposterior (AP) view above the level of the fibular head (Fig. 32.2).

6. **A 45-year-old female presents to your clinic with a complaint of a swollen knee that started 2 days ago after accidentally stepping into a pothole when running a 5K. She notes pain along the posteromedial joint line, especially with getting into and out of the car. She admits to locking of the knee upon standing from a seated position. X-rays are normal. What is the diagnosis?**

Acute medial meniscus tear. Locking of the joint, intermittent swelling, and pain with weight-bearing twisting motions are typical of a meniscal injury. On exam, the patient is generally tender along the joint line with occasional inability to fully extend the knee. Thessaly test has a higher sensitivity and specificity in detecting a meniscal tear on exam compared to McMurray test. X-rays typically show no acute abnormality, and MRI will confirm the diagnosis. Inability to fully extend the knee is concerning for displaced "bucket handle" meniscal tear, and the patient should remain non–weight-bearing until seen by orthopedics. Treatment of other meniscal injuries will depend on the patient's symptoms, age, comorbidities, and imaging studies.

Table 32.1. Differential Diagnosis of the Acutely Swollen Knee

TRAUMATIC	NONTRAUMATIC
Ligamentous injury	Osteoarthritis
Meniscal injury	Infection (Lyme, bacterial, fungal, tuberculosis)
Knee dislocation	Crystal deposition
Patellar dislocation	Rheumatic disease
Intraarticular fracture	Tumor
Tendon rupture (quad/patellar)	Idiopathic synovitis/capsulitis
Prepatellar bursitis	Baker cyst
Baker cyst	

7. **What is the most common mechanism for isolated posterior cruciate ligament (PCL) rupture?**
   A direct blow to the anterior proximal tibia with a flexed knee or a fall onto a flexed knee with the foot plantarflexed. Most of these injuries will occur as a result of a dashboard injury in a motor vehicle accident or a high-energy collision in sport. Examination will be positive for posterior drawer test and possibly tibial sag test.

8. **How are isolated PCL injuries treated?**
   Many will be treated conservatively with protected weight-bearing and therapy for range of motion and strengthening of the affected knee.

9. **What is a pathognomonic sign on radiographs for intraarticular fracture?**
   Lipohemarthrosis (fat-fluid level) seen on the lateral view (Fig. 32.3).

10. **Who is susceptible to patellar dislocations and subluxations?**
    Patients with Down syndrome, Ehlers-Danlos syndrome, Marfan syndrome, cerebral palsy, generalized ligamentous laxity, and anatomical malalignment. Patients will generally be able to tell you that they felt their kneecap shift or slide out. On exam, patients will have a positive patellar apprehension sign and difficulty with a straight leg raise. Initial treatment should consist of immobilization of the knee.

11. **An 85-year-old male presents to your clinic complaining of progressive swelling of the left knee without injury or trauma. He describes stiffness in the morning and medial joint line pain made worse with any weight-bearing activity. What will you likely see on his weight-bearing radiographs?**
    The etiology of this gentleman's knee pain and swelling is osteoarthritis. His x-rays will show medial joint space narrowing with subchondral cysts and osteophyte formation. Typically, effusions secondary to osteoarthritis will recur after aspiration; therefore, treating the underlying cause in a progressive conservative approach is preferred. Stepwise progressive approach includes acetaminophen, NSAIDs, therapy, bracing, corticosteroid injection, viscosupplementation injections for mild to

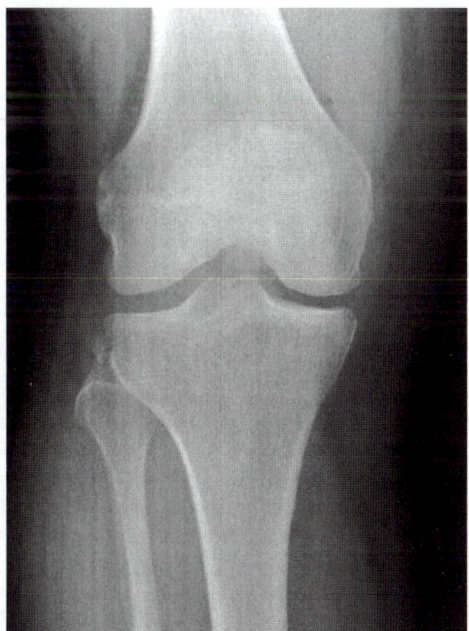

Fig. 32.2. Segond Fracture with Associated ACL Rupture. *(http://radiopaedia.org/cases/segond-fracture-3)*

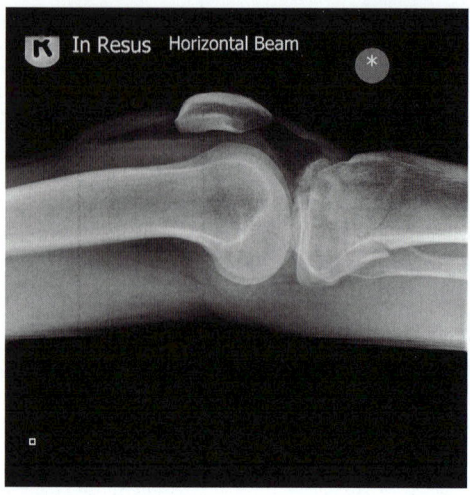

Fig. 32.3. Lipohemarthrosis with Tibial Plateau Fracture. *(http://radiopaedia.org/cases/lipohaemarthrosis-3)*

moderate arthritis, and referral to a surgeon for joint replacement. Don't forget about weight loss in overweight and obese patients! One pound of weight loss results in a fourfold load reduction across a weight-bearing joint. It is reasonable to aspirate the knee if the effusion is severe enough to cause debilitation, such as limited range of motion and pain.

12. **What are some causes of a nontraumatic, hot, painful swollen knee?**
Septic arthritis, gout, pseudogout, idiopathic synovitis/capsulitis, Lyme arthropathy, and rheumatoid arthritis. All of these disease entities can present with an acutely swollen knee that is erythematous, painful, and warm to the touch.

13. **What is the preferred diagnostic tool for a red, hot, painful, and acutely swollen knee?**
Arthrocentesis to analyze the synovial fluid. Serum lab markers including complete blood count (CBC), erythrocyte sedimentation rate (ESR), C-reactive protein (CRP), and blood cultures can be helpful in the workup of an acutely swollen knee; however, joint fluid analysis is the most sensitive investigation. Synovial fluid should be sent for the following analyses: cell count and differential, Gram stain, culture, crystals, and Lyme polymerase chain reaction (PCR). Based on these results, a more accurate diagnosis and treatment plan can be made (Table 32.2). When possible, treatment should be withheld until joint fluid aspiration is performed.

14. **What is the gold standard for diagnosing a septic joint?**
The overall impression of an experienced clinician is the gold standard in diagnosing a septic joint. The presence of normal laboratory and radiologic studies does exclude the diagnosis of septic arthritis. If septic arthritis is suspected, advice from a musculoskeletal specialist should be sought as soon as possible, and treatment with antibiotics should not be delayed. Delayed or inadequate treatment can lead to irreversible joint damage and disability with a significant mortality rate of 11%.

15. **What is the most common bacterial pathogen in septic arthritis?**
Staphylococci and *Streptococci* account for the majority of cases of bacterial arthritis. *Neisseria gonorrhoeae* is the most common pathogen in younger, sexually active individuals.

16. **What is the recommended treatment of septic arthritis?**
Parenteral antibiotics and debridement of the joint. Gram stain results of the joint aspirate should guide initial antibiotic choice. If the Gram stain is negative but there is a strong clinical suspicion for bacterial arthritis, broad spectrum antibiotics such as vancomycin and ceftazidime should be started until the synovial fluid culture has returned.

Table 32.2. Synovial Fluid Analysis

DIAGNOSIS	COLOR	TRANSPERANCY	VISCOCITY	WBC PER mm³	PMN %	GRAM STAIN	CULTURE	PCR TEST	CRYSTALS
Normal	Clear	Transparent	High/thick	<200	<25	Negative	Negative	Negative	Negative
Noninflammatory	Straw	Translucent	High/thick	200–2,000	<25	Negative	Negative	Negative	Negative
Inflammatory: crystalline disease	Yellow	Cloudy	Low/thin	2,000–100,000	>50	Negative	Negative	Negative	Positive
Inflammatory: noncrystalline disease	Yellow	Cloudy	Low/thin	2,000–100,000	>50	Negative	Negative	Negative	Negative
Infectious: Lyme disease	Yellow	Cloudy	Low	3,000–100,000	>50	Negative	Negative	Positive	Negative
Infectious: gonococcal	Yellow	Cloudy-opaque	Low	34,000–68,000	>75	Variable	Positive	Positive	Negative
Infectious: nongonococcal	Yellow-green	Cloudy	Very low	>50,000	>75	Positive	Positive	-	Negative

Horowitz D, Horowitz S: Approach to Septic Arthritis. *Am Fam Physician* 84(6):653-660, 2011.

17. **Can *Borrelia burgdorferi* be cultured in synovial fluid?**
No; however, synovial fluid PCR testing can be used as a confirmatory test in patients with Lyme arthritis. The diagnosis of Lyme arthritis is made with a two-step serologic testing process involving enzyme-linked immunosorbent assay, followed by confirmation with a Western blot or immunoblot test. Treatment includes 28 days of oral doxycycline.

18. **What is a characteristic sign of crystalline arthropathy on radiographic imaging?**
Chondrocalcinosis (Fig. 32.4).

19. **How do crystals of gout and pseudogout differ?**
The urate crystals of gout appear as strongly negative birefringent rods or needles when examined with a polarizing microscope; calcium pyrophosphate crystals of pseudogout are weakly positive birefringent rectangles or rhomboids.

20. **What is the treatment for an acute gouty or pseudogout attack?**
NSAIDs, colchicine, or oral corticosteroids. With diagnosis of gout, it is important to counsel the patient on dietary modifications, including alcohol restriction and decreased intake of foods high in purine.

21. **What are some common x-ray findings suggestive of rheumatoid arthritis?**
Joint space narrowing, bony erosions, and periarticular osteopenia. Severe deformity of the joint can be seen in more advanced disease.

22. **What types of bony tumors are associated with knee effusions?**
Both benign and malignant tumors can present as knee effusions. Plain radiographs will usually rule out a bone lesion. Based on the patient's history and lesion characteristics on radiographs, further evaluation with gadolinium enhanced MRI may be warranted.

23. **Do Baker cysts need to be aspirated?**
No. A Baker cyst is a benign swelling in the popliteal fossa that arises from the synovium of the knee. It is generally associated with osteoarthritis or occasionally a meniscal tear. Treatment should be directed toward the underlying cause. Unless the cyst is large enough to cause pain due to a mass effect on surrounding structures, it does not require aspiration.

KEY POINTS

1. In the absence of trauma, do not jump directly to MRI of the knee.
2. Always start your knee exam by checking neurovascular status.
3. The best diagnostic tool for an acute nontraumatic knee effusion is arthrocentesis for synovial fluid analysis.
4. Detailed history and comprehensive exam are imperative when working up an acutely swollen knee.
5. Crystalline disease can coexist with septic arthritis; positive fluid analysis for crystals does not exclude infection.

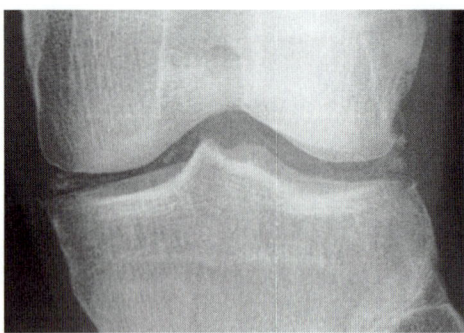

Fig. 32.4. Chondrocalcinosis Seen in Crystalline Arthropathies. *(http://radiopaedia.org/articles/chondrocalcinosis)*

BIBLIOGRAPHY

Gupte C, St Mart JP. The acute swollen knee: diagnosis and management. *J R Soc Med*. 2013;106:259–268.

Guyver PM, Arthur CH, et al. The acutely swollen knee. Part two—management of traumatic pathology. *J Royal Naval Medicine Service*. 2014;100(2):186–192.

Guyver PM, Arthur CH, et al. The acutely swollen knee. Part two—management of traumatic pathology. *J Royal Naval Medicine Service*. 2014;100(1):24–33.

Horowitz D, Horowitz S. Approach to septic arthritis. *Am Fam Physician*. 2011;84(6):653–660.

Johnson M. Acute knee effusions: a systematic approach to diagnosis. *Am Fam Physician*. 2000;61(8):2391–2400.

Messier S, Gutekunst D, et al. Weight loss reduces knee-joint loads in overweight and obese older adults with knee osteoarthritis. *Arthritis and Rheumatism*. 2005;52(7):2026–2032.

Sillanpää PJ, Kannus P, et al. Incidence of knee dislocation and concomitant vascular injury requiring surgery: a nationwide study. *J Trauma Acute Care Surg*. 2014;76(3):715.

CHAPTER 33

ACUTE FINGER AND WRIST INJURIES

Ariel Nassim, DO, Timothy Gill, MD, Timothy Salkauskis, MD, Thomas Trojian, MD

Some of the most common acute hand and wrist injuries include scaphoid fracture, distal radius fracture, boxer's fracture (fifth metacarpal neck fracture), mallet finger, jersey finger, skier's thumb, and proximal interphalangeal (PIP) joint dislocations. This chapter reviews these injuries with emphasis on initial management and treatment.

Case: A 26-year-old male was trying to impress his girlfriend while ice skating and attempted to skate backward. In doing so, he slipped and fell, trying to catch himself with an outstretched hand with the wrist in extension. (Needless to say, he did not impress her at all!) He presents with pain, swelling, and tenderness in his right wrist. This type of injury is called a FOOSH (fall on outstretched hand) and can lead to hand or wrist injuries.

1. **How does a scaphoid fracture occur?**
   The scaphoid is the most commonly fractured carpal bone, accounting for 15% of acute wrist injuries. This often results from a force on an extended wrist, which places a tensile force at the volar scaphoid and a compression force at the dorsal scaphoid. The other mechanism in which scaphoid fractures occur is with a longitudinally directed axial force across the wrist.

2. **What are the physical examination findings for a patient with a scaphoid fracture?**
   Wrist range of motion is usually only slightly reduced, but pain is reproduced with extremes of flexion and extension. Patients will generally have pain in the anatomic snuffbox in neutral or with the wrist in ulnar deviation. Associated injuries may cause symptoms of median nerve compression (paresthesias).

3. **When should radiographs be used to evaluate the injury?**
   Radiographs are always indicated in evaluation of suspected scaphoid fracture! Posteroanterior (PA), lateral, scaphoid, and 45-degree pronated views are helpful in assessing for possible fracture. Magnetic resonance imaging (MRI) is most sensitive in determining fractures and ligament injuries.

4. **What if x-ray findings are negative but the patient has snuffbox tenderness?**
   Snuffbox tenderness should be treated as a scaphoid fracture regardless of negative radiographs on the initial evaluation (Fig. 33.1).

5. **What if radiograph findings at 2 weeks are negative?**
   Radiographs may continue to be negative at 2 weeks. If tenderness persists over the scaphoid, further imaging is indicated (see Fig. 33.1).

6. **When are referrals for surgical evaluation needed?**
   Surgical referral is needed for unstable fractures. Proximal pole fractures are particularly at risk for nonunion given their avascular nature, so these fractures should be referred for internal fixation. Additionally, displacement >1 mm, comminuted fractures, and radiolunate angle >15 degrees should be referred for surgical evaluation. Nondisplaced fractures may be referred for internal fixation if quicker return to sport is required. Surgical fixation leads to 90%–95% union rates. Given the risk of these fractures to progress to nonunion and subsequent pain and disability, these fractures should be managed by physicians trained in the management of scaphoid fractures.

7. **Length and type of immobilization. (Table 33.1)**

8. **What is the typical length of injury/healing time? (Table 33.1)**

9. **What is a boxer's fracture?**
   A boxer's fracture is a fracture of the fifth metacarpal neck. This results from an impaction injury with an axial load to the fifth metacarpal. Ironically this injury is less common in boxers but more common

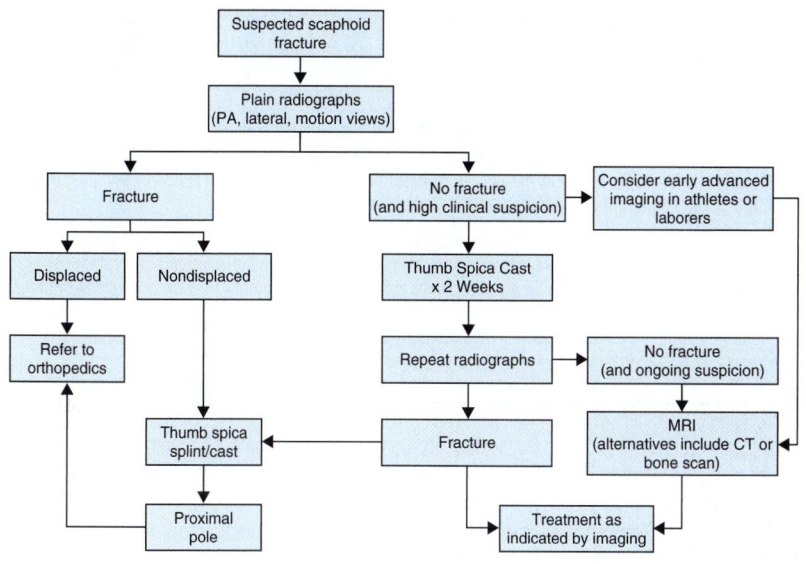

Fig. 33.1. Algorithm for snuffbox tenderness.

Table 33.1. Treatment of Suspected/Nondisplaced Scaphoid Fractures

	SUSPECTED	DISTAL	MIDDLE	PROXIMAL
		Initial Treatment		
			Fracture Location	
Splint type and position	Short-arm thumb spica cast or splint	Short arm-thumb spica cast with slight wrist extension	Long arm-thumb spica cast/splint with slight wrist extension	
Follow-up	2 weeks	1–2 weeks		
Patient education	Ice and elevate for 24–48 hours Maintain finger and shoulder range of motion			
Follow-Up Care				
Splint type and position	Short-arm thumb spica cast or splint	Short arm-thumb spica cast with slight wrist extension	Long arm-thumb spica cast/splint with slight wrist extension for weeks 1–6; then short arm-thumb spica cast/splint	
Immobilization time	Until diagnosis confirmed	4–6 weeks	10–12 weeks	12–20 weeks
Healing time		6–8 weeks	12–14 weeks	18–24 weeks
Follow-up interval	Every 2 weeks until diagnosis confirmed	Every 2–3 weeks until union confirmed		
Repeat radiographic interval	Every 2 weeks until diagnosis confirmed	Every 2–3 weeks until union confirmed		
Patient education	Maintain finger and shoulder range of motion			
Indications for orthopedics referral	Proximal pole fractures due to high risk of avascular necrosis Displaced fractures Nonunion Concern for early signs of avascular necrosis			

in individuals not trained in throwing punches. Metacarpal fractures account for 40% of all hand injuries, and the fifth metacarpal is the most commonly fractured.

10. **What symptoms will a patient with a boxer's fracture have?**
Individuals often present with pain, swelling, and ecchymosis at the area over the fifth metacarpal dorsally. Despite this, most individuals are able to maintain a full functional status of the hand and fingers, unless there is an open wound along with the fracture.

11. **What findings should I look for on physical examination for a boxer's fracture?**
Attention should be given to any obvious bony step-off or deformity. More importantly, rotational angulation of the fracture can be assessed with closed fist assessment of the distal phalanx of the fifth digit. Normal orientation of the fifth digit should have it pointing toward the scaphoid bone. Ulnar deviation may indicate further angulation of the fracture. Loss of the bony knuckle at the metacarpophalangeal (MCP) joint is frequently seen with these fractures.

12. **When should imaging be used to evaluate a boxer's fracture?**
Radiographs should be ordered with any suspicion of a metacarpal fracture. Standard anteroposterior (AP), lateral, and oblique views are the most appropriate used to evaluate. Advanced imaging is generally not needed. A computed tomography (CT) scan may be considered if there are multiple carpometacarpal (CMC) dislocations, a complex metacarpal head fracture, or inconclusive CMC findings.

13. **When are referrals for surgical evaluation needed for metacarpal fractures?**
Indications for surgery of a metacarpal fracture include intraarticular fractures, significantly displaced fractures >40 degrees in the fifth metacarpal (>30 degrees in ring finger, >20 degrees in index and long fingers). Other indications include rotational malalignment and multiple shaft fractures. Fractures of the base of the fifth metacarpal are inherently unstable and nearly always require internal fixation. Additionally, patients with evidence of ulnar nerve damage should be promptly referred to an orthopedic surgeon. If any degree of residual angulation is unacceptable to the patient, referral for internal fixation is indicated.

14. **How do I manage a boxer's fracture?**
For patients with stable fractures, no significant displacement, angulation, or shortening, nonoperative management is the initial treatment of choice. The best method of nonoperative management for these injuries has not been universally determined; however, initial treatment is an ulnar gutter splint. For metacarpal fractures, the wrist should be placed in 30 degrees of extension, MCP joint should be immobilized at 70–90 degrees of flexion, and remain in a cast for 4 weeks. Follow-up at 5–7 days should be recommended at the time of initial evaluation. Minimally angulated fifth metacarpal neck fractures without evidence of angulation may adequately be treated with buddy taping and soft wrap around the hand.

15. **When can individuals return to play/normal activity after a boxer's fracture?**
Individuals typically require 4–6 weeks for recovery. This includes the 4 weeks of immobilization. The bone will typically heal enough to return to sport by 6 weeks, although continued bone remodeling can occur for up to one year.

16. **How does a mallet finger occur?**
A mallet finger is the result of a forced flexion of the extended fingertip and occurs most commonly with sports (think ball hitting directly onto an extended fingertip). This is the most common closed tendon injury of the finger. Forced flexion of the distal interphalangeal (DIP) joint results in a disruption of the terminal extensor tendon from the dorsum of the base of the distal phalanx, with or without a bony avulsion. The long finger is most commonly injured.

17. **What are the symptoms of a mallet finger?**
Pain is the most common symptom that patients experience, while many will have swelling present. With these injuries, patients often maintain use of the hand, so there may be a delay in seeking treatment. Patients will often present with an "extensor lag," ranging from a 5- to 20-degree loss of extension in partial tears, to over 50–60 degrees of extensor lag in complete ruptures. Physical examination will reveal a loss of active extension at the DIP joint, while full passive range of motion (ROM) is maintained.

18. **When should imaging be used to evaluate a mallet finger?**
Anteroposterior, lateral, and oblique views of the affected finger should be obtained. If no apparent fracture is seen, a pure tendon avulsion may have occurred. More commonly, a small avulsion fracture may be seen. In more complicated cases, a volar subluxation of the distal fragment may be visualized.

19. **When are referrals for surgical evaluation needed for a mallet finger?**
Indications for early surgical referral include volar subluxation of the distal phalanx, inability to fully extend DIP joint passively, avulsion fracture involving >30% of the articular surface, or a swan neck deformity (hyperextension of PIP joint and flexion of DIP joint). Surgery may also be considered if the injury becomes chronic and the joint is healthy. Attempts for tendon reconstruction are only successful in approximately 50% of cases.

20. **How are mallet finger injuries treated?**
Most patients with mallet finger should be treated conservatively with prolonged splinting of the DIP joint in slight hyperextension. Extension splinting of the DIP joint is used for 6–8 weeks followed by 2–3 weeks of nighttime-only splinting. Essential to appropriate treatment is educating the patient that the DIP joint must not drop into flexion at any point in the treatment period. The tip of the distal phalanx should be supported when the splint is being changed. Depending on severity of the lag and the time to presentation, or if significant lag persists after the initial 6- to 8-week splinting period, some patients may require a longer period of immobilization, up to 12 weeks.
Many different splints can afford good outcomes. Stack splints, dorsal padded aluminum splints, or a volar unpadded splint can all be used for placing the DIP joint in slight hyperextension.

21. **What is the typical length of injury for a mallet finger? When can individuals return to play/normal activity?**
After the 6–12 weeks of extension splinting, individuals can start rehabilitation for finger flexion. Many athletes can return to play with the injured finger in a splint. Most individuals recovery fully; however, some may maintain a mild to moderate extensor lag, more common in those who presented for treatment late after the initial injury or older individuals. Even in these cases, patients will typically have full function of the finger.

22. **Are there any special considerations in the pediatric mallet finger?**
In the pediatric population, the growth plate is weaker than the surrounding bone but provides the ability for growth and remodeling that can correct an initially displaced fracture.

23. **What is a "Seymour" fracture?**
An often undiagnosed or overlooked injury in the pediatric population is a distal phalanx physeal fracture, which may appear as a nail bed injury. This type of fracture, a variant of a Salter Harris type I and II fracture, is also known as a "Seymour" fracture. A mallet finger that presents with blood in the nail bed should be considered an open fracture. This is an avulsion of the proximal edge of the nail from the eponychial fold. A true lateral radiograph is required to evaluate the fracture. The difference between a Seymour fracture and mallet finger is the displacement through the physis instead of at the DIP joint. Late presentations of a Seymour fracture include infection, growth arrest, or persistent deformity. Management of a Seymour fracture includes debridement, nail removal, irrigation, reduction as needed, nail replacement, and antibiotics. These fractures should be referred to orthopedics for ongoing management.

24. **How does a jersey finger occur?**
A jersey finger is an avulsion injury of the flexor digitorum profundus (FDP). It most commonly occurs during athletic competition, specifically tackling sports such as football or rugby. This occurs when a player is grasping an opponent who attempts to pull away, resulting in forced extension while the DIP is held in flexion. The result is a volar avulsion of the FDP tendon at the base of the distal phalanx. The ring finger is the most commonly affected finger due to it being more prominent in a grip than other fingers in 90% of patients.

25. **What symptoms will a patient with a jersey finger have?**
Patients will have pain and often swelling over the volar aspect of the distal phalanx. The finger will lie in slight extension in relation to other fingers when at rest. The patient will be unable to actively flex the finger at the DIP joint. The retracted tendon may be palpable along the flexor sheath.
(Remember: you must isolate the DIP joint when testing FDP function by stabilizing the PIP joint and the middle phalanx and asking the patient to flex the DIP joint.)

26. **When should imaging be used to evaluate a jersey finger?**
Lateral and oblique views are always necessary in the evaluation of a suspected jersey finger. As with mallet fingers, radiographs are useful in determining if there is an avulsion fracture.

Table 33.2. Jersey Finger Classification		
Leddy and Packer Classification		
TYPE	**DESCRIPTION**	**TREATMENT**
I	Flexor digitorum profundus (FDP) retracts into palm with disruption of vascular supply	Surgical repair within 7–10 days
II	FDP retracts to proximal interphalangeal (PIP) joint	Surgical repair within 21 days post injury, but may be repaired up to 2–3 months
III	Large avulsion fracture with limited retraction to distal interphalangeal (DIP) joint	
IV	Avulsion fracture with complete disruption of FDP tendon from fragment and retraction into palm ("double avulsion")	Surgical repair with Open reduction and Internal Fixation (ORIF) of avulsed osseous fragment and subsequent reattachment of tendon

27. **When are referrals for surgical evaluation needed for a jersey finger?**
Always! Prompt diagnosis and early referral to orthopedic or hand surgery are vital to the treatment of this injury. A jersey finger is not amenable to conservative or nonoperative treatment. Timing for surgery can vary and is based on the classification of the injury, as noted in Table 33.2.

28. **What should be done to protect the jersey finger injury from further damage?**
Unlike many of the other injuries, this injury typically requires an urgent surgical evaluation. Prior to surgery, splint the affected finger in slight flexion at the DIP and PIP joints to avoid further injury; this, along with ice and pain medication as needed, can be helpful.

29. **What is the typical length of recovery for a jersey finger injury? When can individuals return to play/normal activity?**
After surgery, it takes 2–3 months before the hand can be used without protection. Even with this, it may take another 1–2 months before the hand can be used with force. Return to play (tackling sports) typically takes 4–6 months. Early rehabilitation after surgery to improve range of motion and function is important for best outcomes.

30. **How is the jersey finger injury different in the pediatric population?**
Avulsion of the FDP does occur in adolescents; in this population, a Salter Harris IV fracture can be seen (avulsion of the metaphysis along with a portion of the physis). This avulsion fragment is usually tethered at the A-4 pulley, similar to type III injury in adults. This injury should have the DIP and PIP splinted in slight flexion and should be referred promptly to a hand surgeon.

31. **How does a skier's thumb (ulnar collateral ligament [UCL] of the thumb) injury occur?**
A skier's (or gamekeeper's) thumb results from an injury to the UCL of the MCP joint of the thumb. A skier's thumb refers to a more acute injury, whereas a gamekeeper's thumb refers to a chronic UCL injury. The injury results from increased valgus stress (abduction injury) usually on a hyperextended thumb.

32. **What symptoms will a patient with UCL injury of the thumb have?**
Patients will have pain localized to the ulnar aspect of the thumb at the MCP joint (web space between thumb and index finger). They may complain of difficulty pinching or grasping objects with the thumb. Palpation of the thumb may reveal focal swelling from the torn ligament, or a bony avulsion fragment. Stress testing of the ligament should be performed once an avulsion fracture has been ruled out with radiographs (stress testing can potentially convert a nondisplaced fracture to a displaced one). Instability may be seen with radial deviation of the thumb in neutral (indicating accessory UCL injury) or at 30 degrees of flexion (indicating a proper UCL injury). Instability in both positions indicates a complete rupture. It is essential to test the contralateral thumb for laxity, as there is great variety in ligamentous laxity from person to person.

33. **When should imaging be used to evaluate the UCL injury?**
Radiographs should be obtained when you suspect a UCL injury to evaluate for avulsion fractures. AP, lateral, and oblique view of the thumb should be ordered. Stress radiographs, in adults, can also

be obtained to assess stability. Ultrasound or MRI may aid in the diagnosis if exam is equivocal or if suspicion of Stener lesion is present.

34. What is a Stener lesion?
A Stener lesion is an avulsed ligament, with or without bony attachment, displaced above the adductor aponeurosis. This interposition of soft tissue of the adductor aponeurosis between the torn ends of the UCL is called a "Stener lesion": it prevents primary healing in cases of complete rupture of the ligament. Stener lesions generally require surgical repair.

35. When are referrals for surgical evaluation needed for UCL injury?
Operative management is recommended for acute injuries with >35 degrees opening on valgus stress, fractures displaced >2 mm, fractures involving >20% articular surface, concern for a Stener lesion, or symptomatic chronic injury. Surgical repair within 2–3 weeks affords better results than delayed reconstruction.

36. What is done to protect the UCL injury from further damage?
Nondisplaced avulsion injuries and UCL injuries without joint laxity do well with nonoperative management. They are treated initially with immobilization in a thumb spica splint (or cast) with the thumb in slight extension for 4–6 weeks.

37. What is the typical length of injury recovery for gamekeeper's thumb? When can individuals return to play/normal activity?
For nonoperative cases, patients are able to begin rehabilitation 3–4 weeks after diagnosis. For surgical cases, the patient will be immobilized for 4–5 weeks followed by a 1- to 2-week period with occasional time out of the splint for ROM activity. Full return to play occurs in 6–8 weeks for surgical and nonsurgical cases; however, some authors recommend protecting the thumb from excessive abduction during work or sports with a removable splint for 2–3 months after the injury.

KEY POINTS

1. Scaphoid fractures often do not show on initial radiographs.
2. Angulation of metacarpal fractures that indicate surgical intervention varies by metacarpal.
3. Mallet fingers often are treated nonoperatively, but jersey fingers need surgical referral.
4. UCL of thumb injuries (gamekeeper's thumb) need to determine if a Stener lesion exists.

BIBLIOGRAPHY

Eiff MP, Hatch R. *Fracture Management for Primary Care*. 3rd ed. Philadelphia: Elsevier Saunders; 2012:36–101.
Leggit J, Meko C. Acute finger injuries: Part I: tendons and ligaments. *Am Fam Physician*. 2006;73:810–816, 823.
Leggit J, Meko C. Acute finger injuries: Part II: fractures, dislocations, and thumb injuries. *Am Fam Physician*. 2006;73:827–834, 839.
Phillips TG, Reibach A, Slomiany WP. Diagnosis and management of scaphoid fractures. *Am Fam Physician*. 2004;70:879–884.
Clifford R, Wheeless. *Wheeless' Textbook of Orthopedics*: Hand/Wrist Chapter. Available at http://www.wheelessonline.com/ortho/wheeless_textbook_of_orthopaedics_6. Accessed on 19.05.16.

CHAPTER 34

FOOSH (FALL ON OUTSTRETCHED HAND) INJURIES

Alicia Kenton, MD, Bret C. Jacobs, DO, MA

1. **What are the most common upper extremity joints affected by a fall on outstretched hand (FOOSH) injury?**
Joints commonly affected by a FOOSH injury include elbow, wrist, and hand.

2. **What is the most common mechanism for an upper extremity fracture in a child?**
   - Fall on an outstretched hand while playing.
   - Children are typically more likely to have an upper extremity fracture than a lower extremity fracture.
   - The distal radius is the most commonly fractured bone.

3. **List the three most common clinical signs to suggest a forearm shaft fracture after a FOOSH injury.**
Visible deformity, tenderness, and decreased range of motion are the most common clinical signs to indicate a fracture.

4. **Name a risk factor that can lead to decreased bone mineral density and can increase the risk of fracture in the pediatric population after a FOOSH injury.**
   - Obesity in childhood and adolescence has been shown to decrease bone mineral density.
   - Obese and overweight children also tend to fall more frequently with activity due to balance difficulties.
   - Maintaining a healthy body weight can reduce the fracture risk from a FOOSH injury in the pediatric population.

5. **Name the most common pediatric fracture, which is often related to a FOOSH injury.**
   - Clavicle fractures are the most common pediatric fractures and frequently the result of a FOOSH injury.
   - The majority of these injuries occur at the middle-third of the clavicle.

6. **What x-ray views are necessary to evaluate a clavicle fracture?**
Shoulder x-rays including anteroposterior (AP) and outlet views, along with dedicated clavicle views, should be obtained when there is a suspicion of a clavicle fracture.

7. **Describe treatment options for children and adults with a clavicle fracture as a result of a FOOSH injury.**
   - After diagnosing a clavicle fracture, patients can use a sling for 2 to 3 weeks to help with pain, if necessary. Early motion is also allowed if tolerated.
   - A figure-of-eight brace can also be used, although a sling is typically more comfortable and less cumbersome to put on.

8. **When assessing a patient with a FOOSH injury, what are the pertinent history items that need to be considered?**
Pertinent historic items when assessing a FOOSH include:
   - Mechanism of injury: How did the patient land? What was the direction and magnitude of the force to the extremity?
   - History of prior injury.
   - Any other associated signs or symptoms.

9. **Which nerve needs to be assessed when evaluating a proximal humerus fracture sustained from a FOOSH injury?**
   - The axillary nerve needs to be assessed with a proximal humerus fracture. Carefully assess deltoid function and sensation over the lateral aspect of the proximal humerus.
   - Any signs of neurovascular compromise should necessitate urgent evaluation with an orthopedic surgeon.

10. **What injury should be considered in a pediatric patient who presents with a painful elbow and decreased range of motion following a FOOSH injury?**
    - Supracondylar fractures account for 60% to 80% of all pediatric elbow fractures, with the most common mechanism being FOOSH injury with elbow in hyperextension.
    - Typically, these patients will have pain and swelling. Visible deformity may be present. These patients will often be quite uncomfortable when any physical examination is attempted.

11. **Why are supracondylar humerus fractures the most common elbow fractures in children?**
    Supracondylar humerus fractures typically occur in children aged 5–10 years because it is one of the weakest parts of the elbow joint, with thin bony architecture and ligamentous laxity.

12. **Name the x-ray views necessary to evaluate for a supracondylar elbow fracture.**
    - Standard elbow x-rays, including an AP and lateral view with elbow flexed at 90 degrees, typically are sufficient to visualize a supracondylar elbow fracture.
    - Comparison views to unaffected side may be helpful to diagnose subtle abnormalities.
    - Also consider imaging shoulder and wrist for associated injuries.

13. **Describe the radiographic findings that are indicative of a supracondylar fracture, even if no fracture line is clearly visible.**
    - A fracture may still be present despite the absence of a clear fracture line.
    - The presence of a posterior fat pad or an anterior fat pad is indicative of an intraarticular fracture with associated effusion and hemarthrosis.

14. **When a supracondylar humerus fracture is clearly visible on x-ray, does the distal fracture fragment typically displace anteriorly or posteriorly?**
    The distal fragment displaces posteriorly in >95% of cases. Posterior displacement of the capitellum is often best visualized on lateral radiographs.

15. **What is the best splint to immobilize a supracondylar fracture?**
    To immobilize a supracondylar fracture, use a long arm posterior splint with elbow flexed to 90 degrees.

16. **What are the common complications of a supracondylar humerus fracture?**
    - Cubitus varus angulation can form with loss of normal carrying angle, which is mostly secondary to malreduction or loss of reduction.
    - Nerve injury to radial or median nerve, which is usually a neurapraxia (impairment in nerve conduction), that will resolve within a few weeks.

17. **Name the carpal bone most commonly fractured in a FOOSH injury.**
    - The scaphoid is the most common carpal bone fractured in a FOOSH injury.
    - Scaphoid fractures account for 60%–70% of all carpal fractures.

18. **Describe the typical distribution of fractures within the scaphoid following a FOOSH injury.**
    Of scaphoid fractures, 80% occur at the scaphoid waist; 10% affect the proximal pole, and 10% affect the distal pole. Waist fractures and proximal pole fractures have the highest risk of avascular necrosis.

19. **Describe common physical examination findings for a patient with a scaphoid fracture.**
    - Patients with a scaphoid fracture may have radial-sided wrist pain with associated swelling. Typically, these patients have localized tenderness over the anatomic snuffbox. The snuffbox is located on the dorsal wrist between the tendons of the extensor pollicis longus medially and the extensor pollicis brevis and abductor pollicis longus laterally.
    - Tenderness over the anatomic snuffbox is the most sensitive physical examination finding. Sensitivity ranges from 0.87 to 1.00 (Fig. 34.1).

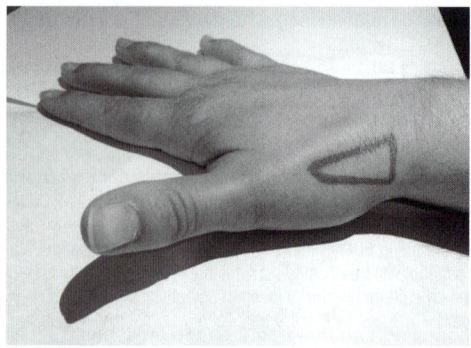

Fig. 34.1. Location of anatomic snuffbox.

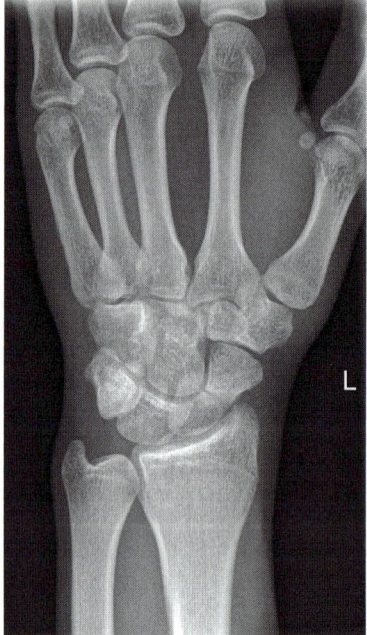

Fig. 34.2. X-ray of scaphoid fracture.

20. **How useful are plain radiographs for the diagnosis of scaphoid fracture after a FOOSH injury (Fig. 34.2)?**
    - Reported sensitives for plain radiographs for scaphoid fracture range from 70% to 86%.
    - With clinical concern for scaphoid fracture on initial presentation, the patient should be placed in a thumb spica splint and have follow-up radiographs in 1–2 weeks.
    - If follow-up radiographs are normal and there is still high suspicion for scaphoid fracture, a computed tomography (CT) scan or magnetic resonance imaging (MRI) may be necessary to confirm suspected scaphoid fracture.

21. **Name a long-term complication of a scaphoid fracture that makes it so important to diagnose correctly.**
    Nonunion and avascular necrosis are long-term complications of a scaphoid fracture. The scaphoid is susceptible to these complications because it receives its blood supply in a retrograde fashion from branches of the radial artery.

22. **Describe a common injury of the distal forearm sustained by adults following a FOOSH injury.**
    - Adults are more likely to sustain a distal radius fracture (Colles fracture) after a FOOSH injury.
    - A Colles fracture is a fracture of the distal radius with posterior displacement of the distal fragment.

23. **What age group has the highest incidence of distal radius fractures following a FOOSH injury?**
    - Children and adolescents are at a higher risk for distal radius fractures, with higher rates in boys. Recent studies have suggested the peak age of incidence for boys is 11–14 years and for girls is 8–11 years.
    - Pediatric patients are more susceptible to this injury, in part because of rapidly developing skeletal structure with smaller increases in bone mineralization.
    - Adults have a lower incidence of this fracture, but it is still the most common fracture seen in young adults.

24. **What is the best imaging for diagnosis of a distal radius fracture?**
    Plain radiographs are the mainstay in diagnosing distal radius fractures. Standard views should include PS, lateral, and oblique views. These views can be used to assess ulnar variance and contour of the articular surface and to provide visualization of the dorsal ulnar cortex.

25. **Distal radius fractures from FOOSH injuries may include torus fractures or bicortical fractures. Explain the difference between a torus fracture and a bicortical fracture.**
    - Torus fractures, also known as buckle fractures, are common injuries of childhood. They are incomplete cortical fractures that result from compression along one side of the bone. They are stable fractures that can be treated conservatively with immobilization in a short arm cast or removable wrist splint for 3 weeks.
    - Bicortical fractures of the metaphysis are complete fractures through the cortex. These may include transverse, oblique, or spiral fractures and can present with significant displacement. These occur because of bending, rotational, or shear forces sustained at the wrist. Maligned displaced fractures should be reduced and splinted. Definitive treatment includes closed reduction with cast immobilization.

26. **What are the indications for conservative treatment for a distal radius fracture after a FOOSH injury?**
    Indications for conservative treatment are incomplete fractures, nondisplaced complete fractures, and displaced extraarticular fractures, which can be reduced to stable fractures.

27. **When should distal radius fractures be referred for surgical treatment?**
    Indications for surgical treatment are displaced extraarticular fractures with unstable reduction, displaced unstable intraarticular fractures, shortening of distal radius more than 2 mm, and comminuted extraarticular fractures with a small extraarticular fragment not reduced after closed reduction.

28. **What are the common associated injuries related to distal radius fractures from FOOSH injuries?**
    Associated injuries can occur to the distal radius ulnar joint and triangular fibrocartilage complex. Ulnar styloid, carpal, metacarpal, or phalangeal fractures can also occur. Always be sure to assess joints above and below a fracture, as there may be associated injuries.

29. **Name an important potential complication of distal radius fracture in pediatric patients.**
    Pediatric patients with distal radius fracture may experience distal radius growth arrest. Growth arrest occurs in approximately 4% of pediatric patients with a distal radius fracture. If deformity persists, a corrective osteotomy can be performed after skeletal maturity is attained.

30. **What are the two common locations for fractures of the proximal radius following a FOOSH injury?**
    Fractures of the proximal radius usually occur at the radial head through the physis or just distal to the physis at the radial neck (Fig. 34.3).

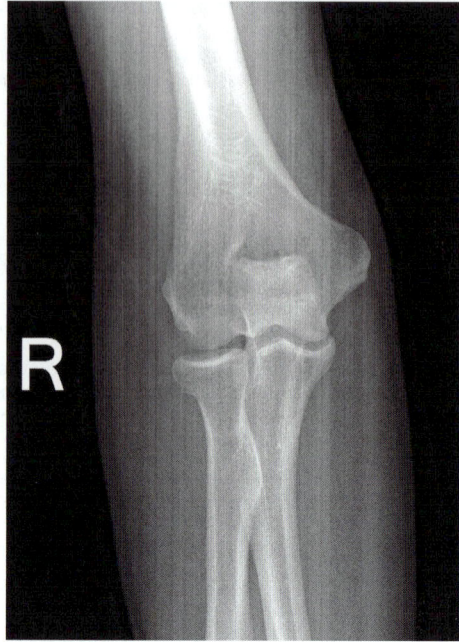

Fig. 34.3. X-ray of radial head fracture.

31. **True or False. Proximal radius fractures are among the most common elbow fractures in children.**
    False. They are among the least common elbow fractures in children. They commonly occur in children aged 9–10 years. In adults, they make up approximately 33% of elbow fractures.

32. **What four factors affect treatment of proximal radius fractures?**
    Treatment depends on degree of angulation, amount of displacement, age of child, and associated fractures.

33. **What degree of angulation of the radial head and neck with the radial shaft is usually acceptable for splinting and early range of motion after a proximal radius fracture?**
    Angulation up to 30 degrees can be treated conservatively.

34. **What are the indications for surgical referral for proximal radius fractures?**
    Complete displacement of the radial head, irreducible angulation over 45 degrees, or displaced Salter Harris IV fracture.

35. **What is the most common complication of proximal radius fractures treated conservatively?**
    Loss of motion, specifically the inability to extend the elbow fully, is the most common complication with conservative therapy.

36. **Following a both-bone forearm fracture of the radius and ulna, what is the accepted alignment after anatomic reduction?**
    Accepted alignment is related to the age of the patient, with not more than 10–50 degrees of angulation accepted in children less than 8 years old and 5–10 degrees of angulation accepted in children 8 years old and older.

37. **What is a common complication of both-bone forearm fractures?**
    Residual loss of motion in the forearm is a common complication seen in nearly 60% of children. This complication is related to length discrepancy, residual malangulation, malrotation deformity, and narrowing of the interosseous space.

KEY POINTS

1. A fall on an outstretched hand can lead to injuries of the hand, wrist, forearm, elbow, arm, and shoulder.
2. Supracondylar humerus fractures are the most common elbow fractures in pediatric patients following a FOOSH injury.
3. Clavicle fractures are the most common pediatric fractures following a FOOSH injury.
4. The scaphoid is the most common carpal bone fractured in a FOOSH injury.
5. Scaphoid fractures may not appear on plain x-rays immediately after an injury.

BIBLIOGRAPHY

Arora R, et al. Pediatric upper-extremity fractures. *Pediatr Ann*. 2014;43(5):196–204.

Bae D, Waters P. Pediatric distal radius fractures and triangular fibrocartilage complex injuries. *Hand Clin*. 2006;22: 43–53.

Basu S, Khan SHM. Radiology of acute wrist injuries. *Br J Hosp Med*. 2010;71(6):M90–M93.

Black W, Becker J. Common forearm fractures in adults. *Am Fam Physician*. 2009;80:1096–1102.

Zorilla S de Neira J, Prada-Canizares A, Marti-Ciruelos R, et al. Supracondylar humeral fractures in children: current concepts for management and prognosis. *Int Orthop*. 2015;39:2287–2296.

Kocher M, Waters P, Micheli L. Upper extremity injuries in the paediatric athlete. *Sports Med*. 2000;30:117–135.

Mallee WH, Henny EP, van Dijk CN, et al. Clinical diagnostic evaluation for scaphoid fractures: a systematic review and meta-analysis. *J Hand Surg Am*. 2014;39(9):1683–1691.

Schneppendahl J, Windolf J, Kaufmann R. Distal radius current concepts. *J Hand Surg*. 2012;37:1718–1725 (A).

Shrader MW. Pediatric supracondylar fractures and pediatric physeal elbow. *Orthop Clin North Am*. 2008;39:163–171.

Sinikumpu J, Serlo W. The shaft fractures of the radius and ulna in children: current concepts. *J Pediatr Orthop*. 2015;24:200–206.

Taljanovic MS, Karantanas A, Griffith JF, et al. Imaging and treatment of scaphoid fractures and their complications. *Seminars in Musculoskeletal Radiology*. 2012;16:159–174.

Tang J. Distal radius fracture: diagnosis, treatment, and controversies. *Clin Plast Surg*. 2014;41:481–499.

Tiel-van Buul MM, van Beek EJ, Borm JJ, Gubler FM, et al. The value of radiographs and bone scintigraphy in suspected scaphoid fracture. A statistical analysis. *J Hand Surg Br*. 1993;18:403–406.

Townsend D, Bassett G. Common elbow fractures in children. *Am Fam Physician*. 1996;53:2031–2041.

CHAPTER 35

WHEN TO IMAGE FOR SPORTS-RELATED COMPLAINTS

Heath C. Thornton, MD, CAQSM, Lindsay A. Smith, MD, Crystal M. Higginson, MD

1. **In an acutely injured athlete, what should I look for to decide if x-ray imaging might be needed?**
Focal swelling, point tenderness over bony prominences or growth plates, gross deformity, inability to move a joint, and traumatic mechanism of injury are all signs of potential fracture. Any concern for fracture would justify proceeding with radiographic imaging.

2. **When ordering plain radiographs, how many views should be requested?**
A good rule of thumb is two views for long bones and three views for joints.

3. **Are there any special views I should consider for pediatric injuries given growth plates and ossification centers?**
Contralateral imaging in addition to the area of concern for pediatric injuries will allow comparison of the injury to the patient's "normal." This can help in determining if the growth plates or ossification centers are asymmetric. Any asymmetry that correlates with injury and/or tenderness on exam justifies treatment and follow-up.

4. **A middle-aged male sustains an injury to his ankle. He is unable to bear weight immediately after the event. Upon evaluation in the office he is able to walk four steps and has no tenderness on palpation of the foot or ankle. Is imaging indicated at this time?**
Given the patient is able to ambulate and has no tenderness on exam, he does not require imaging at this time.

5. **What guideline can be applied to help determine if imaging is indicated after a foot or ankle injury?**
The Ottawa ankle rules (Table 35.1) were created to encourage judicious use of radiography in acute midfoot and ankle injuries. These rules can be useful in ruling out fracture due to their high sensitivity.

6. **In what scenarios do the Ottawa ankle rules not apply?**
These rules should not be applied to patients less than 5 years old or ankle injury greater than 10 days old. The rules should also not be applied to patients with intoxication, skin injuries, head injury, or decreased sensation in the lower extremities.

7. **A patient presents with an acute knee injury. Is there a decision rule that can be used to help rule out fracture in acute knee injury?**
Both Ottawa knee rules and Pittsburgh knee rules can be used to rule out fracture in acute knee injury (Table 35.2). Pittsburgh knee rules have been found to have a sensitivity of 99%–100% with a slightly better specificity than the Ottawa rules. While the Ottawa rules initially were validated in adults, the Pittsburgh criteria were described in patients of all ages.

8. **Can the Ottawa knee rules be applied to children?**
In a systematic review and meta-analysis in 2009, the Ottawa knee rules were found to have high sensitivity (99%) and adequate specificity (46%) for children over 5 years of age.

9. **What exclusion criteria exist for the Ottawa and Pittsburgh knee rules?**
Decision rules for imaging in knee injuries should not be applied to patients with skin injuries surrounding the knee, multiple injuries, injuries greater than 1 week old, altered consciousness or intoxication, head injury, decreased sensation in the lower extremities, or history of previous surgery or fracture on the affected knee.

Table 35.1. Ottawa Ankle Rules

ANKLE SERIES IF ANY CRITERIA BELOW ARE MET	FOOT SERIES IF ANY CRITERIA BELOW ARE MET
• Bony tenderness of the distal 6 cm of the posterior edge of the lateral malleolus • Bony tenderness of the distal 6 cm of the posterior edge of the medial malleolus	• Bony tenderness of the base of the fifth metatarsal • Bony tenderness of the navicular bone

Inability to bear weight for four steps both immediately following the injury and upon presentation to the physician's office or emergency room

Table 35.2. Comparison of Ottawa and Pittsburgh Criteria

OTTAWA KNEE RULES	PITTSBURGH KNEE RULES
One or more of the following: • Age >55 years • Tenderness of patella • Tenderness over fibular head • Limited knee flexion to 90 degrees • Inability to bear weight	Blunt trauma or fall **plus** either of the following: • Age <12 or >50 years • Inability to bear weight

10. **What fractures seen on plain films of the knee are concerning for associated ligament and meniscal tears requiring further evaluation with MRI?**
Segond fracture, tibial spine fracture, fibular head avulsion fracture, and posterior tibial plateau fracture.

11. **A patient presents after a traumatic event with inability to move the left arm and severe pain. On exam, his arm is held in adduction and internal rotation. You suspect anterior shoulder dislocation. What imaging test do you obtain to confirm the diagnosis?**
Plain radiograph is used to verify the diagnosis and rule out fracture. Anteroposterior (AP), axillary, and lateral scapular views should be obtained. These images are also important to rule out associated humeral and glenoid fractures.

12. **After verifying the anterior dislocation by radiograph, you reduce the shoulder. What image can be used to confirm reduction of anterior dislocation?**
Axillary plain radiograph can be used to confirm reduction in anterior dislocations.

13. **What additional radiographs can be obtained to identify common associated bony injuries with recurrent dislocations and instability?**
The West Point axillary view may be used to identify a fracture of the anterior glenoid rim, also known as a bony Bankart lesion. Additionally, a Stryker notch view may be used to identify a Hill-Sachs lesion in the posterosuperior portion of the humeral head, caused by recurrent contact of the humeral head with the glenoid rim.

14. **Is there an indication for plain radiographs in the diagnosis of elbow dislocation?**
In order to facilitate timely reduction of elbow dislocations, diagnosis is often based on evidence of obvious deformity with the elbow held in varus position and the forearm supinated on physical exam. If diagnosis is unclear, confirmation with anteroposterior and lateral plain radiographs is appropriate.

15. **Should imaging studies be completed after reduction of an elbow dislocation?**
Postreduction anteroposterior and lateral radiographs should be obtained to verify reduction and identify any associated fractures, such as a coronoid process avulsion.

16. **Can head imaging be a useful tool in diagnosing concussion?**
Concussion is a clinical diagnosis. Structural neuroimaging should be normal in patients with concussion and is not necessary for diagnosis. Imaging may be indicated to evaluate for more serious traumatic brain injury in patients with certain symptoms.

Table 35.3. Canadian Head Computed Tomography Rules: Risk Factors

HIGH-RISK FACTORS	MEDIUM-RISK FACTORS
Glasgow Coma Scale Score <15 at 2 hours after injury	Amnesia before impact >30 minutes
Any sign of basilar skull fracture: • Hemotympanum • Raccoon eyes • Cerebrospinal fluid otorrhea or rhinorrhea • Battle sign	Dangerous mechanism: • Pedestrian struck by motor vehicle • Occupant ejected from motor vehicle • Fall from 3 or more feet or down five stairs
Suspected open or depressed skull fracture	
Two or more episodes of vomiting	
Age 65 or older	

17. **What imaging guidelines could be applied to determine the need for computed tomography (CT) after minor head injury?**
Canadian Head Computed Tomography Rules can be applied to patients with minor head injury who present with a Glasgow Coma Scale (GCS) of 13–15 after witnessed loss of consciousness, amnesia, or confusion.

18. **How are the Canadian Head Computed Tomography Rules used to determine need for imaging?**
Computed tomography of the head is recommended if any of the risk factors are met (Table 35.3). In a study completed in 2001, high-risk factors had 100% sensitivity for predicting neurologic intervention and medium-risk factors had 98.4% sensitivity and 49.6% specificity for predicting clinically important brain injury.

19. **What exclusion criteria exist for the Canadian Head Computed Tomography Rules?**
Canadian Head Computed Tomography Rules should not be used for patients with GCS score less than 13, age less than 16 years, obvious open skull fracture, seizure after injury, bleeding disorder, or use of anticoagulation.

20. **If you are concerned for facial fracture, what type of imaging is most useful?**
Computed tomography is superior to conventional radiography and magnetic resonance imaging (MRI) in detection of facial fractures.

21. **A patient presents with neck pain after falling off her bike while road cycling. She is sitting up and comfortable. What rules could you use to help decide whether to get imaging?**
Two decision-making rules are commonly used: National Emergency X-Radiography Utilization Study (NEXUS) (Box 35.1) and Canadian C-Spine Rule (Box 35.2). Both have been well studied and found to be highly sensitive.

KEY POINTS

1. In general, imaging is not indicated in the setting of concussion unless criteria for Canadian Head CT Rules are met.
2. There are several imaging guidelines that can assist in the decision to obtain radiographic imaging for ankle, knee, and neck injuries.
3. Ottawa Ankle Rules do not apply to patients less than 5 years old or ankle injury greater than 10 days old.
4. After reduction of a dislocation, radiographic imaging is generally recommended to evaluate for associated fractures.

BIBLIOGRAPHY

American College of Radiology Appropriateness Criteria. <https://acsearch.acr.org/list>; Accessed 06.07.16.
Bachmann L, Haberzeth S, Steurer J, et al. The accuracy of the Ottawa knee rule to rule out knee fractures: a systematic review. *Ann Intern Med.* 2004;140(2):121–124.

Box 35.1. NEXUS Criteria

- No midline cervical tenderness
- No focal neurologic deficit
- Normal alertness
  - Glasgow Coma Scale of 15
  - No disorientation to person, place, time, or events
  - Ability to remember three objects in 5 minutes
  - Appropriate response to external stimuli
- No intoxication
- No painful, distracting injury
  - Examples: long bone fractures, visceral injury requiring surgical consultation, large lacerations, crush injuries, or large burns

Data from Hoffman JR, Wolfson AB, Todd K, et al: Selective Cervical Spine Radiography in Blunt Trauma: Methodology of the National Emergency X-Radiography Utilization Study (NEXUS). *Ann Emerg Med* 32(4):461, 1998.

Box 35.2. Canadian C-Spine Rules

- Is there any high-risk factor that mandates radiography?
  - Age 65 years or older
  - Dangerous mechanism
  - Fall from 1 m (or five stairs)
  - Axial load to the head (e.g., diving accidents)
  - Motor vehicle collisions at high speed (>100 km/h)
  - Motorized recreational vehicle accident
  - Ejection from a vehicle
  - Bicycle collision with an immovable object
  - Paresthesias in extremities
- Is there any low-risk factor that allows safe assessment of range of motion? Patients who do not have any of the following low-risk factors should be radiographed and are not suitable for range of motion testing:
  - Simple rear-end motor vehicle collision
  - Sitting position in emergency department
  - Ambulatory at any time since injury
  - Delayed onset of neck pain
  - Absence of midline C-spine tenderness
- Range of motion testing
  - Is the patient able to actively rotate neck 45 degrees to the left and right (regardless of pain)? If so, imaging is not indicated.

Data from Stiell IG, Wells GA, Vandemheen KL, et al: The Canadian C-spine rule for radiography in alert and stable trauma patients. *JAMA* 286(15):1841, 2001.

Dowling S, Spooner C, Liag Y, et al. Accuracy of Ottawa ankle rules to exclude fractures of the ankle and midfoot in children: a meta-analysis. *Acad Emerg Med.* 2009;4(4):277–287.

Kanwar R, et al. Emergency department evaluation and treatment of cervical spine injuries. *Emerg Med Clin N Am.* 2015;33:241–282.

Kobayashi A, Kobayashi T, Kato K, et al. Diagnosis of radiographically occult lumbar spondylolysis in young athletes by magnetic resonance imaging. *Am J Sports Med.* 2013;41(1):169–176.

Masci L, Pike J, Malara F, et al. Use of the one-legged hyperextension test and magnetic resonance imaging in the diagnosis of active spondylolysis. *Br J Sports Med.* 2006;40(11):940–946.

Seaberg D, Yealy D, Lukens T, et al. Multicenter comparison of two clinical decision rules for the use of radiography in acute, high-risk knee injuries. *Ann Emerg Med.* 1998;32(1):8–13.

Stiell I, Clement C, Grimsaw J, et al. A perspective cluster randomized trial to implement the Canadian CT head rule in emergency departments. *CMAJ.* 2010;182(14):1527–1532.

Stiell I, Wells G, Vandemheen K, et al. The Canadian CT Head Rules for patients with minor head injury. *Lancet.* 2001;357(9266):1391–1396.

Vijayasankar D, Boyle A, Atkinson P. Can the Ottawa knee rule be applied to children? A systematic review and meta-analysis of observational studies. *Emerg Med J.* 2009;26(4):250–253.

CHAPTER 36

ENVIRONMENTAL EMERGENCIES

Ayesha Abid, MD, Matthew L. Silvis, MD

COLD INJURIES

1. What causes injuries from cold exposure?
Injuries from cold exposure are due to low air temperatures, water immersion, rain, and wind, which all affect a body's ability to maintain normothermic temperature. They are divided into low core temperature (hypothermia), freezing (frostbite), and nonfreezing (chilblains, trench foot) injuries.

2. How do you prevent cold injuries?
C- Keep area **clean** and **covered** (cover head and neck as they are areas of high heat loss)
O- Avoid **overheating** (remove layers as necessary)
L- Wear **loose** clothing and in **layers** (wicking fabric such as wool with wind-blocking garment)
D- Keep skin **dry** to prevent heat loss from moisture (waterproof outer layer)

3. What are the common symptoms and signs of cold exposure injuries?
See Table 36.1.

4. Who is at high risk?
Individuals younger than 2 years of age or older than 60 years are at highest risk. Elderly persons are especially prone due to age-related decrease in sympathetic nervous system–mediated vasoconstriction, reduced function of sweat glands, and comorbidities. Younger individuals have larger surface area/mass ratios and exhibit greater heat loss. Homelessness and sports activity in inclement environments pose the greatest risk. Specific risk factors include intoxicants (alcohol), psychiatric illness, wet clothing, bare skin, malnutrition, dehydration, fatigue, and sleep deprivation.

5. What temperatures do cold injuries occur at?
Hypothermia is defined as body temperature less than 95°F (35°C) rectally and occurs when heat loss exceeds heat production. Hypothermia can occur at higher temperatures, especially when clothing is wet. Most cold exposure injuries can occur within minutes, depending on the temperature, wind, duration, evaporation, and direct exposure. The Wind-Chill Equivalent Index (WCEI) can be used to assess heat loss from exposed skin.

6. How should you assess and begin management for hypothermia?
If there is concern for hypothermia, begin by removing all wet clothing. Assess mental status, airway, and breathing. If patient is breathing, provide oxygen, obtain vital signs, and place an intravenous (IV) line if able. An accurate core temperature is crucial and ideally is obtained rectally with a thermometer scaled for hypothermia. The core temperature guides treatment, classified as mild, moderate, or severe (Table 36.2). If there is no concern for hypothermia based on core temperature and observation, assess exposed areas and treat.

7. What is the difference between frostnip and frostbite?
Frostnip is the formation of superficial ice crystals (affects the epidermis only) and causes no tissue damage. Mild frostbite penetrates the dermis, and deep frostbite affects all layers of the skin (permanent damage may occur). Frostbite is due to a localized tissue response whereby electrolyte shifts lead to water crystallization in temperatures below 32°F (0°C), leading to tissue damage. These injuries occur in minutes to hours and typically affect the face, ears, fingers, and toes.

8. What are the major considerations in frostbite injury?
Remove wet, constrictive clothing and assess for hypothermia. If there is a concern for tissue refreezing, do not attempt initial thawing as tissue necrosis may occur (extended freeze preferred to refreeze). Provide adequate anesthesia. Do not massage open blisters or expose area to open heat (stoves, flame, steam, heat packs). Consider transfer for emergency care, especially when affected area is large. The injured body part should be protected with a bulky splint for transport. See Fig. 36.1.

Table 36.1. Common Symptoms and Signs of Cold Exposure Injuries

EARLY	LATE
Shivering	"Stumbles, grumbles, mumbles"
Numbness	Decreased or no shivering
Pain, burning	Sluggish, poor judgment, confusion
Erythema, edema, blistering	Frozen tissue (stiff to touch)
Fatigue	Shallow breathing

Table 36.2. Core Temperature Treatment Guide

HYPOTHERMIA	TEMPERATURE (RECTAL)	SYMPTOMS	MANAGEMENT
Mild	32°C–35°C (89.6°F–95°F)	Shivering, muscle spasms, lethargy, slurred speech, pallor, low pulse, usually normal blood pressure	- Remove wet clothing, move indoors - Passive external rewarming with blanket or wrap - Warm liquids by mouth (if able)
Moderate	28°C–32°C (82.4°F–89.6°F)	+/- shivering, cyanosis, disorientation, decreased motor skills, muscle stiffness, decreased respiration, low or irregular pulse, low blood pressure	- Rapid transport to medical facility for active core re-warming (+/- active external rewarming) - Avoid active external rewarming (fires, hot water bottles, heating pads) until active core rewarming has begun to avoid life-threatening risk of core temperature after drop - Warmed humidified oxygen if available - Monitor for arrhythmias
Severe	<28°C (82.4°F)	Loss of consciousness, rigidity, pulse not palpable, depressed respirations, dilated pupils, pulmonary edema, arrhythmias	- Rapid transport to a medical facility for active core rewarming (warmed IV fluids, warmed humidified oxygen, and/or peritoneal/thoracic/gastric lavage). Monitor for ventricular fibrillation or cardiac arrest while awaiting transport.

9. **What causes chilblain and trench foot injuries?**

Chilblains and trench foot are both nonfreezing injuries (Table 36.3). Prolonged water exposure or sweating from wet-cold conditions (rain, snow, immersion) causes an exaggerated inflammatory response. This causes increased vascular permeability and fluid leakage. Feet (wet socks, footwear) and hands are commonly affected. Wet and constrictive clothing should be removed. Avoid weight-bearing, friction, lotions, or exposing area to extreme heat.

10. **What is the role of radiologic studies?**

There is no role for any imaging unless a fracture is suspected.

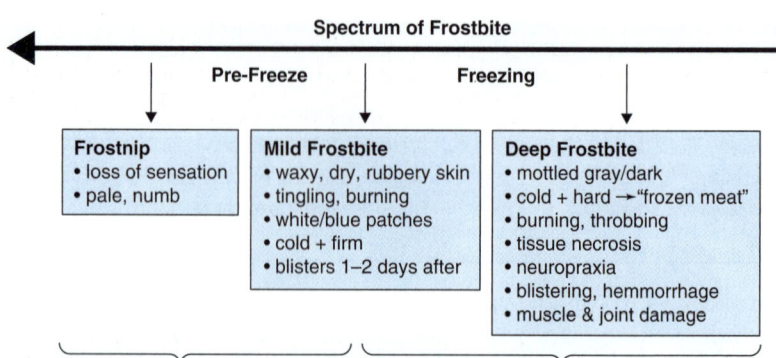

Fig. 36.1. Spectrum of Frostbite.

Table 36.3. Spectrum of Heat Illness

	CHILBLAIN (PERNIO)	TRENCH FOOT (IMMERSION FOOT)
Etiology	- Local skin lesions (vesicles, bullae, plaques) typically on hands/feet - Exposure at 33°F–60°F for 1–5 hours - Superficial (can be freezing)	- Frequent and prolonged immersion of body part in cold water (typically feet) - Exposure at 32°F–50°F for >12 hours - Soft tissues, nerves, blood vessels
Presentation	- Edema, erythema, cyanotic, tender, pruritic, numbness, burning, tingling, sloughing - No symptom resolution with rewarming	- Edema, erythema, cyanotic or blotchy skin, blistering, bleeding, skin fissures, maceration, shooting pain, infection, gangrene
Management	- Wash and dry affected area - Elevate, cover with loose, warm, dry clothing. Use dry bandages if needed - Usually no permanent sequelae and resolves within 2–3 weeks	- Treatment as per chilblains with following additions: apply warm packs or soak in warm water (102°F–110°F) for 5 minutes - Often requires prolonged wound care as healing can take 3–6 months - Consider transfer to facility

11. **What is the role of epinephrine pens in cold-induced urticaria?**
Mediated by histamine, cold-induced urticaria is an allergic response to cold exposure. The response can present as hives, angioedema, or, rarely, anaphylaxis. When localized to the skin, symptoms may be controlled with oral antihistamines and low concentration, short-term corticosteroids. Topical antihistamines can provide pruritus relief. If the reaction is anaphylaxis, epinephrine should be administered and the individual transferred to a medical facility. Treat underlying disorder, if present. The only prevention known is to avoid cold exposure.

12. **What is the management of cold-induced bronchoconstriction?**
Cold-induced bronchoconstriction causes airway surface liquid (ASL) to evaporate faster than it can be replaced, causing cooling and drying. This may trigger a reflex response of coughing and bronchial narrowing. Inhaled β_2-adrenergic agonists (albuterol) can be used 15–30 minutes before exercise. In the setting of regular exercise in the cold, mast cell stabilizers (cromoyln), leukotriene receptor antagonists, and inhaled corticosteroids are capable of attenuating cold air–provoked bronchoconstriction.

HEAT INJURIES

13. **What causes heat injuries?**
Heat injuries are caused by failure of thermoregulatory mechanisms (evaporation, radiation, conduction, convection), resulting in impaired heat production and heat loss. They can be caused by metabolic and/or environmental effects. High temperatures can result in impaired blood flow to vital organs, and death. The spectrum of heat illness is depicted in Table 36.3. Heat edema, rash, and heat cramps are mild heat illnesses. Heat syncope and heat exhaustion are medical urgencies; heat stroke is an emergency.

14. **What are the risk factors for heat-related injuries and who is at risk?**
   - High temperatures; heat waves
   - Obesity
   - Dehydration
   - Sickle cell trait, cystic fibrosis, and comorbidities
   - Burns (e.g., sunburn)
   - Alcohol consumption
   - Children, elderly, athletes
   - Certain medication/supplement use*
   - Certain skin conditions (eczema, psoriasis)
   - Low physical fitness
   - History of heat illness or febrile illness
   - Sleep deprivation, fatigue
   - Garments that don't allow ventilation
   - Lack of acclimatization
      * Tricyclic antidepressants, anticholinergics, antihistamines, benzodiazepines, diarrheal agents, typical antipsychotics, antihypertensives, neuroleptics, thyroid agonists, stimulants, caffeine, diuretics.

15. **What is the difference between classic and exertional heat stroke?**
Classic heat stroke is environmental in origin, such as heat waves, and most commonly affects the elderly with predisposed medical conditions. Exertional heat stroke occurs due to dysfunction of heat dissipation, can occur in all weather conditions, and commonly affects the healthy and young.

16. **What are the symptoms and signs of heat injuries?**
Signs
   - Sweating
   - Decreased performance
   - Lethargy
   - Changes in mental status
Symptoms
   - Muscle cramps
   - Thirst
   - Vision changes
   - Nausea/vomiting
   - Headache
   - Feeling faint/fatigue

17. **What are the steps to approaching an athlete with a heat illness?**
Assess airway, breathing, and circulation (ABCs). Transport to a cooler location, and initiate cooling with ice bags and/or fan mist. Assess for appropriate mentation. If mentation is appropriate, provide fluids and electrolyte replacement by mouth. If not mentating well, remove

excess clothing, initiate rapid cooling, and alert emergency medical services (EMS). After doing so, obtain a rectal temperature by inserting a thermometer with the metal tip 1–2 inches into the rectum. Obtain vital signs, blood glucose, and sodium levels. Obtain IV access if able. Transfer the patient to a medical facility.

18. What is the role of laboratory studies?

The differential for heat illness is broad and includes hypoglycemia, seizures, hyponatremia, thyroid storm, neuroleptic malignant syndrome, drug ingestion, and closed head trauma. Laboratory assessment may include:

- Basic Metabolic Profile (BMP) for electrolytes, glucose, creatinine
- Arterial blood gases (ABG) for respiratory alkalosis
- Creatine phosphokinase (CPK) for rhabdomyolysis
- Chest x-ray for pulmonary edema
- Others: lactate (↑), calcium (↓), phosphorous (↓)
- Eelectrocardiogram and troponins for cardiac abnormalities
- Fibrinogen, fibrin-split products for disseminated intravascular coagulation (DIC)
- Liver function tests (LFTs) for hepatic injury
- Urine analysis and output (for myoglobin)

19. What are the types of heat injuries and what is the management?

Remember: Cool if able, then transport. The goal is to lower the core body temperature to 37.5°C–38°C as soon as possible. See Table 36.4.

20. What are the complications of heat stroke?

- Seizures
- Rhabdomyolysis
- Pulmonary edema, acute respiratory distress syndrome (ARDS)
- Arrhythmias
- Hypotension
- Organ damage (liver, heart, kidney)
- DIC
    * Shivering and seizures can be treated with benzodiazepines. Arrhythmias often resolve with improvement in temperatures.

21. How are heat injuries prevented?

- Fluid and electrolyte replacement before and during exercise
- Acclimatize prior to extreme exercise
- Balanced nutrition, may need high-sodium and high-potassium diet
- Wear temperature-appropriate clothing (loose, lightweight, light colored, moisture wicking)
- Educate civilians and athletes
- Frequent rest periods

22. What medications should be avoided in patients with heat-related illness?

Avoid alpha agonists and anticholinergic agents as they can cause peripheral vasoconstriction and prevent sweating.

23. When can an athlete return to play after suffering a heat illness?

Generally, an athlete can return after 24 hours with adequate hydration if illness is mild. However, if suffering from heat exhaustion or heat stroke, all vital signs should be normalized, and patient should be asymptomatic. Athletes are often instructed to wait at least 1 week after discharge from medical care before returning to play. A follow-up physical exam and laboratory testing in 1 week following return to play should be considered. When returning to play, athletes should slowly increase heat exposure and length and intensity of exercise over a 2-week period. If heat tolerance is demonstrated, they can be cleared within 2–4 weeks.

KEY POINTS

1. Severe hypothermia is a medical emergency, requiring immediate transfer to a hospital.
2. In cold exposure injuries, do not allow thawed skin to refreeze and do not use excess heat, cold, or massage or provide direct heat.
3. If a patient has a temperature >104°F, persistent vomiting, or altered mental status, alert emergency medical services for immediate transfer.

Table 36.4. Heat Injury Management

CONDITION	SIGNS/SYMPTOMS	MANAGEMENT AND COMMENTS
Heat Edema	Swelling in dependent areas (typically hands, lower extremities) *Occurs due to body's attempt at heat loss by peripheral vasodilation Commonly seen in elderly and unacclimatized *Rule out organic cause of heat edema (heart/kidney failure)	Compression stockings. Generally condition resolves on its own within 1–2 weeks. Diuretics will worsen the condition and deplete intravascular volume.
Heat Rash (miliaria rubra)	Papulovesicular skin eruptions, typically on covered areas of skin (i.e., trunk, groin). May cause pruritus *Sweating causes clogged skin eccrine sweat glands which may predispose to infection	Condition is self-limited. Pruritus can be managed by topical or oral antihistamine agents. Infection is managed with antibiotics based on severity.
Heat Cramps (CT normal or ↑ but <40°C)	Muscle spasms or cramps (i.e., quadriceps, calves, abdomen), sweating *Involuntary painful skeletal muscle contractions	Fluids, electrolyte solutions with sodium, stretching and massaging muscles, cooling with ice. IV normal saline in severe or rebound cases can be used. **Most common in individuals with heavy sodium in sweat
Heat Syncope (normal core temperature*)	Weakness, faint feeling, improvement in symptoms when supine	Place patient in supine position, provide fluids **Occurs due to orthostatic hypotension from peripheral vasodilation
Heat Exhaustion (CT 37°C–40°C) *Body's attempt to maintain normothermia	Headache, lethargy, hypotension, tachycardia, nausea, vomiting, +/- sweating, cold clammy skin, oliguria, normal mental status	Remove excess clothing, elevate legs, rapid cooling with ice cloths to neck, torso, axilla, and groin. Hydration with cool fluids. Legs propped above heart level. Use IV if needed (Dextrose-0.5NS). Consider transfer to a medical facility.
Heat Stroke (CT usually ≥40°C) *Body can no longer maintain normothermia	Hypotension, tachycardia, loss of sweating, constricted pupils, warm and dry skin, oliguria, tachypnea, mental status changes, convulsions, coma *Lactic acidosis, DIC, acute renal failure, hypokalemia and rhabdomyolysis are typically seen in exertional heat stroke	"Cool first, transport second" Remove excess clothing, elevate legs, rapid cooling with ice packs or cold towels over neck, axilla, groin (think major vessels). Apply cool water to bare skin and start fan for evaporative cooling. Ice-water immersion if able. Initiate IV fluids (NS). Transfer to a medical facility for possible peritoneal lavage, internal cooling, ECMO (extracorporeal membrane oxygenation), and vasopressors (dobutamine) if needed.

CT, Core temperature.

BIBLIOGRAPHY

Barrow MW, Clark KA. Heat-related illnesses. *Am Fam Phys.* 1998;58:749–756.

Brown CH, Brown MT, Tyler WB, Cruz S. Environmental factors affecting human performance. In: *Medical Manual.* International Association of Athletics Federation; 1990. [chapter 11].

Cappaert TA, Stone JA, Castellani JW, et al. National Athletic Trainer's Association position statement: environmental cold injuries. *J Athl Train.* 2008;43(6):640–658.

Casa D, Armstrong L, Kenny G, et al. Exertional heat stroke: new concepts regarding cause and care. *Curr Sports Med Rep.* 2012;11(3):115–123.

Casa D, DeMartini J, Bergeron M, et al. National Athletic Trainer's Association position statement: exertional heat illness. *Journal of Athletic Training.* 2015;50(9):986–1000.

Castellani JW, Young AJ, Ducharme MB, et al. American College of Sports Medicine position stand: prevention of cold injuries during exercise. *Med Sci Sports Exerc.* 2006;8(11):2012–2029.

Claudy A. Cold urticaria. *J Investig Dermatol Symp Proc.* 2001;6:141–142.

Corris EE, Ramirez AM, Durme DJ. Heat illness in athletes: the dangerous combination of heat, humidity and exercise. *Sports Med.* 2004;34:9–16.

Dammann GG, Boden BP. On-the-field management of heat stroke: sports medicine update. *AOSSM Newsletter (May-June).* 2004:4–7.

Glazer JL. Management of heatstroke and heat exhaustion. *Am Fam Phys.* 2005;71:2133–2140.

Howe AS, Boden BP. Heat-related illness in athletes. *Am J Sports Med.* 2007;35(8):1384–1395.

Inter-Association Task Force on Exertional Heat Illnesses Consensus Statement. National Athletic Trainers' Association, June 2003.

Kazman JB, Heled Y, Lisman PJ, et al. Exertional heat illness: the role of heat tolerance testing. *Curr Sports Med Rep.* 2013;12(2):101–105.

Koester MC. Cold-related illness. In: *Sports Medicine Handbook.* 4th ed. National Federation of State High School Associations; 2011:40–43.

Koskela HO. Cold air-provoked respiratory symptoms: the mechanisms and management. *Int J Circumpolar Health.* 2007;66(2):91–100.

Krafczyk MA, Asplung CA. Exercise-induced bronchoconstriction: diagnosis and management. *Am Fam Physician.* 2011;84(4):427–434.

McMahon J, Howe A. Cold weather issues in sideline and event management. *Curr Sports Med Rep.* 2012;11(3):135–141.

NCAA 2014-2015. Sports Medicine Handbook. Indianapolis, IN: National Collegiate Athletic Association <www.ncaa.org.>; Accessed 12.05.16.

Raducan A, Tiplica GS. Chillblains and frostbite. *J Eur Acad Dermatol Venereol.* 2013;6(1):60–64.

U.S. Army Research Institute of Environmental Medicine. Prevention and management of cold weather injuries. Technical Bulletin Material 508. Washington, DC: Department of the Army.

CHAPTER 37

THE ACUTELY INJURED SHOULDER

Craig F. Betchart, MD, Mark Mirabelli, MD

1. **What is the differential diagnosis for an acute shoulder injury?**
   - A thorough differential is dependent on an understanding of shoulder anatomy. The shoulder is a girdle consisting of four articulations: glenohumeral, acromioclavicular, sternoclavicular, and scapulothoracic. These articulations are supported by muscles, tendons, and ligaments.
   - Fractures, sprains, dislocations, and soft tissue tearing are all common ways to injure the shoulder.
   - The focus of this chapter will be to outline the evaluation and management of clavicle fracture, proximal humerus fracture, glenohumeral dislocation, AC separation, and acute rotator cuff sprain/tear.
   - In a young patient with a direct fall onto the shoulder, the most common injuries are AC separation and clavicle fracture.

2. **What imaging is useful for the acutely injured shoulder?**
   - Typical x-ray views for any acute shoulder injury include a standard AP, true AP, and axillary view.
   - Additional views may be useful if certain injuries are suspected. This will be described in more detail later in the chapter.

Case: A 24-year-old hockey player is skating mid-ice and collides with a player from the opposing team. He loses his balance and falls on his right shoulder. He gets up and skates to the bench, where he complains to his athletic trainer of right anterior shoulder pain. He tries to lift his arm forward and has significant pain.

CLAVICLE FRACTURE

3. **What are the acute exam findings in a clavicle fracture and how does this injury present?**
   Patients often appear to have a sagging shoulder. There is pain with palpation (often with crepitus) over the clavicular injury. There may be bruising, swelling, or tenting of the skin over the fracture site. There is pain with shoulder elevation.

4. **What are the best x-ray views if a clavicle fracture is suspected?**
   The acute shoulder series will typically be enough for diagnosis. For clavicle fractures, the addition of a full AP clavicle for bilateral comparison as well as 45-degree cephalic and caudal views in order to determine displacement are useful.

5. **Will this patient require surgery?**
   - Clavicle fractures are divided into three groups: medial, middle, and lateral. All nondisplaced middle fractures can be managed nonoperatively with rest and a sling for comfort. Displaced, comminuted, or fractures with >2 cm shortening should be referred to orthopedics for definitive management. Fractures of the clavicle that are lateral to the CC ligament are at high risk for displacement and should warrant surgical referral. Recurrent clavicle fractures should also be referred for surgical intervention. Displaced medial fractures are rare but can be associated with neurovascular injury and are considered an emergency.
   - Complications of clavicle surgery include skin erosion, pain, and hardware breakage.

AC SEPARATION

6. **The case above could also result in an AC separation. How does an AC separation/sprain present?**
   Shoulder pain after a direct blow or fall onto the shoulder. On exam there is pain to palpation over the AC joint. There is usually pain with overhead shoulder movement and pain with the cross arm test. In a shoulder separation, there may be a step-off deformity.

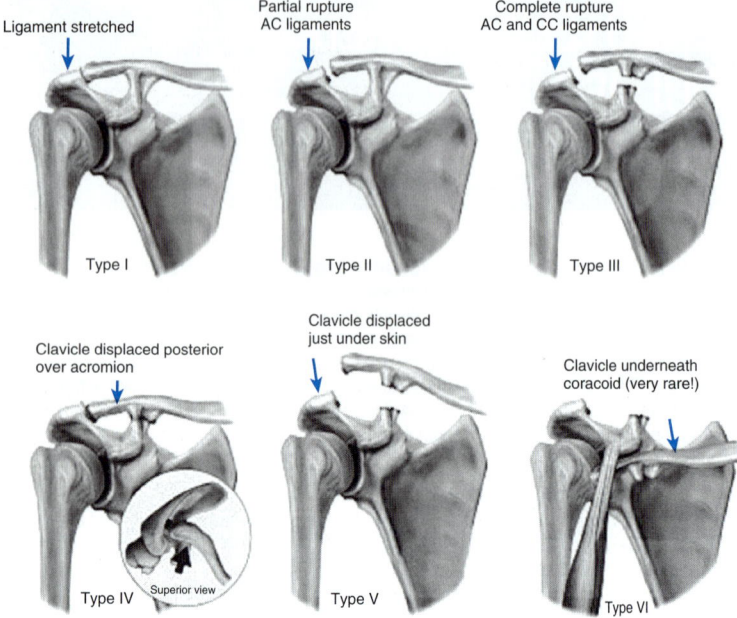

Fig. 37.1. Classification of AC Injuries. *(From Rockwood Jr., Charles A., et al. Rockwood and Green's Fractures in Adults: Fourth Edition. Vol. 3. Set. Philadelphia/New York; Raven Publishers, 1996.)*

7. **Are there any special x-ray views that are helpful for looking at the AC joint?**
   A standard shoulder series is usually adequate (Fig. 37.1). A direct AP of the AC joint may provide greater resolution. Weighted films are no longer recommended as they do not significantly change treatment.

8. **How are AC injuries managed? Who needs orthopedic follow-up?**
   - Fig. 37.2 and Table 37.1 outline appropriate treatment for AC injuries. Nonoperative treatment consists of pain control and sling.
   - Anesthetic injection can be used for acute pain control in situations when the patient needs short-term use of the arm (i.e., participation in a single game).

   Case: A 63-year-old retired female was outside gardening. She fell while carrying pots to her garden and landed on her outstretched arm. She reports she heard a "pop" and felt immediate pain.

ROTATOR CUFF TEAR

9. **What is the common presentation of an acute rotator cuff tear?**
   Patients will complain of pain and weakness with overhead and reaching activities following trauma or high demand use.

10. **What are the exam findings?**
    The most common finding is weakness with abduction (supraspinatus tear). Weakness with internal or external rotation would indicate subscapularis or infraspinatus/teres minor tear, respectively.

11. **What special tests are helpful?**
    Supraspinatus: positive drop arm. Infraspinatus: positive external rotation lag sign. Subscapularis: positive lift-off test. Teres minor: positive horn blowers.

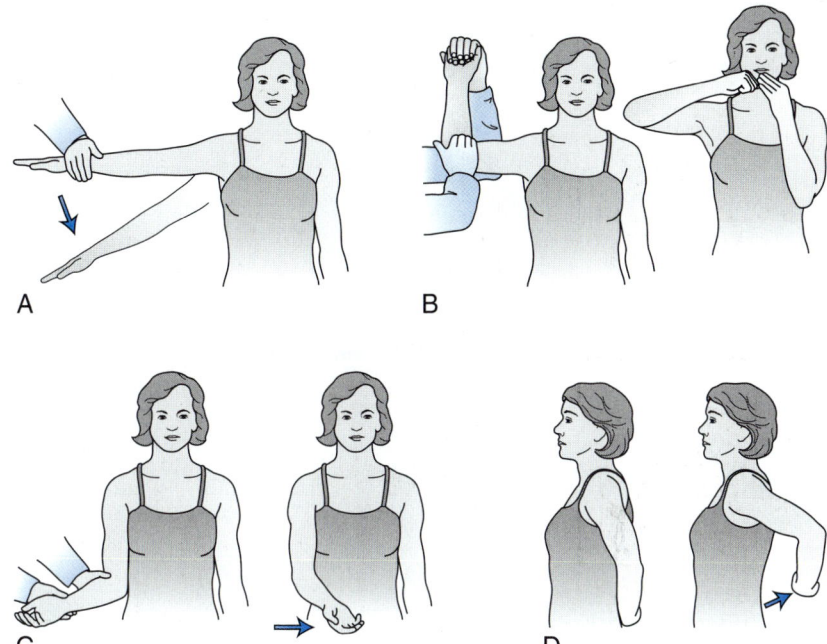

Fig. 37.2. Special Tests for Rotator Cuff Tears. A, Drop arm sign. B, Hornblower's sign. C, External rotation lag. D, Lift off test.

Table 37.1. The Rockwood Classification for AC Injuries and Typical Treatments

	AC	CC	DISPLACEMENT	TREATMENT
Type I	Sprain	Sprain	None	Non-op
Type II	Tear	Sprain	<25% CC displace	Non-op
Type III	Tear	Tear	25%–100% CC displace	Usually non-op
Type IV	Tear	Tear	Posterior displacement	Operative
Type V	Tear	Tear	>100% CC displace	Operative
Type VI	Tear	Tear	Clavicle under coracoid	Operative

12. **What imaging tests are useful?**
    - Standard shoulder series x-rays are recommended to rule out bony abnormalities. MRI or ultrasound can provide a definitive diagnosis.
    - It is important for the clinician to be aware that partial rotator cuff tearing is a common finding in older asymptomatic patients.

13. **Is there a way to clinically differentiate complete versus partial tears?**
    Rotator cuff tears exist on a spectrum from partial to full width and from partial to full thickness and may involve one or more tendons (Fig. 37.3). As such, there is no perfect test. The described special tests can be useful in identifying tears that are large enough to cause substantial weakness. If pain interferes with the exam, a subacromial lidocaine injection followed by repeat exam can allow

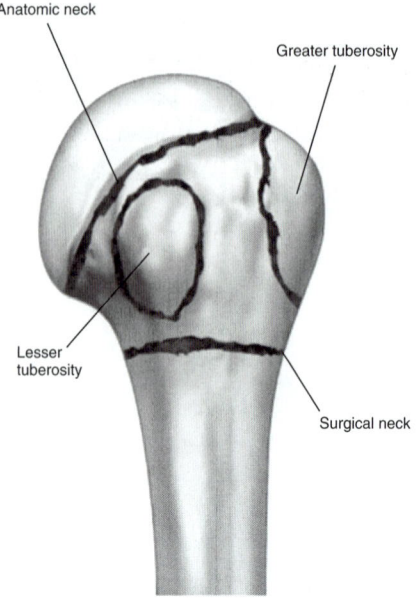

Fig. 37.3. Fracture Planes in the Proximal Humerus. *(From Sanders TG, Jersey SL. Conventional radiography of the shoulder.* Semin Roentgenol *40(3):207-222, 2005.)*

pain-free muscle activation. Be aware that injections of lidocaine may result in a false-positive tear or bursitis seen on subsequent MRI if done shortly after the injection due to the iatrogenic introduction of fluid.

14. **How are tears managed?**
    Most partial tears can be managed nonoperatively. Acutely, the best treatment is rest, followed by rehabilitation. A sling may be used for comfort for a short time, but early mobilization is important to avoid atrophy and risk of adhesive capsulitis. Corticosteroid injection can be considered for pain relief after the acute phase. Early surgical repair (<6 to 8 weeks) should be considered for large/complete tears. Young patients and patients with high physical demands may also be referred at an earlier time to an orthopedic surgeon to discuss possible surgical options.

PROXIMAL HUMERUS FRACTURE

15. **Are there special considerations when examining patients with proximal humerus fractures?**
    - In any acute shoulder injury, it is important to check neurovascular function. In proximal humerus fractures, as well as shoulder dislocation, checking the function of the deltoid (axillary nerve) is essential.
    - Ruling out dislocation is essential. Posterior dislocation is not easily seen on AP views of the shoulder.

16. **What imaging views should be obtained?**
    The acute shoulder series plus the scapular Y view are helpful to evaluate the extent of the fracture, angulation, and displacement. The axillary view is essential to rule out dislocation.

17. **How are proximal humerus fractures managed?**
    - Most fractures are nondisplaced and can be managed nonoperatively with sling immobilization and pain medication.

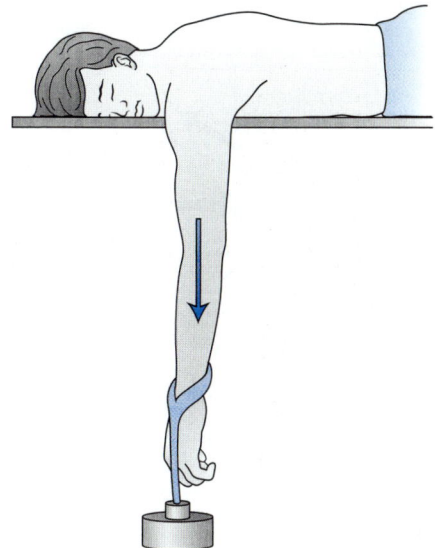

Fig. 37.4. Methods for Acute Shoulder Reduction. Gravity traction. (Общая хирургия [General Surgery] by Гостищев ВК (Hostishev VK) (2002).)

- Orthopedic referral is recommended for fractures with >1 cm of displacement or >45 degrees of angulation as this increases the chance of necrosis and nonunion. Young patients and patients with multipart (three- or four-part) fractures should also consider surgical management.

18. What is a multipart fracture?
See Fig. 37.4. The most common classification system for proximal humerus fractures was developed by Neer. There are four common fracture sites: the anatomic neck, the surgical neck, the greater tuberosity, and the lesser tuberosity.

19. What are the common complications of proximal humerus fractures?
Secondary rotator cuff syndrome and secondary osteoarthritis of the glenohumeral joint.

Case: An 18-year-old wrestler is brought in urgently following a wrestling match. He reports his shoulder was abducted and externally rotated forcefully. He felt a pop, followed by pain and the inability to use his shoulder. He has never dislocated his shoulder before but does report that during prior matches he has felt his shoulder "slide out and slide back in." (See Figs. 37.5 and 37.6.)

GLENOHUMERAL (GH) DISLOCATION/INSTABILITY

20. Who gets dislocated shoulders?
- The above case is a classic presentation. Shoulder dislocation and subluxation are more common in young males and the elderly.
- Patients with a genetic predisposition (Ehlers-Danlos syndrome).

21. What imaging views are helpful?
- The standard shoulder series views are helpful for dislocation. The axillary view is essential to diagnose posterior dislocation.
- Imaging should always be repeated following relocation. Additional postreduction views should include internal and external rotational AP. Stryker notch and West Point views are helpful to evaluate for Hill-Sachs (Fig. 37.7) and Bankart lesions.

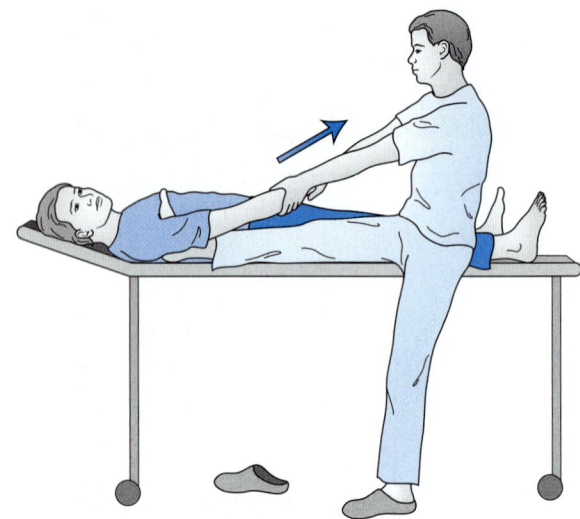

Fig. 37.5. Methods for Acute Shoulder Reduction. Assisted traction. *(From Regauer M, Polzer H, Mutschler W. Neurovascular complications due to the Hippocrates method for reducing anterior shoulder dislocations. World J Orthop 5(1):57-61, 2014. http://www.wjgnet.com/2218-5836/full/v5/i1/57.htm)*

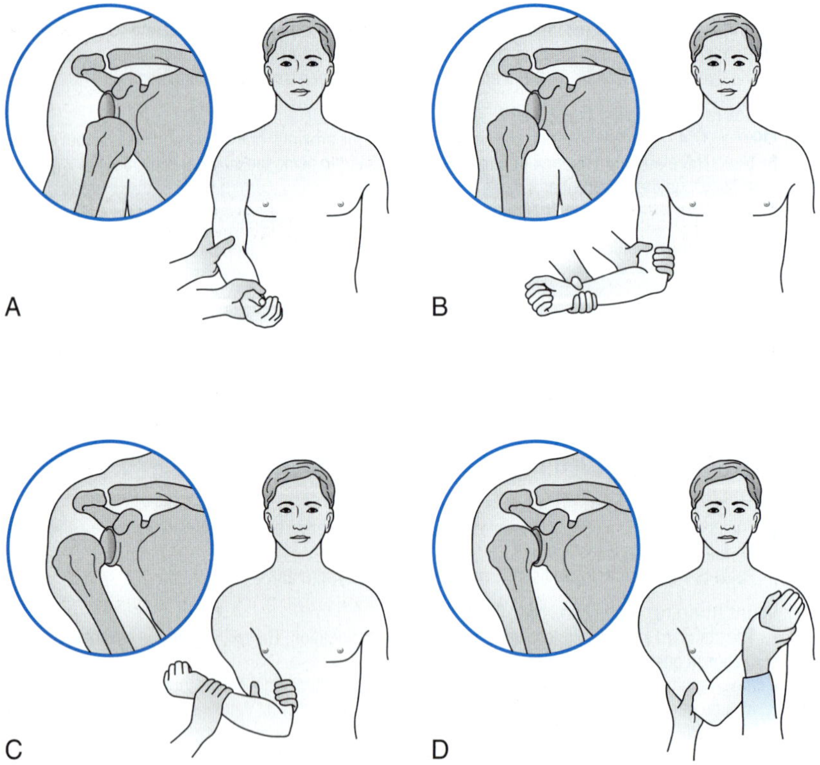

A

B

C

D

Fig. 37.6. Methods for Acute Shoulder Reduction. Kocher method (A) adduction (B) externally rotate (C) flex arm forward (D) internally rotate. (Общая хирургия [General Surgery] by Гостищев ВК (Hostishev VK) (2002).)

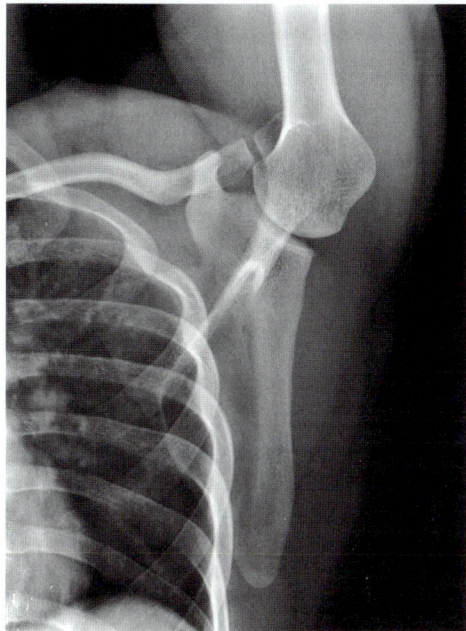

Fig. 37.7. Hill-Sachs Lesion on a Stryker Notch View. *(From Patel, MS. Stryker notch view radiograph.* http://radiopaedia. org/cases/stryker-notch-view-radiograph*)*

22. How are GH dislocations managed?
- Urgent relocation is required. A variety of relocation techniques have been described. See Figs. 37.4 - 37.6 for details.
- Immediate single attempt at reduction can be tried in the field if diagnosis is certain. Otherwise, imaging should be performed followed by intraarticular injection of anesthetic and/or oral pain medication prior to attempted reduction.
- The longer the duration between dislocation and relocation, the more challenging the procedure is due to muscle spasm and pain, and patients may require sedation. In rare cases, dislocations will require operative reduction.
- Following relocation, treatment involves sling immobilization for 2 to 4 weeks followed by strengthening and rehabilitation.
- There is a high recurrence rate among young men (>90% lifetime in military studies of young men), and surgical repair can be considered even after a single dislocation if the patient is a young athlete who places high demand on the shoulder.
- Recurrent dislocations, persistent instability, mechanical symptoms, and chronic pain are other indications for surgical stabilization.

23. What complications occur with dislocation?
- Dislocation in the elderly is often concomitant with fracture or rotator cuff tear. Shoulder dislocation may also result in labral tearing, intraarticular fractures, and axillary nerve injury.
- Bankhart lesions (breaks of the glenoid) and Hill-Sachs lesions (cortical crush fractures of the humeral head; see Fig. 37.7) are common in dislocations.

24. In what directions can shoulders dislocate?
- Anterior-inferior (most common), inferior, and posterior.

25. Who gets posterior dislocations?
- These classically are described from seizures and electrocution.

KEY POINTS

1. In any acute shoulder injury, it is important to check neurovascular function. In proximal humerus fractures, as well as shoulder dislocation, checking the function of the deltoid (axillary nerve) is essential.
2. All nondisplaced middle clavicle fractures can be managed nonoperatively with rest and a sling for comfort.
3. Acutely, the best treatment for a partial rotator cuff tear is rest, followed by rehabilitation. A sling may be used for comfort for a short time, but early mobilization is important to avoid atrophy and risk of adhesive capsulitis.
4. Bankhart lesions (breaks of the glenoid) and Hill-Sachs lesions (cortical crush fractures of the humeral head) are common in glenohumeral joint dislocations.

BIBLIOGRAPHY

Abbasi D, Badylak J. Acromio-clavicular injuries (AC separation). <http://www.orthobullets.com/sports/3047/acromio-clavi cular-injuries-ac-separation>.

Banerjee R, Waterman B, Padalecki J, Robertson W. Management of distal clavicle fractures. *J Am Acad Orthop Surg.* 2011;19(7):392–401.

Beim GM. Acromioclavicular joint injuries. *J Athl Train.* 2000;35(3):261–267.

Bencardino JT, Gyftopoulos S, Palmer WE. Imaging in anterior glenohumeral instability. *Radiology.* 2013;269(2):323–337.

Burkhart KJ, Dietz SO, Bastian L, et al. The treatment of proximal humeral fracture in adults. *Dtsch Arztebl Int.* 2013;110(35-36):591–597.

Cutts S, Prempeh M, Drew S. Anterior shoulder dislocation. *Ann R Coll Surg Engl.* 2009;91(1):2–7.

Hébert LJ, Moffet H, McFadyen BJ, Dionne CE. Scapular behavior in shoulder impingement syndrome. *Arch Phys Med Rehabil.* 2002;83(1):60–69.

Hsu J, Keener JD. Natural history of rotator cuff disease and implications on management. *Oper Tech Orthop.* 2015;25(1):2–9.

Lasbleiz S, Quintero N, Ea K, et al. Diagnostic value of clinical tests for degenerative rotator cuff disease in medical practice. *Ann Phys Rehabil Med.* 2014;57(4):228–243.

Lin A, Yannopoulos P, Warner J. Joint injuries and pain. <http://bostonshoulderinstitute.com/patient-resources/modules/ac-joint-injuries/>.

Motamedi D, Everist BM, Mahanty SR, Steinbach LS. Pitfalls in shoulder MRI: Part 1—normal anatomy and anatomic variants. *AJR Am J Roentgenol.* 2014;203(3):501–507.

Paladini P, Pellegrini A, Merolla G, Campi F, Porcellini G. Treatment of clavicle fractures. *Transl Med UniSa.* 2012;2:47–58.

Patel, MS. Stryker notch view radiograph. <http://radiopaedia.org/cases/stryker-notch-view-radiograph>.

Sanders TG, Jersey SL. Conventional radiography of the shoulder. *Semin Roentgenol.* 2005;40(3):207–222.

Savoie III FH, O'Brien MJ. Anterior instability in the throwing shoulder. *Sports Med Arthrosc.* 2014;22(2):117–119.

van der Meijden OA, Gaskill TR, Millett PJ. Treatment of clavicle fractures: current concepts review. *J Shoulder Elbow Surg.* 2012;21(3):423–429.

Warth RJ, Martetschläger F, Gaskill TR, Millett PJ. Acromioclavicular joint separations. *Curr Rev Musculoskelet Med.* 2013;6(1):71–78.

CHAPTER 38

CONCUSSION

Adae Amoako, MD, Thomas Trojian, MD

1. **During a soccer game, a 12-year-old girl collides (head to head) with the opponent while jumping for the ball. After the incident, she complains to the athletic trainer of a headache, nausea, and some dizziness. She is evaluated by the trainer, who decides to sit her out of the game on suspicion of a concussion. Her mother asks, "What is a concussion?"**

   Concussion is a disruption to the normal function of the brain secondary to a force such as a blow or punch to the head, which may be manifested by neurologic or cognitive symptoms.

2. **The patient's mother indicates she has seen several players collide with each other who were not diagnosed with concussion, and therefore she wants to know how common concussions are.**

   There are approximately 300,000 sports-related concussions and as many as 3.8 million sports and recreation–related concussions seen annually.

3. **What are some of the risk factors for a concussion?**

   Athletes playing in high-risk sports such as American football are at greater risk, but athletes in any sport can and do get concussions. A major determinant of sustaining a sports-related concussion is a prior history of a concussion. For comparable sports females have more concussions than males. Females tend to have more symptoms and require more time to recover. Attention-deficit disorder, psychiatric disorders, or a history of headaches/migraines can impact concussion recovery time (lengthen).

4. **What sports or activities have high concussion rates?**

   Concussion can occur in almost any type of sport but more commonly contact sports. Heading a soccer ball incorrectly, a hit to the head with a ball/puck, and player-to-player contact are the most common mechanisms of sustaining a concussion. Sports such as wrestling, ice and field hockey, lacrosse, football, rugby, soccer, basketball, baseball, and softball are examples of sports with high concussion rates.

5. **What are the symptoms and signs of a concussion?**

   The symptoms and signs of a concussion are divided into physical, cognitive, emotional, and sleep.
   - **Physical** manifestations of concussion include nausea, dizziness, imbalance, visual problems, and sensitivity to light and sound.
   - **Cognitive** impairments include mental fogginess, memory difficulties, difficulty with concentration, and confusion about recent events.
   - **Emotional** symptoms of concussion include sadness, irritability, personality changes, depression, and nervousness.
   - **Sleep** disturbances include difficulty initiating sleep, decreased sleep, and increased drowsiness.

6. **What red flag symptoms suggest a more severe injury in concussion?**

   Prolonged loss of consciousness (LOC) and amnesia may indicate severe brain injury.

   Recognized red flag signs are the athlete complains of neck pain, deteriorating conscious state, increasing confusion or irritability, severe or increasing headache, repeated vomiting, unusual behavior change, seizure or convulsion, double vision, and weakness or tingling/burning in arms or legs.

7. **What do you do with a patient who is suspected of having severe injury or persistent red flag symptoms?**

   Athletes with longer than brief LOC or persistent red flag symptoms should be transferred to the emergency department.

8. **How quickly do concussion symptoms appear?**

   The symptoms of concussion are generally apparent after an injury but can be delayed often 5 to 10 minutes; presentations up to 24 hours after impact have been reported.

9. **You are at a college football game, and a receiver is hit while running with the ball. After the play, he reports feeling "slow" and has difficulty remembering the events leading up to the hit and after the impact. What are three basic steps you should do to evaluate the injury?**
   - Remove the athlete from the game or practice to a quiet location.
   - Take away a piece of essential equipment (i.e., helmet).
   - Ask questions about symptoms and perform a full cognitive and neurologic examination.

10. **What should be included in the sideline neurologic exam?**
    Assess for amnesia and check for cranial nerves, peripheral sensation, extremity strength, and coordination.

11. **What are some of the cognitive tools available for evaluation of concussion on the sideline?**
    Some of the cognitive assessment tools available include:
    - **Balance Error Scoring System (BESS):** Consists of three tests lasting 20 seconds each, performed on a firm surface, with the eyes closed, and scored based on the number of errors across trials.
    - **Sport Assessment Concussion Tool 3 (SCAT3):** Combines three tests, the Standard Assessment of Concussion (SAC), Maddock's questions, and the BESS. The SAC and Maddock's questions focus on orientation, immediate memory, concentration, and delay recall.
    - **King-Devick (KD) test:** Measures how fast an athlete can read aloud single-digit numbers from three test cards. Captures attention, language, and eye movement impairments.

12. **What is the role of neuropsychological testing in concussion?**
    Neuropsychological testing has become commonplace in the diagnosis of concussion but cannot be independently used to determine if a concussion has occurred. There remains concern about reliability and positive predictive value.

13. **What types and examples of commercial neuropsychological testing tools are available?**
    Neuropsychological testing is available in written and computerized formats. Some of the neuropsychological written tests currently available are the Hopkins Verbal Learning Test, the Symbol Digit Modalities Test, and the Trail Making Parts A and B.

14. **How does evaluation of concussion in an urgent care facility differ from the sideline?**
    Evaluation in the urgent care is similar in terms of current symptoms and the tools used; however, considering the incident was not witnessed, a thorough history of symptoms and signs during the activity until the time of evaluation should be explored.

15. **What is the value of computed tomography (CT) scan or magnetic resonance imaging (MRI) in the evaluation of concussion?**
    These imaging modalities are used to rule out other causes of altered mental status (i.e., subdural hematoma). Neuroimaging in sports-related concussion is usually not recommended as a concussion is a functional and not structural injury; therefore, no abnormalities are expected with standard imaging.

16. **When should neuroimaging be considered?**
    Neuroimaging should be considered when there is a suspicion for intracranial bleed as seen in those patients with persistent red flag symptoms.

17. **What are some of the signs and symptoms of intracranial injury?**
    Focal neurologic findings on exam; repeated emesis; seizures; significant drowsiness or difficulty walking; poor orientation to person, place, or time; and slurred speech. In addition, athletes with worsening symptoms and prolonged (30 seconds or more) loss of consciousness should be considered for neuroimaging.

18. **What is the main treatment for concussion?**
    There is no single recommended treatment for concussion; however, physical and cognitive rest for 48 hours followed by a slow progressive increase in cognitive activity until symptoms resolve is widely accepted practice. Physical activity should be curtailed until symptoms resolve.

19. What does physical rest entail?

Physical rest includes removal of the athlete from activities that place him/her at risk for repeat impact and removal from aerobic conditioning and strength training to avoid overexertion. Strict bed rest is not recommended and has been shown to offer no additional benefit over usual care.

20. What does cognitive rest entail?

Cognitive rest includes minimizing or cessation of activities that input stimuli to the brain. Examples include watching television, using a computer, looking at presentation screens, playing video games, doing schoolwork, reading and writing, using a cell phone (with emphasis on texting), and avoiding areas with increased sensitivity to light and noise. Using a cognitive activity scale can be helpful to increase activity in a stepwise manner.

21. What is the role of medication in the management of concussion?

Symptomatic management of concussion is widely practiced with different medications depending on the patient's symptoms. There is no evidence that any one particular medicine is effective in specifically treating or altering the course of sports-related concussion.

22. What are the treatments for some of the common symptoms of concussion?

See Table 38.1.

23. When is the appropriate time to return to school or work?

There is no universal recommendation for when one can return to work or school because of the heterogeneity of concussion symptoms. The goal should be to disrupt life as little as possible and return to school or work as soon as possible.

24. What are some reasonable accommodations that may be needed for concussive patients?

Reduced academic load at school or duties at the workplace, which may include shortened or altered schedules, should be considered. In the student athlete, adjustments may include excused school absences or lighter homework load, scheduled rest breaks during the day, extended time to complete homework assignments and projects, and extended time on tests.

25. When is the appropriate time to return to play for athletes after sustaining a concussion?

- Athletes should never return to play the same day as diagnosis.
- Return to play should be considered when the concussed patient is asymptomatic with a normal exam for 24 hours.
- Return to play should follow a stepwise progression for a minimum of 5 days.

26. What is the recommended stepwise progression for return to play?

Return to play should begin with light aerobic activity followed by sport-specific activity, noncontact training drills, full contact practice, and ultimately full return to play.

If any symptom recurrence occurs during this process, the athlete should return to the previous asymptomatic level and begin the progression again.

Table 38.1. Some Accepted Treatments for Common Symptoms of Concussions

SYMPTOM	TREATMENT	COMMENTS
Headache	1. NSAID and acetaminophen 2. Ice, massage, manual therapy for concomitant neck pain in acute setting 3. Dim, quiet environment 4. Amitriptyline	• NSAIDs should be avoided acutely as they can theoretically increase bleeding risk • Rebound headaches have been reported with frequent NSAID use
Sleep disturbances	1. Amitriptyline 2. Melatonin	Good sleep hygiene should be encouraged
Balance, vertigo, and ocular dysfunction	Vestibular rehabilitation	Focus on vestibular-ocular exercises, smooth pursuit, gaze stabilization, and balance training

27. **What is the role of provocative testing such as the Buffalo Concussion Treadmill Test in return to play decisions?**

Provocative exercise testing provides the opportunity to access physiologic response to exercise in a concussed patient using parameters of symptom exacerbation such as heart rate and blood pressure. This helps to identify the athlete who is not ready to return to play but also to determine at what level an athlete may exercise without provoking symptoms.

28. **What is postconcussion syndrome?**

Postconcussion syndrome is a poorly defined condition referring to symptoms and/or signs of concussion that persist for weeks or months after the concussion.

29. **A 15-year-old football player is diagnosed with concussion. His mother asks why his helmet and mouth guard did not protect against the concussion. What do you say to her?**

Despite advances in helmet technology, there is no evidence to suggest helmets or mouth guards reduce the incidence of concussion in football. However, they reduce dental, facial, and head injuries such as skull fractures.

30. **In what ways can concussion be prevented?**

Rule changes in sports have been shown to reduce the incidence of concussion. Examples include banning spear tackling in American football, eliminating back checking in ice hockey, and limiting elbow-to-head contact in soccer. Sport-specific techniques need to be taught correctly to athletes.

KEY POINTS

1. Immediately remove the athlete from the game or practice when concussion is suspected.
2. Seize key equipment to ensure the athlete does not return to the game or practice.
3. Do not return the athlete to the game, practice, or physical activity the same day as diagnosis.
4. Consider reduced academic load at school or duties at the workplace after the diagnosis of a concussion.

BIBLIOGRAPHY

Cantu RC. Posttraumatic retrograde and anterograde amnesia: pathophysiology and implications in grading and safe return to play. *J Athl Train.* 2001;36(3):244–248.

Darling SR, Leddy JJ, Baker JG, et al. Evaluation of the Zurich guidelines and exercise testing for return to play in adolescents following concussion. *Clin J Sport Med.* 2014;24(2):128–133.

Gammons MR. Helmets in sport: fact and fallacy. *Curr Sports Med Rep.* 2013;12(6):377–380.

Harmon KG, Drezner JA, Gammons M, et al. American Medical Society for Sports Medicine position statement: concussion in sport. *Br J Sports Med.* 2013;47(1):15–26.

Kelly JP. Loss of consciousness: pathophysiology and implications in grading and safe return to play. *J Athl Train.* 2001;36(3):249–252.

Leddy JJ, Baker JG, Kozlowski K, Bisson L, Willer B. Reliability of a graded exercise test for assessing recovery from concussion. *Clin J Sport Med.* 2011;21(2):89–94.

McCrory P, Meeuwisse W, Aubry M, et al. Consensus statement on concussion in sport - The 4th International Conference on Concussion in Sport, Zurich, November 2012. *Phys Ther Sport.* 2013;14(2):e1–e13.

McGuine TA, Hetzel S, McCrea M, Brooks MA. Protective equipment and player characteristics associated with the incidence of sport-related concussion in high school football players: a multifactorial prospective study. *Am J Sports Med.* 2014;42(10):2470–2478.

Scorza KA, Raleigh MF, O'Connor FG. Current concepts in concussion: evaluation and management. *Am Fam Physician.* 2012;85(2):123–132.

US Department of Health and Human Services, Centers for Disease Control and Prevention. Heads Up: Facts for Physicians About Mild Traumatic Brain Injury (MTBI). <http://www.cdc.gov/headsup/basics/concussion_whatis.html>; Accessed 20.05.16.

CHAPTER 39

OVERUSE APOPHYSEAL INJURIES

Jayson Loeffert, DO, Cayce Onks, DO, MS, ATC

1. What is apophysitis?

Apophysitis is an injury secondary to overuse, seen in young, skeletally immature athletes. It is believed to result from repetitive microtrauma from forceful contractions by surrounding musculature. In the immature athlete, the area surrounding the growth plate, or apophysis, is relatively weak compared to attached tendons. Chronic tension from these attachments causes bony disruption and may lead to avulsion of the secondary ossification centers. As this area continues to grow, ossify, and enlarge, it may result in fibrous nonunion or union with bony enlargement. These areas of bony disruption may become painful and persist during an athlete's growing years. Pain will generally resolve after athletes complete their growth; however occasional individuals may complain of chronic pain into adulthood.

The aim of this chapter is to educate on the presentation of various apophysitides, offer guidance that can be provided to patients, and provide some structure and ideas for treatment. The following chapter is limited to overuse apophyseal injuries.

2. In patients with Osgood-Schlatter disease, will continued play result in long-term knee problems?

Background: Osgood-Schlatter disease (OSD), sometimes referred to as Osgood-Schlatter syndrome, is one cause of anterior knee pain in young athletes. OSD was first described by Robert Osgood and Carl Schlatter in 1903. Due to chronic tension from the quadriceps muscle and patellar tendon, the apophyseal cartilage of the tibial tuberosity becomes separated from the anterior aspect of the tibia.

Presentation: The age of presentation is 12–15 years in boys, and 8–12 years in girls, with boys more commonly affected. History of pain is generally vague and progressive and located over the area of the tibial tuberosity. Pain typically worsens with activities, including running, jumping, squatting, kicking, and kneeling, and is relieved with rest. Risk factors for developing OSD include increased sporting activity in young individuals, family history of OSD, and quadricep and hamstring muscle tightness.

Physical examination: On physical examination, patients will have tenderness to palpation over the tibial tuberosity and a bony enlargement may be visualized. Pain with resisted knee extension may also be noted. The diagnosis of OSD is best made clinically.

Imaging: Radiographic imaging can be used for unilateral cases to rule out diagnoses such as fracture, infections, or tumor. Radiographs may demonstrate separation of the apophysis from the tibial tuberosity; however, this will not alter management. Magnetic resonance imaging (MRI) or computed tomography (CT) offer little in terms of establishing the diagnosis or treatment and should be reserved for refractory cases that do not respond to conservative management. Ultrasound is an inexpensive and safe option to assess the tibial tuberosity and may distinguish stages of disease; however, more research is needed.

Treatment: OSD is generally a self-limiting condition and will resolve after the patient has completed growth. Approximately 90% will improve with conservative treatment. Patients may be treated with ice, nonsteroidal antiinflammatory drugs (NSAIDs), and knee padding. Physical therapy may be beneficial for strengthening and improving flexibility of the quadriceps, hamstring, and gastrocnemius muscles and iliotibial band. High-intensity quadriceps strengthening should be avoided in early rehabilitation. If an athlete complains of mild pain and no weakness, activity may continue as tolerated. The patient may initially require modification of activity to continue pain-free participation. If the athlete continues to have pain despite modifying activities, then complete rest is necessary, which can be guided by individual pain levels. The importance of rest should not be underestimated as nonadherence may increase the risk of pain continuing into adulthood. Time of rest is variable and may require anywhere from 2 to 10 months. Surgical intervention is the last line of treatment and should be reserved for only those who are skeletally mature and continue to have symptoms despite appropriate conservative therapy. Corticosteroid use for this condition should be avoided due to risk of subcutaneous atrophy and tendon damage.

3. **Are radiographic images necessary to diagnose Sever disease?**
   Background: Another location of pain seen in young athletes from apophysitis is in the posterior heel. This was first described by Haglund in 1907and then Sever in 1912. This condition is believed to result from traction of the Achilles tendon on the secondary ossification center of the calcaneus.

   Presentation: The average age of onset is 11–15 years in boys and 8–13 years in girls. Boys are more commonly affected. Risk factors include high levels of athletic activity, obesity, increased height, and decreased ankle dorsiflexion. Pain is routinely described as "non-specific" and aggravated by activity.

   Physical examination: The diagnosis of Sever disease is best made clinically. Edema, erythema, and warmth will be absent. There will be tenderness at the posteroplantar aspect of the calcaneus. Research demonstrates the most reliable physical examination findings are positive squeeze test (lateral compression over the calcaneal tubercle) and barefoot one-leg heel standing. These have the highest sensitivity (97% and 100%, respectively) and specificity (each 100%) for making the diagnosis.

   Imaging: Imaging for suspected Sever disease is low yield. Abnormalities over the calcaneus in a young athlete are neither sensitive nor specific. No radiographic sign has been found to be pathognomonic, and changes can be seen in asymptomatic, healthy individuals. For these reasons, radiographs should be reserved for ruling out pathologic abnormalities in recalcitrant cases. A lateral view provides the highest benefit. Ultrasound has also been investigated with some promise; however, further studies are needed.

   Treatment: Calcaneal apophysitis is self-limited. Treatment options include rest, orthotics, physical therapy, ice, and NSAIDs. Although several treatment options are available, it does not appear they have a large impact on time to resolution, as pain improves within 3 months. Heel lifts may be recommended as those patients admitted to improved satisfaction with treatment; however, this comes with financial implications. Over-the-counter heel lifts would be desirable over custom orthotics, as their use should be short term.

4. **Do athletes with pelvic apophysitis face any risks should they continue to play in spite of pain?**
   Iliac crest apophysitis: There are many growth plates that can be affected in the pelvis; the most common is the iliac crest. Ossification of the iliac crest occurs from anterior lateral to posterior and typically takes 1 year to complete. This process begins in females around age 13 and males around age 15. Apophysitis of the iliac crest occurs anteriorly and more commonly affected than posteriorly due to repeat traction from the external oblique, transversus abdominis, and tensor fascia lata muscle attachments. High-risk activities include running and gymnastics. Patients may report pain with coughing or sneezing. Physical examination reveals tenderness to palpation along the iliac crest, as well as tightness of the iliotibial band, hip flexors, and rectus femoris. The patient may have pain with resisted hip abduction. Radiographs may demonstrate slight widening of the iliac apophysis. Treatment consists of rest until pain resolves, which may take several weeks. When pain free, the athlete can begin a hip abductor rehabilitation program. There is a risk for complete avulsion if the patient returns to intense activity too early. Fig. 39.1 demonstrates an iliac crest avulsion fracture.

   Ischial apophysitis: Another affected growth center in the pelvis is the ischial apophysis, site of hamstring insertion. Repetitive contraction of the hamstrings can cause the apophysis to become inflamed. It occurs between the ages of 13 and 25. Athletes complain of vague pain, with or without injury. Examination will show tenderness over the ischium and pain with straight leg raising. Progression to avulsion is a relatively common occurrence. Discussion of treatment in the literature is limited, however. A period of rest and refraining from sports is currently accepted. Conservative treatment should include partial weight bearing with use of crutches until pain free and then therapy aimed at hamstring rehabilitation. Further treatment is controversial, but surgical referral should be considered if bony displacement is greater than 1–2 cm or no symptom improvement occurs with 2 months of rest.

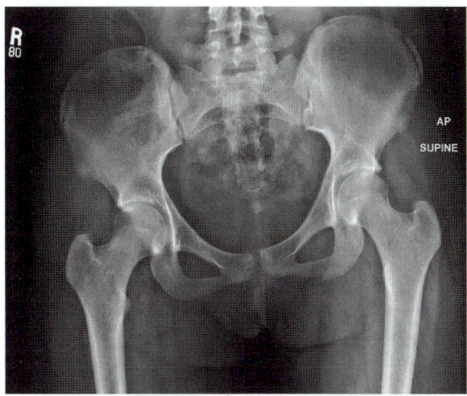

Fig. 39.1. Iliac crest avulsion fracture. There is a displaced ossification center of the left ilium. In apophysitis, the patient will complain of similar pain; however, the growth plate will remain unchanged. Comparison can be made to the right side. *(From Duryea D, Penn State radiology archive.)*

Other key areas of apophysitis: Other areas of the pelvis that are subject to apophyseal injury are the anterior superior iliac spine (ASIS), anterior inferior iliac spine (AIIS), and the lesser trochanter. The origin of the sartorius muscle is the ASIS, and injury can be due to sprinting. The rectus femoris, which is attached to the AIIS, is commonly injured by kicking in soccer. The lesser trochanter, which is attached to the iliopsoas tendon, can be injured from active hip extension and knee flexion. Due to the complexity of the hip anatomy, plain radiographs are important in confirming the diagnosis and ruling out avulsion. More advanced imaging, such as CT or MRI, is commonly unnecessary. Treatment is generally conservative, including nonweight bearing, then transitioning to routine activities with therapy progression focusing on the strength and flexibility of the offended muscle. Apophysitis in these areas can progress to acute avulsion fractures. For this reason, a suggested timeline for treatment includes 1 week of nonweight bearing followed by 2–3 weeks of limited activity and partial weight bearing, before initiating a therapy progression.

5. **In a young athlete with lateral foot pain, does a radiolucency parallel to the shaft and across the tubercle at the base of the fifth metatarsal raise concern for fracture?**
Background: Apophysitis of the fifth metatarsal head was first described in 1912 by Dr. H. Iselin. The apophysis is present at the attachment of the peroneus brevis, on the plantar aspect of the base of the fifth metatarsal.
Presentation: The timing of occurrence for this injury is generally between ages 10 and 12 for girls and 12 and 14 in boys. This apophysitis occurs secondary to repeat tension from the peroneus brevis or by inversion injuries.
Physical examination: Physical examination will reveal tenderness to palpation at the attachment site of the peroneus brevis and pain with resisted eversion or passive extreme plantar and dorsiflexion. An enlarged tuberosity, with edema or erythema, compared to the uninvolved side, may also be appreciated.
Imaging: Radiographs are not necessary to make the diagnosis; however, oblique films may visualize the ossification center and reveal a small bone piece at the plantar-lateral edge of the tuberosity or enlargement of the apophysis. The apophysis crosses the tubercle parallel to the shaft, whereas fractures occur more transverse. This distinction may help to prevent misdiagnosis on radiographs (see Fig. 39.2, for example). With a history of an acute inversion injury, radiographs should be obtained to make this differentiation.
Treatment: Treatment is conservative with a period of rest, nonweight bearing, NSAIDs, bracing, and physical therapy. A walking boot for 1 month before progressing to physical therapy, rather than the use of crutches, could also be considered.

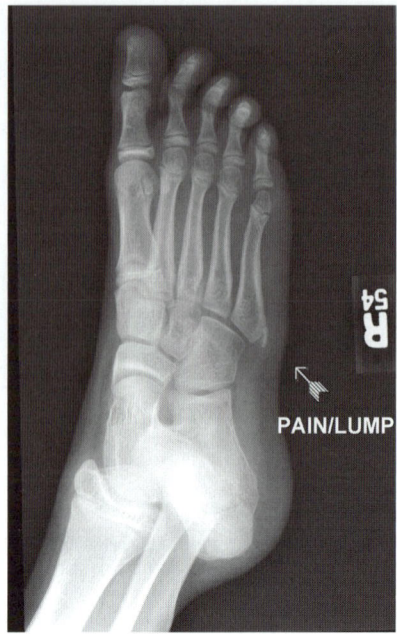

PAIN/LUMP

Fig. 39.2. Iselin's apophysitis. The bony irregularity at the proximal fifth metatarsal is parallel with the shaft. This differs from a fracture to this area as the fracture will occur more transverse, across the shaft. *(From Duryea D, Penn State radiology archive.)*

6. **In patients with medial epicondyle apophysitis, are there any shoulder mechanics that make them more susceptible to this injury that could be addressed and improved through physical therapy?**

Background: Apophysitides of the upper extremity are rare due to its general lack of weight bearing. For this reason, sports such as gymnastics increase the risk of injury. Overhead throwers also put enough stress on their elbow to cause injury. Throwers are more likely to injure their medial epicondylar apophysis (little league elbow) as the greatest amount of stress is transferred through this side of the joint. This is due to valgus extension overload and can also occur from tennis or swimming.

    Presentation: Patients complain of medial sided elbow pain and decreased throwing distance. History of overuse is quite common. For pitchers, the numbers and types of pitches thrown are important components of the history. Breaking pitches are thought to be exceptionally dangerous and should generally be avoided in the skeletally immature pitcher.

    Physical examination: Physical examination demonstrates tenderness to palpation over the medial epicondyle and possible bony enlargement.

    Imaging: Ossification center enlargement or detachment may be seen on radiograph.

    Treatment: Treatment is rest from throwing for 4–6 weeks. After athletes are pain free, they may slowly progress their throwing activities as tolerated. It is also important to address concomitant skeletal abnormalities, such as scapular dyskinesis, weak core strength, and spinal posture. These abnormalities can increase the force being transmitted through the elbow, increasing risk of injury. If the athlete is not compliant with a progression, decreasing pitch counts, and avoiding aggravating pitch mechanics, bony avulsion can occur. Surgery may be required in these circumstances.

    Olecranon apophysitis: A similar apophyseal injury can occur at the location of the olecranon from repeated triceps contraction. Patients will elicit tenderness to palpation over the olecranon and pain with resisted elbow extension. A period of 4–6 weeks' rest is advised, and activity can gradually resume when the patient is pain free. Radiographs may take 10 months to demonstrate bone consolidation. Return to play is determined clinically.

KEY POINTS

1. Individuals with Osgood Schlatter disease may continue to play sports in spite of pain; however, they should use pain as their guide. An athlete should discontinue activities and rest if modification of activities does not alleviate pain.
2. Sever disease can be expected to improve within 3 months of diagnosis, regardless of therapeutic treatment.
3. Contrary to most other areas of apophysitis, concern around the pelvis should be evaluated with radiographs to rule out avulsion fracture.
4. Use caution when viewing radiographs in Iselin's disease, as fractures can look similar to apophysitis.
5. If rest is not performed for little league elbow, the injury may progress to an avulsion fracture and could require surgical intervention.

BIBLIOGRAPHY

Canale S, Williams K. Iselin's disease. *J Pediatr Ortho.* 1992;12(1):90–93.

Frush T, Lindenfeld T. Peri-epiphyseal and overuse injuries in adolescent athletes. *Sports Health.* 2009;1:3.

Gholve P, Scher D, Khakharia S, et al. Osgood Schlatter syndrome. *Curr Opin Pediatr.* 2007;19.

Hasgoren B, Koktener A, Dilmen G. Ultrasonography of the calcaneus in Sever's disease. *Indian J Pediatr.* 2005;42(8): 801–803.

Hermans G, De Jonghe B, Bruyninckx F, et al. Clinical review: critical illness polyneuropathy and myopathy. *Crit Care.* 2008;12:238.

James A, Williams C, Luscombe M, et al. Factors associated with pain severity in children with calcaneal apophysitis (Sever disease). *J Pediatr.* 2015;2:167.

Kose Ozkan. Do we really need radiographic assessment for the diagnosis of nonspecific heel pain (calcaneal apophysitis) in children? *Skeletal Radiol.* 2010;39(4):359–361.

Kujala U, Dvist M, Heinonen O. Osgood-Schlatter's disease in adolescent athletes; retrospective study of incidence and duration. *Am J Sports Med.* 1985;4:13.

Launay F. Sports-related overuse injuries in children. *Orthop Traumatol Surg Res.* 2015;1:101.

Leahy I, Schorpion M, Ganley T. Common medial elbow injuries in the adolescent athlete. *J Hand Ther.* 2015;28(2):201–210.

Nakase J, Goshima K, Numata H, et al. Precise risk factors for Osgood-Schlatter disease. *Arch Orthop Trauma Surg.* 2015;135(9):1277–1281.

Perhamre S, Lazowska D, Papageorgiou S, et al. Severs injury: a clinical diagnosis. *J Am Podiatr Med Assoc.* 2013;5:103.

Pointinger H, Munk P, Poeschl G. Avulsion fracture of the anterior superior iliac spine following apophysitis. *Br J Sports Med.* 2003;37(4):361–362.

Rachel J, Williams J, Sawyer J, et al. A novel approach to treatment for chronic avulsion fracture of the ischial tuberosity in three adolescent athletes: a case series. *J Pediatr Orthop.* 2011;31(5):548–550.

Schoensee S, Nilsson K. Is radiographic evaluation necessary in children with a clinical diagnosis of calcaneal apophysitis (Sever disease). *Int J Sports Phys Ther.* 2014;7:9.

Wiegerinck J, Zwiers R, Sierevelt I, et al. Treatment of calcaneal apophysitis: wait and see versus orthotic device versus physical therapy: a pragmatic therapeutic randomized clinical trial. *J Pediatr Orthop.* 2015;36(2):162–157.

Yanagisawa S, Osawa T, Saito K. Assessment of Osgood-Schlatter disease and the skeletal maturation of distal attachment of the patellar tendon in preadolescent males. *Orthop J Sports Med.* 2014;2:7.

CHAPTER 40

THE ACUTELY LIMPING CHILD

Eric Requa, DO, Mark Lavallee, MD

1. **Why is an acutely limping child a serious concern?**
   A child who presents with an acute onset of limping can have a serious, sometimes life-threatening diagnosis and must have a comprehensive evaluation. Delays in diagnosis and treatment can result in significant morbidity and mortality. Often the child is too young to communicate symptoms. Historical clues and a comprehensive physical examination combined with laboratory studies and imaging are often needed to arrive at a final working diagnosis (Fig. 40.1). It is important to develop a stepwise approach to treating the acutely limping child. The differential diagnosis of limp in a child is extensive as described in Table 40.1.

2. **What exactly is a limp?**
   A limp typically will come from an antalgic gait. During an antalgic gait, the stance phase on the affected side will be shortened to prevent pain on that side. Assessing a limp is difficult because most children do not have a rhythmic, steady gait until after 7 years of age, so an acute change in the gait cycle that is typically observed by the parents becomes essential to help evaluate gait.

3. **What is a normal gait pattern for a child?**
   It is important to accurately analyze a child's gait. By the age of 3, a mature gait pattern is typically established and by the age of 7, a child's gait emulates that of an adult.

4. **What is the key factor in forming the differential diagnosis for an acutely limping child?**
   The differential can be narrowed based on age upon presentation. For example, slipped capital femoral epiphyses (SCFE) are more common in overweight boys over the age of 11, while Legg-Calvé-Perthes (LCP) is more common in those between 4 and 10 years of age (Table 40.2). An atraumatic limp in a child up to 3 years of age is most commonly septic arthritis, developmental dysplasia of the hip (DDH), or toddler's fracture.

5. **What components of the physical examination are essential when evaluating a limping child?**
   When evaluating a limping child, you must include the following in your physical examination: core and limb temperature, observed gait, knee (question of effusion), passive hip flexion with internal rotation, foot/ankle, forward bending test, abdomen, and testicles (to rule out testicular torsion).

6. **What modality of imaging is useful in evaluating a limping child?**
   Imaging should begin with frog-leg lateral radiographs, which will be useful in diagnosing DDH, LCP, and SCFE. Ultrasound is highly sensitive for detecting hip effusion but is not very sensitive for differentiating among hemorrhagic, sterile, and purulent fluid accumulations. Ultrasound is also preferred when suspecting septic arthritis as it may also facilitate hip aspiration. Magnetic resonance imaging (MRI) is highly sensitive and specific for visualizing the joint, soft tissue, and cartilage. This makes it the preferred method for diagnosing osteomyelitis and stress fractures.

7. **What is DDH?**
   Present since birth, DDH can go undetected until ambulatory. Patients will have a painless limp, Trendelenburg gait if unilateral, waddling gait if bilateral. They may also have leg shortening, abnormal skin creases in the leg, and limited hip abduction. Ortolani and Barlow maneuvers can be performed to aid in diagnosis and are more sensitive in infants <2 months of age. All cases of DDH should be referred promptly for orthopedic consultation.

8. **What is a toddler's fracture?**
   A toddler's fracture is a spiral, oblique, nondisplaced fracture of the distal tibial shaft in children 9 months to 3 years of age. They are caused by rotational or twisting force through the tibia while on a planted foot. If there is unclear history, this should raise suspicion for child abuse. Plain x-ray is only 53% sensitive for detecting fracture. Bone scan can be useful if diagnosis is unclear. Current treatment includes long leg cast for 3–5 weeks, followed by short leg cast for 6 weeks.

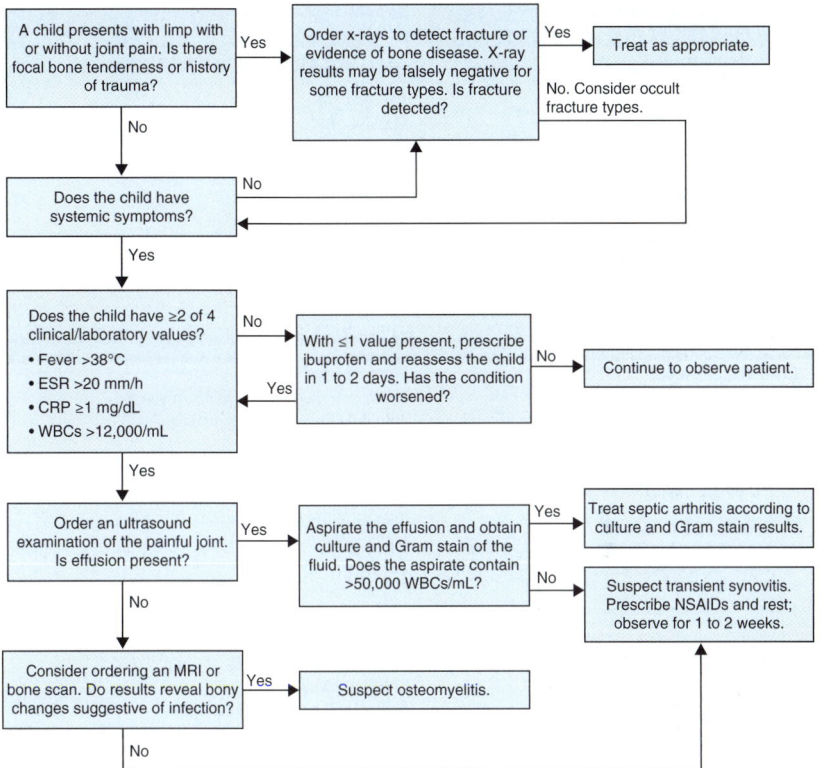

Fig. 40.1. Algorithm for approaching acutely limping pediatric patient. *(From: Hill D, Whiteside J. Limp in children: differentiating benign from dire causes. J Fam Pract. 60(4):193–197.)*

Table 40.1. Possible causes of limp in a child

Traumatic/Mechanical	Fractures, developmental dysplasia, slipped capital femoral epiphysis, tarsal coalition, child abuse, overuse injury, leg length discrepancy, clubfoot, osteochondritis desiccans, Sever disease, Blount disease
Infectious	Septic arthritis, osteomyelitis, Lyme disease, psoas abscess, diskitis, appendicitis
Inflammatory	Transient synovitis, Reiter syndrome, lupus, juvenal rheumatoid arthritis, ankylosing spondylitis
Vascular	Legg-Calvé-Perthes disease, osteonecrosis, sickle cell disease
Neoplastic	Leukemia, lymphoma, Ewing sarcoma, osteogenic sarcoma
Metabolic	Rickets, hyperparathyroidism
Neuromuscular	Muscular dystrophy, cerebral palsy, peripheral neuropathy

9. What is the most common cause of pediatric hip pain in general?

The most common cause of pediatric hip pain up to 10 years of age is idiopathic transient synovitis. It is most common in boys 4–8 years of age. The cause is unclear but is proposed to relate to a viral agent. This condition typically resolves in 1–2 weeks without long-term sequelae. Treatment is generally symptomatic including rest, nonsteroidal antiinflammatory drugs (NSAIDs), and reassurance.

Table 40.2. Differential Diagnosis of Limping in Children

AGE GROUP	DIAGNOSTIC CONSIDERATIONS
Early walker: 1 to 3 years of age	*Painful Limp* Septic arthritis and osteomyelitis Transient monarticular synovitis Occult trauma ("toddler's fracture") Intervertebral diskitis Malignancy *Painless Limp* Developmental dysplasia of the hip Neuromuscular disorder Cerebral palsy Lower extremity length inequality
Child: 3 to 10 years of age	*Painful Limp* Septic arthritis, osteomyelitis, myositis Transient monarticular synovitis Trauma Rheumatologic disorders Juvenile idiopathic arthritis Intervertebral diskitis Malignancy *Painless Limp* Developmental dysplasia of the hip Legg-Calve-Perthes disease Lower extremity length inequality Neuromuscular disorder Cerebral palsy Muscular dystrophy (Duchenne)
Adolescent: 11 years of age to maturity	*Painful Limp* Septic arthritis, osteomyelitis, myositis Trauma Rheumatologic disorder Slipped capital femoral epiphysis: acute; unstable Malignancy *Painless Limp* Slipped capital femoral epiphysis: chronic; stable Developmental dysplasia of the hip: acetabular dysplasia Lower extremity length inequality Neuromuscular disorder

From Walter, Kevin D and Tassone, J Channing. "Orthopedic Assessment." Nelson Essentials of Pediatrics. By Karen J. Marcdante and Robert M. Kliegman. 7th ed. Philadelphia: Elsevier, 2015. 667-69. Print.

10. What is the most life-threatening cause of acute limp in pediatric patient?

Septic arthritis of the hip is very serious, and diagnosis should be made quickly. If the diagnosis is delayed, the patient is at risk of sepsis, growth arrest, permanent loss of joint function, and osteonecrosis. The presentation is similar to transient synovitis; however, the patient is often more toxic appearing and may have temperature elevation. This can occur in neonates, young infants, and children. Patient may hold their leg in a flexed and abducted position and have irritability with passive movement of the hip.

11. What clinical features help distinguish and predict septic arthritis?

Refusal to bear weight, pain with passive hip movement, temperature >101.3°F, erythrocyte sedimentation rate (ESR) >44 mm/hr, white blood cell count (WBC) >12,000, C-reactive protein (CRP) level >2.0 (Table 40.3).

Table 40.3. Laboratory tests for diagnosis in a limping child

TEST	CONDITION	EXPECTED FINDING
ANA	SLE	Positive
Blood culture	Septic arthritis	Positive
Bone culture	Osteomyelitis	Positive
CBC	Infection Malignancy	Increased WBC/platelets Cytopenia
CRP	Infection/inflammation/malignancy	Increased CRP
ESR	Infection/inflammation/malignancy	Increased ESR
Lyme titer	Lyme disease	Positive
Synovial fluid analysis	Septic arthritis Transient synovitis	Turbid, WBC 50–100 K/mm PMNS >75% Clear yellow, WBC 5–15 K/mm PMNs <15%
Synovial fluid culture	Septic arthritis Transient synovitis	Positive Negative
Urethral, cervical, pharyngeal cultures	Gonococcal arthritis	*Neisseria gonorrhoeae*
Urethral and stool cultures	Reactive arthritis	Chlamydia (urethral) *Salmonella, Shigella, Campylo-bacter* in stool cultures

From: The timping child: a systematic approach to diagnosis. *Am Fam Physician* 79(3):215–224, 2009.

12. What is the gold standard for diagnosing septic arthritis?

Hip aspiration, the gold standard for diagnosing septic arthritis, should be performed whenever this diagnosis is suspected. Aspirated fluid should be analyzed for culture/sensitivity, Gram stain, glucose, and WBC count. Ultrasound is recommended over plain films because it may also facilitate aspiration. Treatment includes surgical drainage, antibiotics for a minimum of 3 weeks to cover *Staphylococcus*, *Streptococcus*, and *Neisseria* pathogens. Approximately 25% of patients will have long-term sequelae even after appropriate treatment with antibiotics.

13. What is the pathophysiology of LCP?

LCP is more common in 8-year-old boys. This disease results from interruption of the blood supply to the still-growing femoral head causing avascular necrosis. LCP occurs in children 2–12 years of age and is most common in children 4–9 years of age. LCP presents with hip pain and an atraumatic limp; it is more common in boys (male-to-female ratio 4:1). It often presents as a painless limp; if pain is present, it may be referred and present as knee or back pain. Common physical findings include leg-length discrepancies, limited abduction and internal rotation, and the presence of a Trendelenburg gait. When ordering radiographs, anteroposterior (AP) and frog-leg lateral views are essential. X-rays typically reveal sclerosis of the proximal femur with joint space widening. An MRI confirms osteonecrosis but is often unnecessary. A common long-term consequence is early onset hip arthritis.

14. How is LCP treated?

Initial treatment of LCP includes rest, typically with crutches, with concomitant physical therapy to help maintain range of motion. For severe cases, pediatric orthopedic referral is required.

15. What is the most common cause of hip pain in boys older than 11 years?

SCFE occurs when the proximal femoral epiphysis slips posteriorly and inferiorly on the femoral neck through the growth plate. SCFE is often misdiagnosed, because the symptoms are frequently vague. It is the most common hip disorder in early adolescence, 9–15 years of age. Peak age is 13 for boys and 11 for girls during rapid growth spurts. It occurs more often in boys, with African Americans and Pacific Islanders having a higher rate of involvement, possibly due to increased levels of obesity in these population groups. SCFE occurs bilaterally 25%–40% of the time, and very often the pain is vague and poorly localized.

16. How does SCFE typically present?

The typical presentation is a limping child who may have pain in the groin, hip, thigh, or knee. The hallmark of SCFE on examination is limited internal rotation of the hip. The child presents with the hip slightly flexed and externally rotated. Specific to SCFE is the even greater limitation of internal rotation when the hip is flexed to 90 degrees. No other pediatric condition has this physical finding, which makes this maneuver very useful in children with lower extremity pain. Whitman's sign is obligatory external rotation of the involved hip when the hip is passively flexed to 90 degrees. Orthopedic consultation is advised if SCFE is suspected. Radiographs should include frog-leg lateral views and AP views of both hips. Definitive treatment is operative internal fixation. Chronic complications can develop from severe displacement including avascular necrosis and leg length discrepancy.

17. What condition involves a growth disturbance of the medial tibial physis?

Blount's disease or tibia vara is common in obese children, ages 10–14, but can also occur as young as 2 years of age. This disease is most common in African Americans. This condition is typically described as a chronic progressive limp and should be considered whenever evaluating a limping child. Often these children have a leg length discrepancy and tenderness at the medial tibial physis. Plain radiographs are best for diagnosis. Referral to a pediatric orthopedic surgeon is indicated for surgical intervention.

KEY POINTS

1. In a young child, knee pain is hip pain until proven otherwise.
2. Consider abuse if a child presents with fracture after an unwitnessed trauma and the story does not match the injury pattern.
3. A mid-shaft tibia fracture may be an indication of child abuse.
4. A child with septic arthritis will usually appear more ill than those with transient synovitis.
5. *Staphylococcus aureus* is the most common pathogen isolated in patients with septic arthritis.
6. Hip aspiration is the gold standard for diagnosing septic arthritis and should be performed whenever this diagnosis is suspected.
7. Transient synovitis is the most common cause of a limping child.
8. SCFE is more common in boys >11 years of age and can be diagnosed with plain x-ray.
9. LCP is more common in boys <10 years of age and can be diagnosed with plain x-ray.

BIBLIOGRAPHY

Hill D, Whiteside J. Limp in children: differentiating benign from dire causes. *J Fam Pract.* 2011;60(4): 193–197.

Madden Christopher C, Frank H. Netter: *Netter's Sports Medicine*. Philadelphia: Saunders/Elsevier; 2010.

Peck D. Slipped capital femoral epiphysis: diagnosis and management. *Am Fam Physician.* 2010;82(3):258.

Perry Daniel C. Bruce Colin: evaluating the child who presents with an acute limp. *BMJ.* 2010;341:c4250.

Storer SK, Skaggs DL. Developmental dysplasia of the hip. *Am Fam Physician.* 2006;74(8):1310–1316.

Smith E, Anderson M, Foster H. The child with a limp: a symptom and not a diagnosis. *Arch Dis Child Educ Pract Ed.* 2012;97:185–193. http://dx.doi.org/10.1136/archdischild-2011-3012.

Sawyer JR, Kapoor M. The limping child: a systematic approach to diagnosis. *Am Fam Physician.* 2009;79(3):215–224.

CHAPTER 41

ANKLE SPRAINS

Duron A. Lee, MD, Peter H. Seidenberg, MD

GENERAL INFORMATION

1. **What is an ankle sprain?**
   Ligaments serve to provide mechanical stability, directed motion, and proprioceptive information for the joint. An ankle sprain occurs when one or more ligaments stretch beyond their limits. They range from mild to severe, depending on how much damage there is to the ligament (e.g., stretching, partial rupture, or complete rupture). This chapter focuses on lateral and high ankle sprains.

2. **What are the different types of ankle sprains?**
   There are three major classifications of ligamentous ankle injuries: lateral, medial (deltoid), and syndesmotic (high) ankle sprains.

3. **What is the incidence of ankle sprains?**
   - Ankle ligament injuries are among the most common orthopedic injuries encountered in the primary care office and emergency department.
   - The incidence of ankle sprains in the United States is 2.15 per 1,000 person-years, with teenagers and young adults (15–19 years of age) having the highest rates, with a peak incidence of 7.2 per 1,000 person-years.
   - Acute ankle sprains result in an estimated annual aggregate health care cost of $2 billion.

4. **Is there a difference in ankle sprains between populations?**
   - No difference in the incidence of ankle sprains between men and women.
   - Slight preponderance in Caucasians and African Americans compared with other ethnicities.
   - Approximately half of acute ankle sprains occur during athletic activity, most commonly basketball.
   - Increased incidence in those who were near overweight and overweight (body mass index [BMI] >25).

5. **What is the greatest risk factor for ankle sprains?**
   The greatest risk factor for ankle sprain is a previous ankle sprain that has not been appropriately rehabilitated.

6. **What are the signs and symptoms of acute ankle sprain?**
   - Pain
   - Swelling
   - Tenderness
   - Ecchymosis
   - Difficulty with weight bearing

7. **What are the long-term effects of repeated ankle sprains?**
   Repeated ligamentous injuries may result in chronic instability, degenerative bony changes, and chronic pain.

ANATOMY

8. **Describe the bony anatomy of the ankle joint.**
   The ankle joint is a hinge-type synovial joint that forms the articulation between the lower leg and foot composed of three articulations. The **talocrural joint** is the articulation between the tibia and fibula proximally and the talus distally. The **tibiofibular joint** (syndesmosis) is the distal articulation between the medial side of the fibula and the lateral side of the tibia. The **subtalar (talocalcaneal) joint** is the articulation between the inferior talus and the superior calcaneus.

9. **What is the ankle mortise?**
   The mortise is a three-sided, rectangular socket formed by the tibial plafond, the medial malleolus, and lateral malleolus.

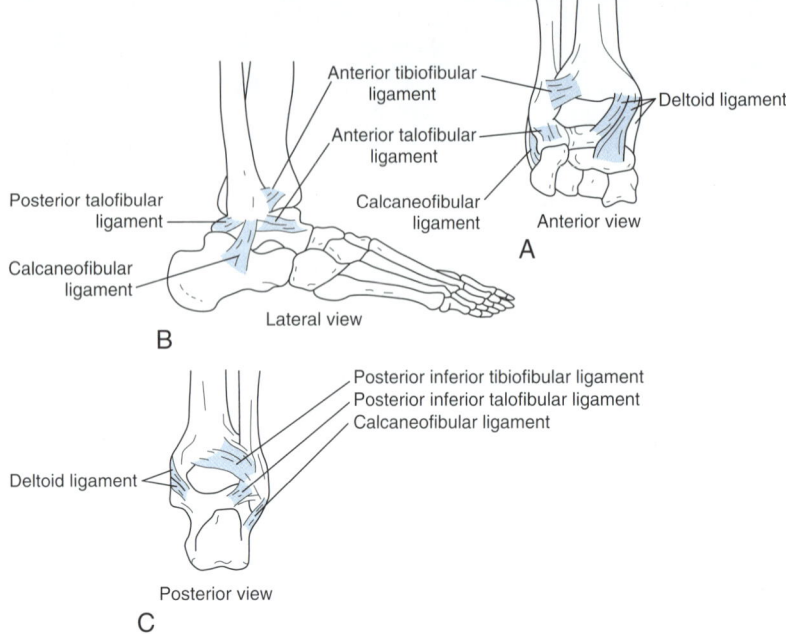

Fig. 41.1. Ligamentous anatomy of the ankle. (A) Anterior view. (B) Lateral view. (C) Posterior view. *(Adapted from Pommering TL, Kluchursky L, Hall SL. Prim Care Clin Office Pract. 2005;32:133.)*

10. Describe the ligamentous anatomy of the ankle joint.
The ligamentous complexes of the ankle include the lateral, deltoid, and syndesmotic ankle ligaments, which in addition to the surrounding musculotendinous structures provide dynamic stability to the ankle joint (Fig. 41.1).

11. What comprises the lateral ligamentous complex of the ankle joint?
The lateral ankle ligamentous complex is composed of the anterior talofibular (ATFL), calcaneofibular (CFL), and posterior talofibular (PTFL) ligaments.

12. Describe the anatomy and function of the anterior talofibular ligament (ATFL).
The ATFL is a flat band that extends anteromedially from the anterior border of the lateral malleolus and inserts onto the lateral neck of the talus. It is taut in plantar flexion and loose in dorsiflexion and prevents internal rotation and adduction of the talus. It is relatively weak and has the lowest load to failure among the other lateral ankle ligaments and is thus the most commonly injured ankle ligament.

13. Describe the anatomy and function of the calcaneofibular ligament (CFL).
The CFL is a round, cord-like, extracapsular ligament that is confluent with the peroneal tendon sheath. It passes posteroinferiorly from the distal tip of the lateral malleolus and inserts onto the lateral calcaneus. The CFL is slack in plantar flexion and tense in dorsiflexion, preventing adduction of the talus within the talocrural joint.

14. Describe the anatomy and function of the posterior talofibular ligament (PTFL).
The PTFL is a capsular ligament that extends from the posteromedial aspect of the lateral malleolus and inserts onto the posterolateral aspect of the body of the talus. It has maximal tension in ankle dorsiflexion and prevents external rotation of the ankle while dorsiflexed.

15. What is the syndesmosis?
The distal tibiofibular joint is a fibrous syndesmotic articulation consisting of the concave surface of the distal tibia and convex shape of the distal fibula. The syndesmotic ligamentous complex connects the tibia and fibula through four ligamentous structures.

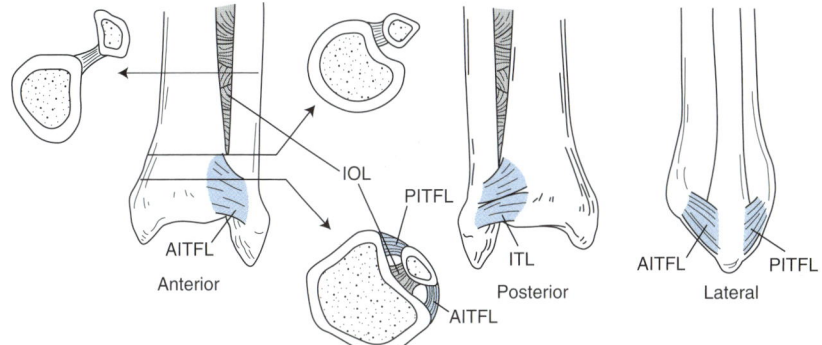

Fig. 41.2. Anterior, posterior, and lateral views (from left to right) of syndesmosis anatomy demonstrating location and relationship of the anterior inferior talofibular ligament (AITFL), interosseous ligament (IOL), inferior transverse tibiofibular ligament (ITL), and posterior inferior tibiofibular ligament (PITFL). *(Adapted from Hsu AR, Garras DN, Lee S.* Oper Tech Sports Med. *2014;22:270.)*

16. Describe the four ligamentous structures that make up the syndesmosis.

The interosseous ligament (IOL) extends from the fibular notch of the tibia to the medial surface of the distal fibula. It travels superiorly with the interosseous membrane running the length of the tibia and fibula and forms the principal connection between them. It is strengthened by the anterior-inferior tibiofibular ligament (AITFL) and posterior-inferior tibiofibular ligament (PITFL), which extend from the fibular notch of the tibia to the anterior and posterior surfaces of the lateral malleolus, respectively. The deep, inferior portion of the PITFL is called the inferior the transverse ligament (ITL) and functions to reinforce the posterior capsule of the ankle joint (Fig. 41.2).

17. What is the function of the syndesmosis?

The four syndesmotic ligamentous structures combined play a critical role in providing stability of the ankle mortise and serve to prevent dissociation of the tibia and fibula, as well as preventing posterolateral bowing of the fibula during activities that stress the fibula. Between 40% and 45% of the resistance to diastasis comes from the PITFL and ITL, 35% from the AITFL, and 20%–25% from the interosseous membrane.

LATERAL ANKLE SPRAIN

18. What is a lateral ankle sprain?

A lateral ankle sprain is a sprain of the lateral ligamentous complex of the ankle. They account for approximately 88% of all ligamentous ankle injuries, 50% of all sport-related injuries, and 25% of all injuries of the musculoskeletal system.

19. What are the mechanisms of injury for lateral ankle sprain?

Lateral ankle sprains usually result from excessive inversion of the foot combined with external rotation of the leg. The ATFL is most commonly injured, placing increased stress on the remaining ligaments. Combined ruptures of the ATFL and CFL occur in 20% of cases, whereas isolated CFL rupture is rare. Injury to the PTFL is also rare in ankle sprains but is more commonly associated with ankle fractures and/or dislocations.

20. What is the classification scheme for lateral ankle sprains and the associated signs and symptoms?

Each ligament is graded according to its individual severity of injury.

Grade I: Mild sprain resulting from ligamentous stretch without macroscopic tearing. Mild swelling or tenderness. No mechanical instability. No loss of function or motion.

Grade II: Moderate sprain resulting from partial macroscopic tearing of the ligaments. Moderate swelling, ecchymosis, and tenderness. Mild to moderate instability. Slight loss of motion. Moderate pain with weight bearing and ambulation.

Grade III: Severe sprain resulting from complete ligamentous rupture. Severe swelling, ecchymosis, tenderness, and pain. Significant mechanical instability. Loss of function and motion. Inability to bear weight.

21. **What are some of the other injuries associated with ankle sprains?**
    - Osteochondral defects
    - Peroneal tendon injuries
    - Avulsion fracture
    - Epiphyseal injuries
    - Loose bodies
    - Posterior tibialis injury

HIGH ANKLE SPRAIN

22. **What is a high ankle sprain?**
    A high ankle sprain (syndesmotic injury) is a sprain of the distal syndesmotic ligaments that connect the tibia and fibula in the lower leg. They occur less frequently in the general population, comprising approximately 0.5% of ankle sprains without fracture and 13% of all ankle fractures. They occur more commonly in collision sports, including football, ice hockey, and soccer.

22. **What is the classification scheme for high ankle sprains?**
    Several classification schemes have been developed without consensus based on time duration of symptoms, the number of ligaments involved, the level of diastasis, clinical findings, and radiographic and magnetic resonance imaging (MRI) criteria.

23. **Describe stable versus unstable acute high ankle sprains.**
    A stable injury is characterized by a lesion of the AITFL (with or without IOL rupture) and without involvement of the deltoid ligament. An unstable ankle sprain is classified as latent or frank diastasis. Latent diastasis involves rupture of the AITFL with or without IOL and the deltoid ligament rupture. It can be detected on stress radiographs, MRI, and/or arthroscopic assessment. Frank diastasis involves rupture of all syndesmotic and deltoid ligaments. It can be detected on the mortise view of standard ankle radiographs.

24. **What is the mechanism for high ankle sprain?**
    Several mechanisms of injury have been proposed for the cause of high ankle sprains, including pronation-abduction, pronation-eversion, supination-eversion, external rotation, supination-abduction, and dorsiflexion. The typical mechanism of injury is hyper-dorsiflexion and external rotation of the foot in relation to the tibia. They are often associated with further soft tissue injury and fractures, which may lead to significant ankle instability.

25. **How do you test for high ankle sprain?**
    Various stress tests are used to clinically evaluate the integrity of the syndesmosis: External/Lateral Rotation Test (Kleiger's Test), Squeeze Test (Hopkin's Test), Fibular Translation Test, and Cotton (Magee) Test. These tests are used to induce displacement and/or elicit pain as an aid to diagnosis. Other provocative tests include the Crossed Leg Test, Dorsiflexion Compression Test, Dorsiflexion Maneuver, and Heel Thump Test.

26. **What are the radiographic signs of syndesmotic injury?**
    X-ray radiographs with anteroposterior (AP), lateral, and mortise views can be used to assess syndesmotic injury.
    - Decreased tibiofibular overlap (normal >6 mm on AP view and >1 mm on mortise view).
    - Increased medial gutter clear space at the distal talus and medial malleolus (normal ≤4 mm).
    - Increased tibiofibular clear space at 1 cm above the tibial articulation (normal <6 mm on both AP and mortise views) or a difference >2 mm when compared to the contralateral ankle.

27. **What are the long-term sequelae of high ankle sprain?**
    Syndesmosis injuries generally require significantly more time to heal compared with patients who have lateral ankle sprains. Early diagnosis and appropriate management is necessary to avoid long-term sequelae, including reinjury, discomfort due to impingement from scar tissue, articular degeneration, increased risk of osteoarthritis, chronic instability, formation of heterotopic ossification, and deformity of the ankle joint.

DIAGNOSIS

28. What are the physical examination tests for diagnosing ankle sprains (Table 41.1)?

Table 41.1. Physical examination tests for diagnosing ankle sprains

TESTS	DESCRIPTION	INJURY
Anterior Drawer Test	Anterior translation force applied to the ankle by grasping the plantar heel and holding the foot in neutral position (plantar flexed 10–15 degrees and slightly inverted) while stabilizing the distal leg. Anterior translation indicates a positive test.	ATFL
Talar Tilt Test	Inversion stress applied to the ankle with the foot held in neutral position and the distal leg stabilized. The degree of inversion is compared to the uninjured side.	CFL
External Rotation Test	External rotation and dorsiflexion of the foot with the knee flexed at 90 degrees and the ankle in neutral position. Pain indicates a positive test.	Syndesmotic Complex
Squeeze Test	Medial and lateral compression of the leg at the mid-calf level. Pain at the ankle indicates a positive test.	Syndesmotic Complex
Fibular Translation Test	Anterior and posterior translation force applied to the distal fibula with the tibia stabilized. Pain and increased translation of the fibula indicates a positive test.	Syndesmotic Complex
Cotton Test	Lateral translation force applied to the talus within the ankle mortise by grasping the plantar heel and stabilizing the proximal ankle. Pain indicates a positive test.	Syndesmotic Complex

29. What are the guidelines for obtaining ankle radiographs?
    The Ottawa Ankle Rules are guidelines indicating that x-ray studies should be obtained if there is pain in the malleolar zone and A) bony tenderness at the distal 6 cm of the fibula –or– B) bony tenderness at the distal 6 cm of the tibia –or– inability to take 4 steps immediately after injury. The Ottawa Foot Rules indicate that x-rays should be obtained if there is pain in the midfoot zone and: C) bony tenderness at the base of the fifth metatarsal –or– D) bony tenderness at the navicular bone tibia –or– inability to take 4 steps immediately after injury (Fig. 41.3).

TREATMENT

30. Describe the initial treatment for acute ankle sprains.
    The treatment of ankle sprains in the acute phase of injury focuses on minimizing swelling, pain control, protection from further injury, and promotion of healing. The essential components of treatment include PRICEMMMS (an extension of RICE).

31. What is PRICEMMMS?
    Protection from further injury by restricting inversion and eversion stress (e.g., ankle stabilizing brace, air cast) and employing crutches, depending on the ability of the individual to bear weight.
    Rest to avoid further exacerbation of pain.
    Ice applied to the ankle as needed is effective for decreasing swelling.
    Compression (e.g., ACE wrap, compression stockings) aids in edema resorption.
    Elevation above the level of the heart will improve venous return and decrease swelling.
    Medications (e.g., NSAIDs, analgesics) may aid in reducing pain and inflammation.
    Modalities (e.g., electrical stimulation, ultrasound) may be used for pain control, maintenance of strength, and range of motion.
    Mobilization should begin early and include active, pain-free plantarflexion and dorsiflexion.
    Strength training should begin early, focusing on the peroneal and gastrocnemius muscles.

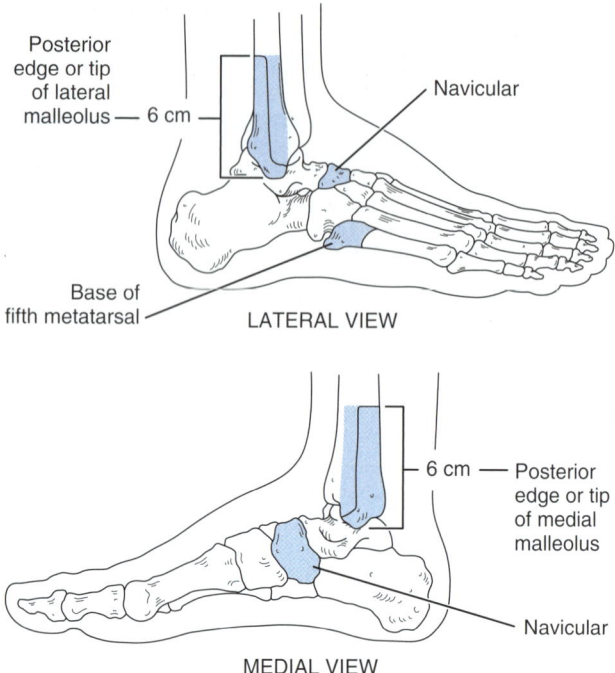

Fig. 41.3. Sites of palpation for the Ottawa Ankle and Foot Rules. Tenderness over the shaded areas warrants further radiographic evaluation. *(Adapted from Seidenberg, et al (eds).* Sports Medicine Resource Manual, *Philadelphia, 2008, W.B. Saunders, p. 358.)*

32. Describe the process of functional rehabilitation in the treatment of ankle sprain.
The primary goals of rehabilitation are regaining normal function and strength, while preventing future reinjury. Functional rehabilitation is an extension of traditional elements of physical therapy with the purpose of slowly progressing the patient in a step-wise fashion from simple activities (e.g., walking or jogging) back to highly complex movement patterns that require refined levels of proprioceptive acuity (e.g., sports, athletics).

33. What are the stages of functional rehabilitation?
Functional rehabilitation progresses through three general stages: the acute stage, early rehabilitation, and late functional rehabilitation stage.

34. Describe the acute stage of functional rehabilitation.
The acute stage focuses on minimizing inflammation, pain reduction, promotion of healing, and protection from further injury. It typically lasts 1–3 days and includes PRICEMMS.

35. Describe the early rehabilitation stage of functional rehabilitation.
The early rehabilitation stage focuses on early mobilization to reestablish full range of motion (e.g., ankle pumps), regain strength (e.g., resistance exercise bands), normalize neuromuscular control, restore proprioception and balance (e.g., balance board), improve endurance, and maintain cardiovascular fitness (e.g., strength training, water jogging, swimming, and cycling). It aims for a safe return to physical activity and typically lasts from several days to weeks.

36. Describe the late rehabilitation stage of functional rehabilitation.
The late functional rehabilitation stage includes advanced-phase rehabilitation activities that focus on regaining normal function and includes exercises specific to those performed during athletics or sports (e.g., sport-specific drills) accelerated in a gradual fashion. Lack of proper, gradual, step-wise

rehabilitation places the patient at risk for recurrent, more severe ankle injury with the potential to develop into chronic functional instability.

37. What are some of the common therapeutic modalities?

Common therapeutic modalities used for ankle sprain rehabilitation include ultrasound, contrast baths, neuromuscular electrical stimulation, massage, taping, phonophoresis, iontophoresis, and cryotherapy.

38. What are the mechanical, functional, and degenerative causes of chronic ankle instability?

Acute ankle sprains may lead to mechanical, functional, or degenerative deficits resulting in chronic ankle instability, persistent pain, and mechanical signs. Mechanical causes include pathologic laxity, arthrokinetic restriction, synovial changes, and degenerative changes. Functional causes include proprioception abnormalities, loss of neuromuscular control, impairment in postural control, and strength deficits. Degenerative causes include osteochondral lesions of the talus, impingement, loose bodies, painful ossicles, adhesions, chondromalacia, and osteophyte formation.

39. How do you prevent or decrease the incidence of ankle sprains?

Evidence suggests that a well-structured, preseason conditioning that focuses on agility, balance, coordination, and flexibility decreases injury risk. Warming up should precede all intensive physical activity, and patients with sprained ankles should complete rehabilitation before resuming athletics. The use of orthotics, ankle bracing, or high-top shoes may prevent recurrence of ankle sprain, while the use of proprioceptive/kinesthetic training (e.g., balance board training or equivalent) may also substantially reduce the risk and occurrence of ankle sprains.

40. When do you refer ankle injuries?

Indications for immediate referral include (1) structurally significant fracture (opposed to small avulsion fractures), (2) an obvious deformity, (3) evidence of neurovascular compromise, (4) a penetrating wound into the joint space, (5) a sudden locking of the ankle, (6) suspicion of grade III strain (tendon rupture), and (7) a syndesmotic injury.

KEY POINTS

1. The ankle joint is composed of three articulations: the talocrural joint, the tibiofibular joint (syndesmosis), and the subtalar (talocalcaneal) joint.
2. There are three major classifications of ligamentous ankle injuries: lateral, medial (deltoid), and syndesmotic (high) ankle sprains.
3. The ATFL is the most commonly injured ligament in lateral ankle sprains.
4. A high ankle sprain is a sprain of the distal syndesmotic ligaments that connect the distal tibia and fibula.
5. PRICEMMMS (Protection, Rest, Ice, Elevation, Medications, Modalities, Mobilization, and Strengthening) is employed during the acute phase of treating ankle sprains.

BIBLIOGRAPHY

Amendola A, Williams G, Foster D. Evidence-based approach to treatment of acute traumatic syndesmosis (high ankle) sprains. *Sports Med Arthroscop.* 2006;14(4):232–236.

Clanton TO, Matheny LM, Jarvis HC, Jeronimus AB. Return to play in athletes following ankle injuries. *Sports Health.* 2012;4(6):471–474.

Czajka CM, Tran E, Cai AN, DiPreta JA. Ankle sprains and instability. *Med Clin North Am.* 2014;98(2):313–329.

Ferran NA, Maffulli N. Epidemiology of sprains of the lateral ankle ligament complex. *Foot Ankle Clin.* 2006;11(3):659–662.

Hergenroeder AC. Diagnosis and treatment of ankle sprains. *Am J Dis Child.* 1990;144(7):809–814.

Kemler E, van de Port I, Backx F, van Dijk CN. A systematic review on the treatment of acute ankle sprain. *Sports Med.* 2011;41(3):185–197.

McCriskin BJ. Management and prevention of acute and chronic lateral ankle instability in athletic patient populations. *WJO.* 2015;6(2):161–12.

Mattacola CG, Dwyer MK. Rehabilitation of the ankle after acute sprain or chronic instability. *J Athl Train.* 2002;37(4):413–429.

van Dijk CN, Longo UG, Loppini M, et al. Classification and diagnosis of acute isolated syndesmotic injuries: ESSKA-AFAS consensus and guidelines. *Knee Surg Sports Traumatol Arthrosc.* 2016;24(4):1200–1216.

Witt BL, Witt SL. Acute ankle sprains: a review of literature. *Osteopath Fam Physician.* 2013;5(5):178–184.

CHAPTER 42

ACUTE INFECTIOUS DISEASES AND THE ATHLETE

Ryan Cudahy, MD, George G.A. Pujalte, MD, FACSM

UPPER RESPIRATORY TRACT INFECTIONS

THE COMMON COLD

1. **How does the common cold present?**
   Also known as a viral syndrome or upper respiratory tract infection (URI), the common cold is the leading cause of missed school or work days in the United States, often leading to missed athletic participation. Presenting symptoms typically include rhinorrhea and cou, and occasionally fever may be present.

2. **What are the risk factors for getting the common cold?**
   Risk factors that may be concerning for more severe disease include young age, low birth weight, prematurity, chronic disease, immunodeficiency, malnutrition, and crowding.

3. **How do you diagnose and manage a common cold?**
   For the most part, the common cold does not require confirmatory testing or further workup when at the top of the differential diagnosis list. The gold standard of confirmation, however, is viral culture, rarely indicated. A complete blood count (CBC) may show a leukocytosis with a left shift. The mainstay of treatment is symptomatic management. Many agents have been studied in the treatment of the common cold, with antihistamines and decongestants proven to have the highest efficacy. Patients with the common cold should be provided precautions even though the course is commonly benign and self-limited as more serious complications such as acute bacterial sinusitis (which occurs in 2.5% of patients after a viral URI), pneumonia, or asthma exacerbations may result. Exercise and return to play is permitted as tolerated.

SINUSITIS

4. **How does sinusitis present?**
   Also among the most commonly diagnosed illnesses in the United States, acute sinusitis affects 16% of the adult population annually. Patients present with significant nasal congestion, purulent nasal discharge, maxillary tooth discomfort, headaches, fever, and facial pain/pressure in an acute (<4 weeks), subacute (4–8 weeks), or chronic (>8 weeks) manner.

5. **How do you differentiate viral versus bacterial sinusitis?**
   When distinguishing between viral and bacterial infections, it is important to note that bacterial infections are less common, last longer than the usual 7- to 10-day course for a viral infection, and are associated with a history of persistent purulent rhinorrhea and facial pain. History and physical examination are key as further diagnostic workup is typically not indicated. Purulent nasal discharge and/or colored rhinorrhea, history of maxillary pain or sinus tenderness on exam, and poor response to decongestants have been shown to increase the likelihood of acute bacterial sinusitis.

6. **What diagnostic tests may be helpful in diagnosing sinusitis?**
   Gold standard for diagnosis, though not routinely done in the outpatient setting, is sinus aspirate culture. Computed tomography (CT) scanning is preferred over other imaging modalities if a diagnosed sinusitis does not respond to initial therapies.

7. **How is sinusitis treated?**

Antibiotics are typically indicated for acute bacterial sinusitis when symptoms have not improved over 10 days or for severe illness. Amoxicillin should be the initial choice in children and adults with uncomplicated disease for 10–14 days of treatment. Symptomatic management may also include antihistamines, decongestants, and nasal steroids, but studies have not proven efficacy to date and their use is not routinely recommended. Exercise and return to play are permitted as tolerated.

PHARYNGITIS

8. **How is pharyngitis assessed?**

Responsible for approximately 2% of all ambulatory visits in the United States, acute pharyngitis is caused by an equal proportion of viral and bacterial pathogens. The most commonly treated etiology is group A streptococcus (GAS), but this only accounts for ~10% of adult cases. Centor criteria are used in an attempt to differentiate viral causes from bacterial, especially GAS. These include tender anterior cervical adenopathy, tonsillar exudates, fever by history, and absence of cough. In a large study of 206,870 patients, 7% of patients with one Centor criterion, 21% of patients with two Centor criteria, 38% of patients with three Centor criteria, and 57% of patients with four Centor criteria tested positive for GAS.

9. **What diagnostic tests may be helpful?**

Throat cultures are the gold standard of diagnosis but can take 24–48 hours to become positive and therefore are not as readily useful for same-day management. The rapid streptococcal antigen test (RSAT) is the first test of choice with a good sensitivity and specificity and is available in minutes.

10. **How is pharyngitis treated?**

If positive, treatment for GAS is warranted, with penicillin V being the first-line antibiotic. Otherwise, symptomatic management is typically sufficient. Athletes who are sexually active may warrant suspicion and workup for gonococcal infection as a cause of pharyngitis, which is easily treatable with antibiotics. We treat pharyngitis to prevent the risk of rheumatic fever, acute glomerulonephritis, and supportive complications. Important to remember, athletes with acute bacterial pharyngitis must be held from play and are considered contagious until treated with an antibiotic for 24 hours. After this time has passed, activity as tolerated is recommended.

INFECTIOUS MONONUCLEOSIS

11. **How does infectious mononucleosis present?**

More commonly known as "mono" or "the kissing disease," this illness occurs commonly at the high school and collegiate level and is spread primarily by the passage of saliva. It is caused by the Epstein-Barr virus (EBV), which can persist in the oropharynx for up to 18 months after clinical recovery. Classical presentation includes the triad of fever, tonsillar pharyngitis, and posterior cervical lymphadenopathy. Typical pharyngitis in mono is described as white or gray exudate. This is often accompanied by severe fatigue and splenomegaly.

12. **What diagnostic tests are useful?**

Diagnostic evaluation usually starts and stops with the Monospot test, which detects heterophile antibodies that appear within 1 week of the onset of clinical symptoms and may persist at low levels for up to 1 year. EBV-specific antibodies can also be detected and are commonly used in athletes to determine acuity of illness. A peripheral smear, although not always warranted, will show a mild leukocytosis on occasion with a predominance of lymphocytes, with more than 10% of these being atypical.

13. **How is "mono" treated?**

Treatment for infectious mononucleosis is supportive care. It is especially important in these patients to stress adequate nutrition, hydration, and rest.

14. **When can athletes return to play after a bout of "mono"?**

Return to play guidelines for athletes with mono has been heavily disputed and is largely based on the prevention of splenic rupture, which occurs most commonly in 1–2 per 1,000 patients 4–21 days after onset of symptoms. For this reason, gradual return to play may be started after 3 weeks but typically contact and vigorous exercise are prohibited for the first 4 weeks after onset of symptoms. It is also important to ensure the athlete is afebrile and without pharyngitis, the spleen is not enlarged or painful, and liver enzymes are at baseline.

PULMONARY INFECTIONS
PNEUMONIA

15. How does pneumonia present?
Athletes with pneumonia will typically be classified as community-acquired (CAP), and common pathogens in this population include streptococcal pneumonia, legionella, chlamydia, and influenza. Patients will present with cough, sputum production, shortness of breath, and/or chest pain. Other associated symptoms may include malaise, anorexia, headache, myalgias, fever, and chills. Physical examination is very important in diagnosis, and vital signs will often be abnormal including fever, tachycardia, tachypnea, hypoxemia, or hypotension. Exam may reveal dullness to percussion of the chest, tactile fremitus, or egophony. Auscultation can be positive for crackles, rales, or bronchial breath sounds.

16. What diagnosis tests may be helpful?
Gold standard for diagnosis includes a chest radiograph showing an infiltrative lesion. Other workup may include complete blood count (CBC) showing leukocytosis, sputum cultures with Gram stain, and urine antigens for streptococcus or legionella.

17. How is pneumonia treated?
The pneumonia severity index is often used to help determine whether outpatient management is appropriate, but clinician judgment is the final word. Typically, a patient with unstable vital signs, including hypoxemia, or inability to maintain hydration or oral intake requires inpatient hospitalization. Treatment usually consists of a macrolide, such as azithromycin, for 7–10 days. If athletes are short of breath for extended periods of time despite adequate antibiotic therapy and resolution of other symptoms, they may have developed a transient reactive airway disease and would benefit from a short course of inhaled bronchodilator therapy. Continued fevers should warrant suspicion for other complications such as empyema, abscess, sepsis, or secondary lung infection.

18. When can an athlete return to play?
Although there are few studied recommendations for return to play in these patients, the athlete should be afebrile and returned to participation in a gradual and progressive fashion.

ACUTE BRONCHITIS

19. How does acute bronchitis present?
Accounting for more than 10 million office visits yearly, bronchitis is characterized by cough lasting up to 3 weeks and concurrent upper airway infection. Most commonly caused by viral infection, less than 10% of patients with bronchitis have a bacterial etiology. Examination is nonspecific, and patients may have pharyngeal erythema, lymphadenopathy, rhinorrhea, and less commonly fever. It is a clinical diagnosis and should be suspected in patients with prolonged cough after resolution of other URI symptoms. Postnasal drip, sinusitis, asthma, and GERD are often in the differential diagnosis.

20. How is acute bronchitis treated?
Acetaminophen, ibuprofen, and nasal decongestants are commonly used. As with pneumonia above, these patients may also develop a reactive airway disease or worsening of asthmatic symptoms and may benefit from short-term inhaled bronchodilator therapy. Exercise and return to play is permitted as tolerated.

PERTUSSIS

21. How does pertussis (also known as "whooping cough") present?
"Whooping cough" is caused by the gram-negative coccobacillus *Bordetella pertussis* and is a highly contagious infection transmitted by droplets. For this reason, it is important not to miss this diagnosis in the training room or when working with athletes in constant close contact. Athletes present with a persistent cough with URI symptoms, which may have a paroxysmal quality lasting more than 2 weeks, posttussive emesis, and/or inspiratory whooping.

22. How is pertussis diagnosed and managed?
Diagnosis is confirmed by nasopharyngeal culture and/or polymerase chain reaction (PCR). The Centers for Disease Control and Prevention (CDC) recommends reporting and treating pertussis

even prior to laboratory confirmation, however, when clinical suspicion is high. Treatment, including prophylaxis for athletes in close contact with a suspected case of pertussis, includes 500 mg erythromycin four times a day for 14 days.

23. How is the spread of pertussis prevented?

Athletes with pertussis need to be isolated from participation for 5 days from the start of treatment. Routine preventive measures in the general population are recommended by means of Tdap vaccine for 11- to 18-year-olds who require a booster dose as well as a single dose for adults 19–64 years of age. After isolation for 5 days, athletes must be monitored for further complications of pertussis such as reactive airway disease, pneumonia, dehydration, weight loss, and sleep disturbances prior to return to play.

INFLUENZA

24. How does influenza present?

Usually presenting in the winter months, these athletes may complain of abrupt onset of fever, headache, myalgia, malaise, nausea, vomiting, cough, and/or sore throat. Physical exam findings may include minimal cervical lymphadenopathy, oropharyngeal hyperemia, eye lacrimation or redness, or dehydration.

25. How is influenza diagnosed and managed?

Rapid viral diagnostic tests completed with the use of nasal or throat swabs can be helpful in the outpatient setting. Influenza A and B can be treated with the neuraminidase inhibitors zanamivir and oseltamivir, whereas influenza A alone can be treated with amantadine and rimantadine. Studies have shown a 2- to 3-day shortening of symptoms when these antiviral medications are given within the first 24–30 hours of symptoms. Symptomatic treatment is the mainstay of therapy for patients presenting outside of that initial 1–2 days of symptom onset and includes acetaminophen or ibuprofen, cough suppressants, and adequate sleep and hydration.

26. How is influenza prevented, and when can athletes return to play?

Annual vaccine is important for all athletes for prevention of illness. Similar to the recommendations for pertussis, athletes with influenza should be isolated for 5 days after which they should be monitored for fever, dehydration, or dyspnea prior to return to play.

CARDIAC INFECTIONS

MYOCARDITIS

27. How does myocarditis present?

In the typical athlete, the most common cause of myocarditis is viral illness, but this can also be caused by drug hypersensitivity, radiation, or chemical agents. It is a difficult diagnosis to make as its presentation can mimic a URI or flulike syndrome, or athletes may simply be asymptomatic. Typical presentation includes chest pain and/or symptoms of heart failure that may be associated with fever, malaise, or arthralgias. Physical examination may show tachycardia, a muffled first heart sound, and/or third heart sound, which can be associated with a mitral regurgitation murmur, edema, and pulmonary crackles. URI symptoms may also remain.

28. What diagnostic tests may be helpful?

When clinical suspicion is high, echocardiography is useful and may show decreased global ventricular function. Cardiac MRI can demonstrate myocardial edema and myocyte damage, but definitive diagnosis requires histologic evidence of mononuclear cellular infiltrates, myocyte necrosis, and disorganized myocardiac cytoskeleton on endomyocardial biopsy.

29. How is myocarditis treated, and when can athletes return to play?

If presuming a viral myocarditis, treatment is supportive care, and most patients will recover completely. Athletes with myocarditis are at an increased risk for heart failure, cardiomyopathies, arrhythmias, associated pericarditis, and sudden cardiac death. Thus it is important to withdraw these athletes from participation in sports for 6 months and only return to play once left ventricular (LV) function and wall motion return to normal, arrhythmias are absent on ambulatory Holter monitoring, serum markers of inflammation and heart failure have normalized, and echocardiogram (EKG) has normalized.[33]

PERICARDITIS

30. How does pericarditis present?
Similar to myocarditis, pericarditis is most commonly infectious or idiopathic with a similar presentation. Athletes will present with retrosternal, pleuritic chest pain, typically exacerbated by coughing, that may radiate to the back. Classically this chest pain is exacerbated when lying down and relieved by sitting forward. Fever, cough, fatigue, myalgias, or arthralgias are not uncommon. The cardinal physical exam finding is the pericardial friction rub, and in more severe cases signs of cardiac tamponade may be evident.

31. What diagnostic tests may be helpful?
Multiple laboratory values may be abnormal including elevations in erythrocyte sedimentation rate (ESR), C-reactive protein (CRP), leukocyte count, and cardiac enzymes. EKG must be obtained in initial evaluation and may show diffuse t-wave inversion. Echocardiogram is ordered to rule out pericardial effusion.

32. How is pericarditis treated, and when can athletes return to play?
Nonsteroidal antiinflammatory drugs (NSAIDs) or colchicine are first-line therapy for the management of pericarditis, and athletes may be treated in the outpatient setting in the absence of the following: subacute onset, leukocytosis, cardiac tamponade, fever, acute trauma, immunosuppression, large pericardial effusion, anticoagulation, or failure to respond to NSAIDs within 7 days. These athletes must be excluded from participation from all competitive sports until there is no evidence of effusion on echocardiogram and normalized serum inflammatory markers.

ENDOCARDITIS

33. How does endocarditis present?
This diagnosis requires a high clinical suspicion in athletes with structural heart disease such as bicuspid aortic valves, mitral valve prolapse, or rheumatic heart disease. Fever is the most common presenting symptom and may be associated with chills, night sweats, anorexia, dyspnea, cough, chest pain, and myalgias. Physical exam may reveal mitral or aortic regurgitation murmurs and classically will reveal peripheral manifestations such as petechiae, splinter hemorrhages, Osler nodes, Janeway lesions, or Roth spots.

34. How is endocarditis diagnosed and managed?
Laboratory evaluation is nonspecific and may be positive for elevations in ESR and CRP and leukocytosis. The Duke criteria are commonly used for evaluating these patients with concern for infective endocarditis. Parenteral antibiotics such as penicillin and gentamycin are started, then narrowed based on blood culture results, and typically are continued for 2–6 weeks. If the athlete remains afebrile after completion of the antibiotic course, repeat blood cultures remain negative, and repeat echocardiography is performed to establish a new baseline, then they may be gradually reintroduced to competition depending on any residual aortic (AR) or mitral regurgitation (MR) as follows: mild to moderate AR/MR may participate in all competitive sports, severe AR/MR and LV enlargement (>65 mm) should not participate, and symptomatic athletes with mild to moderate disease should also be excluded from competition.

BACTERIAL DERMATOSES
COMMON BACTERIAL SKIN INFECTIONS

35. What are the common bacterial skin infections, and how do they present?
Impetigo, folliculitis, furuncles, abscesses, cellulitis and erysipelas, keratolysis, and erythrasma are among the many common skin infections affecting athletes today. Impetigo is known for its classic "honey-crusted" lesions that typically begin as isolated vesicular or pustular lesions and progress to the mature bullous or nonbullous form. These lesions are commonly mistaken for contact dermatitis such as poison ivy or acne.

36. How are common bacterial skin infections diagnosed and treated?
Treatment is topical mupirocin BID for 10 days and/or systemic antibiotic treatment with a cephalosporin or macrolide for larger areas of skin infection. Folliculitis, or inflammation of the superficial portion hair follicles, typically occurs as a small pustule on an erythematous base.

Confirmatory diagnosis can be made by shaving an entire lesion superficially and placing it on culture media. Lesions are typically seen in areas of shaved skin, underneath thigh pads, or occluded areas under a bathing suit and can be pruritic, urticarial, erythematous, and mildly painful. Folliculitis is typically treated with oral antibiotics, and cephalexin or erythromycin are commonly used first line. Topical antibacterial soaps may also help prevent recurrence.

Furuncles and abscesses are larger, more painful, erythematous, fluctuant, and circumscribed masses that may initially resemble erysipelas or cellulitis but quickly progress. The most common sites include the groin, axilla, and posterior thighs due to friction. Incision and drainage is always the first-line therapy for easily accessible lesions although warm compresses and antibiotics are intermittently used for enclosed abscesses.

Erysipelas and cellulitis present with the triad of erythema, edema, and pain and are distinguished by depth of infection, with cellulitis involving the subcutaneous tissue. Fever or lymphadenopathy may accompany these lesions. Diagnosis is made clinically, and treatment usually includes a first-generation cephalosporin or macrolide.

Pitted keratolysis, or "sweaty sock syndrome," presents as hyperhidrosis, malodor, and a general sliminess of the skin, with general pitting of the soles of the feet as a classic distinguishing feature. Diagnosis is clinical, and treatment always commences with frequent drying, use of moisture-wicking synthetic socks, and antibiotic therapy with topical erythromycin or clindamycin.

Erythrasma, caused by *Corynebacterium* sp. and known as the most common bacterial infection of the foot, presents as patchy, erythematous, and irregular plaques usually seen in the interdigital spaces of the feet. These lesions can be diagnosed under a Wood light examination with coral-red fluorescence. Multiple treatments have been used including topical and/or oral erythromycin or clindamycin, topical miconazole, oral clarithromycin, and red-light photodynamic treatment.

37. When can athletes typically return to play?

Return to play guidelines are the same for most of the bacterial dermatoses and range from 48 to 72 hours of systemic antibiotics with no moist, oozing, or exudative lesions and no new onset of lesions in the past 48 hours.

METHICILLIN-RESISTANT *STAPHYLOCOCCUS AUREUS* (MRSA) INFECTIONS

Community-acquired MRSA infections in athletes most commonly involve the skin and soft tissues, often occurring at turf-abrasion sites or other open lesions. These infections require prompt treatment and monitoring as they will often progress to an abscess. For this reason, any abscess in an athlete or skin or soft tissue infection that does not respond to initial antibiotic therapy should raise concern for MRSA.

Wound culture is imperative, especially when MRSA is suspected by appearance of the lesion or by history, such as knowledge of an infected team member.

Incision and drainage of any accessible abscess are usually recommended in addition to presumptive, systemic antibiotics. Trimethoprim-sulfamethoxazole and doxycycline are first-line agents, and clindamycin is commonly used second line due to potential resistance. Intravenous (IV) vancomycin is typically used in the inpatient setting for severe infections.

Return to play guidelines are the same as for most of the bacterial dermatoses and range from 48 to 72 hours of systemic antibiotics with no moist, oozing, or exudative lesions and no new onset of lesions in the last 48 hours.

VIRAL CUTANEOUS INFECTIONS: HERPES SIMPLEX

Also known as herpes gladiatorum in wrestlers or "scrumpox" in rugby players, this infection is transmitted by skin-to-skin contact and causes lesions that appear as a group of vesicles that may ulcerate and leave a painful, shallow ulcer on an erythematous base. Common locations include the lips, face, hands, body, and genitalia.

Diagnosis is clinical and may be confirmed by a Tzanck smear or viral culture. First-line therapy includes acyclovir and valaciclovir, with the latter often being preferred for its twice a day dosing compared to five times daily with acyclovir.

Athletes must complete oral antiviral treatment for at least 120 hours, have no new lesions for at least 72 hours, and remain free of systemic symptoms for 72 hours.

GASTROINTESTINAL INFECTIONS

VIRAL

Noroviruses are the leading cause of acute, epidemic gastroenteritis in adults and older children in the United States and worldwide. Transmitted by the fecal–oral route, most outbreaks are from fecal contamination of food or water by a handler, and athletes are contagious until 48 hours after diarrhea resolves.

Symptoms typically include nausea, vomiting, abdominal cramping, and diarrhea.

Diagnosis is clinical and workup is not commonly required.

Treatment is supportive and can be limited to simple rehydration for the average athlete.

BACTERIAL

Campylobacter sp., *Escherichia coli, Salmonella* sp., and *Shigella* sp. are among the most common causes of bacterial, infectious diarrhea in the United States, and presenting symptoms typically include moderate to severe diarrhea, which may progress to bloody diarrhea, abdominal pain, nausea/vomiting, and fever. Transmitted by the fecal–oral route, athletes are typically contagious for 48 hours following the final episode of diarrhea.

Diagnosis requires stool evaluation including culture, microscopy, Gram stain, and/or specific toxin testing.

Once diagnosed, treatment varies depending on organism, but supportive care with electrolyte-rich hydration is always first line.

Antibiotics should not be used in *E. coli* as this has not been shown to be effective and may increase risk of hemolytic uremic syndrome. *Campylobacter* sp. infection is usually self-limited, but salmonellosis and shigellosis can be treated with trimethoprim-sulfamethoxazole or ciprofloxacin for moderate to severe disease or to shorten the course of illness.

Training staff may need to observe and/or teach proper handwashing technique if teams travel to endemic areas with poor hygiene.

FOODBORNE

Bacterial toxins, typically the culprits of "food poisoning," cause illness by the GI tract's reaction to the toxin when ingested. The most common examples include *Bacillus* sp., *Campylobacter* sp., *Clostridium* sp., *Salmonella* sp., *Shigella* sp., *Listeria* sp., *E. coli,* and *Staphylococcus* sp.; these organisms are typically responsible for the outbreaks on cruise ships.

Safe practices in endemic areas include avoidance of tap water, iced drinks, or raw fruits and vegetables and only eating food served at appropriately hot temperatures.

These illnesses are self-limited, but chemoprophylaxis has been used in athletes not able to miss participation; typically, ciprofloxacin 500 mg daily is used.

KEY POINTS

1. When distinguishing between viral and bacterial upper respiratory tract infections, it is important to note that bacterial infections are less common, last longer than the usual 7- to 10-day course for a viral infection, and are associated with a history of persistent purulent rhinorrhea and facial pain.
2. Most acute bronchitis cases are secondary to a viral etiology; less than 10% of patients have a bacterial cause.
3. Once a gastrointestinal tract infection is diagnosed, treatment varies depending on the organism, but supportive care with electrolyte-rich hydration is always first line.

BIBLIOGRAPHY

Abramowicz M. The choice of antibacterial drugs. *Med Lett Drugs Ther.* 2001;43:69–78.
Adams BB. Sports dermatology. *Dermatol Nurs.* 2001;13(5):347–363.
Anon JB, Jacobs MR, Poole MD, et al. Sinus and Allergy Health Partnership. Antimicrobial treatment guidelines for acute bacterial rhinosinusitis. [Published correction appears in *Otolaryngol Head Neck Surg* 130:794–796, 2004]. *Otolaryngol Head Neck Surg.* 2004;130(suppl 1):1–45.
Arroll B, Kenealy T. *Antibiotics for the common cold and acute purulent rhinitis. In The Cochrane Library.* Chichester (UK): John Wiley & Sons, Ltd. [issue 2]; 2005.
Baddour LM, Wilson WR, Bayer AS, et al. AHA scientific statement on infective endocarditis diagnosis, antimicrobial therapy, and management of complications. *Circulation.* 2005:e394–e428.
Baldwin DR, Macfarlane JT. Community-acquired pneumonia. In: Cohen J, Powderly WG, eds. *Cohen & Powderly: Infectious Diseases.* 2nd ed. St. Louis: Mosby; 2004:369–380.

Barton SE, Ebel CW, Kirchner JT, et al. The clinical management of recurrent genital herpes: current issues and future prospects. *Herpes*. 2002;9:15–20.

Becker KM, Moe CL, Southwick KL, et al. Transmission of Norwalk virus during a football game. *N Engl J Med*. 2000;343:1223–1227.

Braman SS. Chronic cough due to chronic bronchitis: ACCP evidence-based clinical practice guidelines. *Chest*. 2006;129(suppl):S104–S105.

Brown MO, St. Anna L, Ohl M. Clinical inquiries. What are the indications for evaluating a patient with cough for pertussis? *J Fam Pract*. 2005;54:74–76.

Centers for Disease Control and Prevention. *Nonspecific Upper Respiratory Tract Infection*; 2006. <cdc.gov/getsmart>.

Centers for Disease Control and Prevention. Prevention and control of influenza: recommendations of the Advisory Committee on Immunization Practices (ACIP). *MMWR Recomm Rep*. 1999;48:1–28.

Centor RM, Witherspoon JM, Dalton HP, et al. The diagnosis of strep throat in adults in the emergency room. *Med Decis Making*. 1981;1:239.

Chow AW. Acute sinusitis: current status of etiologies, diagnosis, and treatment. *Curr Clin Top Infect Dis*. 2001;21:31–63.

Cohen PR, Kurzrock R. Community-acquired methicillin-resistant *Staphylococcus aureus* skin infection: an emerging clinical problem. *Clin Infect Dis*. 2005;4:100–107.

Cooper RJ, Hoffman JR, Bartlett JG, et al. Principles of appropriate antibiotic use for acute pharyngitis in adults: background. *Ann Intern Med*. 2001;134:509.

Darras-Vercambre S, Carpentier O, Vincent P, et al. Photodynamic action of red light for treatment of erythrasma. *Photodermatol Photoimmunol Photomed*. 2006;22(3):153–156.

Feldman AM, McNamara D. Myocarditis. *N Engl J Med*. 2000;343:1388–1398.

Felker GM, Boehmer JP, Hruban RH, et al. Echocardiographic findings in fulminant and acute myocarditis. *J Am Coll Cardiol*. 2000;36:227–332.

Finch SC. Laboratory findings in infectious mononucleosis. In: Carter RL, Penman HG, eds. *Infectious Mononucleosis*. Boston: Blackwell Scientific Publications; 1969:47–52.

Fine MJ, Smith MA, Carson CA, et al. Prognosis and outcomes of patients with community acquired pneumonia. A meta-analysis. *JAMA*. 1996;275:134–141.

Gwaltney Jr JM: Acute community-acquired sinusitis. *Clin Infect Dis*. 1996;23:1209.

Gwaltney Jr JM, Hendley JO. Transmission of experimental rhinovirus infection by contaminated surfaces. *Am J Epidemiol*. 1982;116:828.

Habif T. *Clinical Dermatology*. 4th ed. Philadelphia: Mosby; 2004:264–306.

Houck PM, MacLehose RF, Niederman MS, et al. Empiric antibiotic therapy and mortality among Medicare pneumonia inpatients in 10 western states: 1993, 1995, and 1997. *Chest*. 2001;119:1420–1426.

Hueston WJ. A comparison of albuterol and erythromycin for the treatment of acute bronchitis. *J Fam Pract*. 1991;33: 476–480.

Imazio M, Demichelis B, Parrini I, et al. Day-hospital treatment of acute pericarditis: a management program for outpatient therapy. *J Am Coll Cardiol*. 2004;43:1042–1046.

Johnson MA, Cooperberg PL, Boisvert J, et al. Spontaneous splenic rupture in infectious mononucleosis: sonographic diagnosis and follow-up. *AJR Am J Roentgenol*. 1981;136:111.

Kazakova SV, Hageman JC, Matava M, et al. A clone of methicillin-resistant *Staphylococcus aureus* among professional football players. *N Engl J Med*. 2005;352(5):468–475.

Lange RA, Hillis D. Acute pericarditis. *N Engl J Med*. 2004;351:2195–2201.

Lung EE. Acute diarrheal diseases. In: Friedman SL, McQuad KR, Grendell JH, et al, eds. *Current Diagnosis and Treatment in Gastroenterology*. 2nd ed. New York: McGraw-Hill; 2003:414–418.

Maron BJ, Zipes DP, Ackerman MJ, et al. 36th Bethesda Conference: eligibility recommendations for competitive athletes with cardiovascular abnormalities. *J Am Coll Cardiol*. 2005;45:1313–1375.

Mason JE. Techniques for right and left ventricular endomyocardial biopsy. *Am J Cardiol*. 1978;41:887–892.

Moe CL, Christmas WA, Echols LJ, et al. Outbreaks of acute gastroenteritis associated with Norwalk-like viruses in campus settings. *J Am Coll Health*. 2001;50(2):57–66.

Mylonakis E, Calderwood SB. Infective endocarditis in adults. *N Engl J Med*. 2001;345:1318–1328.

NCAA Rules Committee: Appendix D: skin infections. In Wrestling: 2006 Rules and Interpretations. <http://www2.ncaa.org/media_and_events/ncaa_publications/playing_rules/>; Accessed 30.11.05.

Niederman MS, Bass Jr JB, Campbell GD, et al. Guidelines for the initial management of adults with community-acquired pneumonia: diagnosis, assessment of severity, and initial antimicrobial therapy. *Am Rev Respir Dis*. 1993;148:1418–1426.

Nieman DC. Current perspective on exercise immunology. *Curr Sports Med Rep*. 2003;2(5):239–242.

O'Connell JB, Mason JW. Diagnosing and treating active myocarditis. *West J Med*. 1989;150:431–435.

O'Dell ML. Skin and wound infections: an overview. *Am Fam Physician*. 1998;57(10):2424–2432.

Piccirillo JF. Clinical practice. Acute bacterial sinusitis. *N Engl J Med*. 2004;351:902.

Procop GW, Cockerill F. Enteritis caused by *Escherichia coli* & *Shigella* & *Salmonella* species. In: Wilson WR, Sande MA, eds. *Current Diagnosis and Treatment in Infectious Diseases*. New York: McGraw-Hill; 2001:483–486.

Rea TD, Russo JE, Katon W, et al. Prospective study of the natural history of infectious mononucleosis caused by Epstein-Barr virus. *J Am Board Fam Pract*. 2001;14:234.

Reed SL. Amebiasis: an update. *Clin Infect Dis*. 1992;14(5):1161–1162.

Roush S, Birkhead G, Koo D, et al. Mandatory reporting of diseases and conditions by health care professionals and laboratories. *JAMA*. 1999;282:164–170.

See DM, Tilles JG. Viral myocarditis. *Rev Infect Dis*. 1991;13:951–956.

Teichtahl H, Buckmaster N, Pertnikovs E. The incidence of respiratory tract infection in adults requiring hospitalization for asthma. *Chest*. 1997;112:591.

Williams Jr JW, Simel DL, Roberts L, et al. Clinical evaluation for sinusitis: making the diagnosis by history and physical examination. *Ann Intern Med*. 1992;117:705–710.

Woodwell DA, Cherry DK. *National Ambulatory Medical Care Survey: 2002 summary, no. 346*. Hyattsville, MD: National Center for Health Statistics. Advance data from Vital and Health Statistics; 2004.

World Health Organization. Prevention of Foodborne Disease: Five Keys to Safer Food, 2006. <http://www.who.int/foodsafety/consumer/5keys/en/index2.html>; Accessed 10.10.06.

Wright SW, Edwards KM, Decker MD, et al. Pertussis infection in adults with persistent cough. *JAMA*. 1995;273:1044–1046.

WOUND ASSESSMENT, BURNS, AND ANIMAL BITES

John A. Park, MD, Lilia Reyes, MD

CHAPTER 43

WOUND ASSESSMENT

1. Why does wound assessment matter?

Traumatic wounds are a common presenting complaint to acute care centers. Nearly 12 million wounds are treated in U.S. emergency departments annually, with about one third of those in patients under the age of 18. Wound care accounts for approximately 10% of all procedures performed in emergency departments, with literally millions more wounds assessed yearly that do not require procedural intervention.

Each wound is different, necessitating individualized treatment based on clinical assessment. Without appropriate treatment, patients with acute wounds may suffer complications such as poor healing and infections.

2. How do we begin wound assessment?

In assessment of any patient in the acute care setting, patient resuscitation and stabilization always take precedence and should proceed according to pediatric advanced life support (PALS), advanced trauma life support (ATLS) protocols. Assuming the patient is stable and requires only management of minor wounds, assessment may progress. Careful history taking and examination are essential to appropriate assessment and treatment of wounds. Documentation should include the mechanism described by the family as well as a clear description of the wound and assessment of whether or not the wound is consistent with the mechanism described by the caregiver.

3. What types of wounds may be appropriately treated in the urgent care setting?

- Appropriate: Minor cuts, lacerations, and abrasions.
- Not Appropriate: Any penetrating, complex, or severe traumatic injury should be referred to an emergency department (ED) for definitive management after ensuring patient stability for transfer. Any wounds concerning for nonaccidental trauma should also be referred to the ED.

4. What are the goals of wound management?

- Establishing hemostasis
- Minimizing the risk of infection
- Optimizing cosmetic results
- Returning function to normal
- Minimizing pain

5. Are there different types of wounds?

- Abrasions: Caused by force applied in opposite directions that scrapes away layers of skin or underlying tissue.
- Lacerations: Wounds where there is a separation between tissues. Different types of force can generate different subtypes.
  - Cuts: Caused by shearing forces in injuries such as knife wounds, which are often "cleaner" in appearance with sharp edges or margins.
  - True lacerations: Caused by compressive or tensile forces and often have somewhat rough, jagged, or torn edges and may be associated with contusion.
  - Puncture wounds: Penetrating injuries with a small surface opening and depth that cannot be directly visualized. Susceptible to infection because of the enclosed environment, caused by a combination of forces.
  - Avulsions: Tissue is separated either completely or nearly so from its base. Caused by shearing and tensile forces.
- Burns: Result in wounds (will be discussed separately)
  Wounds may be a combination of these types.

259

6. **What details of the patient history are key to wound assessment?**
   - How did this happen and what has happened since?
   - When did this happen?
   - Where did this happen? (Any exposure to soil, natural bodies of water, or animals or insects that bite can cause wounds that are at increased risk of infection.)
   - Immunization and immune status
   - Does story make sense and fit with the presenting injury? (If it does not or there is any doubt, appropriate steps to investigate nonaccidental injury should be taken.)

7. **What aspects of exam should be focused on?**
   - Examination using clean or sterile gloves and other protective measures such as mask and eye shield.
   - Exam should be conducted in a well-lit area, and additional lamps may be necessary for best visualization of the injury.
   - Measures to control bleeding should be taken and then exam repeated once bleeding is controlled to ensure blood does not obscure any findings.
   - Note extent of injury, any visible contamination, and damage to nearby structures.
   - Neurovascular status in the form of distal perfusion as well as motor and sensory function are important to note and document before the use of any anesthetics.

8. **A 17-year-old male patient presents with a laceration of the left hand that occurred 2 days ago. He states that he wants it "sewn up" so that it will heal faster. Is this laceration too old to be sutured?**
   - There is no absolute time period for when a wound is too old for surgical repair.
   - Studies have demonstrated that many wounds may be closed safely up to 24 hours after injury and this is used as a "golden period" for repair.

9. **A 5-year-old male patient presents with a laceration to the scalp that is bleeding profusely. How can bleeding be controlled?**
   - Apply direct pressure gently but firmly over the wound.
   - Elevate the wound if it is on an extremity.
   - Suturing or stapling of highly vascular areas may be useful for persistent bleeding.
   - Epinephrine, either locally injected into the surrounding soft tissue at a bleeding site or applied topically in a preparation such as LET (Lidocaine, Epinephrine and Tetrocaine) gel may help with hemostasis through vasoconstriction.

10. **A 13-year-old female patient presents for treatment of a laceration on her foot. You decide it requires closure with sutures, but she refuses to allow this, stating she is afraid it will hurt. How can her pain be controlled?**
    - Pain control for minor injuries is often well achieved using local methods such as topical gels or injectable solutions.
    - Generally these methods should be coincidentally given with epinephrine to decrease systemic effects and prolong localized exposure to the medication.
    - Medications such as benzodiazepine given orally, intravenously (IV), intramuscularly (IM), or intranasally (IN) may be useful for anxiolysis as well, particularly prior to attempting wound repair.

11. **Do all lacerations need to be repaired?**
    No. Remembering our goals of wound management, sometimes these are best served by leaving a wound to heal by secondary intent. Many wounds should not be repaired because they will heal well on their own, repair may significantly increase the risk of infection, or for other reasons. The first rule in medicine is do no harm, so repair should only be performed if necessary.

12. **When are antibiotics indicated?**
    Antibiotics should be reserved for complicated wounds such as:
    - Bites
    - Open fractures
    - Tendon or joint involvement
    - Obvious infection or high risk for infection

13. **A 7-year-old male patient presents after stepping on a nail in the backyard. Does he require tetanus immunization or immunoglobulin?**
    See Table 43.1.

Table 43.1. Tetanus Vaccines and TIG for Wound Management

AGE (YEARS)	VACCINATION HISTORY	CLEAN, MINOR WOUNDS	ALL OTHER WOUNDS
0–6	Unknown or not up-to-date on DTaP series based on age	DTaP	DTaP TIG
	Up-to-date on DTaP series based on age	No indication	No indication
7–10	Unknown or incomplete DTaP series	Tdap and recommend catch-up vaccination	Tdap and recommend catch-up vaccination TIG
	Completed DTaP series AND <5 years since last dose	No indication	No indication
	Completed DTaP series AND ≥5 years since last dose	No indication	Td, but Tdap preferred if child is 10 years of age
11 years and older (*if pregnant, see footnote)	Unknown or <3 doses of tetanus toxoid containing vaccine	Tdap and recommend catch-up vaccination	Tdap and recommend catch-up vaccina- tionTIG
	3 or more doses of tetanus toxoid containing vaccine AND <5 years since last dose	No indication	No indication
	3 or more doses of tetanus toxoid containing vaccine AND 5–10 years since last dose	No indication	Tdap preferred (if not yet received) or Td
	3 or more doses of tetanus toxoid containing vaccine AND >10 years since last dose	Tdap preferred (if not yet received) or Td	Tdap preferred (if not yet received) or Td

From http://emergency.cdc.gov/disasters/disease/tetanus.asp

BURN MANAGEMENT

14. What burns can be managed in an urgent care setting?

Children younger than 5 years account for 18% of burns presenting to care in the United States. Of these, the majority are minor, covering <10% of the total body surface area, and the predominant type of injury is a scald. Minor superficial burns are appropriate for treatment in the acute or urgent care setting; however, those affecting larger areas, greater depths, or with other associated injuries should be referred to advanced care centers.

15. How are burns classified?

Burns are generally classified or grouped according to three characteristics: depth of affected tissue, percent of total body surface area affected, and cause of injury (thermal, chemical, electrical, etc.). These classifications are in turn used to determine the severity of a burn and aid in triage toward appropriate treatment (Table 43.2).

Burns are often assigned a "degree" according to depth of affected tissue. Burns affecting only the epidermis are considered first degree or superficial, those affecting dermis as well as epidermis are considered second degree or partial thickness. Burns that damage or destroy all layers of skin are called third degree or full thickness. Some clinicians also consider burns damaging tissue deep to the skin as fourth degree. Burn wounds can change dramatically over the first several days after initial injury and appear more severe than on initial presentation. This occurs in spite of the burn process being arrested and is thought to be part of the pathophysiology of burns.

Table 43.2. Burn Classification

	SUPERFICIAL OR FIRST DEGREE	PARTIAL THICKNESS OR SECOND DEGREE	FULL THICKNESS OR THIRD DEGREE
Tissue depth affected	Epidermis only	Epidermis and dermis	Epidermis, dermis and below
Sensation	Painful	Painful	Diminished
Appearance	Erythematous, hyperemic, intact skin	Blistered, disrupted skin	Skin layers destroyed, deep tissue exposed

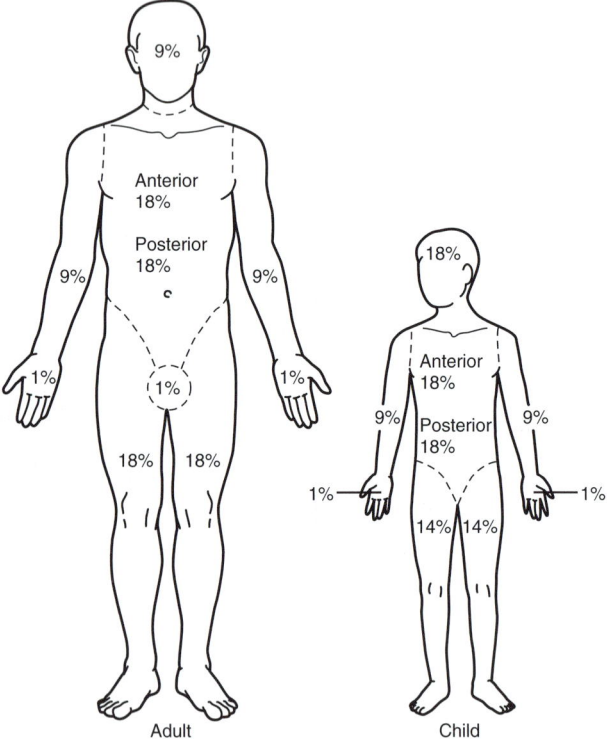

Fig. 43.1. The rule of nines. *(From Ciottone, GR: Ciottone Disaster Medicine, ed 1, Philadelphia, 2005, Elsevier/Saunders.)*

16. **A 2-year-old girl presents to your urgent care with burns to her forearms and the upper portion of her anterior chest wall after pulling her mother's coffee mug from the counter. How would you estimate the percent of total body surface area affected?**
Determining percentage of body surface area affected can be difficult, and although there are many methods utilized by clinicians to estimate this there is no perfect method. The "rule of nines" (Fig. 43.1) is a widespread method and perhaps the oldest in use but is applicable to older pediatric patients and adults. This boils down to each body area roughly equaling a multiple of 9% of the total body surface area (TBSA). This is slightly more complex in children than in adults as various body parts comprise differing percentages of body surface area in children as compared to adults—for example, the head is proportionally much larger in children. Another method used to estimate BSA is the Lund-Browder charts (Fig. 43.2). Similar to the charts illustrating the rule of nines, the charts show percentages of BSA

% Total Body Surface Area Burn

- Be clear and concise
- Do <u>not</u> include erythema

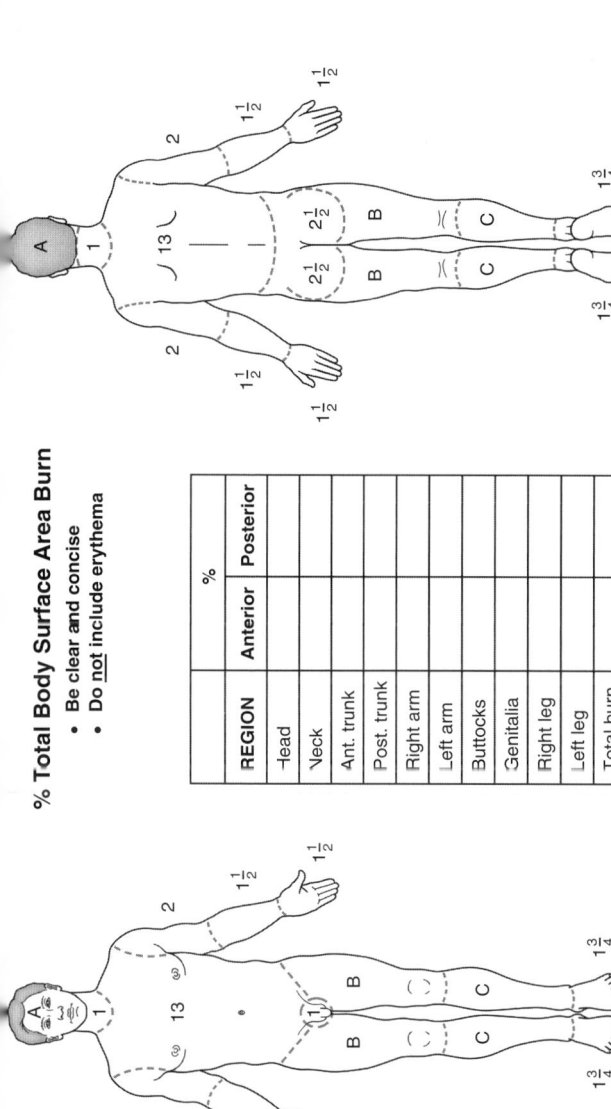

REGION	%	
	Anterior	Posterior
Head		
Neck		
Ant. trunk		
Post. trunk		
Right arm		
Left arm		
Buttocks		
Genitalia		
Right leg		
Left leg		
Total burn		

AREA	Age 0	1	5	10	15	Adult
A = ½ OF HEAD	$9\frac{1}{2}$	$8\frac{1}{2}$	$6\frac{1}{2}$	$5\frac{1}{2}$	$4\frac{1}{2}$	$3\frac{1}{2}$
B = ½ OF ONE THIGH	$2\frac{3}{4}$	$3\frac{1}{4}$	4	$4\frac{1}{2}$	$4\frac{1}{2}$	$4\frac{3}{4}$
C = ½ OF ONE LOWER LEG	$2\frac{1}{2}$	$2\frac{1}{2}$	$2\frac{3}{4}$	3	$3\frac{1}{4}$	$3\frac{1}{2}$

Fig. 43.2. Lund–Browder (LB) Chart. The shape of the burn is drawn onto the chart, excluding simple erythematous areas. Each area is assigned a value of the body surface area percentage, which is entered into the table and the total body surface area affected is then calculated. (Redrawn from Hettiaratchy S, Papini R: Initial management of a major burn: II—assessment and resuscitation, *BMJ* 329:101, 2004.)

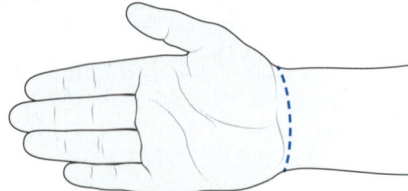

Fig. 43.3. Palm and fingers represent 1% of total body surface area. *(From Kirwan H, Pignataro R: Pathology and Intervention in Musculoskeletal Rehabilitation, ed 2, 2016, pp 25–62.)*

occupied by various body areas. A third way to quickly estimate BSA is by using the palm and fingers of the patient's hand to represent approximately 1% of BSA (Fig. 43.3) and multiplying burn area out from this. No method of BSA estimation is perfect, and clinical judgment should be used in this process.

17. **A 5-year-old male patient presents to care after spilling a cup of hot tea in his lap. After exposing the affected area you note burns encompassing the anterior thighs as well as genitalia and suprapubic area. The burns cover approximately 2%–3% of the boy's TBSA. Is it appropriate to treat this boy as an outpatient?**
   The American Burn Association sets forth criteria for burns necessitating admission as follows:
   1. Partial thickness burns covering greater than 10% total body surface area
   2. Burns involving the face, hands, feet, genitalia, perineum, or major joints
   3. Third-degree burns
   4. Electrical burns
   5. Chemical burns
   6. Inhalation injury
   7. Burns in patients with complicating medical disorders
   8. Burns with concomitant trauma where the burn poses the greater threat to life
   9. Burns in children at hospitals without qualified pediatric providers and facilities
   10. Burns in patients who will require special supportive services or interventions

18. **What comprises the initial outpatient burn care?**
   - Cooling works to help mitigate further injury as well as decrease pain. Irrigation of the wound with room temperature saline or sterile water is effective. Caution should be used with ice as it may cause further thermal injury.
   - Clothing, jewelry, and debris should be removed from the burn area.
   - The wound should be cleaned with a mild antiseptic such as chlorhexidine and irrigated.
   - Blisters are somewhat controversial, with some evidence both for and against rupturing any blisters and removing devitalized tissue. The blister can act as a biodressing, but it has also been reported that devitalized tissue can serve as a nidus for infection.
   - Antibiotic ointment such as bacitracin or Silvadene should be applied to the wound.
   - Nonadhesive dressing should be applied to the wound; if this is unavailable, mesh gauze may be used instead. The wound should then be padded and wrapped with further gauze.
     - If wounds involve the digits of the hand or foot, each digit should be padded and wrapped separately.
     - Some burn wounds may be in areas such as the face that make them difficult to dress. In this case it is acceptable to apply antibiotic ointment in place of dressing and instruct patients to wash the area a few times a day to keep the wound clean, reapplying the ointment after each cleansing.
   - If possible, the wound should be kept elevated to minimize edema.

19. **A 2-year-old male patient with no past medical conditions presents to care with burns on his chest and abdomen. He was reaching up to grab a bowl of hot soup off a table and spilled it on himself after dropping the bowl. He is crying and minimally consolable by parents, and you note a blistered burn about the size of the patient's hand on his torso. After exposing and then cooling the burned area with sterile saline, what is the next step in appropriately treating this patient?**
   Analgesia is a critical component in the treatment of burn wounds. The pain associated with minor burns is often quite severe, and manipulating the wound in the process of examining and dressing the wound can make this pain worse. It is often appropriate to use opiate medication for pain control

during this process. Intravenous intramuscular and intranasal medications should be utilized for their rapid onset and potency of pain control. Oral therapy often takes too long to take effect, limiting the practicality of its use. Local nerve blocks may also be utilized where practical to provide adequate pain control. It is also important to consider pain control after the patient is discharged home.

BITES

20. What makes a cat bite more prone to causing a wound infection?
It causes a deep puncture wound, making it difficult to irrigate, thus subjecting it to having a high infection rate. In a series done in Austria, they were able to observe a six times higher infection rate in cats (48.5%) versus dogs (7.7%) in one study.

21. What are the common pathogens in animal bites, in order of prevalence?
Pasteurella species, staphylococci, streptococci, and anaerobic bacteria.

22. What are the antibiotic options for children after a dog or cat bite?
Amoxicillin-clavulanate 20 mg/kg (amoxicillin component) two times daily (max 875 mg amoxicillin/ 125 mg clavulanic acid per dose). If penicillin allergic, trimethoprim-sulfamethizole (TMP-SMX) 4–5 mg/kg (trimethoprim component) per dose twice daily (max 160 mg trimethoprim per dose) PLUS clindamycin 10 mg/kg three times a day (max 450 mg per dose).

23. For which bites should you initiate antimicrobial therapy?
Moderate or severe bites (i.e., crush injury), puncture wounds, deep or surgically repaired facial wounds, hand and foot bite wounds, genital area bite wounds, wounds in immunocompromised patients, cat bite wounds, and wounds with signs of infections.

24. How many cases of rabies have occurred in the United States after the suspected animal has been observed during the 10-day period?
No case of human rabies in the United States has been attributed to a dog, cat, or ferret that has remained healthy throughout the standard 10-day period of confinement after an exposure. Wildlife animals such as bats, raccoons, skunks, foxes, coyotes, and bobcats are potential sources of rabies infection for humans as well as domestic animals such as dogs, cats, and ferrets. Rabies in small rodents (squirrels, hamsters, guinea pigs) and lagomorphs (rabbits) is rare.

25. A 10-year-old boy was playing basketball with his friends in his driveway when a neighborhood Pitbull bit him. The patient has a deformity in the right distal wrist region with an overlying 3-cm laceration and another 5-cm laceration on his left biceps region. The dog is unknown to the patient and parents. What do you recommend to the family regarding rabies vaccine and immunoglobulin?
In the United States, postexposure prophylaxis consists of a regimen of one dose of immune globulin and four doses of rabies vaccine over a 14-day period. Rabies immune globulin and the first dose of rabies vaccine should be given by the health care provider as soon as possible after exposure. Additional doses of the rabies vaccine should be given on days 3, 7, and 14 after the first vaccination. Human rabies immune globulin (HRIG) is dosed at 20 IU/kg.

26. A 3-year-old girl is brought to the emergency department for evaluation of a bite mark on her arm. Caregiver reports that the bite mark is from a classmate in daycare that occurred earlier in the day. On exam, the child has an ovoid mark with teeth markings on the right radial region without a break in the skin. How can you tell the difference between an adult bite and a child bite on exam?
The measurement of the intercanine distance of the bite will distinguish human adult bites (3–4.5 cm being adult human; 2.5–3 cm being child or small adult; and less than 2.5 cm, child's deciduous teeth). However, this is based on orthodontic data and has not been validated in clinical practice.

27. Human bite wounds tend to become infected with which bacterial species?
Staphylococcus aureus, Streptococcus species, and *Eikenella corrodens*.

28. Why is it recommended to obtain an x-ray on patients after a dog bite, especially bites on the extremities?
Dogs have large, dull teeth and powerful jaws that are capable of inducing a significant amount of damage due to a crush injury. Larger dogs are able to deliver a bite force of greater than 450 pounds per square inch, capable of perforating light sheet metal.

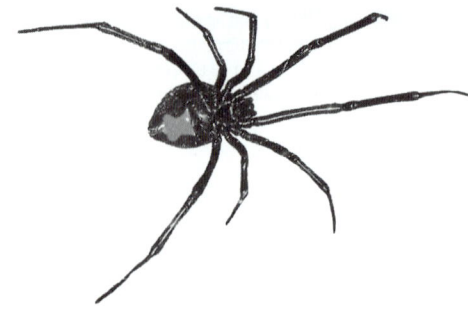

Fig. 43.4. Female black widow spider with a red hourglass marking on the underside of her abdomen. *(From Habif TP: Clinical Dermatology: A Color Guide to Diagnosis and Therapy, ed 5, New York, 2010, McGraw-Hill Companies, pp 581-634.)*

29. **When should a bite wound be repaired surgically, such as with sutures?**
    The decision to repair a bite wound should be made on an individual basis, and there are no hard and fast rules in this regard. Increasing risk for infection associated with repairing the wound must be weighed against the need to improve cosmesis or provide hemostasis in wounds that either gape open, are in highly visible places such as the face, or have persistent bleeding.

INSECTS

30. **What characterizes this spider (Fig. 43.4) as being potentially poisonous?**
    Black widow spiders can be identified by the hourglass pattern (red or orange in color) on the ventral aspect of their shiny, black abdomen. They are located primarily in the southwestern United States. Only female widow spiders are dangerous.

31. **How can a black widow spider bite be identified?**
    The classic *Latrodectus* envenomation starts with a localized reaction that is generally minimal. The bite site quickly develops into a pale central area with surrounding erythema, producing a "target" or "halo" lesion.

32. **What are the expected symptoms after a black widow spider envenomation?**
    Cholinergic symptoms, such as salivation, diaphoresis, tachycardia, hypertension, and bronchorrhea can peak a few hours after the bite. Severe abdominal pain can be seen often. The abdominal pain and associated rigidity of widow spider envenomation can often be mistaken for a surgical abdominal process such as appendicitis.

33. **An 8-year-old boy was brought to the ED by his mother approximately 3 hours after sustaining a black widow spider bite to his right second toe. It is suspected that the spider was in a shoe that the boy put on. The mother had brought the spider to the ED, and it was identified as a female black widow. The patient complained of severe pain that began in his foot and then progressed to his leg, low back, abdomen, and chest.**
    Initial vital signs are blood pressure, 134/92 mm Hg; respiratory rate, 26 breaths/min; heart rate, 130 beats/min; temperature, 97.8°F; pulse oxygen saturation, 96% on room air. He appeared to be in distress secondary to pain. He was diaphoretic. His abdomen was rigid, and he exhibited diffuse guarding. His lungs were clear, and findings on his cardiac examination were normal. There was mild erythema of his right second toe, but there were no identifiable puncture marks. While in the ED, the patient began to complain of difficulty breathing. What would be your treatment for this patient?
    This patient is displaying grade 3 *Latrodectus* spider envenomation (Table 43.3) and would benefit from antivenin treatment. A single vial (2.5 mL) of antivenin *Latrodectus mactans* should be infused intravenously during a 20-minute period.

Table 43.3. Grading Scale for *Latrodectus* Spider Envenomations

GRADE	SIGNS AND SYMPTOMS
1	Normal vital signs, no systemic symptoms, local pain at the bite site
2	Muscular pain in bitten extremity, extension of pain to the chest or abdomen, local diaphoresis at bite site/extremity, normal vital signs
3	Generalized muscle pain to back, chest, and abdomen; diaphoresis distant from bite site/extremity; hypertension/tachycardia; nausea/vomiting; headache

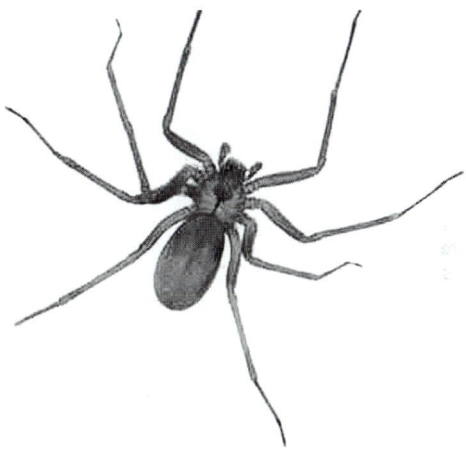

Fig. 43.5. The brown recluse spider. A dark, violin-shaped marking is located on the spider's back. *(From Habif TP: Clinical Dermatology: A Color Guide to Diagnosis and Therapy, ed 5, New York, 2010, McGraw-Hill Companies, pp 581-634.)*

34. A 12-year-old boy reports obtaining a left dorsum of hand spider bite 3 days ago while doing chores in the barn. The wound has a blue-black central area with concentric rings of pallor and erythema. Aside from pain at the site he denies any further symptoms. He happened to take this picture (Fig. 43.5) of the spider with his smartphone. The mother and patient ask what type of spider this is and if there is any further treatment.
This is a brown recluse (*Loxosceles*) spider, which is best identified by its violin-shaped mask marking. Treatment is usually supportive care and local wound management.

35. A 5-year-old female is rock hunting with her sisters on vacation in the Southwest. Her father brings her to the nearest urgent care center because of an acute change in behavior after rock hunting. Patient is complaining of difficulty breathing and father reports that she has been having "dancing eyes." You immediately suspect that your patient has been bitten by what arthropod?
Common symptoms of a scorpion bite include local pain, restlessness, hyperactivity, roving eye movements, and respiratory distress. Treatment is mostly supportive care. Sedative-anticonvulsants can be used to treat hyperactivity, convulsions, and agitation. An equine-derived antivenom made with Fab2 antibodies (Anascorp) can be used for treatment of scorpion envenomation by *Centruroides sculpturatus*.

36. An 8-year-old male is brought to an urgent care center after being stung by a bee. He complains of an itchy throat. On exam, he has some expiratory wheezing, and the bite site has some erythema and swelling. What should be the first intervention?
This patient is experiencing an anaphylactic reaction to the bee sting and should be given epinephrine 1:1000 solution 0.01 mL/kg (max 0.3 mL) intramuscularly x 1. Afterward, the patient may be given antihistamines intravenously or by mouth (IV/PO) and steroids IV/PO. Bee sting patients should be sent to the nearest hospital for a recommended 24-hour observation.

SNAKES

37. **Why does a pediatric patient seem to exhibit severe snakebite envenomation as compared to an adult?**
Because children receive a larger dose of venom per kilogram as compared to adults.

38. **Which pit viper snakes are considered part of the Crotalid family and can account for up to 90% of venomous snakebites in the United States?**
Rattlesnakes, cottonmouths, and copperheads.

39. **A 17-year-old female presents to the emergency department 2 hours after being bitten by a rattlesnake while hiking with her friends. She presents with left lower extremity wound with erythema, edema from the ankle to the knee with palpable pedal pulses. She reports that the wound was originally located at the ankle but has progressed quickly to her knee. The park ranger splinted the extremity, and the patient was brought via Advanced Life Support (ALS) ambulance having received 50 mcg of fentanyl with some relief of pain upon arrival at the emergency department. Upon arrival, the patient reports that she is beginning to feel pain in her left thigh. What are your next steps in the management of this patient?**
Assess the patient's vital signs; if there is evidence of shock begin with resuscitation with normal saline 20 cc/kg according to the PALS recommendation. Treat pain with narcotic analgesia. Keep extremity splinted and elevated. Obtain labs such as complete blood count (CBC) with platelets, prothrombin time, fibrinogen, urine analysis, type and screen, as well as electrolytes. Our patient is exhibiting grade 3 envenomation (see Table 43.2) and would benefit from treatment with Crotalidae polyvalent immune fab (CroFab) (Table 43.4). Initial dose is 4–6 vials of antivenom diluted in 250 mL of crystalloid. May repeat initial dose in 1 hour if no arrest of progression of reaction and return to normal coagulation profile.

40. **What are the indications for CroFab?**
   - Pit viper envenomations
   - Grade moderate to severe within 4 hours
   - Significant local reaction
   - Coagulation abnormalities
   - Cardiovascular instability
      There is a 20% risk of hypersensitivity (anaphylaxis) and 23% risk of serum sickness in giving patient CroFab.

41. **A 16-year-old male presents after being bitten by a red, black, and yellow striped snake. What type of snake is this?**
The animal described could be a coral snake, various species of which can be found in many southern and western areas of the United States, and their bites can be dangerous. There are also many look-alikes for these snakes that are fairly harmless, such as the king snake. A helpful way to pick out coral snakes found in the United States is to look at the banding of color and "if red touches yellow it can kill a fellow" and is probably a coral snake. Note that the yellow bands can be pale and appear white.

42. **What symptoms could a patient bitten by a coral snake display?**
The local wound may progress to extremity paresthesia and weakness. Over a period of hours, the patient may develop malaise, nausea, fasciculations, diplopia, difficulty speaking or swallowing, and generalized weakness.

Table 43.4. Crotalidae Envenomation Grading	
GRADE	**SYMPTOMS**
Minimal	Local swelling and pain without progression
Moderate	Swelling and pain beyond the site of injury with some systemic or laboratory findings
Severe	Severe local, systemic, and laboratory findings

43. How are coral snakebites treated?

Coral snake venom is a potent neurotoxin that can provoke paralysis leading to respiratory failure. Fortunately there are very few of these bites in the United States per year, and they account for less than 1% of all U.S. snakebites. Additionally, the coral snake has very short fangs which often fail to adequately penetrate through clothing and achieve envenomation. Coralmyn is an antivenom similar to CroFab that can be used to treat coral snakebites; however, due to the rarity of these bites it is also rare and difficult to obtain. Any suspected coral snakebite should be emergently referred to advanced care.

MARINE STINGS

44. A 17-year-old male, while swimming in shallow waters, suddenly feels a sharp pain in his leg. He sees the animal swim away, and it appears to be a stingray. He comes to shore and is brought to your urgent care center with a 10-cm laceration on his right leg. How would you manage this wound?

At the scene, the wound should be irrigated with cold saltwater as this can remove much of the venom. Remnants of the integumentary sheath from the stingray's spine should be removed if it can be seen in the wound. The extremity should be placed in hot water (104°F–113°F [40°C–45°C]) for 30–90 minutes. After soaking, the wound should be reexplored, debrided again if necessary, and closed. Pain relief is best achieved with narcotics. Tetanus prophylaxis should be considered and prophylactic antibiotics not needed.

45. An 8-year-old female was playing in the ocean with her sisters on a Florida shore. She saw a shiny "squishy" fish with long legs. She picked up the fish and within a few minutes she began to cry because she was having a burning and painful sensation of her right hand. The nearest urgent care center is within an hour and she begins to have nausea with vomiting. The right hand has erythema extending to her forearm that is pruritic. You suspect a jellyfish sting. What do you do next for this patient?

The sting is often caused by nematocysts located on jellyfish. These nematocysts release a toxin that caused the symptoms in our patient. The unexploded nematocysts can be inactivated with topical application for 30 minutes of 3% acetic acid, a slurry of baking soda, or meat tenderizer (papain). Papain should not be left on for more than 15 minutes. Though being the best disarming agent in jellyfish stings, vinegar is ineffective in Portuguese man-of-war stings. These stings should be washed out with sea water or normal saline. The affected limb should be immobilized. General supportive measures for more systemic reactions can include oral antihistamines, oral corticosteroids, and opiates for pain.

KEY POINTS

1. Appropriate wounds to manage in an urgent care are minor cuts, lacerations, and abrasions.
2. The what, when, where, and why (accidental vs. nonaccidental) of wound occurrence are key pieces of a history.
3. Pain control and anxiolysis are important considerations for treating injured pediatric patients.
4. It is important to assess percent of total body surface area that burns occupy, which can be done by various methods including the "rule of nines," the "hand method," and Lund Browder charts.
5. After the initial A,B,C's, treatment for bites and stings should start with identifying the probable offending species and targeting therapy based on the types of envenomation or injury they cause.

BIBLIOGRAPHY

American Academy of Pediatrics. Red Book Online. <http://aapredbook.aappublications.org>.
American Burn Association. <http://www.ameriburn.org/>.
Centers for Disease Control and Prevention. <http://www.cdc.gov/>.
Jaindl M. Management of bite wounds in children and adults—an analysis of over 5000 cases at a level I trauma centre. *Wien Klin Wochenschr (Dec 11)*. 2015.
Kliegman R, Nelson WE. *Nelson Textbook of Pediatrics*. Philadelphia: Elsevier/Saunders; 2011.
Roberts JR, Custalow CB, Thomsen TW, Hedges JR. *Roberts and Hedges' Clinical Procedures in Emergency Medicine*. 6th ed. Philadelphia: Elsevier/Saunders; 2014.

CHAPTER 44

LACERATION REPAIR

Ruby F. Rivera, MD, Michele Fagan, MD

1. What are important details that one must pay attention to when assessing a laceration?

There are several factors that can affect both the incidence of infection and scar formation.

Laceration factors—mechanism of injury, wound age, possibility of foreign body, and/or contamination, location

Individual factors—underlying medical history/disease state (diabetes, immunocompromised, connective tissue disease, etc.), immunization status

2. Past medical history is important. What questions do we need to ask?

- Do you have any allergies to antibiotics, latex, anesthetics?
- Is there any history of keloid formation?
- Is your tetanus up to date?
- Are you taking any medications currently (i.e., corticosteroids, anticoagulants, nonsteroidal antiin-flammatories, antineoplastic medicine)?

3. How and why are bites managed differently?

Bites, particularly from dogs, are more likely to have components of a crush injury. Crush injuries have devitalized tissue, which is more likely to become infected due to compromised circulation around wound edges. Dog bites have an overall infection rate between 2% and 20%, compared to cat bites with 28%–80% and human bites with 2%–3%. Bite wounds to the hand carry an especially high risk for serious complications because the skin's surface is so close to the underlying bones and joints. One should manage an open wound to the metacarpophalangeal joint from a punch to the mouth as a human bite.

4. What is the concept of the "golden period"?

It is an assumption that bacterial proliferation within wounds is dependent on time from initial insult to repair. Six hours or less was originally designated as the "golden period."

In recent years, this golden period has steadily become longer. This period can range from 6 hours for wounds on the hands and feet to 24 hours or more for clean lacerations on the face.

5. When is primary closure of open lacerations suggested?

In healthy patients who meet all of the following criteria:

- Cosmetically important (e.g., facial lacerations)
- Wounds that are clinically uninfected
- Wounds less than 12 hours old (24 hours on the face)

6. When is delayed closure indicated?

Repair 3 to 5 days postinjury is considered for wounds with high potential for infection—heavily contaminated wounds, selected bite wounds, puncture wounds, and wounds in immunocompromised patients.

7. Does one need to use sterile gloves when performing suture repair?

There is no increased rate of infection seen when nonsterile gloves are used.

8. When should one consider radiographic images?

If one suspects a fracture, a joint disruption, or a foreign body (FB), then radiographic imaging should be considered. A detailed history, exploration with visualization of the base of the wound, and radiography reduce the risk of missing a foreign body but do not eliminate the possibility that one is present. Fragments of glass and metal if larger than 2 mm usually can be identified on plain radiography. Studies show that ultrasound is better to detect plastic, wood, and glass, depending on the operator ability and other confounding factors. Patients should always be told of the possibility of a retained foreign body and what symptoms they should look for.

9. **When should a foreign body be removed?**

   Foreign bodies ideally should be removed; however, one must consider location: intraarticular, intravascular, or close proximity to vital structures.

10. **What should be done about surrounding hair?**

    Hair need not be removed unless it interferes with wound closure. Clipping the hair rather than shaving is preferred as shaving causes small dermal wounds that allow bacteria to penetrate deeper structures and can potentially cause infection. Eyebrows should not be clipped or shaved because they serve as a landmark during repair. In addition, eyebrow growth is unpredictable. Lubrication (i.e., petroleum jelly, bacitracin) can be used to comb the hair away from the laceration.

11. **What type of fluid solution should be used for irrigating a wound?**

    Isotonic (normal) saline is frequently used for irrigation of uncomplicated wounds. Tap water has been shown to be an acceptable alternative solution without increasing risk of infection. Hydrogen peroxide, povidone iodine scrub solution, and chlorhexidine should not be used because of their cytotoxic effects. For contaminated wounds, a 1:10 dilute solution of 10% povidone iodine solution may be used. The area should be anesthetized prior to irrigation. Warming the fluid may also decrease discomfort during wound irrigation.

12. **How much fluid should be used to irrigate a wound?**

    The volume depends on location and mechanism of injury—about 100–200 cc for a clean, uncomplicated 2-cm laceration. Larger volumes may be needed for contaminated wounds. Adequate pressure (5–8 psi) may be obtained by using a 20–50 mL syringe with a splash guard or 19-gauge catheter.

13. **What can be done to reduce pain associated with lidocaine injection?**
    - Use a small gauge needle (27G or 30G).
    - Buffer with sodium bicarbonate.
    - Slow the rate of injection.
    - Warm the local anesthetic.
    - Preanesthetize with topical anesthetic.
    - Infiltrate the anesthetic through the edge of the wound.

         Buffering can be done by adding 1 mL sodium bicarbonate (44 mEq/50 mL) to 9 mL 1% lidocaine. Buffering reduces the shelf life of lidocaine to at least 7 days.

14. **What topical anesthetics are available?**

    Topical anesthetics have the advantage of being administered without using a needle and help reduce pain associated with injection of local anesthetic. There are two topical anesthetics available for laceration repair: lidocaine, epinephrine, tetracaine (LET) and tetracaine, adrenaline, cocaine (TAC). TAC is safe if used properly but has fallen out of favor because it is expensive and contains cocaine, which is a controlled substance. Both LET and TAC are contraindicated for use on mucous membranes as this may result is systemic absorption. LET should not be used on end organs such as tip of the nose, ear, digits, or penis. Other topical anesthetics include eutectic mixture of local anesthetic (EMLA), which contains lidocaine and prilocaine in a cream base, and liposomal lidocaine (LMX). Both are currently approved for use on intact skin and are helpful prior to venipuncture, intravenous (IV) placement, and portacath access.

15. **What are the components of LET and how is it used?**

    LET contains 4% lidocaine, 0.1% epinephrine, and 0.5% tetracaine. It can be mixed with methylcellulose gel or as a solution. About 1–3 mL can be mixed with methylcellulose to make a gel, which then can be applied over the wound and secured with gauze or occlusive dressing (i.e., Tegaderm or OpSite for about 20–30 minutes). It can also be applied by placing solution on a cotton ball, which is then applied over the wound for about 20 minutes. Duration of action lasts 45 to 60 minutes.

16. **A 9-year-old boy comes in with a scalp laceration after hitting his head on a wall while running. There was no loss of consciousness, and on exam he has a 4–5 cm superficial laceration on the right parietotemporal area. What are the options for closure of this laceration?**

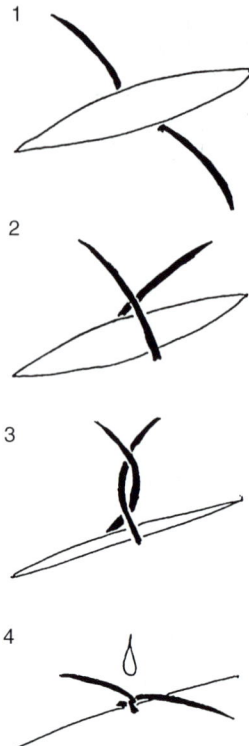

Fig. 44.1. Hair Apposition Technique. Strands of hair on each side are twisted and drop of glue applied. *(From Hock MO, Ooi SB, Saw SM, et al: A randomized controlled trial comparing the hair apposition technique with tissue glue to standard suturing in scalp laceration (HAT study). Ann Emerg Med 40:19-26, 2002.)*

Primary closure is preferred for scalp laceration through the dermis. The wound is anesthetized and irrigated, and options for wound closure include:
- Staples are particularly useful in children.
- Hair apposition technique (Fig. 44.1) involves hair on each side of the scalp being twisted together and then secured with tissue adhesive. This technique is ideal for lacerations that are linear, nonstellate, and <10 cm and in patients with hair >2 cm. Hemostasis is not achieved by this technique, so it should not be used in wounds with significant bleeding.
- Simple interrupted sutures can be used if staples are not available or if hemostasis is required. Absorbable sutures may be used, especially in young children.

17. If the scalp laceration extends into the galea aponeurotica, why is it important to repair the galea?
The scalp consists of five layers: skin, superficial fascia, galea aponeurotica, loose areolar tissue, and pericranium. The galea aponeurotica anchors the frontal muscles; thus, failure to repair galeal lacerations in the frontal scalp may result in abnormalities in facial expression. Large galeal lacerations in other areas of the scalp help prevent hematoma formation and infection.

18. What are tissue adhesives, and what are the indications for their use?
Tissue adhesives provide an alternative method for wound closure that is painless, fast, and does not require a follow-up visit for removal. The most common components of tissue adhesives

are 2-octyl-cyanoacrylate (Dermabond, Surgiseal) and n-2-butyl-cyanoacrylate (Histoacryl Blue, Periacryl). The 2-octyl-cyanoacrylate is preferred because of its plasticity and flexibility. Tissue adhesives are liquid monomers that undergo an exothermic reaction upon exposure to a moist surface (skin), changing to a polymer that forms a strong tissue bond. The wound edges are approximated and two to three layers of tissue adhesive applied. Indications for the use of tissue adhesives include:
- Superficial lacerations
- Length <5 cm
- Low wound tension
- Good wound approximation
- After placement of deep sutures to close skin

19. What are the contraindications for using tissue adhesives?
- Over joints
- Bite wounds
- Eyebrows, hairy areas
- Mucous membranes
- Complex wounds—stellate wounds, crush injuries
- Wounds with increased risk of infection (e.g., puncture wounds, contaminated wounds)

20. What are the complications with tissue adhesive use?
- Infection, especially if the tissue adhesive goes into the wound or if the wound was not adequately cleaned.
- Adhesion of the eye if tissue adhesive gets into the eye. The eye should be protected when using glue near the eye by covering with a gauze impregnated with petroleum. If the tissue adhesive causes adhesion of the eyelids, antibiotic ointment can be applied over the area and manual traction gently applied to open the eye. Ophthalmology should be consulted if this fails to open the eye.
- Glove sticking near site of laceration

21. How do I decide which suture material to use?
There are two types of suture material—absorbable and nonabsorbable. Absorbable sutures are used for deep and subcutaneous repair; nonabsorbable sutures are used to repair superficial skin. However, absorbable sutures (fast-absorbing gut) may be used for closure of facial lacerations, especially in children where suture removal can be a challenge. A recent meta-analysis comparing absorbable and nonabsorbable sutures for skin closure showed no significant difference in postoperative morbidity or cosmetic outcomes. Table 44.1 shows suture material selection by site and depth of laceration.

22. When can adhesive tapes (Steri strips) be used?
- Old contaminated wounds such as dog bites on extremities.
- Superficial, straight lacerations that barely extend through the dermis in areas with low tension.
- Superficial lacerations including flaps in individuals with thin skin (e.g., elderly or those on corticosteroids).
- Adhesive tapes should not be used in hairy areas, oily areas, and over joints.

23. When should an intraoral laceration be repaired?
- When the laceration is greater than 2–3 cm in length.
- When the wound is gaping and is likely to trap food particles.
- When the laceration creates a flap or a free edge or continues bleeding.
- Tongue lacerations involving lateral border.
- Lacerations that involve the Stenson duct should be referred to an oral surgeon. Deep laceration of the cheek anterior to the ear may cause injury to the Stenson duct. On physical examination, bloody discharge may be seen on the buccal mucosa at the level of the second maxillary molar.

24. A 15-year-old boy comes in with a lip laceration involving the vermillion border. What is the most important consideration in repair of this laceration?
Lacerations involving the vermillion border require repair to be done correctly to preserve cosmetic appearance and lip function. As shown in Fig. 44.2, it is important to align the vermillion border first before the rest of the laceration is repaired.

Table 44.1. Wound Closure Type per Anatomic Site

ANATOMIC SITE	LAYER	CLOSURE TYPE	ALTERNATIVES
Scalp	Deep[a]	4-0 Polyglactin 910[b]	4-0 Polyglycolic acid[c]
	Skin	Staples	5-0 Vicryl Rapide
			4-0 Nylon, polypropylene
Face	Deep	5-0 Polyglactin 910	5-0 Polyglycolic acid
	Skin	6-0 Nylon[d]	6-0 Polypropylene[e]
		Wound adhesive (pediatrics)[f]	5-0 Fast-absorbing gut, Vicryl Rapide
Ears	**Skin**	**6-0 Nylon**	**6-0 Polypropylene**
Lip	Muscle/subcutaneous	5-0 Polyglactin 910	5-0 Polyglycolic acid
	Skin	6-0 Nylon	6-0 Polypropylene, Vicryl Rapide
Intraoral	**Mucosa**	**5-0 Chromic gut**	**4-0 Polyglactin 910**
Tongue	Mucosa	4-0 Chromic gut	4-0 Polyglycolic acid
Eyelid	Skin	**6-0 Nylon**	**6-0 Polypropylene**
Neck	Deep	5-0 Polyglactin 910	5-0 Polyglycolic acid
	Skin	5-0 Nylon	5-0 Polypropylene
Trunk	Deep	**4-0 Polyglactin 910**	**4-0 Polyglycolic acid**
	Skin	**4-0 Nylon**	**4-0 Polypropylene, staples[g]**
Arm/forearm	Deep	4-0 Polyglactin 910	4-0 Polyglycolic acid
	Skin	4-0 Nylon	4-0 Polypropylene
Hand	Skin	**5-0 Nylon**	**5-0 Polypropylene, Vicryl Rapide (pediatrics)**
Leg	Deep	3-0 Polyglactin 910	3-0 Polyglycolic acid
	Skin	4-0 Nylon	4-0 Polypropylene staples[g]
Foot	Skin	5-0 Nylon	5-0 Polypropylene
Penis	Skin	5-0 Nylon	5-0 Polypropylene
Scrotum	Skin	**5-0 Chromic gut**	**5-0 Polyglactin 910**
Introitus	Labia majora	5-0 Nylon	5-0 Polypropylene
	Labia minora	5-0 Chromic gut	5-0 Polyglactin 910
	Vagina	5-0 Chromic gut	5-0 Polyglactin 910

[a]Subcutaneous layer.
[b]Polyglactin 910 (Vicryl).
[c]Polyglycolic acid (Down).
[d]Nylon (Ethilon, Dermalon).
[e]Polypropylene (Prolene).
[f]Children.
[g]Avoid weight-bearing surfaces.
From Trott A, editor: *Wounds and Lacerations: Emergency Care and Closure*, ed 4, Philadelphia, 2012, Elsevier Saunders, p 90 [table 8.3].

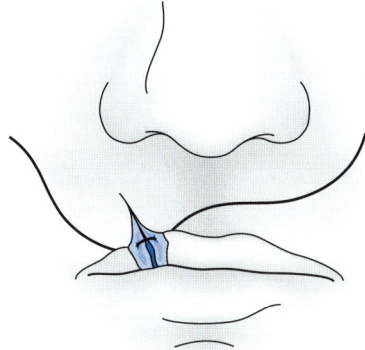

Fig. 44.2. Lip Laceration Involving the Vermillion Border. The vermillion border should be aligned first. *(From Trott A, editor: Wounds and Lacerations: Emergency Care and Closure, ed 4, Philadelphia, 2012, Elsevier Saunders, p 154 [fig. 12.15].)*

25. When should a subungual hematoma be drained?

One should trephinate subungual hematomas that are acute, less than 24–48 hours old, not spontaneously draining, associated with intact nail folds, and painful. Nail removal and primary repair of the laceration are recommended in the event of disruption of the nail matrix (nail fold) or if the nail is partially avulsed. Trephination is easily done by using an electric cautery device or by boring a hole through the nail using a needle. A heated paper clip should not be used as most paper clips are made of aluminum and are difficult to heat sufficiently to penetrate the nail. Anesthesia is usually not needed prior to trephination.

26. If a fingertip is completely cut off, how should the amputated part be taken care of?

- Gently clean the amputated part with water (preferably saline).
- Cover it in gauze wrap.
- Put it in a watertight bag.
- Place the bag on ice.
- Do not put the amputated part directly in ice, to avoid further damage.

27. When should a hand surgeon be consulted?

- Finger fractures (other than tuft fractures)
- Extensive nail bed injury
- Infected wounds
- Fingertip injuries with associated tendon injuries
- Amputation with significant bone exposure

28. When should nasolacrimal duct injury with eyelid laceration be suspected?

- Excessive tearing
- Lacerations medial to the puncta are highly suspicious of canalicular injury

29. When should eyelid lacerations be referred to an ophthalmologist?

- Ptosis in presence of horizontal upper lid laceration—suggests involvement of levator palpebral muscle
- Lid trauma with tissue avulsion
- Periorbital fat exposure
- Full thickness laceration
- Wounds through tarsal plate
- Eyelid margin laceration

30. When are sutures removed?

The timing of suture removal depends on the anatomic location of the wound (Table 44.2).

Table 44.2. Recommended Intervals for Removal of Percutaneous (Skin) Sutures

LOCATION	DAYS TO REMOVAL
Scalp	6–8
Face	3–5
Ear	4–5
Chest/abdomen	8–10
Back	12–14
Arm/leg*	8–12
Hand*	8–10
Fingertip	10–12
Foot	12–14

*Add 2–3 days for joint extensor surfaces.
From Trott A, editor: *Wounds and Lacerations: Emergency Care and Closure*, ed 4, Philadelphia, 2012, Elsevier Saunders, p 289 [table 22.1].

31. **A 33-year-old painter comes in with a puncture wound to the thumb sustained from a high-pressure paint gun. He complains of mild pain, and on physical exam there is a puncture wound on the volar aspect of the proximal phalanx. How should this be managed?**
High-pressure injuries occur due to forceful injection of paint, grease, and liquids through a small high-pressure nozzle. Initially, the patient may be asymptomatic or have mild pain and minimal external injury. However, these materials can cause inflammatory responses and spread throughout the tissues. Delay in diagnosis and management can lead to significant morbidity.

32. **A child comes in having stepped on a sharp object a few days ago. When should one be concerned?**
- Symptoms that are progressive over several days
- Pain with passive movement
- Joint swelling
- Crepitus
- Purulent discharge
- Systemic illness
   Puncture wounds are always deeper than they are wide and impossible to explore well, with an infection rate of 6%–10%.

33. **A 20-year-old patient comes in having stepped on a nail. Is the tetanus vaccine indicated?**
Tetanus prophylaxis depends on the patient's immunization history and the type of wound (Table 44.3). Tetanus-prone wounds include those contaminated with dirt, soil, feces, or saliva; puncture wounds; crush injuries; missile injuries; avulsions; burns; and frostbite. Patients with tetanus-prone wounds and unknown or <3 doses of tetanus immunization should be given tetanus vaccine and tetanus immune globulin. If the patient has had 3 or more doses of tetanus immunization and the last dose is more than 5 years prior, tetanus vaccine should be given. Patients with human immunodeficiency virus (HIV) or other severe immunodeficiency with tetanus-prone wounds should be given tetanus immune globulin regardless of tetanus immunization.

34. **When should one give prophylactic antibiotics?**
Several studies failed to show any benefit for prophylactic antibiotics in simple lacerations.
   General consensus is that antibiotics are not beneficial in clean wounds (even hand injuries).
   Antibiotics should be used in older wounds, human bites, dog bites, cat bites, crush injuries, extensive wounds, exposed cartilage or tendons, puncture wounds through rubbery soles, open fractures, joint cavity violations, moist areas (axilla, perineum), contaminated wounds, and gunshot wounds through clothing and in an immunocompromised host.

Table 44.3. Tetanus Prophylaxis

PRIOR TETANUS TOXOID DOSES	CLEAN, MINOR WOUNDS		ALL OTHER WOUNDS	
	Tetanus Vaccine*	TIG	Tetanus Vaccine*	TIG
Unknown or <3	Yes	No	Yes	Yes
≥3, last <5 yr ago	No	No	No	No†
≥3, last 5–10 yr ago	No	No	Yes	No†
≥3, last >10 yr ago	Yes	No	Yes	No†

Indications for Tetanus Prophylaxis

*Vaccine choice for child <age 7 yr is DTaP, and Tdap if age >7 years (DT or Td if pertussis is contraindicated).
†Any child with HIV infection or who is within the first year after bone marrow transplantation should receive TIG for any tetanus-prone wound, regardless of vaccination status.
Modified from American Academy of Pediatrics: *Red Book: 2012 Report of the Committee on Infectious Diseases*, ed 29, Elk Grove Village, IL, 2012, AAP.
From Engorn B, Flerlage J, editors: *The Harriett Lane: A Handbook for Pediatric House Officers*, ed 20, Philadelphia, 2015, Elsevier Saunders, p 366 [table 16.3].

35. What antibiotics are prescribed?

First-generation cephalosporins cover for *Staphylococcus aureus* and *Streptococcus pyogenes*. For patients with penicillin allergy, clindamycin or azithromycin may be used.

Clindamycin or trimethoprim-sulfamethoxazole is if methicillin-resistant *S. aureus* is a concern.

Amoxicillin-clavulanic acid is the antibiotic of choice for dog and cat bites (contain *Pasteurella multocida, Staphylococcus,* and *Streptococcus*) and human bites (to cover for *Eikenella corrodens, Staphylococcus,* and *Streptococcus*).

36. How should wounds be bandaged after repair?

- Cover the wound for 24–48 hours with a semiocclusive nonadherent dressing and either antibiotic cream or simple petroleum jelly to maintain a moist clean environment.
- Wounds that are closed with tissue adhesives should remain uncovered. Antibiotic ointment should not be used as this may loosen the tissue adhesives.
- Elevate to decrease swelling.
- If a joint is involved, immobilize over the joint with a bulky dressing or splint.
- Apply compression dressing to wounds with potential for hematoma.
- No bathing for 48 hours, then gentle washing with mild soap.

37. When does a wound regain strength?

Between 7 and 10 days after initial injury a wound is prone to dehiscence. Of the wound's ultimate tensile strength, 5% is regained at 2 weeks, 30% at 1–2 months, and full strength at 6–8 months. A scar achieves final appearance at 6–12 months.

38. What are the signs of a wound infection?

- Worsening pain and tenderness
- Erythema
- Warmth
- Swelling
- Discharge
- Fever
- Streaking

39. **An anxious 7-year-old boy has a facial laceration. What are the ways in which to decrease distress associated with the repair procedure?**
    - Apply topical anesthetic prior to the procedure.
    - Explain the procedure using developmentally appropriate terms.
    - During the procedure, find a position of comfort and restrain (i.e., having the patient sit on parent's lap with the parent able to secure arms).
    - Use distraction techniques like videos.

40. **When should we allow wounds to heal by granulation (secondary intention) after appropriate cleaning?**
    - Contaminated with debris that cannot be removed
    - Infected tissue
    - Noncosmetic wounds that come to medical attention late
    - Animal bites in noncosmetic locations
    - Deep puncture wounds that cannot be irrigated well
    - Patients with risk factors (immunocompromised, peripheral artery disease, diabetes mellitus)
    - Superficial wounds involving only the epidermis that will heal well

41. **When should a surgical subspecialist be consulted?**
    - Large deficits
    - Severely contaminated wounds
    - Tendon, nerve, or vessel damage
    - Open fracture, amputation, joint penetration
    - Laceration over site of fracture
    - Compression between two rollers that cause delayed damage
    - Ear lacerations with significant cartilage involvement or tissue loss
    - Paint/grease gun injury
    - Strong concern about cosmetic outcome

KEY POINTS

1. Repair lacerations of the galea aponeurotica to avoid abnormalities in facial expressions.
2. Align the vermillion border first for lip lacerations involving the vermillion border.
3. Eyebrows should not be shaved as hair growth is irregular and the eyebrows serve as important facial landmarks.
4. In young children in whom suture removal may be a challenge, it is reasonable to use absorbable suture material for facial and scalp lacerations.
5. Open wounds involving the metacarpophalangeal joints sustained from punching the mouth should be treated as human bites.

BIBLIOGRAPHY

Armstrong BD. Lacerations of the mouth. *Emerg Clin North Am.* 2000;18(3):471–480.

Bartfield JM, Gennis P, Barbera J, Breuer B, Gallagher EJ. Buffered versus plain lidocaine as a local anesthetic for simple laceration repair. *Ann Emerg Med.* 1990;19:387–389.

Bartfield JM, Homer PJ, Ford DT, Sternklar P. Buffered lidocaine as a local anesthetics: an investigation of shelf life. *Ann Emerg Med.* 1992;21:16–19.

Brown DJ, Jaffe JE, Henson JK. Advanced laceration management. *Emerg Clin N Am.* 2007;25:83–99.

DeBoard RH, Rondeau DF, Kang CS, Sabbaj A, McManus JG. Principles of basic wound evaluation and management in the emergency department. *Emerg Med Clin N Am.* 2007;25:23–39.

Fernandez R, Griffiths R. Water for wound cleansing. *Cochrane Database Syst Rev.* 2012;2. CD003861.

Garcia-Gubern CF, Colon-Rolon L, Bond MC. Essential concepts of wound management. *Emerg Med Clin N Am.* 2010;28:951–967.

Jaindl M, Grunauer J, Platzer P, et al. The management of bite wounds in children—a retrospective analysis at a level 1 trauma centre. *Injury.* 2012;43(12):2117–2121.

Karaduman S, Yuruktumen A, Guryay SM, Bengi F, Fowler JR. Modified hair apposition technique as the primary closure method for scalp lacerations. *Am J Emerg Med.* 2009;27:1050–1055.

Singer AJ, Hollander JE, Quinn JV. Evaluation and management of traumatic lacerations. *N Eng J Med.* 1997;337(16):1142–1148.

Trott AT, ed. *Wounds and Lacerations: Emergency Care and Closure.* 4th ed. Philadelphia: Elsevier Saunders; 2012.

Xu B, Xu B, Wang L, et al. Absorbable versus nonabsorbable sutures for skin closure: a meta-analysis of randomized controlled trials. *Ann Plast Surg.* 2016;76:598–606.

FRACTURE AND DISLOCATION REACTIONS

Daniel M. Fein, MD, Maya Haasz, MD

CHAPTER 45

1. **When is an emergent reduction of a fracture or dislocation indicated?**
   The majority of fractures and dislocations can either be reduced in a nonemergent fashion in the urgent care center, splinted and stabilized for future reduction, or, in the case of certain fractures, not require reduction. However, if there are any signs of neurovascular compromise, emergent reduction is indicated. Symptoms of neurovascular compromise include absent or diminished pulses, cyanosis, pallor, and/or loss of sensation or motor function distal to the fracture.

2. **A 17-year-old girl has not been able to close her mouth since yawning 1 hour ago. What is another mechanism for this injury?**
   Mandibular dislocation can occur after prolonged or extreme mouth opening, or following a direct blow to an open mouth. Either of these mechanisms stretches the ligaments, allowing the mandibular condyles to move anterior to the articular eminence. The dislocation can be either unilateral or bilateral.

3. **Why is sedation useful prior to reduction of a mandibular dislocation?**
   In addition to providing anxiolysis and analgesia, sedation helps to overcome the muscle spasm that prevents the patient from closing her mouth. Benzodiazepines may be particularly helpful in this respect.

4. **How does one reduce a mandibular dislocation?**
   After wrapping his thumbs in gauze to protect them, the provider should apply downward pressure to the molars. Backward pressure to the chin or molars may also be required. This allows the condyles to slip below the articular eminence and back into the mandibular fossa.

5. **What postreduction care is indicated for this patient?**
   The patient should be counseled to eat a soft diet and should have follow-up with otolaryngology or a maxillofacial surgeon.

6. **A 20-year-old female presents after sustaining an injury to her left shoulder while playing basketball when she attempted to block a shot. X-rays confirm an anterior shoulder dislocation. How does an anterior shoulder dislocation most commonly occur?**
   Anterior shoulder dislocations are most commonly caused by sudden external rotation of the shoulder while in abduction (e.g., getting hit on the volar aspect of the arm while reaching for a loose ball).

7. **What complications can occur during a shoulder dislocation?**
   A Bankhart lesion occurs when the inferior labrum is avulsed from the glenoid rim. A Hill-Sachs lesion occurs when the posterior aspect of the humeral head sustains trauma as it strikes the anterior glenoid rim. Rotator cuff tears are also common.

8. **What nerve is at risk of injury from a shoulder dislocation? How do you test its function?**
   The axillary nerve is at risk, and its function can be tested by assessing for deltoid muscle function and sensation over the lateral aspect of the shoulder.

9. **How do I best provide analgesia for reduction of a dislocated shoulder?**
   In addition to providing the patient with either oral or parenteral analgesia as soon as possible, additional medication may be necessary for the reduction itself, as it can be a painful procedure that requires significant force. Choices for procedural analgesia include conscious sedation or intraarticular lidocaine.

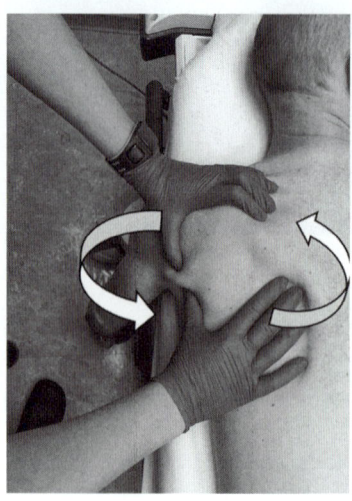

Fig. 45.1. Scapular manipulation to reduce an anterior shoulder dislocation. The inferior aspect of the scapula is rotated toward the spine while the patient is lying in the prone position.

10. **What are some common mechanisms to reduce an anterior shoulder dislocation?**
There are many different mechanisms available for reducing a shoulder dislocation. They include (but are not limited to) external rotation, scapular manipulation, and traction–countertraction.

11. **How does one reduce a shoulder using the external rotation method?**
The patient lies supine or sits supported with the affected arm completely adducted and elbow flexed to 90 degrees. The elbow is then supported while the arm is slowly rotated externally. The arm is then slowly flexed at the shoulder. The technique is completed by then rotating the shoulder internally. Relocation may occur during either external or internal rotation.

12. **Describe the scapular manipulation method of anterior shoulder dislocation reduction.**
The patient lies prone, with the affected arm hanging off the side of the bed. A weight is taped or strapped to the affected wrist to provide axial traction, or a second clinician can provide traction manually. The inferior aspect of the ipsilateral scapula is pushed medially, toward the spine, while the superior aspect is rotated laterally, away from the spine (Fig. 45.1).

13. **What is the traction–countertraction method of shoulder reduction?**
The patient is placed supine with the affected arm abducted and elbow flexed to 90 degrees. A sheet is wrapped around the clinician's waist and the affected forearm with the clinician stabilizing the forearm. A second clinician places a sheet around his or her waist and the patient's trunk just below the axilla. The clinicians both lean backward, providing slow, steady traction (and countertraction), until reduction is achieved (Fig. 45.2).

14. **How do I know that my reduction was successful?**
Reduction of a dislocated shoulder is not subtle. There is usually an audible "clunk" as the humeral head returns to the glenoid fossa. Additionally, the shoulder regains its normal contour and the patient has decreased pain and increased range of motion.

15. **What should I do after successful reduction of a dislocated shoulder?**
Patients are at risk of redislocation as the integrity of the rotator cuff is not the same after a dislocation. The arm should be placed in a sling and the patient should have follow-up with an orthopedic surgeon.

16. **When is reduction of an anterior dislocation contraindicated?**
Reduction of an anterior shoulder dislocation is contraindicated if there is an associated fracture.

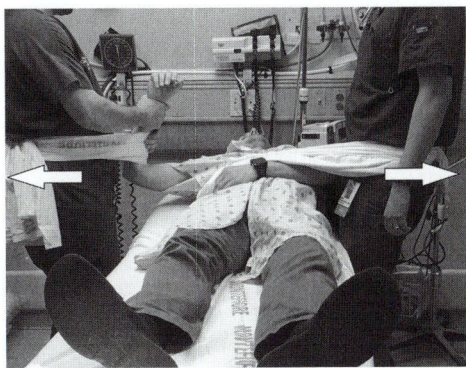

Fig. 45.2. Traction–countertraction to reduce an anterior shoulder dislocation. The clinicians lean backward, providing steady traction until reduction is achieved.

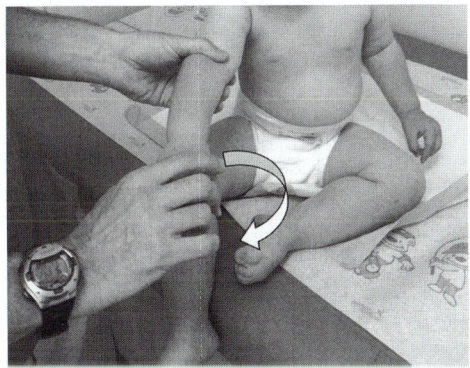

Fig. 45.3. Hyperpronation for reduction of a nursemaid's elbow. The forearm is slowly rotated into hyperpronation, with the stabilizing hand situated to feel the reduction at the radial head.

17. **A 3-year-old girl is brought to your urgent care center for a right arm injury. Her mother was holding her hand when she tripped and fell, and she has not moved her arm since. On exam, her arm is immobile in slight flexion and pronation. What injury did this child likely sustain?**
    "Nursemaid's elbow" is the most common joint injury in children less than 5 years of age, frequently resulting from traction on an outstretched and slightly pronated hand. This causes displacement and slightly entrapment of the annular ligament at the radial head.

18. **What are options for reduction of a nursemaid's elbow?**
    The two options for reduction are:
    a. Supination-flexion: The arm is held in flexion at the elbow with the provider's thumb over the radial head and the other hand holding the patient's hand. Applying mild longitudinal traction, the provider then supinates the forearm while flexing at the elbow.
    b. Hyperpronation: The affected arm is stabilized at the elbow with the provider's thumb over the radial head and the other hand holding the patient's hand. Applying mild longitudinal traction, the hand can then be hyperpronated (Fig. 45.3).

19. **How do you know if you are successful in reducing a nursemaid's elbow?**
    In either technique, the provider may feel a click when the reduction is successful. As this is not always the case, the provider should observe the child to ensure function returns.

20. **Is one reduction method preferable to the other?**
A number of studies suggest that hyperpronation is more effective and less painful than the supination-flexion method, with success rates in one study nearly 96% in the former and only 68% in the latter (Gunaydin); however, both are commonly accepted methods of reduction.

21. **How long after reduction should return of function be expected?**
Function typically returns rapidly, within the first 10–15 minutes after reduction. This may take longer for a more remote injury.

22. **What should the provider do if function does not return within a reasonable time frame?**
If the history and physical exam are convincing for a nursemaid's elbow, the initial maneuver may be reattempted or the alternate maneuver may be employed. If repeated attempts are unsuccessful or the diagnosis is not certain, the provider should consider imaging to evaluate for a fracture. In the absence of another injury, the arm should be placed in a sling and the child referred for outpatient orthopedic follow-up.

23. **A 24-year-old playing basketball went up to grab a rebound; however, the ball bounced off the tip of his finger, resulting in significant pain and an obvious deformity. An x-ray shows a dorsal dislocation of the proximal interphalangeal (PIP) joint. What is the nomenclature used for finger dislocations?**
The distal aspect of the finger is described relative to the proximal aspect. For example, in a dorsal dislocation of the PIP joint, the distal and middle phalanges are located dorsal to the proximal phalanx.

24. **What is the proper analgesia for reduction of finger fractures or dislocations?**
Proper analgesia can typically be obtained by performing a digital nerve block.

25. **How is a digital nerve block preformed?**
A classic digital nerve block involves injection of local anesthetic without epinephrine into the web spaces on both sides of the digit immediately distal to the metacarpophalangeal (MCP) joint. This should provide anesthesia for the entire digit as the dorsal and palmar digital nerves run alongside the phalanx traversing the web spaces.

26. **How do I reduce a dislocated interphalangeal (IP) joint?**
Reduction of a dislocated IP joint begins with application of longitudinal traction of the dislocated phalanges. Dorsal dislocations are reduced with subsequent hyperextension of the dislocated phalanx with gentle pressure at the dorsal aspect of the base of the dislocated phalanx, pushing it back into place. Volar dislocations are reduced with hyperflexion of the dislocated phalanx with gentle pressure at the volar aspect of the base of the dislocated phalanx, pushing it back into place. Lateral dislocations are reduced with radial or ulnar pressure in the direction that will move the distal phalanx back to midline.

27. **What are the common complications of an IP joint reduction?**
Complications are rare when reducing IP joints; however, it is possible that there is an inability to reduce the dislocation. This is more common with volar dislocations as the dislocated phalanx can get entrapped in the extensor tendons. Inadequate stabilization can lead to recurrent dislocation.

28. **How do you reduce a dorsally dislocated MCP joint?**
Reduction of a dorsal MCP joint dislocation can typically be reduced by flexing the wrist to relax the flexor tendon, hyperextending the digit and applying volar pressure on the dorsal aspect of the proximal phalanx.

29. **How is a finger splinted after reduction of a dislocation or fracture?**
The key to splinting a finger depends on the location of the dislocation or fracture. For fractures that were reduced, stabilization of the joints proximal and distal to the fracture are necessary. For dislocations, it suffices to stabilize the joint that was reduced. Fractures of the distal or middle phalanges and dislocations of the distal IP joint are stabilized with a finger splint. Proximal phalanx fracture reductions and proximal IP joint or MCP reductions require stabilization of the proximal IP and MCP joints, which can be obtained with an ulnar or radial gutter splint, volar splint, or thumb spica, depending on the digit involved.

30. **What should be done after splinting the reduction?**
Obtain postreduction films to ensure proper alignment and have the patient follow up with a hand surgeon.

31. **What is a mallet finger? Why is it important to recognize it?**
A mallet finger is caused by avulsion of the extensor tendon that inserts on the base of the distal phalanx. It results in an inability to extend the distal phalanx and occurs in association with a Salter-Harris I or II fracture in a child or Salter-Harris III fracture in adolescents. While the fracture does not typically need reduction, it is crucial to splint the distal phalanx in slight hyperextension.

32. **A 34-year-old male comes to the urgent care center after punching a wall with a closed fist. The distal ulnar aspect of his hand is swollen and tender. An x-ray shows an angulated fracture of the neck of the fifth metacarpal with volar angulation of the metacarpal head. How does one reduce a boxer's fracture?**
The first step is providing adequate analgesia—typically with a hematoma block or an ulnar nerve block. Once adequate analgesia is obtained, the fifth digit is flexed to 90 degrees at the MCP joint. Reduction is performed by applying pressure to the dorsal aspect of the metacarpal proximal to the fracture and upward pressure to the volar aspect of the metacarpal distal to the fracture. Alternatively, if the MCP and PIP joints are both flexed to 90 degrees, dorsally angled pressure can be applied at the PIP joint while volarly directed pressure is applied to the fifth metacarpal proximal to the fracture (Fig. 45.4).

33. **How do you splint a reduced boxer's fracture?**
A reduced boxer's fracture is immobilized with an ulnar gutter splint.

34. **A 15-year-old boy was at bat during a baseball game, and as he swung at the ball he developed abrupt onset of right knee pain and inability to bear weight. On your exam, his knee is edematous and the patella appears to be laterally displaced. What physical exam findings are suggestive of this injury?**
Patients with patellar dislocation typically present with the knee held in slight flexion, edema of the knee, and tenderness along the medial patellar retinaculum at the medial superior aspect of the patella. If not spontaneously reduced, the laterally displaced patella is clinically evident.

35. **Is sedation indicated for reduction of patellar dislocation?**
Depending on the patient, sedation may be needed for reduction. At times, the injury will reduce spontaneously after administration of a benzodiazepine alone.

36. **How does one reduce a lateral patellar dislocation?**
Hold the ipsilateral hip in flexion with the upper leg stabilized by an assistant. Slowly extend the knee, applying gentle medial pressure to the patella.

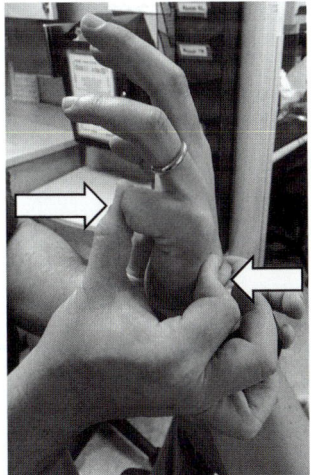

Fig. 45.4. Reduction of a boxer's fracture. Pressure is applied to the PIP joint, which is flexed to 90 degrees with simultaneous pressure to the dorsal aspect of the proximal fifth metacarpal.

37. **What is the "apprehension test"?**
   In the apprehension test, the provider holds the knee slightly flexed while applying lateral pressure to the patella. The test is positive if the patient expresses pain or anxiety that the patella will dislocate, either verbally or by sudden contraction of the quadriceps. This indicates that the patient had a patellar dislocation that has spontaneously reduced.

38. **Why is postreduction imaging indicated for these patients?**
   Postreduction x-rays are required to rule out concomitant fracture of the lateral femoral condyle or medial patellar facet.

39. **What postreduction care is indicated for this patient?**
   The patient should be placed in a knee immobilizer and referred for orthopedic follow-up in approximately 1 week.

KEY POINTS

1. A benzodiazepine can be used to overcome muscle spasm in mandibular dislocations, greatly facilitating reduction.
2. Reduction of an anterior shoulder dislocation can be accomplished by many different maneuvers; however, they can be painful and require appropriate analgesia.
3. Reduction of a dislocated phalanx requires longitudinal traction and pressure at the base of the dislocated phalanx, gently pushing it back into place.
4. Patellar dislocations may reduce spontaneously prior to presentation; this can be assumed if the patient becomes anxious when lateral pressure is applied to the patella.

BIBLIOGRAPHY

Aronson PL, Mistry RD. Intra-articular lidocaine for reduction of shoulder dislocation. *Pediatr Emerg Care*. 2014;30:358.
Borchers JR, Best TM. Common finger fractures and dislocation. *Am Fam Physician*. 2012;85:805.
Cutts S, Prempeh M, Drew S. Anterior shoulder dislocation. *Ann R Coll Surg Engl*. 2009;91:2.
Gunaydin YK, Katirci Y, Duymaz H, et al. Comparison of success and pain levels of supination-fexion and hyperpronation maneuvers in childhood nursemaid's elbow cases. *Am J Emerg Med*. 2013;31:1078.
Johnson FC, Okada PJ. Reduction of common joint dislocations and subluxations. In: King C, Henretig FM, eds. *Textbook of Pediatric Emergency Procedures*. 2nd ed. Philadelphia: Wolters Kluwer; 2008:962–990.
Mailhot T, Lyn ET. Hand. In: Mar JA, ed. *Rosen's Emergency Medicine*. 8th ed. Philadelphia: Elsevier-Saunders; 2014:534–569.

CHAPTER 46

SPLINTING AND CASTING

Todd A. Mastrovitch, MD, Yashas Nathani, MD

1. What is the purpose of casting and splinting?

To decrease pain, for mechanical stabilization, to prevent soft tissue contractures, to decrease further injury. Splints should be noncircumferential, somewhat loose, and applied in a position of function.

2. What materials are needed for splinting?

- Gauze roll or elastic ACE bandage (Fig. 46.1A)
- Cotton stocking material (stockinette)
- Soft cotton roll (Webril) (Fig. 46.1B)
- Fiberglass roll (Ortho glass) or plaster roll
- Measuring tape/scissors/water

3. What are the layers of a splint, from inner to outer layer?

- Stockinette (optional)
- Soft cotton bandage/undersplint material (e.g., Webril padding), especially at bony prominences (Fig. 46.2)
- Plaster or fiberglass placed to maintain position of immobilization
- Outer layer of ACE bandage

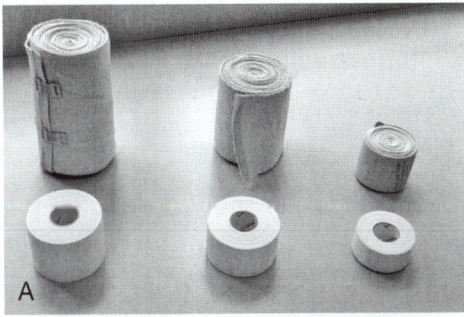

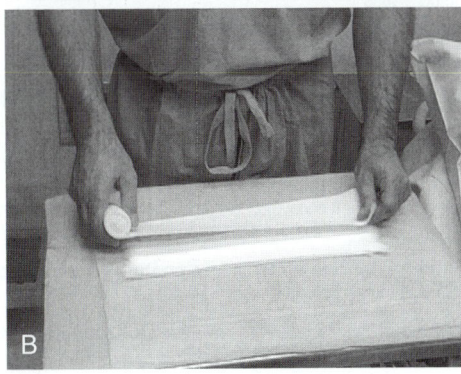

Fig. 46.1. A, Tape (foreground) and ACE bandage (background). *(From Garza D: Taping and bandaging. In: Auerbach PS, Cushing TA, Harris NS (eds):* Auerbach's Wilderness Medicine. *Philadelphia, 2016, Elsevier.)* B. Webril/cotton soft padding. *(From Ramirez MA: Procedures Consult. General Splinting Techniques, 2007, Philadelphia, 2017, Elsevier.)*

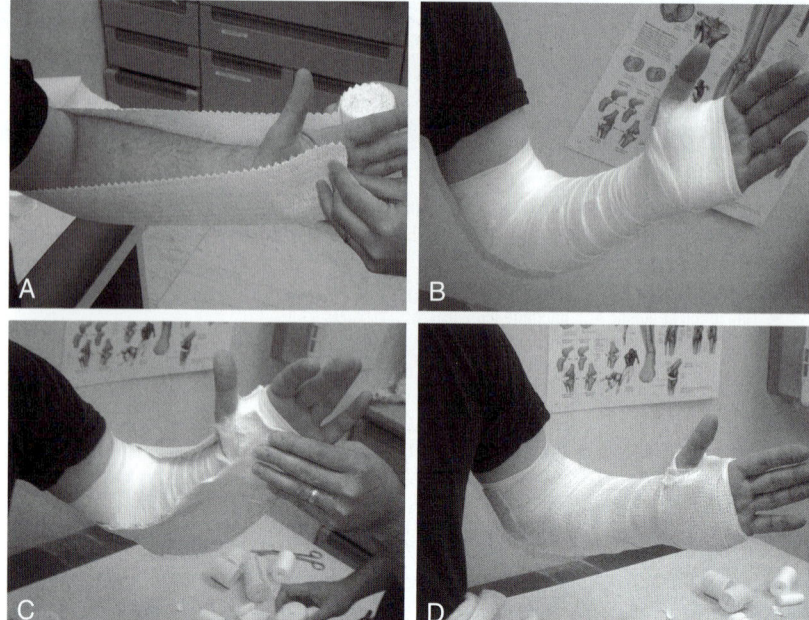

Fig. 46.2. Webril (B) and plaster splint application (A,C,D) for a sugar tong wrist splint. *(From Mazzola T: Splinting and casting. In: Seidenberg P, Beutler A (eds): The Sports Medicine Resource Manual. Philadelphia, 2008, Saunders, Fig. 16-3.)*

4. **What are the disadvantages of splinting?**
   - Motion at the injury site
   - Patient noncompliance (taking off the splint)

5. **What are the complications of casting an orthopedic injury in the acute phase?**
   - Compartment syndrome
   - Pressure sores
   - Thermal injury
   - Joint stiffness
   - Skin infection and dermatitis

6. **Is sedation required for splinting or casting?**
   Closed reduction for displaced fractures should always be done under sedation.

7. **What are the indications for surgical management of clavicular fractures?**
   Open fracture, >100% displacement; complicated comminuted fractures; neurovascular/airway compromise.

8. **What is a dreaded complication of forearm fractures?**
   Compartment syndrome. Significant ecchymosis is a risk factor for compartment syndrome in forearm fractures.

9. **What are the contraindications for long arm posterior splint placement?**
   Complex and unstable distal forearm fractures

10. **What is the proper splint to immobilize the wrist for fracture/sprain?**
    Volar (Fig. 46.3) or dorsal splint with the following:
    LENGTH = proximal fingers to proximal forearm
    WIDTH = as wide or slightly wider than the surface of the forearm

11. **What are the different methods of casting/splinting of the upper extremities?**
    See Table 46.1.

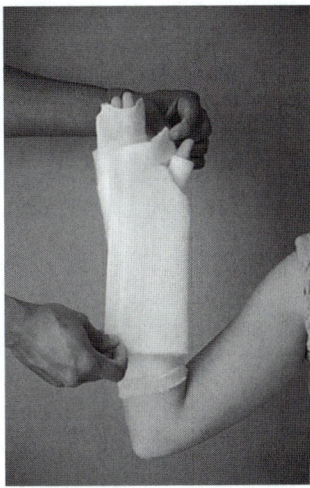

Fig. 46.3. **Volar Wrist Splint.** *(From Cromer DA: Splinting and casting. In: Rynders SD, Hart JA (eds):* Orthopedics for Physician Assistants. *Philadelphia, 2013, Saunders, p 373.)*

Table 46.1. Upper Extremity Splinting and Casting

Proximal or middle phalanx: stable and nondisplaced	Buddy taping
Distal phalangeal fracture	Aluminum U-shaped splint
Carpal bone fractures (excluding scaphoid and trapezium)	Volar/dorsal splint
Scaphoid (nondisplaced)	Thumb spica
First metacarpal and thumb fracture (nondisplaced)	Thumb spica
Second or third metacarpal or corresponding proximal/middle phalangeal shaft fracture (nondisplaced/nonrotated)	Radial gutter
Third or fourth metacarpal or corresponding proximal/middle phalangeal shaft fracture (nondisplaced/nonrotated)	Ulnar gutter
Acute distal radial/ulnar fractures	Sugar tong, long arm posterior splint
Proximal humeral/humeral shaft fractures	Simple sling or coaptation splint for severely displaced fractures
Distal humeral, proximal (supracondylar Type I Gartland)/middle forearm, and nonbuckle wrist fractures	Long arm posterior cast
Supracondylar (Type II, III Gartland)	Surgical reduction with pin fixation
Lateral condylar fracture	Surgical fixation
Medial condylar fracture (nondisplaced <3–5 mm)	Long arm posterior splint
Clavicle (middle 1/3, distal 1/3, medial 1/3)	Figure-of-eight splint or simple sling (need clavicle-specific x-rays)

12. Is there a difference in treating younger versus older children's femur fractures?
Yes. There is a trend to treat younger children nonoperatively with suspension traction and spica casting. The trend in older children is to treat the femur fracture with sliding hip screw fixation/plate fixation.

13. Which lower extremity problems need splinting?
- Ankle sprain
- Distal tibia/fibula fracture
- Metatarsal fracture

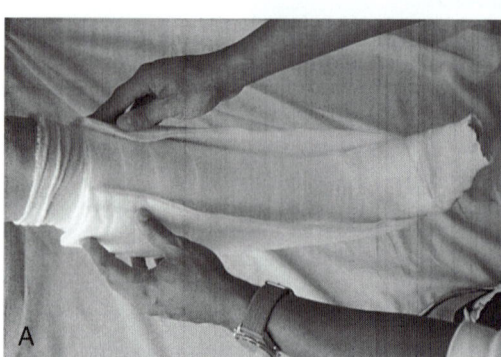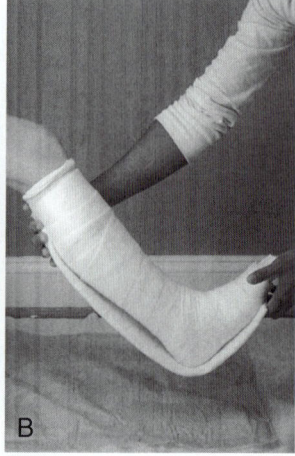

Fig, 46.4. A, Sugar tong ankle splint. **B,** Posterior ankle splint. *(From Cromer DA: Splinting and casting.In: Rynders SD, Hart JA (eds): Orthopedics for Physician Assistants. Philadelphia, 2013 Saunders, pp 379–381.)*

Table 46.2. Lower Extremity Splinting and Casting	
Hip fracture	Hip spica cast
Femur fracture	Spica cast
Tibular/fibular fracture	Long leg splint or long leg cast
Ankle fracture (nondisplaced)	Short leg posterior splint or short leg cast
Fifth metatarsal fracture (Jones fracture)	Bulky Jones dressing and postoperative shoe or non–weight-bearing short leg cast
Spiral fracture, fifth metatarsal neck (dancer's fracture)	Short leg cast
Toe fracture (nondisplaced)	Buddy taping

14. What is the proper splint to immobilize the above problems in question 13?
Sugar tong (Fig. 46.4A)/Posterior (Fig. 46.4B) splint with the following:
LENGTH = fibular head to base of toes *or* fibular head around heel to below the medial knee
WIDTH = half the circumference of the lower leg

15. Is it appropriate to manage an open toe fracture with splinting only?
No. Open toe fractures, in which the germinal matrix of the proximal nail bed is trapped in the fracture site:
- Need external repair and antibiotics
- If severe, may need Open Reduction Internal Fixation surgery with K-wire repair and intravenous antibiotics

16. What are the different methods of casting/splinting the lower extremities?
See Table 46.2.

KEY POINTS

1. Splinting is a potential treatment for nondisplaced, closed fractures or sprains.
2. Contraindications to splinting include open fractures, fractures involving the joint, severe fractures (displaced, angulated, or overlapping fractures), Salter-Harris V fractures, severe plastic fractures (greenstick, bowing), or evidence of compartment syndrome.
3. Splints should be placed with extremities in their normal position of function.

BIBLIOGRAPHY

Arora R, Fichadia U, Hartwig E, et al. Pediatric upper extremity fractures. *Pediatr Ann*. 2014;5:196–204.
Beaty J, Kasser J, eds. *Rockwood and Wilkins Fractures in Children*. 6th ed. Philadelphia: Lippincott Williams & Wilkins; 2006.
Selbst S. *Pediatric Emergency Medicine Secrets*. 3rd ed. Philadelphia: Elsevier Saunders; 2015.

CHAPTER 47

ABSCESS INCISION AND DRAINAGE

Ee Tein Tay, MD

1. **What is a skin abscess?**
   An abscess is a focal and contained cavity filled with purulent fluid, usually surrounded by inflamed deep subcutaneous tissue.

2. **What causes a skin abscess?**
   Abscesses are usually caused by gram-positive cocci, commonly *Staphylococcus aureus* and group A streptococci. There is now an increase of community-acquired methicillin-resistant *Staphylococcus aureus* (CA-MRSA). Gram-negative bacteria may cause skin abscesses in the buttock and axilla. Infections may occur when the skin barrier is disrupted and bacteria enter the open wound.

3. **What does a skin abscess look like?**
   The skin may appear fluctuant (fluid filled), tender, indurated, and erythematous. There may be an area of skin disruption, such as a punctum or laceration. A "point" may be visible in some abscesses.

4. **What is the difference between an abscess and cellulitis?**
   Cellulitis is a skin infection that usually involves the epidermis, dermis, and superficial subcutaneous tissues and does not have an organized cavity; abscesses have an organized fluid-filled cavity and involve deeper subcutaneous tissues.

5. **How can I tell the difference between an abscess and cellulitis on physical exam?**
   Both the skin of an abscess and cellulitis may be indurated, but abscesses usually are fluctuant on physical exam. Often, it may be difficult to differentiate by visualization and palpation.

6. **Is there a role for ultrasound when evaluating an abscess?**
   Point-of-care ultrasounds have been found to be 90%–97% sensitive and 67%–83% specific in detecting for skin abscesses and have been shown to improve accuracy in abscess diagnosis. Ultrasounds can also be used to measure the size of an abscess, detect loculations, and evaluate surrounding structures such as lymph nodes or blood vessels (Fig. 47.1).

7. **Will discharge be present when examining for an abscess?**
   If an abscess erupts, discharge may be present, but discharge may not necessarily be present during examination.

8. **What is the treatment for an abscess?**
   The treatment of choice is incision and drainage of an abscess. Antibiotics alone, needle aspiration of abscess, and mechanical unroofing of a "point" of an abscess all have high treatment failures.

9. **What type of pain relief is used for incision and drainage?**
   Topical anesthetics can be used to promote drainage through maceration, but local anesthesia is best achieved with lidocaine infiltrate. A "field block" is often injected around the wound of an abscess. Injecting into the wound may not provide adequate local anesthesia. Often, lidocaine is injected over the area of the abscess where the incision is expected.

10. **How is incision and drainage of an abscess performed?**
    After proper local anesthesia is achieved, the wound is cleaned with antiseptic solution. Incision of the abscess along the area of maximum fluctuance is performed by using an 11-blade scalpel through the dermis. The length of the incision depends on the size of the abscess. Once incision is performed, pressure is applied to the surrounding tissue to express the abscess fluid from the incision site.

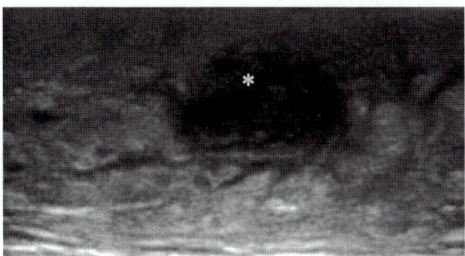

Fig. 47.1. Hypoechoic region (*asterisk*) indicates presence of abscess on ultrasound.

11. Is wound irrigation necessary in the incision site?

Although some providers recommend irrigating the wound after incision to "clean out" the wound, irrigation of an abscess has not been shown to improve wound healing.

12. How do I know if there are septations or loculations within the abscess?

Ultrasounds can potentially detect septations or loculations, but they may not be clinically detectable on physical exam. A hemostat is inserted into the incised wound to explore and break apart any septations and loculations.

13. Are wound cultures performed from the abscess fluid?

Routine swabbing is not recommended for immunocompetent patients without risk factors. Some providers perform wound cultures to survey local resistance patterns or to determine type of antibiotic use.

14. Are blood cultures necessary in a patient with an abscess?

Blood cultures are generally not obtained in immunocompetent patients with skin infections, unless patients have serious or complicated soft tissue infections from surgical or traumatic wounds or require further surgical intervention. The emergence of CA-MRSA increases patients' risks of developing other types of infections such as pneumonia, but generally the incidences of bacteria are low for both immunocompetent patients and patients with CA-MRSA.

15. Does the incision site need to be closed up after the procedure?

Wound healing by secondary intention is generally favored as previous studies have not found a difference in wound healing between primary versus secondary closure following an abscess incision and drainage.

16. Is wound packing necessary after the incision and drainage?

Wound packing following incision and drainage has not been found to impact failure or recurrence rate of an abscess; thus, it is not favored by most providers. Wound packing has been used to assist in wound debridement and to avoid fluid reaccumulation. Packing is removed within 24 to 48 hours, and the wound is reassessed then.

17. What is a wound "stent"?

It is the insertion of a strip of iodoform or Penrose drain to the wound to keep the wound open to promote drainage after the incision and drainage. Its use and impact on wound healing are debatable.

18. What is a loop drain?

A loop drain is the insertion of a rubber vessel loop into the wound and tunneled to a distal healthy tissue and tied to form a loop following incision, drainage, and irrigation of the abscess. The loop remains in place to promote further drainage and is removed between 3 and 10 days. While this is a novel technique, early studies have shown higher healing rate than traditional incision and drainage methods with wound packing.

19. When is procedural sedation necessary during an incision and drainage?

Procedural sedations may assist in the performance of the incision and drainage in patients who may not be cooperative with the procedure. The procedure is often performed in pediatric patients or patients with a large size lesion requiring aggressive manipulation.

20. What medications are often used for procedural sedations during an abscess incision and drainage?

This is generally up to the preference of the provider. Options include ketamine, propofol, or benzodiazepines in oral, intranasal, or intravenous forms.

21. When should consults be called for an abscess drain?

Incision and drainage for simple skin abscesses are generally performed by clinicians in an urgent care setting. Subspecialists such as otolaryngology may be consulted for abscesses involving the face and neck. Gynecology consult may be warranted for patients with abscesses involving the genitalia, such as a Bartholin cyst. In patients with deep and complex lesions, lesions involving the breast, or perianal abscesses, general surgery consult may be necessary.

22. Should patients receive antibiotics after incision and drainage?

Based on the 2014 guidelines provided by the Infectious Diseases Society of America, mild abscesses should be treated with incision and drainage alone without antibiotic use. Antibiotics are recommended in patients with systemic infections, those who are immunocompromised, and those with multiple abscesses, extremes of ages, and lack of response to incision and drainage alone.

23. Which types of antibiotics should be given if the decision was to give antibiotics after incision and drainage?

If antibiotics are recommended, medications against MRSA should be selected. Previous studies have not found any difference in clinical improvement in patients who received antibiotics for coverage against MRSA versus antibiotics for traditional skin flora or placebo, except in patients less than 1 year of age presenting with fever and abscess.

24. Should topical antibiotics be given for abscess treatment?

Topical antibiotics are not helpful in abscesses that require draining.

25. When should patients with abscesses be hospitalized?

Admission may be warranted in patients who appear toxic with systemic symptoms such as fever, diabetic patients, and those who are immunocompromised. Patients with lymphangitis and concomitant rapidly spreading cellulitis should also be hospitalized for intravenous antibiotics.

KEY POINTS

1. Incision and drainage is the treatment of choice for abscesses.
2. Antibiotics after incision and drainage are reserved for patients who are immunocompromised, have systemic symptoms, or have multiple abscesses and patients with persistent symptoms despite incision and drainage.
3. Wound packing after incision and drainage has no impact on wound improvement.

BIBLIOGRAPHY

Chinnock B, Hendey GW. Irrigation of cutaneous abscesses does not improve treatment success. *Ann Emerg Med.* 2016;67(3):379–383.

Fenster DB, Renny MH, Ng C, Roskind CG. Scratching the surface: a review of skin and soft tissue infections in children. *Curr Opin Pediatr.* 2015;27(3):303–307.

Iverson K, Haritos D, Thomas R, Kannikeswaran N. The effect of bedside ultrasound on diagnosis and management of soft tissue infections in a pediatric ED. *Am J Emerg Med.* 2013;30(8):1347–1351.

Kessler DO, Krantz A, Mojica M. Randomized control trial of wound packing to no wound packing following incision and drainage of superficial skin abscesses in the pediatric emergency department. *Pediatr Emerg Care.* 2012;28(6):514–517.

Korownyk C, Allan GM. Evidence-based approach to abscess management. *Can Fam Physician.* 2007;53(10):1680–1684.

Ladde JG, Baker S, Rodgers CN, Papa L. The LOOP technique: a novel incision and drainage technique in the treatment of skin abscesses in a pediatric ED. *Am J Emerg Med.* 2015;33(2):271–276.

Mistry RD. Skin and soft tissue infections. *Pediatr Clin N Am.* 2013;60(5):1063–1082.

Singer A, Taira BR, Chale S, Bhat R, Kennedy D, Schmitz G. Primary versus secondary closure of cutaneous abscesses in the emergency department: a randomized controlled trial. *Acad Emerg Med.* 2013;20(1):27–32.

Stevens DL, Bisno AL, Chambers HF, et al. Practice guidelines for diagnosis and management of skin and soft tissue infections. *Infectious Diseases Society of America.* 2014;59(2):e10–e52.

CHAPTER 48

FOREIGN-BODY REMOVAL

Anne M. O'Connor, MD, MSc, Therese L. Canares, MD

EAR AND NASAL FOREIGN BODIES

1. **What makes foreign-body removal unique in the pediatric patient?**
   The provider must accommodate for the maturity level and behavior of the child and seek input from the parent on the child's ability to tolerate a minor procedure. The provider must explain the procedure to both the parent and the child in language they can understand. Outpatient referral to an otolaryngologist may be warranted if likelihood of success is low based on initial evaluation of the patient.

2. **What behavioral or immobilization techniques can assist in procedures on an uncooperative child?**
   The child may remain in the parent's lap, while giving the parent straightforward instructions on how to assist with holding. An alternative method is laying the child down, swaddling the arms and legs with a bedsheet, with an assistant or parent gently immobilizing the trunk and head.

3. **Should medications be used for ear or nasal foreign-body removal?**
   Lidocaine can be instilled into the ear to assist with anesthesia, or to drown bugs if present; however, it should be avoided if tympanic membrane perforation is suspected. Vasoconstrictors (e.g., oxymetazoline nasal spray) may reduce nasal mucosal swelling and improve success.

4. **Is sedation appropriate for pediatric foreign-body removal?**
   Anxiolysis with intranasal midazolam (0.2–0.4 mg/kg) is the preferred strategy for minor pediatric procedures. A single dose of intranasal midazolam does not induce moderate sedation, and therefore does not require cardiorespiratory monitoring, though pulse oximetry may be used if institutional protocol dictates.

5. **Is there a noninvasive method to remove a foreign body from the nose?**
   In the positive pressure, or "magic kiss," technique, the opposing nostril is occluded and positive pressure is applied through the patient's mouth, either by a parent creating a mouth-to-mouth seal and exhaling forcefully, or using a bag-valve mask.

6. **When is irrigation indicated for foreign-body removal?**
   Irrigation is not indicated for nasal foreign-body removal. Irrigation with warm tap water or saline through the soft catheter of a butterfly cannula can flush a foreign body from the auditory canal. Irrigation should be avoided with organic matter that can swell or injure tympanic membrane, or in button batteries.

7. **When can tissue adhesive (glue) be used to aid foreign-body removal?**
   Tissue adhesive, such as Dermabond, is useful for round, rigid, or smooth objects (e.g., beads) in the ear. The foreign body must be dry and easily visualized. A drop of tissue glue is placed on a thin dowel, such as a cotton swab stick, and applied to make contact with the foreign body. Wait several seconds for the glue to dry, then the object can be extracted. Take caution not to drip tissue adhesive into the ear canal or push the object deeper.

8. **How can a Foley catheter be used to remove foreign bodies from the nose?**
   Apply lubricating jelly to a small Foley catheter bulb (e.g., 6–8 Fr), slide the catheter along the floor of the nare past the foreign body, then inflate the balloon and sweep the object out of the nose (Fig. 48.1).

9. **When are forceps appropriate for foreign-body removal?**
   Forceps are successful for easily visualized, graspable materials with a high level of material integrity and patient cooperation. The risks are canal and mucosal abrasions.

10. **When is a nasal foreign body a medical emergency?**
    Button batteries in any cavity (e.g., ear, nose, esophagus) require immediate removal, due to the risk for liquefaction necrosis, secondary to the battery current discharged when adjacent to mucosal tissue. Two magnets across the nasal septum require emergent removal because they can create ischemic necrosis.

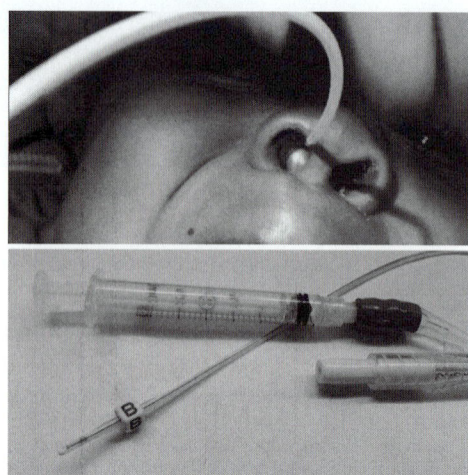

Fig. 48.1. A bead in a 2-year-old's nose, removed with a 6-Fr Foley catheter (*top*). If the bead has a hollow hole, the Foley may be threaded through the hole prior to balloon inflation to aid in removal (*bottom*).

11. **What are the indications for referral to otolaryngology for removal?**
    Indications for referral include need for sedation, development of granulation tissue, signs of trauma, nongraspable or nonvisualized foreign body, sharp objects, objects abutting the tympanic membrane, or unsuccessful extraction attempt.

12. **When are antibiotics needed?**
    Antibiotic coverage is not routinely required after extraction of the acute foreign body, unless there are signs of concomitant infection, such as otitis externa or cellulitis.

FOREIGN-BODY INGESTION OR ASPIRATION

13. **What is the typical profile of a foreign-body ingestion or aspiration in a child?**
    The typical profile of a foreign-body ingestion or aspiration is a toddler to preschool-age child, who was eating or playing with hot dogs, peanuts, seeds, raw carrots, popcorn, coins, toy parts, or balloons and has sudden onset of choking or respiratory distress.

14. **What are the symptoms of foreign-body aspiration or ingestion?**
    Symptoms of a foreign body in the oropharynx or esophagus include throat pain, drooling, gagging, vomiting, or difficulty swallowing. Symptoms of a foreign body in the airway are coughing, choking, stridor, cyanosis, wheeze, or respiratory distress.

15. **What are the x-ray findings of an aspirated foreign body?**
    Secondary signs of an aspirated foreign body may be found on inspiratory and expiratory chest x-rays (or bilateral decubitus views in the uncooperative child). The foreign body causes air trapping, leading to ipsilateral hyperinflation and mediastinal shift to the contralateral side, or segmental hyperlucency or atelectasis. Chest x-ray to identify a foreign body has sensitivity and specificity at 61% and 77%, respectively.

16. **When is a foreign-body aspiration or ingestion considered an emergency?**
    Emergent endoscopic removal is indicated for any foreign-body aspiration, or an ingested object with high risk for perforation, obstruction, or toxicity (Box 48.1). A single, high-powered magnet ingestion is managed expectantly with serial x-rays and removing all nearby magnet sources at home. Management of low-risk objects (e.g., coins) in the stomach includes weekly x-rays to ensure passage. Coins retained in the stomach at 4 weeks may warrant endoscopic removal.

Box 48.1. Indications for Urgent Endoscopic Removal of a Foreign-Body Ingestion

- A sharp and long (>5 cm) object in the esophagus or stomach
- Multiple high-powered magnets
- A disc battery
- Signs of airway compromise
- Signs of obstruction of the esophagus (vomiting and pooling secretions)
- Signs of lower abdominal inflammation or obstruction (fever, abdominal pain, or vomiting)
- Objects containing heavy metals that cause toxicity (e.g., lead, iron)
- Soft tissue swelling visible in the pharyngeal space on neck x-ray

From: Gilger MA, Jain AK, McOmber ME: Foreign Bodies of the Esophagus and Gastrointestinal Tract in Children. UpToDate, 2016.

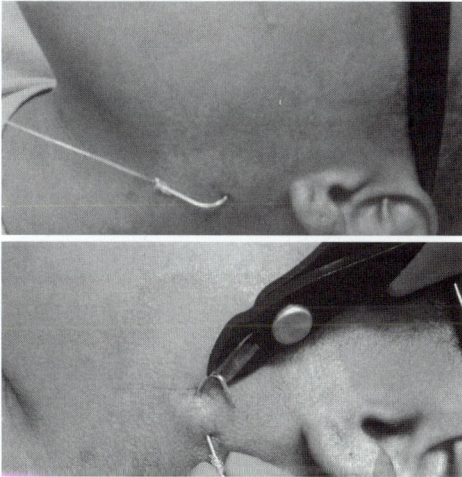

Fig. 48.2. An adolescent boy with a fishhook embedded in his cheek. The hook was removed by the advance and cut method.

FOREIGN BODIES IN THE SKIN

17. **What is the first step in any foreign-body removal from the skin?**
All foreign-body removal from the skin warrants universal precautions for the provider, sterilization of the wound, local anesthesia if indicated, and routine wound care afterwards.

18. **Before removal of a foreign body in the skin, what must the provider examine?**
The provider should determine whether the object has injured deeper structures such as bone, tendon, or vasculature, by performing a thorough neurovasculature exam or x-ray if indicted.

19. **What are the common fishhook removal techniques?**
There are four common techniques to fishhook removal. The advance and cut technique is generally the most successful: Grasp the hook with a needle driver and rotate the hook to emerge the barb, creating an exit wound. Use wire cutters to cut the barb, then remove the hook from the entry site (Fig. 48.2).
Other options include the string-yank (which requires technical experience), retrograde removal (for barbless or superficial hooks), and the needle cover technique.

20. **What are the common techniques for splinter removal?**
A visible wood or plant-based splinter that is parallel to the skin should be removed with caution because simply grasping and pulling can lead to fragmentation. Set a 30-minute time limit for the

procedure, to avoid excess tissue damage or trauma if the object is not found. If the splinter is small and superficial, it may be removed using an 18-gauge needle to gently disrupt the skin over the splinter and then grasping the splinter with forceps. For the deeper, parallel object, use a scalpel to make an incision over the object; or if perpendicular, make an elliptical incision around the object and then remove the core of tissue containing the object.

21. What is the technique for tick removal?
The tick's head is grasped firmly by forceps, as closely to the skin as possible, and constant, vertical traction is applied. Any retained parts can be removed similar to splinter removal.

22. Should chemoprophylaxis be started after tick removal?
Antibiotic prophylaxis after a tick bite is not routinely indicated, due to the low risk of infection (<3%) after a recognized deer tick bite in endemic areas. Prophylaxis of Lyme disease with a single dose of doxycycline can be considered for a child older than 8 years, if it is a high-risk tick bite, within 72 hours of tick removal, if the patient lives in a hyperendemic area, if it was an engorged deer tick, and if duration of attachment is beyond 36 hours. Prophylaxis is not recommended in children under 8 years of age.

23. What vaccinations should be up to date for patients with skin foreign bodies?
For all foreign bodies in the skin, ensure that the patient's tetanus vaccination is up to date.

24. Are antibiotics indicated for a skin puncture wound?
A 3- to 5-day course of prophylactic antibiotics should be considered for injuries that are high risk for infection (Box 48.2). Oral antibiotic selection (Table 48.1) should cover gram-positive skin flora, and expand coverage for aquatic organisms in fishhook injuries, gram negative and anaerobes in dirty wounds, and pseudomonas in punctures through a shoe sole.

Box 48.2. Indications for Prophylactic Antibiotics After Skin Puncture Wounds

- Wounds contaminated with organic matter, dirt, or water organisms (fishhook injuries)
- Deep wounds (including proximity to bone or joint)
- Delicate anatomic sites at risk for infection (e.g., hand, ear)
- Plantar punctures through an intact shoe sole
- Evidence of cellulitis
- Host factors such as immunosuppression or diabetes mellitus

From: Baddour LM, Brown AM: Infectious Complications of Puncture Wounds. UpToDate, 2016.

Table 48.1. Prophylactic Oral Antibiotic Selection After Skin Puncture Wounds

If covering for skin flora:
- Cephalexin OR
- Clindamycin

If exposure to water organisms, add:
- Trimethoprim/sulfamethoxazole OR
- Amoxicillin/clavulanate OR
- Levofloxacin* PLUS
  - Metronidazole for sewage or soil contaminants
  - Doxycycline for seawater exposure

If plantar puncture wounds with risk for *Pseudomonas*:
- Ciprofloxacin or levofloxacin*

If dirty, contaminated wounds, consider:
- Trimethoprim/sulfamethoxazole OR
- Clindamycin OR
- Amoxicillin/clavulanate

*Caution is advised if treating children with fluoroquinolones, due to risk of tendon inflammation or rupture. Advise limited strenuous physical activity and discontinuation at the first sign of musculoskeletal pain or tingling.

From: Baddour LM, Brown AM: Infectious Complications of Puncture Wounds. UpToDate, 2016.

KEY POINTS

1. Nasal foreign bodies can be removed with positive pressure, tissue adhesive, Foley catheter, or forceps.
2. Ear foreign bodies can be removed with irrigation, tissue adhesive, or forceps.
3. Extraction attempts should cease in the event of any tissue damage or inability of the patient to tolerate the procedure.
4. Button batteries in any location or two magnets across the nasal septum are medical emergencies and require immediate removal.
5. Otolaryngology referral for nonemergent foreign bodies is frequently appropriate.
6. Suspect foreign-body aspiration in a child who is toddler to preschool age; was last seen with a small, hard object; and has sudden onset of cough, choke, or wheeze.
7. Chest x-ray with foreign-body aspiration will show air trapping and hyperinflation on the affected side.
8. Low-risk ingested objects can be managed expectantly.
9. Set a 30-minute time limit for the splinter removal procedure, to avoid excess tissue damage or trauma.
10. Tetanus should be up to date for all skin puncture wounds.
11. Antibiotic prophylaxis is indicated for high-risk skin punctures.

BIBLIOGRAPHY

Antonelli PJ, Ahmadi A, Prevatt A. Insecticidal activity of common reagents for insect foreign bodies of the ear. *Laryngoscope*. 2001;111(1):15–20.

Backlin SA. Positive-pressure technique for nasal foreign body removal in children. *Ann Emerg Med*. 1995;25(4):554–555.

Bressler K, Shelton C. Ear foreign-body removal: a review of 98 consecutive cases. *Laryngoscope*. 1993;103(4 Pt 1):367–370.

Committee on Infectious Diseases American Academy of Pediatrics. *Red Book: 2015 Report of the Committee on Infectious Diseases*. 30th ed. Elk Grove Village, IL: AAP; 2015.

Davies PH, Benger JR. Foreign bodies in the nose and ear: a review of techniques for removal in the emergency department. *J Accid Emerg Med*. 2000;17(2):91–94.

Lane RD, Schunk JE. Atomized intranasal midazolam use for minor procedures in the pediatric emergency department. *Pediatr Emerg Care*. 2008;24(5):300–303.

McRae D, Premachandra DJ, Gatland DJ. Button batteries in the ear, nose and cervical esophagus: a destructive foreign body. *J Otolaryngol*. 1989;18(6):317–319.

Safari M, Manesh MR. Demographic and clinical findings in children undergoing bronchoscopy for foreign body aspiration. *Ochsner J*. 2016;16(2):120–124.

Sink JR, Kitsko DJ, Georg MW, Winger DG, Simons JP. Predictors of foreign body aspiration in children. *Otolaryngol Head Neck Surg*. 2016.

Tong MC, Ying SY, van Hasselt CA. Nasal foreign bodies in children. *Int J Pediatr Otorhinolaryngol*. 1996;35(3):207–211.

CHAPTER 49

DENTAL AND ORAL COMPLAINTS AND PROCEDURES

Selena Hariharan, MD, MHSA, Steven Chan, MD

DENTAL INJURIES

1. **In pediatric dental trauma, why is it important to distinguish between primary and permanent teeth?**
   Management strategies and treatment differ depending on whether the injured tooth is a primary or permanent tooth.

2. **A 5-year-old male presents with a dental injury. Your examination reveals a child with an isolated avulsion of his left maxillary central incisor. His mother has the tooth with an intact root in a cup of cold milk. You recall that reimplantation should be performed immediately for avulsed permanent teeth but not for primary teeth. How do you make the distinction whether an injured tooth is a primary or permanent tooth?**
   - Primary teeth
     - Will erupt in a typical pattern depending on the age of the child.
     - Central incisors will erupt as early as 6–8 months of age with a full complement of primary teeth erupted by 3 years of age.
     - Mandibular teeth tend to erupt earlier than their maxillary counterparts.
     - A full complement of primary teeth consists of 10 mandibular and 10 maxillary teeth: 4 central incisors, 4 lateral incisors, 4 canines, and 8 molars.
   - Permanent teeth
     - Similarly, permanent teeth erupt in a typical pattern depending on the age of the child.
     - Central incisors will erupt as early as 6–7 years of age with a full complement of permanent teeth erupted by 16 years of age.
     - A full complement of permanent teeth consists of 16 mandibular and 16 maxillary teeth: 4 central incisors, 4 lateral incisors, 4 canines, 8 premolars, and 12 molars.
   - Answer
     - In this case, the tooth is most likely a primary tooth given the patient's age, and avulsed primary teeth should not be reimplanted. This family should be reassured with recommendations for good oral hygiene.
     - Use the age of the child to help you determine whether the injured tooth is primary or permanent.
       - ALL teeth in children less than 5 years of age are primary.
       - Children 6–12 years of age have mixed dentition.
       - ALL teeth in children older than 13 years of age are permanent.
     - Primary teeth are smaller compared to permanent teeth.
     - The occlusive surface of primary teeth is smooth as opposed to ridged.
     - When in doubt, ask the parents to help distinguish between primary and permanent teeth.

3. **What are the various injuries to primary dentition and how are they managed?**
   - **Fractures** can be classified based on the Ellis classification system.
     - **Enamel fracture (Ellis class I fracture):** fracture through the enamel ONLY
       Treatment: File down sharp edges if present.
     - **Enamel-dentin fracture (Ellis class II fracture):** fracture through the enamel and dentin
       Treatment: Apply sealant with glass ionomer.

- **Crown fracture with exposed pulp (Ellis class III fracture):** fracture through the enamel and dentin WITH exposure of the pulp
  Treatment: Preserve pulp vitality by applying a layer of calcium hydroxide. Tooth extraction is an alternative treatment option.
- **Crown-root fracture:** fracture involving the enamel, dentin, and root structure. The pulp may or may not be exposed. Fragments of tooth may be loose but still attached.
  Treatment: Emergent pediatric dental referral for possible fragment removal or tooth extraction.
- **Root fracture:** fracture involving the enamel, dentin, and root structure. If coronal fragment is displaced, pulp may be exposed.
  Treatment: Emergent pediatric dental referral. If coronal fragment is not displaced, repositioning with splinting can be considered. Otherwise, tooth may need to be extracted.
- **Alveolar fracture:** involving the alveolar bone, usually associated with mobility and dislocation of multiple adjacent teeth with malocclusion.
  Treatment: Emergent referral to a dentist or oral surgeon for reduction, stabilization, and splinting.
- Luxation injuries
  - **Avulsion:** complete displacement of tooth from its socket
    - An avulsed primary tooth should NOT be reimplanted to reduce the risk of further injury to the permanent tooth successor.
    - The apex of the root of the primary tooth lies in close proximity to the permanent tooth germ.
    - Common sequelae can include discoloration and hypoplasia of the permanent tooth.
    - In young children, consider radiographs of the chest/abdomen to rule out aspiration of an avulsed tooth if it cannot be found.
  - **Concussion:** tooth is tender to touch, tooth is not mobile, and there is no evidence of gingival bleeding
    Treatment: Supportive care, soft diet, observation, routine dental follow-up.
  - **Subluxation:** tooth is tender to touch with increased mobility and evidence of gingival bleeding but still within its socket without displacement; "loose tooth"
    Treatment: Gentle mouth care with soft brush, soft diet, supportive care, observation, routine dental follow-up.
  - **Extrusion:** tooth is partially displaced out of its socket, appears elongated, tender to touch, increased mobility, and with gingival bleeding
    Treatment: Depends on degree of displacement.
    - **If <3 mm,** can be carefully repositioned or left to spontaneously align.
    - **If >3 mm or concern for aspiration risk,** consider tooth extraction or emergent referral to a pediatric dentist.
  - **Intrusion:** apex of tooth is displaced into the socket either through the labial bone plate (apical tip can be visualized and the tooth appears shorter) or impinging on the developing tooth bud (apical tip cannot be visualized and tooth can appear elongated)
    Treatment:
    - **If intruded through the labial bone plate,** tooth can be left for spontaneous repositioning.
    - **If apex is displaced into the developing tooth bud,** tooth should be extracted. Consider emergent referral to a pediatric dentist.
  - **Lateral luxation:** displacement of tooth in either palatal, lingual, or labial direction
    Treatment: Soft diet, observation, supportive care, and allow for spontaneous repositioning as long as there is no malocclusion present.
    - Gentle repositioning is warranted if there is occlusal interference.
    - No evidence for prophylactic antibiotics in the treatment of luxation injuries.

4. What is good anticipatory guidance following dental trauma?
- Brush teeth with a soft-bristled toothbrush.
- Use alcohol-free 0.1% chlorhexidine gluconate topically as an oral rinse or apply with a cotton swab twice daily for 1 week to prevent plaque and debris.
- Follow soft diet for 10 days.
- Restrict use of pacifiers or sucking of digits/fingers.
- Avoid flossing.
- Avoid contact sports.
- Provide adequate pain management with acetaminophen and ibuprofen.
- Watch for signs of infection such as fever, redness, swelling, and pain.

5. **How are fractures in permanent teeth managed and treated?**
   - **Enamel fractures:** If tooth fragment is available, it can be bonded to the tooth. Otherwise, the sharp edges of the tooth can be filed down for patient comfort.
   - **Enamel-dentin fractures:** Cover exposed dentin with glass ionomer or composite resin.
   - Emergent pediatric dental referral should be considered for **enamel-dentin-pulp fractures, crown-root fractures, root fractures, and alveolar fractures.** This will be important in preserving pulp vitality. Continued root development, preventing apical periodontitis, and a positive cosmetic outcome.

6. **How are luxation injuries managed and treated in permanent teeth?**
   - **Concussion:** No treatment necessary.
   - **Subluxation:** No treatment necessary, although a flexible splint can be placed to stabilize the tooth for patient comfort.
   - **Extrusion:** Gently reposition tooth back into its socket; stabilize the tooth with a flexible splint.
   - **Lateral luxation:** Gently reposition tooth into its original location. Stabilize with flexible splint.
   - **Intrusion:** If only slightly intruded (<3 mm), can allow for eruption with close follow-up to monitor for movement in case orthodontic repositioning is required. If severely intruded (>7 mm), may require surgical repositioning. Emergent pediatric dental referral would be necessary.
   - **Avulsion:** One of the most serious dental injuries to permanent teeth as the prognosis is dependent on actions taken promptly after the injury takes place.
     - Immediate reimplantation is the treatment of choice in most situations and may ultimately save the tooth.
     - Primary teeth should NOT be reimplanted, only permanent teeth.
     - Dry time of greater than 60 minutes results in irreversible damage to the periodontal ligament cells and decreases the likelihood of tooth viability.
     - Pick up the tooth by the crown.
     - Do NOT touch the root.
     - If the tooth is dirty, wash with cold water briefly before reimplantation.
     - Do NOT scrub the tooth.
     - Gently reimplant tooth into its socket.
     - Instruct patient to bite down on a piece of dry gauze to hold it in position.
     - If reimplantation is not possible, store tooth in a glass of milk or other storage medium (Viaspan, Save-A-Tooth, Hank's Balanced Salt Solution).
     - If patient is conscious and can follow instructions, the tooth can be stored inside the patient's lip or cheeks using saliva as the storage medium.
     - Tap water should NOT be used.
     - Flexible splint is then placed to stabilize the reimplanted tooth.
     - Consider prophylactic antibiotics and tetanus.
       - Penicillin VK or amoxicillin for children under 12 years of age
       - Doxycycline for children older than 12 years of age
     - Pediatric dental follow-up for possible root canal in 7 to 10 days.

7. **A 16-year-old male presents to the urgent care after sustaining a dental injury while playing basketball. On examination, he is revealed to have a fracture of his left mandibular lateral incisor. It is tender to palpation but not mobile and without any bleeding. You notice that the fracture involves the enamel and the dentin without pulp exposure. What is the appropriate treatment for this patient?**
   - This patient has an Ellis II classification dental fracture of a permanent tooth. This type of injury requires application of calcium hydroxide for patient comfort and to maintain pulp vitality and dental follow-up within 48 hours.
   - **Application of calcium hydroxide (Dycal):**
     - Mix equal parts of Dycal base paste with catalyst paste on a padded surface until you achieve a uniform color.
     - Dry the tooth with cotton roll immediately before application.
     - Apply with applicator directly on surface of dentin or exposed pulp of tooth.
     - Apply a thin layer of Dycal (1 mm in thickness).
     - Dycal will harden in 2–3 minutes.

8. A 14-year-old female presents to the urgent care after sustaining a dental injury during soccer practice. On examination, she is found to have an extruded right maxillary lateral incisor. The tooth still appears to be in its socket, is relatively stable, and is elongated about 3 mm. It is tender to palpation, and mobile with some gingival bleeding. What is the appropriate treatment for this patient?
   - This patient has a minor extrusion injury of a permanent tooth. This type of injury requires gentle repositioning of the tooth back into its socket followed by stabilization with a flexible splint and dental follow-up within 48 hours.
   - **Splinting:**
     - Adjust the length of the wire so that it extends one tooth on either side of repositioned tooth.
     - Apply etchant and bonding solution on surface of teeth.
     - Place a dab of composite on the center of teeth to be bonded.
     - Position wire on the composite.
     - Allow composite to set.
     - Add additional composite to cover terminal ends of the wire.
     - Smooth the composite so there are no rough surfaces to irritate the soft tissue.

9. A 5-year-old female presents to the urgent care after falling off a trampoline and sustaining multiple dental injuries. On examination, she is found to have significant extrusion of both her maxillary central incisors with gingival bleeding and tenderness to palpation. They are extremely mobile with the root visible. They are elongated about 5 mm. What is the appropriate treatment for this patient?
   - The patient has significant extrusion of two primary teeth that appear to be very unstable and can put her at risk for aspiration. In this case, extraction of both teeth is warranted with dental follow-up within 48 hours. Since the teeth are significantly extruded, take a dry gauze, grasp the crown, and pull.
   - **Tooth extraction:**
     - Prepare patient with adequate local anesthesia.
     - Elevate the gingival soft tissue attachment.
     - Luxate the tooth with small and large straight elevators.
     - Apply forceps to the crown of the tooth.
     - Continue to luxate tooth with forceps in a buccolingual direction with slight rotation until tooth is removed from socket.

10. A 15-year-old male presents to the urgent care after being assaulted on his way home from school. He reports being punched in the face. On examination, he has multiple subluxed incisors but his dentition is otherwise intact. He denies any malocclusion. He has multiple (<1 cm) superficial lacerations to his buccal mucosa as well as a 1-cm laceration of his tongue that does not involve the lateral border. Bleeding is well controlled. What is the appropriate treatment for this patient?
    - The patient has multiple subluxated permanent teeth that appear stable within their socket without malocclusion. No intervention is required, but placement of a flexible splint for patient comfort is an option.
    - **Buccal mucosal and gingival lacerations:**
      - Minor lacerations in these areas heal very well without intervention.
      - Suture repair should be considered for gaping wounds (>2 cm) or if flaps of tissue are present. For the repair, use absorbable sutures such as 5-0 chromic gut.
      - The patient in this scenario does not need suture repair.
    - **Tongue lacerations:**
      - Minor lacerations to the tongue also heal very well without intervention.
      - Suture repair should be considered for the following situations: gaping wounds (check with the tongue extended), large lacerations (>1.5 cm), actively bleeding, flaps of tissue present, involvement of muscle and involvement of the border of the tongue (particularly the tip of the tongue).
      - Anesthetize with local infiltration without epinephrine.
      - Control the tongue by grasping with dry gauze or throwing a suture through the tip of the tongue and pulling on the suture.
      - Close with absorbable sutures such as chromic gut.

11. A 5-year-old male presents to the urgent care after falling with a pencil in his mouth. He initially cried out in pain and spit out some blood. Since then, he has been calm, playful, is in no acute distress, and the bleeding has stopped. The parents brought the pencil with them. Your examination reveals a puncture wound just lateral to the right tonsillar pillar that is 1 cm in diameter but of unclear depth. There is no active bleeding and no other injuries. What is the appropriate management of this patient?
    - The patient has a puncture wound in an area that puts him at risk for injury to his carotid artery and/or jugular vein. He appears stable and is not actively bleeding, but he should still be referred to a pediatric emergency department for otolaryngology consultation and further imaging, which may include angiography, computed tomography angiogram (CTA), or magnetic resonance imaging arteriogram/venogram (MRA/MRV).
    - Signs of vascular injury include expanding hematoma of the neck or pharynx, continued bleeding, diminished pulses in the neck, and neurologic changes.
    - It is VERY important to rule out a retained foreign body within the puncture wound. In the case here, be sure to inspect the pencil to ensure that it is intact. Otherwise, surgical exploration of the wound may be necessary.
    - Plain radiographs may NOT be helpful to rule out foreign bodies such as pencils or sticks.
    - Children with minor puncture wounds to the central portion of the palate can be sent home with routine mouth care.

DENTAL INFECTIONS

12. Where do dental infections originate?
    Most dental infections occur secondary to cavities or after trauma. They may also be a consequence of periodontal (gum) infection, pericoronitis (inflammation of the soft tissue around a partially erupted tooth, usually the wisdom teeth), or a postoperative complication.

13. Who usually suffers from dental infections?
    Dental infections are most common in healthy people though more severe in chronically ill or immunocompromised individuals.

14. During anatomy, I remember there being a lot of confusing anatomic parts around this area. How can I possibly approach a differential diagnosis?
    - It is helpful to divide the face into sectors.
    - The upper face is the orbits and surrounding structures, maxillary and ethmoid sinuses, ears and surrounding structures, upper buccal areas, and maxillary teeth.
    - The lower face is the mandibular teeth; lower buccal area; and sublingual, submental, and sub-mandibular regions.
    - The neck is everything below the submandibular triangle and above the clavicle.
    - First look at the sector and then at the structures within the sector (soft tissue, muscle, salivary glands, lymph nodes, mucus, bone, skin, or teeth, for example) to determine the origin of infection.

15. A 21-year-old patient presents to the urgent care complaining of excruciating tooth pain. He has been to his dentist repeatedly, and a dental exam and radiographs failed to reveal the cause for his pain. He even had a root canal. He is now on your examining table stating he refuses to leave without an answer. He notices the pain is aching and diffuse and worse when he chews. How will you approach the differential?
    - Not all tooth pain is odontogenic. A careful history and physical can often differentiate non-odontogenic pain referred to the teeth. In this case, pressing on a trigger point on the cheek reproduced the pain, and he was discharged with a muscle relaxant and a referral to physical therapy.
    - Other diagnoses on the differential include neuropathic pain (e.g., trigeminal neuralgia, herpes, injury), idiopathic pain, neurovascular headache, sinus disease, atypical acute myocardial event, psychogenic pain (including drug-seeking behavior), and the ubiquitous "other" like malignancy, temporal arteritis, rheumatologic disease, and bone disease.

16. A 2-year-old with speech delay is brought to the urgent care by her father just prior to closing because she refuses to sleep. With her speech delay, she cannot tell him the source of her discomfort. Not wanting to miss closing time, he has not given her any pain medicine. She is afebrile but did not eat dinner. She is, however, sucking on her bottle with vigor. You are convinced she is going to have an ear infection and are disappointed to note her ears are totally normal. What is another potential and common source for her pain and what are the clues in the history?
    - Overlooking the fact that this is a chapter on dental complaints, dental caries are a common source of infection and pain in children.
    - Caries are caused by a continuous process of bacteria and nutrients interacting and creating fluctuations in pH on the surface of the teeth. These fluctuations result in changes in the surface mineralization of the tooth. If the net mineralization change is a loss, then caries eventually form.
    - Clues to a dental source of pain for this child are refusing to eat (pain with mastication); pain when lying down (referred pain to the ears); and still drinking from a baby bottle and using it at night (baby bottle caries). If you take a close look at what is in the bottle, it is likely to be milk, juice, or soda.
    - For tonight, you can offer pain control with acetaminophen or ibuprofen, give recommendations for oral hygiene, ensure there is not an evolving dental abscess, facial cellulitis, or airway involvement, and provide a referral for dental care.

17. What are the most common bacteria found in the oral cavity?
    - When a baby is born, the bacteria in the mouth are mostly aerobic.
    - The teeth provide a surface for anaerobes to proliferate.
    - As dental hygiene diminishes and cavities increase, acidic bacteria increase.
    - There are gram-positive cocci, most importantly streptococci, peptostreptococci, and staphylococci.
    - There are gram-negative cocci that are less recognized: *Veillonella, Neisseria,* and Branhamella.
    - There are gram-positive rods collectively known as diphtheroids and branched filaments known as the *Actinomyces* species.
    - There are anaerobes: *Bacteroides, Capnocytophaga, Eikenella, Fusobacterium.*
    - An organism specific to juvenile periodontitis is *Aggregatibacter actinomycetemcomitans.*
    - Finally, there are a variety of spirochetes, fungi, yeast, viruses, and protozoa.
    - These organisms usually live in harmony, but when the oral environment gets out of balance, any one or several of them adhere to the mucous membranes, overcome host defenses, and create an infection.

18. An adolescent female presents complaining of tooth pain. She has a dentist, but it is Saturday, and she does not want to wait to be seen on Monday. When you look in her mouth, you notice diffuse gingivitis and an area of purulence above her canine. She has no facial swelling, erythema, or fever and can tolerate oral intake. How should this patient be treated? Does she need to be transferred from the urgent care to an emergency department?
    - As this patient does not have any systemic symptoms or evidence of facial cellulitis at this time, she can be treated in the urgent care as long as the family will ensure follow-up with her primary physician or, preferably, her dentist.
    - The noted abscess should be incised and drained.
    - Anesthesia can be achieved using a nerve block (to be reviewed in a later section) or using a topical or locally injected anesthetic if the abscess is localized and circumscribed.
    - The patient should be discharged on antibiotics and antibacterial mouthwash. She does not need to be transferred to an emergency department for further evaluation.

19. What antibiotics should the patient from question 18 be prescribed?
    - In an urgent care, it is unlikely the provider will identify the exact organism causing infection.
    - Rather, the provider should use general principles when choosing an antibiotic.
    - Dental infections are usually polymicrobial and a mix of aerobic and anaerobic bacteria.
    - The aerobic bacteria are overwhelmingly some variety of *Streptococcus*.
    - The anaerobic pathogens are multiple and varied.
    - First choice antibiotics for uncomplicated dental infections are the penicillins, cephalosporins, tetracyclines, or clindamycin after taking into consideration age, allergies, and previous drug history.
    - She can also be discharged with a mouthwash such as chlorhexidine swish and spit.

20. **Should the patient from question 18 have radiographs done at this visit?**
    For uncomplicated dental caries or an abscess without deep tissue spread, radiographs are not needed.

21. **The adolescent from question 18 returns Sunday night complaining of eye pain and a fever to 101°F. Her cheek is swollen and warm. She did not fill the prescription for the penicillin you gave her as she had a school event last night and slept in this morning. What do you do now?**
    - She should be transferred to an emergency department for further evaluation, imaging, and admission.
    - Risks of dental infections that spread along facial and fascial planes include facial cellulitis, periorbital cellulitis, orbital cellulitis, airway compromise, mediastinitis, intracranial infections, and death.

22. **Should you do any imaging of the patient from question 18 at the urgent care prior to transfer?**
    - There is a role for imaging in dental infections, though not in this case as the eye pain and rapid progression of fever suggest urgent transfer and initiation of therapy will benefit the patient most.
    - Computed tomography (CT) and magnetic resonance imaging (MRI) are considered the gold standard for soft tissue imaging for facial cellulitis or abscess.
    - Plain x-ray films are effective in diagnosing dental caries and local trauma that may be a source of infection but are relatively ineffective for diagnosing infection or inflammation in soft tissue.
    - Dental experts rely on a panoramic x-ray, which also is good at delineating bony abnormalities but is not effective at diagnosing soft tissue infection.
    - CT and MRI machines are prohibitive for urgent cares; however, ultrasound is increasingly being used to effectively diagnose soft tissue infections of odontogenic origin.

23. **Fortunately, when you call for follow-up of the patient from question 18, the doctor on the night shift tells you a CT in the emergency department showed periorbital cellulitis but no orbital cellulitis. You ask, "What is the protocol at this hospital for treatment of such patients?"**
    - These patients are admitted for intravenous antibiotics (either a penicillin derivative or clindamycin, depending on previous therapy and medical history).
    - Dental or oromaxillofacial surgery is consulted as an inpatient.
    - The infected tooth (or teeth) is extracted as soon as possible.

24. **Are the characteristics of bacterial odontogenic infections changing significantly?**
    - A study compared patients hospitalized with odontogenic infections in the 1980s and the 1990s.
    - Patient characteristics did not change.
    - Bacteria isolated in the 1990s were more likely to show emerging resistance to commonly used antibiotics.
    - Responsible antibiotic stewardship and narrow spectrum use when possible are recommended to prevent further resistance.

25. **An adolescent male presents with fever, trismus, and a firm, tender neck swelling originating in the submandibular space. When you are finally able to coax him to open his mouth, you notice his tongue is elevated and resting on a firm, tender, sublingual mass. What is your concern?**
    - This description should immediately raise concern for Ludwig angina, a potential airway emergency.
    - Ludwig angina is an infection of the submandibular, submental, and sublingual spaces.
    - It was first fully described by Wilhelm Friedrich von Ludwig in 1836 and recognized as frequently fatal.
    - The term "angina" was added as it gave a feeling of suffocation.
    - Dental infection is usually the cause.
    - Preventive care and antibiotics have reduced mortality significantly.

26. **What should you do?**
    - First, ensure the patient's airway is intact and arrange for critical care transport if available; use ALS if critical care is not available.

- If the airway is not intact, you must intubate. This should be considered a difficult airway, and you should consider using video laryngoscopy and airway adjuncts and avoiding sedatives and muscle relaxants. Due to the massive neck edema and distortion of the anatomy in Ludwig angina, even airway experts are often unsuccessful. While tracheostomy was once considered standard, with the advancements in available airway technology, this is no longer the case.
- If the child is stable, establish intravenous access and start broad-spectrum antibiotics as the infection is polymicrobial.
- The adolescent male in question 25 is successfully transferred to a tertiary care hospital, where he is intubated by an otolaryngologist in the operating suite. The infection was surgically drained, he received intravenous antibiotics for several weeks, and he had extensive dental extractions done.

27. **A 10-year-old girl presents to the urgent care with a fever to 104°F. She recently had dental work done and has been complaining of continued tooth pain for the last 5 days. Her mother treated her fever with acetaminophen and ibuprofen, but over the last 6 hours, she noted her daughter had developed vomiting, rigors, and pallor and was increasingly difficult to arouse. On your exam, her heart rate is 140 beats per minute, her blood pressure is 75 systolic over 30 diastolic, and she is ill appearing and very sleepy. The only time she seems to wake up and respond is when you palpate the left side of her neck, when she cries, and when you percuss her left lower molars. What are you thinking?**
    - Most likely you are wishing you had drawn a different schedule for the month!
    - Since that did not happen, your mind reaches into its far recesses, and you recall reading a case study about Lemierre syndrome. However, as you recall, Lemierre syndrome is usually the consequence of pharyngitis and not dental infection.
    - After stabilizing the patient by treating her sepsis with aggressive fluid resuscitation, broad spectrum antibiotics, respiratory support, and transfer to a pediatric center with a critical care unit, you take a moment to read about Lemierre syndrome.
    - Dental infections account for only about 2% of cases, but it is a virulent complication.
    - An oropharyngeal infection causes septic thrombophlebitis of the internal jugular vein and, ultimately, hematogenous spread of the infection via septic emboli, resulting in multisystem abscesses and organ failure.
    - Common presenting symptoms are fever, chills, rigors, and sore throat that progress to trouble swallowing and trismus, due to deep neck space infection. Ultimately, symptoms of distal infection develop, such as chest pain, tachypnea, and tachycardia. Finally, if unrecognized, the patient will develop severe sepsis and die. Mortality has diminished significantly since the advent of penicillin. Death is often due to mediastinitis.
    - Patients may also develop intracranial infections from the septic emboli.
    - In the urgent care, while awaiting transfer of this patient, ultrasound may detect jugular thrombosis. However, ultrasound lacks the diagnostic certainty of contrast CT or MRI and should not be used as the sole diagnostic modality. Further, the attempt to image the internal jugular in the urgent care should not delay aggressive resuscitation or transfer of the patient.
    - Treatment ultimately consists of sepsis management, antibiotics, controlling the airway, and surgical debridement.

28. **What are other common complications of pediatric dental infections?**
    - The jaw bone structure makes children more prone to osteomyelitis and subsequent facial deformity.
    - The permanent teeth can be damaged.
    - Tetracyclines commonly used in dental infections can cause tooth discoloration and hypoplasia to developing teeth of both small children and fetuses.
    - Abscesses are more likely to create a fistula to the skin that necessitates repeated surgery and results in permanent deformity.

29. **A 13-year-old girl presented to the urgent care complaining of tooth pain. She has multiple caries but no evidence of abscess, facial cellulitis, or systemic symptoms. The family does not feel that ibuprofen is providing adequate pain control, and you are uncomfortable prescribing narcotics for this family who**

presents frequently with various complaints of pain. You decide to offer a dental nerve block instead. What are the various approaches?

- Infraorbital nerve block
  - Anesthetizes the anterior and middle superior alveolar nerves by the infraorbital foramen denervating the anterior maxillary teeth.
  - The patient should be semi- or fully reclined.
  - Palpate the supraorbital and infraorbital notches. About 0.5 cm below the infraorbital notch there is a depression. Retracting the upper lip, insert the needle with the syringe of local anesthetic anterior to the first premolar and direct the tip toward the depression without entering the foramen to avoid nerve damage.
  - Potential complications include excessive advancement into the orbit, improper angle of insertion, prevention of adequate anesthesia, and nerve damage as a result of direct damage from needle puncture.
- Inferior alveolar nerve block
  - Anesthetizes all the mandibular teeth, the skin of the chin and the lower lip, and usually the tongue on the side of the block.
  - The block is placed in the mandibular sulcus.
  - To inject, picture the inside of the mandible as a rectangle. Draw a horizontal line through the rectangle marked by the occlusal plane of the teeth and a vertical line marked by the midpoint of the rectangle. Where these intersect is the point of injection.
  - Grasp the ramus of the mandible with the thumb inside the mouth and the finger behind the ramus of the mandible, approach the nerve from the opposite side of the mouth over the primary molars, and inject.
  - Potential complications include nerve damage and excessive pain.

KEY POINTS

1. If immediate reimplantation of an avulsed permanent tooth is not possible, it should be stored in a suitable culture media such as cold milk.
2. Most lacerations of the buccal mucosa, gingiva, and tongue heal well without intervention.
3. Penicillin, clindamycin, and tetracylines provide appropriate antimicrobial activity against the most common oropharyngeal bacteria.
4. If a dental infection is localized and there are no systemic symptoms of disease, the patient can be treated with oral antibiotics, antimicrobial mouthwash, and pain control. If there are systemic symptoms of disease, the patient should be stabilized and transferred to a medical center with the ability to admit the patient and manage potential airway and cardiovascular compromise.
5. Dental pain can be managed with oral pain medications or with a dental block that targets nerve groups that include the affected tooth.

BIBLIOGRAPHY

Andersson L, Andreasen JO, Day P, et al. International Association of Dental Traumatology guidelines for the management of traumatic dental injuries: 2. avulsion of permanent teeth. *Dent Traumatol.* 2012;28(2):88–96.

Bassiony M, Yang J, Abdel-Monem TM, Elmogy S, Elnagdy M. Exploration of ultrasonography in assessment of fascial space spread of odontogenic infections. *Oral Surg Oral Med Oral Pathol Oral Radiol Endod.* 2009;107:861–869.

Diangelis AJ, Andreasen JO, Ebeleseder KA, et al. International Association of Dental Luxations Traumatology guidelines for the management of traumatic dental injuries: 1. fractures and of permanent teeth. *Dent Traumatol.* 2012;28(1):2–12.

Heimdahl A, Nord CE. Treatment of orofacial infections of odontogenic origin. *Scand J Infect Dis Suppl.* 1985;46:101–105.

Kassutto Z, Helpin ML. Orofacial anesthesia techniques. In: Henretig FM, King C, eds. *Textbook of Pediatric Emergency Procedures.* Baltimore: Williams & Wilkins; 1997:713–723.

Malmgren B, Andreasen JO, Flores MT, et al. International Association of Dental Traumatology guidelines for the management of traumatic dental injuries: 3. injuries in the primary dentition. *Dent Traumatol.* 2012;28(3):174–182.

Noy D, Rachmiel A, Levy-Faber D, Emodi O. Lemierre's syndrome from odontogenic infection: review of the literature and case description. *Ann Maxillofac Surg.* 2015;5:219–225.

Thikkurissy S, Rawlins JT, Kumar A, Evans E, Casamassimo PS. Rapid treatment reduces hospitalizations for pediatric patients with odontogenic-based cellulitis. *Am J Emerg Med.* 2010;28:668–672.

Topazian RG, Goldberg RH, eds. *Odontogenic Infections and Deep Fascial Space Infections of Dental Origin.* 2nd ed. Philadelphia: WB Saunders Co; 1987.

Yatani H, Komiyama O, Matsuka Y, Wajima K, Muraoka W, Ikawa M, Heir GM. Systematic review and recommendations for nonodontogenic toothache. *J Oral Rehabil.* 2014;41:843–852.

CHAPTER 50

ANALGESIA AND SEDATION

R. Blake Windsor, MD

CASE 1

A 6-year-old boy with a history of sickle cell disease presents to urgent care for pain in his right lower leg. He describes the pain as severe (Numeric Rating Scale [NRS] 9/10), "sharp and throbbing," and similar to his typical vaso-occlusive episodes. He has not had fevers, dyspnea, cough, limp, or joint swelling. He is intermittently crying and guarding his right leg.

1. What is pain?

Pain is a complex sensory and emotional experience. It is unpleasant by definition and inherently subjective. *Nociception* is the perception of painful, actual or threatened, tissue damage. In response to painful stimuli, people exhibit *pain behaviors* that are influenced by age, developmental status, comorbid conditions, and other biopsychosocial factors.

2. What are various age-appropriate ways to measure pain?

Many validated scales exist to measure nociception or pain behaviors.

- FLACC: A commonly used pain scale for infants, children, and people with cognitive impairment who have trouble communicating. FLACC is an abbreviation and mnemonic for **F**aces, **L**egs, **A**ctivity, **C**ry, and **C**onsolability. Each section is scored 0–2 for a possible total of 10 points.
- Wong-Baker FACES scale: An instrument validated for children as young as 3 years, as well as children and adults with cognitive delay. Six faces (scores of 0–5) of progressive discomfort are displayed, and patients pick the face that corresponds to their pain. To extrapolate the scale, the score is doubled to create a 10-point scale.
- Numeric Rating Scale (NRS): The most commonly used self-report scale; patients pick a number on a scale from 0 ("no pain") to 10 ("the worst pain imaginable"). This is validated in children as young as 5 years who have a concept of numbers (i.e., "5 is larger than 1").

3. What is the difference between acute and chronic pain?

Pain can be divided into acute pain and chronic pain. Acute pain is defined by self-limited pain of <3–6 months' duration. Chronic pain is defined as pain lasting longer than 3–6 months, or longer than expected for the mechanism of injury. The approaches to acute and chronic pain differ, and an in-depth approach to treating chronic pain is beyond the scope of this chapter.

4. How can classifying pain help guide treatment?

Pain descriptors and patterns can help discern the underlying injury. There are many taxonomies of pain; however, they are broadly classified as *nociceptive, neuropathic, psychogenic,* and *mixed.* Nociceptive pain is pain associated with tissue injury (e.g., surgery or fracture), inflammation (e.g., rheumatoid arthritis or ankle sprain), or tumor. Neuropathic pain is broadly classified to involve both direct nerve injury (i.e., amputation or trauma), central nervous system (CNS) injury (i.e., spinal cord injury or post-stroke pain), or altered nerve activity (i.e., functional pain). Psychogenic pain is pain existing without discovered anatomic tissue injury and in a distribution inconsistent with other functional causes. Most types of acute pain are nociceptive, and most causes of chronic pain have mixed etiologies.

5. What is the general approach to acute pain?

Acute pain is best treated with medications that target the underlying cause of pain. Effective treatments include nonsteroidal antiinflammatory drugs (NSAIDs), acetaminophen, local anesthetics, general anesthetics, muscle relaxants, and opioids. The World Health Organization (WHO) pain ladder (Fig. 50.1) is an effective framework for treating acute and cancer-related pain. For pain with a predictable trajectory, scheduled dosing of nonopioid medications is preferred. These strategies can help prevent opioid use, or reduce total opioid dose if they are required. This concept is called *opioid-sparing strategies.*

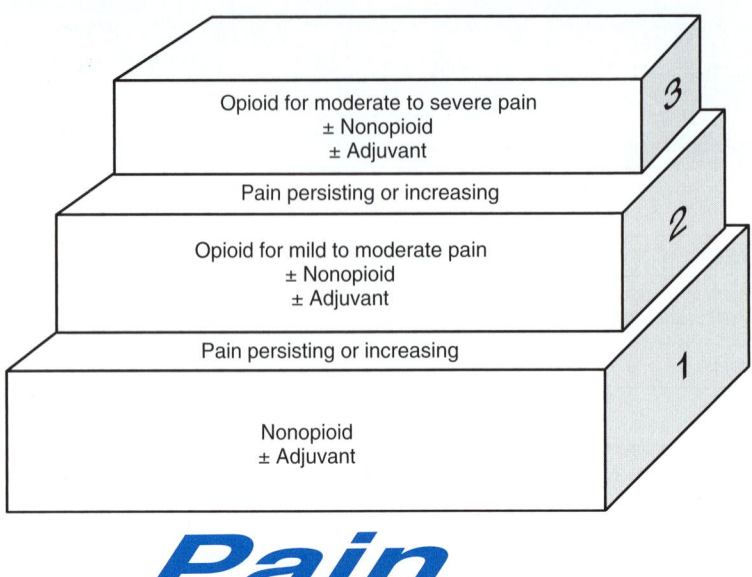

Fig. 50.1. **World Health Organization (WHO) Pain Relief Ladder for Adults.** A useful strategy is to continue weak analgesics when stepping up to stronger medications. Weak analgesics can be scheduled to reduce the need and total dose of opioids.

Table 50.1. Select COX-2/COX-1 Ratios (Higher Value Indicates Higher Proportion of COX-2 Inhibition)	
Celecoxib	30
Meloxicam	18
Ibuprofen	1.5
Naproxen	0.7
Indomethacin	0.02

6. How do NSAIDs work?

NSAIDs inhibit the enzyme cyclooxygenase (COX), which produces prostaglandins that contribute to inflammation. This causes pain by sensitizing nerve terminals to injury. Thus, NSAIDs are useful for decreasing inflammation and are generally considered weak analgesics. COX-1 and COX-2 are differentially produced. Most tissues constitutively produce COX-1, and COX-2 is induced by inflammation.

7. What are the differences between NSAIDs?

NSAIDs are more similar than they are different. Nonselective NSAIDs have similar predictable side effect profiles based on their COX-2/COX-1 inhibition. Also, NSAIDs differ in their duration of action. COX-2 inhibitors ("Coxibs") were designed to minimize the long-term side effect profile of this medication class, but unfortunately were associated with a possible increase in the risk of myocardial infarction and thrombotic strokes with prolonged use. The only COX-2 inhibitor currently approved for use in the United States is celecoxib.

8. What are the principal adverse effects of long-term NSAID therapy?

The frequency of side effects is often associated with COX-2/COX-1 inhibition (Table 50.1):
- Gastrointestinal (GI) effects: Gastritis, peptic ulcer disease (Table 50.2), diarrhea, GI hemorrhage

Table 50.2. Cumulative Prevalence of GI Ulcers after 12 Weeks of NSAID Therapy without GI Protection

Celecoxib (200 mg bid)	8.5%
Naproxen (500 mg bid)	40.7%
Ibuprofen (800 mg tid)	28.5%

bid, Twice a day; *GI*, gastrointestinal; *NSAID*, nonsteroidal antiinflammatory drug; *tid*, three times a day.

Table 50.3. Suggested Dosing and Useful Notes for Common NSAIDs

DRUG	DOSE (MG/KG)	DURATION	ROUTES	NOTES
Ibuprofen	400–800 mg (4–10 mg/kg)	4–8 h	IV, PO	PO form inexpensive and available OTC. For use >6 months old
Naproxen	250–500 mg (5 mg/kg)	8–12 h	PO	Inexpensive often started with a loading dose in adults
Diclofenac	50 mg (1 mg/kg)	8 h	PO, TOP	Inexpensive; often used with a loading dose in adults. Topical gel available.
Ketorolac	15–30 mg IV, 60 mg IM once (0.5 mg/kg IV or 0.1 mg IM once)	8 h	IV, IM, PO	Potent analgesic; use for <5 days. PO generally used only for IV continuation. Consider 50% dose reduction in critical illness. For use >8 months and 8 kg.
Indomethacin	25–50 mg (0.5–1 mg/kg)	6–12 h	PO	Max dose of 200 mg/day for adults, 4 mg/kg for children. Use in children limited; alternative use is preferred.
Meloxicam	5–10 mg (0.125 mg/kg)	24 h	PO	Capsules and tablets are not interchangeable, even if dose is equal.
Celecoxib	100–200 mg 10–25 kg–50 mg 25–50 kg – 100 mg	12–24 h	PO	Best GI profile and use with platelet disorders. May increase risk of thrombosis and myocardial infarction.

IM, Intramuscularly; *IN*, intranasally; *IV*, intravenously; *NSAIDs*, nonsteroidal antiinflammatory drugs; *OTC*, over the counter; *PO*, orally; *TOP*, topical.

- Renal effects: Decreased renal blood flow, decreased glomular filtraon rate (GFR), salt and water retention, acute papillary necrosis, chronic interstitial nephritis
- Hematologic effects: Inhibition of platelet aggregation, increased bleeding time
- Pulmonary effects: Bronchospasm
- Hepatic effects: Elevated aspartate aminotransferase/alanine aminotransferase (AST/ALT), drug-induced hepatitis
- Idiopathic reactions: Vasomotor rhinitis, angioedema, hypotension, drug-induced rash

9. **Which is the best NSAID to use?**
   - No NSAID is clearly better than another, although subtle differences may make one more preferable for a specific reason. Table 50.3 lists typical doses and useful notes about select NSAIDs. Factors that influence choice include route of administration, desired dosing interval, COX selectivity, and special considerations.
   - Intravenous (IV) ketorolac is very potent, and therapeutic doses are often described as producing analgesia equivalent to typical doses (10 mg or 0.1 mg/kg) of IV morphine. This is accompanied with a higher than typical adverse effect profile, and use should not exceed 5 days.

10. **How is acetaminophen different from typical NSAIDs?**
    Acetaminophen has an unclear mechanism of action and different elimination and side effect profile. However, it also contains both analgesic and antipyretic activity. It can be safely used in combination with all NSAIDs.

11. **What side effects are associated with acetaminophen?**
    Acetaminophen is not associated with the GI or renal effects of NSAIDs. The most concerning side effect is hepatotoxicity. Acetaminophen-induced hepatotoxicity can be life threatening. It is influenced by dose, duration of use, and comorbid conditions such as hepatic disease or malnutrition.

12. **What are the safe dose ranges for acetaminophen?**
    Acetaminophen is safe and effective at doses of 650–1,000 mg every 4–6 hours in adults, and 10–15 mg/kg for infants and children. Rectally administered acetaminophen should be dosed as 15 mg/kg due to reductions in bioavailability. The maximum recommended daily dose is 4 g/day for adults and 75 mg/kg/day for infants and children.

13. **What are toxic doses of acetaminophen?**
    Toxicity depends on multiple factors, including dose, duration of use, and comorbid conditions. Single dose toxicity is unlikely at doses below 7.5–10 g for adults or 150 mg/kg for infants and children. Chronic administration can produce toxicity at any dose at or above the maximum recommended daily dose.

14. **What diseases influence acetaminophen toxicity?**
    Comorbid conditions that decrease hepatic glucuronidation (i.e., liver disease, malnutrition, or alcoholism) and states of induced cytochrome P-450 (i.e., alcoholism, medications) lead to increased production of NAPQI. NAPQI is a toxic metabolite that can lead to oxidative hepatic injury. In these states, the daily acetaminophen dose should be reduced or avoided entirely.

15. **When are opioids indicated?**
    Opioids, a useful and versatile class of medications, are broadly indicated for surgical conditions, trauma, procedural sedation, cancer-related pain, and severe pain. Unfortunately, opioid prescriptions have increased due to multiple factors and have resulted in an epidemic of substance abuse disorders and deaths.

16. **What general guidelines should be followed when prescribing opioids?**
    Opioids are best prescribed when there is a clear endpoint to their use. Opioids are not first-line therapy for chronically painful conditions except in palliative care or atypical conditions. Multimodal therapies should be used whenever possible to limit opioid dose to the minimal effective dose.

17. **What are opioid-sparing strategies?**
    Strategies include maximizing multimodal therapy, such as scheduling use of acetaminophen, NSAIDs, topical therapies, and disease-specific therapies (i.e., muscle relaxant for muscle spasms or anticonvulsants for neuropathic pain). Opioids should not be prescribed for longer than 3–7 days by a clinician with a single point of contact, such as an emergency or urgent care environment. Variations from this practice should be supported in documentation. If needed for longer-term therapy, opioids are best prescribed by clinicians with continuity of care and advanced training in evidence-based practice and opioid monitoring.

18. **What does PRN mean?**
    PRN is a Latin abbreviation that stands for *pro re nata* (loosely translated "as the circumstances arise"). In practice, it often means "Pain Relief Nil." Telling patients to take a weak analgesic "as needed" often results in a medication not being taken. A useful strategy is to tell patients to take a weak analgesic on a schedule for a few days and to use an opioid "as needed." This strategy can reduce opioid use.

19. **How do opioids work?**
    Major opioids bind to opioid receptors, primarily mu-, kappa-, and delta-receptors. These are located both centrally (spine and brain) as well as peripherally and are responsible for the analgesic, euphoric, and adverse effects of opioid medications.

20. **What are the differences between opioids?**
    Major opioids are agonists of their receptors. Newer opioids have been developed that are partial agonists, mixed agonists/antagonists, and antagonists. Combination agonist and antagonist products are also available in an attempt to limit substance abuse. Mu agonists should be used if analgesia is the primary goal (i.e., procedural sedation or surgical process). Partial agonists/antagonists typically

Table 50.4. Suggested Dosing and Useful Notes for Common Opioids

| SELECT MEDICATIONS | Usual Starting Doses and Intervals for Analgesia in Opioid-Naïve Patients | | NOTES |
	CHILD <50 KG	CHILD >50 KG AND ADULTS	
Morphine IV: PO: IR	0.05–0.1 mg/kg IV every 4–6 h 0.3 mg/kg every 4–6 h	2.5–5 mg every 4–6 h 10–30 mg every 4–6 h	Traditional initial choice for opioid. Contraindicated in renal failure due to accumulation of toxic metabolite.
Hydromorphone IV: PO: IR	0.01–0.02 mg/kg every 4–6 h 0.04–0.08 mg/kg every 3–4 h	0.2–1 mg every 4–6 h 2–4 mg every 4–6 h	More rapid onset of CNS effects (analgesia, sedation) compared to morphine. Evidence for better adverse effect profile is mixed. Safer for use in renal failure.
Fentanyl IV: IN:	0.5–2 mcg/kg every 30–60 min 2 mcg/kg as initial load	25–50 mcg every 30–60 min 100 mcg as initial load	Considered hemodynamically neutral. Rapid onset of 2–3 minutes. Can be dosed intranasally for rapid analgesic load prior to IV access. For children, dose volume should not exceed 1 mL per nostril. Transbuccal, sublingual, and transdermal forms also available.
Oxycodone PO:	0.1–0.2 mg/kg every 4–6 h	5–15 mg every 4–6 h	Good choice for opioid rotation. Possibly enhanced effect on visceral pain due to increased kappa agonism.

CNS, Central nervous system; *IN*, intranasally; *IR*, immediate release; *IV*, intravenously; *PO*, orally.

provide less analgesia and should be used for patients with moderate pain that does not respond to conservative therapy, for patients with relative contraindications to opioid use (including substance abuse history), or in an attempt to limit typical opioid adverse effects. Most partial agonists/antagonists have limited use in children and generally should be avoided.

21. **What are some of the expected effects of opioids?**
 • CNS: Analgesia, mood changes (positive or negative), sedation
 • Eyes: Miosis
 • Respiratory: Respiratory depression, hypercapnea
 • Cardiac: Hypotension, bradycardia (high doses)
 • GI: Nausea, vomiting, delayed gastric emptying, constipation
 • Skin: Pruritus
 • Urinary: Urinary retention

22. **Is any major opioid better?**
 No particular opioid is inherently superior or stronger than another. Medications vary in potency, but when dosed appropriately (Table 50.4), they typically provide equal analgesia. Patients with frequent opioid exposures often express preferences, most often due to adverse effect profiles. This is thought to be due to complex interactions between an individual's opioid receptor subtypes and the opioid's selectivity for those subtypes. Additionally, certain opioids have clear advantages in select situations.

23. **What is opioid tolerance?**
 Chronic administration of opioids can lead to tolerance. Tolerance is defined as the need for an increased dose of medication to achieve the same effect. Tolerance develops to all effects of opioids except constipation. Patients may or may not have miosis if taking their usual dose of opioids.

24. How is tolerance different than dependence?

Tolerance is a prerequisite for dependence. Tolerance demonstrates neurologic changes that reduce the inhibitory effects of the opioid dose. Dependence is the state where abrupt discontinuation leads to rebound neurologic excitation and development of a withdrawal syndrome. Opioid dependence does not indicate addiction or substance abuse.

25. How are opioids dosed when someone is opioid tolerant?

Knowing the patient's history of opioid exposure is helpful. If that information is unavailable, one option is to start at the upper range of usual dosing and reassess every 5–10 minutes (for IV morphine and hydromorphone) until captured. When patients demonstrate tolerance to the analgesic effects of opioids, they are typically also tolerant to the respiratory depression.

26. Why do opioids cause respiratory depression?

Opioids act directly on the brainstem to affect respiration. The respiratory rhythm is the most sensitive and leads to an initial hypopnea with increased tidal volume. With higher doses, the tidal volume also decreases and leads to apnea. Opioids also shift the sensitivity of the medullary chemoreceptors to CO_2 and lead to hypercapnea. Natural sleep and co-administration of medications, such as benzodiazepines and other sedatives, can potentiate respiratory depression. Pain and stimulation can reduce respiratory depression.

27. How is iatrogenic opioid-induced respiratory depression treated?

Treatment is context dependent. With oversedation and hypopnea in an otherwise stable patient, stimulating the patient is the first treatment. Low-dose naloxone can be titrated to increase respiratory rate without affecting analgesia. An ampule of 0.4 mg of naloxone is diluted with 10 mL of saline, and 0.04–0.08 mg (1–2 mL) is given every 1–2 minutes to desired effect. To achieve the same effect in children, 0.01 mg/kg of naloxone can be given every 2 minutes until desired effect. Naloxone typically lasts 20–40 minutes, and respiratory depression may return as the naloxone is eliminated. Close monitoring is required.

28. How is opioid-induced constipation treated?

Opioids act on intestinal smooth muscle to decrease peristalsis. Because of this, stool softeners are not appropriate monotherapy to prevent constipation. Pro-motility agents, such as senna, bisacodyl, and lactulose, are the mainstay of treatment because they improve peristalsis. Softeners, such as polyethylene glycol, docusate, or magnesium hydroxide, can be added.

29. What is methylnaltrexone?

Methylnaltrexone is a peripherally acting opioid antagonist that is approved to reverse opioid-induced constipation without affecting analgesia. It rapidly reverses ileus from opioids, which may be painful if peristalsis occurs against desiccated stool.

30. How do opioids cause nausea and how is it treated?

Opioids can cause delayed gastric emptying and directly stimulate both the vestibular system and the chemoreceptor trigger zone of the area postrema.

31. How do opioids cause itching and how is it best treated?

Opioid-induced pruritus is caused by histamine. It is best treated by a peripheral opioid antagonist, such as nalbuphine, or low-dose naloxone. Antihistamines, such as diphenhydramine, can potentiate the sedating effects of opioids.

32. What is an opioid rotation?

An opioid rotation is an empiric trial of a different opioid in an attempt to obtain better analgesia with fewer adverse effects.

33. How is someone transitioned to a different opioid?

Typically, a total daily dose of the opioid is calculated and then converted to morphine equivalents (either IV or orally [PO]). This morphine equivalent dose is then converted to the daily dose of the chosen opioid. The daily dose of the chosen opioid is then divided and administered on a frequency consistent with its duration of action. New opioids should be reduced by 20%–50% to account for incomplete cross-tolerance, although there is no need to go below the typical starting dose for an opioid. Multiple free calculators are available on the internet to reduce calculation errors.

CASE 2

An 8-year-old girl presents to urgent care for wrist pain and deformity after a fall during soccer practice. X-ray reveals a greenstick fracture with 30-degree angulation. Orthopedics is consulted and recommends closed reduction and immobilization.

34. What is the general approach to procedural sedation?

Most importantly, sedation should be performed only by a clinician experienced in airway management. A safe sedation requires a clinician dedicated to monitoring the patient's safety, pain, and anxiety and capable of intervening as necessary. Reversal medications, oxygen, and airway equipment should be immediately available.

35. What equipment is needed for procedural sedation?

A helpful mnemonic for setting up a room for sedation is "SOAP-ME."

S – Suction

O – Oxygen source (including face mask, nonrebreather)

A – Airway equipment (including bag-mask and endotracheal tube)

P – Pharmacy (sedation medications, reversal agents, code medications)

M – Monitors (cardiac monitor, oximetry, capnography)

E – Equipment for procedure (fluoroscopy, peripherally inserted central catheter [PICC], etc.)

36. What are the special considerations for pediatric sedations?

Pediatric sedations require appropriately sized equipment. This is especially true of airway equipment, particularly mask size, and multiple endotracheal tube or laryngeal mask airway sizes. Children receive weight-based dosing of medications. Comorbid conditions, such as craniofacial abnormalities, genetic syndromes, and viral infections, are relatively common in children who require sedation and need special consideration.

37. What are the red flags for procedural sedation?

- Craniofacial abnormality or high-risk airway on examination
- History of difficult sedation or airway
- Active vomiting or severe, uncontrolled gastroesophageal reflux disease (GERD)
- Active viral upper respiratory infection
- Obstructive sleep apnea
- Symptomatic asthma
- Young age or history of extreme prematurity

38. What are the typical medication doses for procedural sedation?

Typical doses and useful notes are listed in Table 50.5.

CASE 3

A 25-year-old man presents to urgent care after a crush injury to the nail of his right index finger. He is in significant pain, with a nail matrix laceration, and has developed a subungual hematoma. There is no neurovascular compromise and x-rays reveal no fracture.

39. How do local anesthetics provide analgesia?

Local anesthetics bind to sodium channels most tightly in the open and inactivated states. When deposited into tissue near a nerve, the local anesthetic diffuses across the hydrophobic cell membrane and inactivates the sodium channel. The pKa of the medication determines its ionization, which ultimately determines its onset and duration of action. Other factors that affect local anesthetic kinetics include tissue acidity, vascularity, and proximity to nerve.

40. What is the maximum total dose of select common local anesthetics?

Table 50.6 provides basic dosing information for some commonly used local anesthetics. Local anesthetic toxicity is extremely rare in the urgent care setting as most nerve blocks require only a few milliliters of anesthetic. However, when injecting infants or with multiple planned injections, attention to the total dose is crucial.

Table 50.5. Suggested Dosing and Useful Notes for Common Procedural Sedation Medications

MEDICATION	DOSE	ONSET/DURATION	NOTES
Midazolam	IN: 0.5 mg/kg (max 10 mg) PO: 0.5 mg/kg (max 20 mg) IV: Max 2 mg/dose 6 mo–5 y – 0.05–0.1 mg/kg/dose 6–12 y – 0.025–0.05 mg/kg/dose >12 y – initial 2 mg/dose, titrate with 1 mg prn	IN: 1–3 min/60 min PO: 15–30 min/60–90 min IV: 1–3 min/45–60 min	Peak IN/IV effect after 20 minutes May cause paradoxical effect in children Given over 10–20 seconds
Fentanyl	IN: 2 mcg/kg (max 100 mcg/dose) IV: Max 100 mcg/dose 1–2 mcg/kg/dose q3min prn	IN: 3–5 min/30 min IV: 2–3 min/30 min	Give over 10–20 s
Ketamine	IV: Initial dose of 1–2 mg/kg/dose (max 100 mg/dose), repeat with 0.5 mg/kg (max 50 mg/dose) q5–10 min prn IM: 4–5 mg/kg/dose, repeat 2–4 mg/kg after 10–20 min	IV: 0.5–1 min/5–15 min IM: 3–5 min/15–30 min Recovery: 60–150 min	Dissociative anesthetic with all or no response May cause laryngospasm, hallucinations, vocalization, recovery agitation Contraindicated in obstructive hydrocephalus, active respiratory infection, poorly controlled asthma
Propofol	IV Induction: 0–4 y – 2 mg/kg 5–10 y – 1.5 mg/kg >10 y – 1 mg/kg* Maintenance: 50–200 mcg/kg/min to effect	IV: <1 min/5–15 min	Associated with hypotension, bradycardia, apnea, and infusion pain For infusion pain: apply tourniquet proximal to IV, give lidocaine 1% IV 1 mg/kg (max 25 mg), remove after 60 s and flush with propofol bolus

*May require additional 0.5 mg/kg bolus every 60–90 s for induction
IN, Intranasally, *IV*, intravenously, *PO*, oral.

Table 50.6. Basic Dosing and Useful Notes for Commonly Used Local Anesthetics

MEDICATIONS	ONSET	DURATION	TOXIC DOSE
Lidocaine 1% (10 mg/mL)	1–2 min	1–1.5 h	4.5 mg/kg
Lidocaine 1% with 1:100,000 epinephrine	1–2 min	2–6 h	7 mg/kg
0.25% bupivacaine (2.5 mg/mL)	5 min	2–8 h	2 mg/kg
0.2% ropivacaine (2 mg/mL)	5 min	2–8 h	3 mg/kg

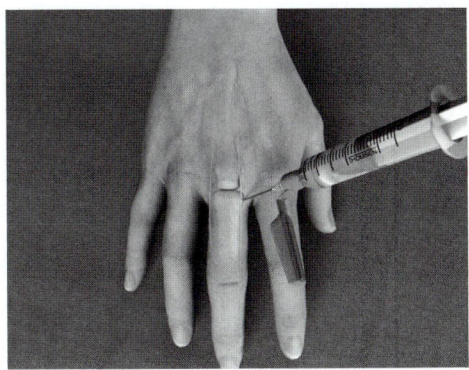

Fig. 50.2. Traditional Digital Nerve Block. Prepare the skin using antiseptic technique. Using a 25-, 27-, or 30-g needle, the needle is advanced to bone and withdrawn a few millimeters as shown. One or 2 mL of local anesthetic is injected to the dorsal and volar surfaces of the finger. A similar process is performed on the opposite side of the finger to numb both palmar nerves. Traditionally, epinephrine should not be used when injecting digits. *(From: Thomsen TW, Setnik GS: Digital Nerve Block, figure 7. Procedure Consult [serial online]. 2008. Available at:* http://www.proceduresconsult.com/medical-procedures/digital-nerve-block-EM-053-procedure.aspx. *Last accessed: 7/26/2016.)*

41. What does local anesthetic toxicity look like?

Local anesthetics are nonselective sodium channel blockers and can also affect myocytes and CNS neurons. Local anesthetic toxicity can be life threatening. CNS effects generally occur first, including tinnitus, drowsiness, altered taste, seizures, altered mental status, and coma. Cardiac effects include increased tachycardia, T-wave changes, P-R interval and QRS duration, reentrant tachyarrhythmias, ventricular arrhythmias, and torsades de pointes.

42. How is local anesthetic toxicity treated?

Local anesthetic toxicity can be very challenging to treat. Strategies include maintenance of Airway, Breathing, and Circulations using Advanced Cardiovascular Life Support and Pediatric Advanced Life Support protocols, as well as benzodiazepines for seizures. Intralipid 20% is used as an "antidote." It is thought to act as a hydrophobic "sink" and sequester the local anesthetic. It is administered at 1.5 mL/kg over 1 minute, followed by an infusion of 0.25 mL/kg/min. Boluses can be repeated every 3–5 minutes.

43. What equipment is needed for local anesthetic infiltration?

Syringe, large bore drawing needle, injection needle (25, 27, or 30 gauge), local anesthetic of choice, antiseptic.

44. What are the special considerations for local anesthetics?

Buffered lidocaine at a mixture of 1 mL of 8.4% bicarbonate to 10 mL of lidocaine can reduce injection pain. Additionally, warming lidocaine to body temperature reduces the burning sensation. Accidental intravascular administration of local anesthetic should be avoided by a careful aspiration prior to injection. It is a medical maxim never to inject lidocaine with epinephrine into the ears, fingers, penis, or toes, although this has recently been called into significant question by multiple studies.

45. What are the common nerve blocks performed in urgent care?

Common nerve blocks in the urgent care are the digital nerve block (Fig. 50.2), infraorbital nerve block (Fig. 50.3), and mental nerve blocks (Fig. 50.4). These blocks are useful because they are painful locations with clear nerve territories. An effective nerve block can eliminate the need for procedural analgesia, although procedural anxiolysis may still be needed for younger or needle-phobic patients. The infraorbital and mental nerve blocks are particularly useful for repair of the vermillion border because injection of local anesthetic into the damaged lip can make repair of the vermillion border extremely challenging.

KEY POINTS

1. Distinguishing acute from chronic pain and categorizing pain mechanisms can help drive treatment choices.
2. Multimodal treatments should always be used to treat pain without opioids or to reduce the opioid to the minimum required dose.

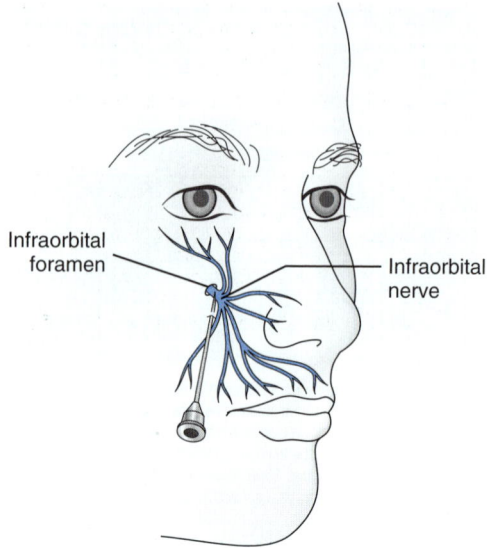

Fig. 50.3. Extraoral Infraorbital Nerve Block. Prepare the skin using antiseptic technique. Using a 25-, 27-, or 30-g needle, insert the needle as shown. After a negative aspiration, 1–2 mL of local anesthetic is injected. This block produces analgesia to the face in the region shown. It is especially useful for upper lip lacerations because local infiltration can affect the repair of the vermillion border. *(From: Waldman, S: Infraorbital nerve block, Figure 17-3. In: Waldman S (ed): Atlas of Interventional Pain Management, ed 4. Philadelphia, 2015, Elsevier Saunders, pp 61–64.)*

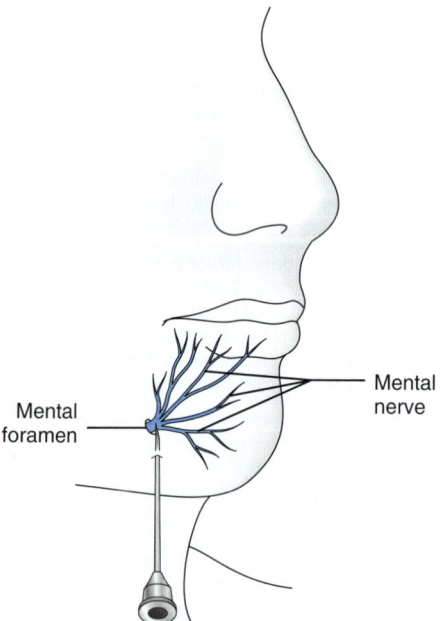

Fig. 50.4. Extraoral Mental Nerve Bock. Prepare the skin using antiseptic technique. Using a 25-, 27-, or 30-g needle, insert the needle as shown. After a negative aspiration, 1–2 mL of local anesthetic is injected. This block produces analgesia to the face in the region shown. It is especially useful for lower lip lacerations because local infiltration can affect the repair of the vermillion border. *(From: Figure information: Waldman, S: Mental nerve block, Figure 19-3. In: Waldman S (ed): Atlas of Interventional Pain Management, ed 4. Philadelphia, 2015, Elsevier Saunders, pp 68–71.)*

3. The WHO analgesic ladder is an effective treatment approach for acute and cancer-related pain.
4. Scheduling weak analgesics for a few days around an injury can improve pain control and reduce the need for opioids.
5. Procedural sedation should be performed by a clinician experienced in managing airways, and with appropriate emergency equipment and medications immediately available.

BIBLIOGRAPHY

Berde CB, Sethna NF. Analgesics for the treatment of pain in children. *N Engl J Med*. 2002;14:347.

Birmingham B, Buvanendran A. Nonsteroidal anti-inflammatory drugs, acetaminophen, and COX-2 inhibitors. In: Benzon H, Raj PP, Rathmell JP, et al., ed. *Practical Management of Pain*. 5th ed. Philadelphia: Mosby; 2014:553–568, 697–715.

Cortazzo MH, Copenhaver D, Fishman SM. Major opioids and chronic opioid therapy. In: Benzon H, Raj PP, Rathmell JP, et al., ed. *Practical Management of Pain*. 5th ed. Philadelphia: Mosby; 2014:697–715.

Feldon L, Walter C, Harder S, et al. Comparative clinical effects of hydromorphone and morphine: a meta-analysis. *Br J Anaest*. 2011;3:107.

World Health Organization: WHO's Pain Relief Ladder. Available at: http://www.who.int/cancer/palliative/painladder/en/. Accessed July 26, 2016.

CHAPTER 51

ADULT EMERGENCIES PRESENTING TO URGENT CARE CENTERS

Jeffrey Rixe, MD, Alexander Y. Sheng, MD

GENERAL APPROACH

1. **What are the main priorities of an urgent care center in a true emergency?**
   In a true emergency, where delays can lead to increased risk of morbidity and mortality, the priorities of an urgent care facility are rapid recognition and disposition.
   Recognition: Quickly identifying patterns is a necessity in urgent care medicine. Seeing a patient clutching the chest in pain, in respiratory distress, or unable to move half of his or her body should prompt immediate action.
   Disposition: True emergencies require an emergency department. Call 911 or the closest possible ambulance to rapidly transport the patient to the nearest hospital.

2. **How can an urgent care provider rapidly identify "sick" patients among many stable patients?**
   Recognition of "sick" versus "well" is a skill honed through experience and practice. Nevertheless, Table 51.1 shows some simple features to look out for.

3. **What is an approach to stabilization and disposition of "sick" patients at an urgent care center presenting with common adult emergencies?**
   Stick to C-A-B (circulation, airway, breathing), according to Basic Life Support guidelines. Establish peripheral intravenous access and give fluids if patient is hypotensive. Hold pressure on any sites of ongoing bleeding. Give oxygen if the patient is in respiratory distress. Perform advanced cardiovascular life support and/or advanced airway techniques only if you and your staff are trained and experienced in doing so. If you cannot quickly stabilize the patient for transport to the nearest hospital, call 911 for additional assistance.

CHEST PAIN WITH DISTRESS

4. **What are the main priorities when a patient presents to urgent care with chest pain?**
   Any patient who appears acutely ill and complains of chest pain needs to be taken seriously. Focus on the basics first: Does the patient have a pulse? Is the patient talking and maintaining an airway? Is the patient breathing spontaneously? (In other words, perform C-A-B.) Next, obtain a set of vital signs. Finally, the most important step, quickly obtain a 12-lead electrocardiogram (ECG). If the patient has no contraindication (i.e., severe allergy), give 325 mg of aspirin. Call for immediate transportation to an emergency department.

5. **What are the potentially life-threatening causes of chest pain?**
   Pulmonary embolism (PE), myocardial infarction (MI), pneumothorax, hemothorax, aortic dissection, esophageal rupture, and cardiac tamponade can cause life-threatening chest pain.

6. **What are the criteria for ST-segment elevation myocardial infarction on ECG?**
   An ST-segment elevation myocardial infarction (STEMI) (Fig. 51.1) is identified by ST-segment elevation in two or more contiguous leads. Threshold values vary based on age and gender, but in general, if the elevation is >1 mm in two leads on the ECG, there is a high index of suspicion for STEMI.

Table 51.1. Differentiating Sick vs. Not Sick

	SICK	NOT SICK
Vital Signs	• Tachycardia/bradycardia • High or low respiratory rate • Hypoxia • Hypotension, severe hypertension	• Within normal range
General Appearance	• Pale • Diaphoretic • Vomiting • Not communicating • Not walking	• No acute distress

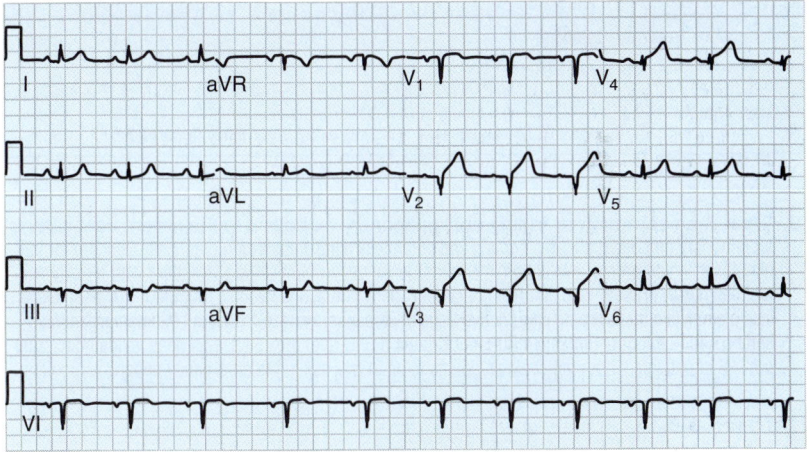

Fig. 51.1. Anterior ST-segment Elevation Myocardial Infarction.

7. What actions should be taken for a patient with chest pain and a STEMI on ECG?

Arrange transportation to the nearest hospital with a cardiac catheterization laboratory (cath lab), where percutaneous coronary intervention (PCI) can be performed. Call ahead to the hospital to alert them of the incoming patient. Give a full 325-mg aspirin. Give nitroglycerin sublingual, and morphine to alleviate pain. Place the patient on a cardiac monitor for rapid transport.

8. What are the historical features that are more concerning for acute coronary syndrome (ACS)?

According to a large systematic review, the following features have the highest specificity for ACS in patients presenting with chest pain:

Symptoms:

Radiation to both arms: Sensitivity 11%, Specificity 96%
Diaphoresis: Sensitivity 24%–28%, Specificity 79%–82%
Exertion: Sensitivity 38%–53%
Vomiting: Specificity 77%–80%

Risk factors:

Prior abnormal stress test: Specificity 96%
Peripheral arterial disease (PAD): Specificity 97%

Box 51.1. Pulmonary Embolism Rule-out Criteria

Rules out PE if no criteria are present and pretest probability is <15%

Age ≥50
HR ≥100
O_2 sat on room air <95%
Prior history of venous thromboembolism
Trauma or surgery within 4 weeks
Hemoptysis
Exogenous estrogen
Unilateral leg swelling

Table 51.2. FAST Signs and Symptoms Concerning for Stroke or TIA

F	Face drooping
A	Arm weakness
S	Speech difficulty
T	Time to call 911/Arrange rapid transport to the emergency department

9. **What is an approach to "ruling out" pulmonary embolism in the urgent care setting?**
   A pulmonary embolism (PE) is a serious and potentially a life-threatening diagnosis. Concern for this diagnosis should prompt evaluation in an emergency department setting. A patient with a pulmonary embolism may present with pleuritic chest pain, tachycardia, and hypoxia, but often the diagnosis is less clear. While there are no prospective trials of screening tools to "rule out" PE in an urgent care setting, the Pulmonary Embolism Rule-out Criteria (PERC rule) (Box 51.1) has been validated to "rule out" PE in patients whom the clinician deems to be at low risk in the emergency department setting.

TIA/STROKE

10. **What is a stroke or cerebrovascular accident (CVA)?**
    A stroke or CVA is defined as brain cell death due to blockage or rupture of a blood vessel that supplies that area of brain. There are two types of strokes. Ischemic stroke is caused by a clot obstructing the flow of blood to the brain. Hemorrhagic stroke is due to rupture of a blood vessel preventing blood flow to the brain.

11. **What is a transient ischemic attack (TIA)?**
    Traditionally, TIA was defined as focal neurologic symptoms or signs lasting less than 24 hours. However, in recent years, magnetic resonance imaging (MRI) has found infarction in a significant portion of patients diagnosed with TIA.
    The new definition of TIA is a transient episode of neurologic dysfunction caused by focal brain, spinal cord, or retinal ischemia, without acute infarction. TIA is important as a diagnosis because affected patients have up to nearly 15% risk of stroke within 90 days.

12. **What are the most important pieces of history to ask regarding a patient with suspected stroke?**
    In addition to gathering the history of recent events and symptoms the patient is experiencing, the exact time that the patient was last noted to be feeling at baseline (last known normal) is a crucial piece of information that affects treatment. This is because within 3 hours, and up to 4.5 hours of last known normal, treatment with thrombolytics may have improved outcomes for patients diagnosed with ischemic stroke.

13. **What are the signs and symptoms concerning for a stroke or TIA?**
    See Table 51.2. Other symptoms and signs of stroke or TIA include vision changes, vertigo, nausea, vomiting, ataxia, and altered mental status.

Table 51.3. Seizure Types and Mimics

Convulsive status epilepticus	Clonic (repetitive, rhythmic movements) and tonic (stiffening) phases, lasting >5 minutes with associated loss of consciousness
Tonic-clonic seizures	Initial body and extremity stiffening followed by rhythmic contractions of muscle groups
Absence seizures	Staring episodes or an arrest in behavior
Myoclonic Clonic	Brief sudden muscular contractions Repetitive jerks
Simple partial seizure Complex partial seizure	Commonly motor or sensory symptoms isolated to one body part (facial twitching, unilateral arm clonus) Simple partial seizure + change in consciousness
Seizure mimics Syncope Psychogenic nonepileptiform events (pseudoseizures) Breath-holding spells	Sudden, brief loss of consciousness. Can be associated with brief episode of stiffening or jerking motions. Eyes closed, patient talking through the event, movements nonrhythmic, appear purposeful Children shaking/twitching after breath holding or crying

Table 51.4. Common Causes of Seizures

- Hypoglycemia
- Hyponatremia
- Eclampsia
- Alcohol withdrawal
- Benzodiazepine withdrawal
- Intracranial hemorrhage
- Brain tumor
- Meningitis or encephalopathy

14. What are common stroke "mimics"?

Hypoglycemia, seizure, syncope, intracranial mass, complex migraine, psychiatric disorder, metabolic disorder, peripheral vertigo, sepsis, encephalopathy, transient global amnesia, drugs, alcohol, and dementia.

15. What are the priorities in the management of a patient with suspected stroke or TIA in urgent care?

Rule out hypoglycemia by checking fingerstick glucose. After initial stabilization, if patient's last known normal was within 4.5 hours, arrange emergent transport to the nearest emergency department capable of administering thrombolytics or stroke center, whichever is closer. If patient's last known normal was more than 4.5 hours ago, once stabilized, arrange for the patient to be urgently transported to the nearest stroke center.

SEIZURES

16. What are the commonly encountered seizure types, and what do these look like to an observer?

Not all seizures look the same, and urgent care providers should be able to identify the common seizure patterns and mimics described in Table 51.3.

17. What are the common causes of seizures?

While many of these seizure types can look similar, it is important to recognize that not all seizures are caused by epilepsy. Other common causes of seizures are listed in Table 51.4.

18. How can you help a patient who is actively seizing in urgent care?

Taking care of a seizing patient can provoke anxiety among health care providers. First make sure the patient has a patent airway (not choking on blood, tongue, secretions), is breathing spontaneously with equal breath sounds, and has an appropriate peripheral pulse. Then use any of the formulations of benzodiazepines shown in Table 51.5, in the dose appropriate for the patient.

Table 51.5. Benzodiazepine Formulations and Routes of Administration

Lorazepam (Ativan)	IV, IM, rectal, intranasal
Diazepam (Valium)	IV, rectal
Midazolam (Versed)	Buccal

Table 51.6. Delirium vs. Dementia

DELIRIUM	DEMENTIA
Acute onset (hours-days)	Chronic
Fluctuating course	Slowly worsening (months-years)
Inattention, distractibility	Normal level of consciousness
Disorganized thinking, illogical ideas	
Alteration in consciousness	

Table 51.7. Differential Diagnosis for Altered Mental Status

A	Alcohol, Acidosis
E	Endocrine, Electrolytes
I	Infection
O	Opiates, Overdose
U	Uremia
T	Trauma
I	Insulin
P	Poisoning/Psychosis
S	Seizure, Stroke, Syncope

ALTERED MENTAL STATUS

19. **What is an approach to assessing mental status in a patient "altered from baseline"?**
    The most important part of an altered mental status workup is a focused history and physical exam. Find a family member, friend, or health care worker who knows the patient well and has seen him or her recently. Get an idea of the patient's prior functional baseline. Then ask: What behaviors specifically have changed, and when did the changes occur? The physical exam should be thorough with focus on mental status and an appropriate neurologic exam. Mental status encompasses alertness (person/place/time), cognition (attention/memory), and behavior (psychosis/suicidal/agitation). Importantly, a front line provider needs to decide if this process is acute, chronic, medical, or psychiatric.

20. **What are the differences between delirium and dementia?**
    Both delirium and dementia are common in the elderly population. The features in Table 51.6 can help distinguish the two diseases.

21. **What is a common differential diagnosis for a patient presenting with altered mental status?**
    Changes in mental status can arise from multiple organ systems outside the central nervous system and can be caused by medications or toxins. A useful mnemonic to recall all of these possible causes is AEIOU TIPS (Table 51.7).

Table 51.8. Differentiating Syncope vs. Seizure

SYNCOPE	SEIZURE
No aura	Aura
Post loss of consciousness jerks	Pre loss of consciousness jerks
Asynchronous jerks	Synchronous jerks
Tongue bite at the tip	Tongue bit lateral
Flaccid	Stiff
Quick recovery	Postictal
No anion gap acidosis	Transient anion gap acidosis

22. **What is the appropriate disposition for a patient with altered mental status?**
Patients with altered mental status should be evaluated in an emergency department. A large portion of them should be admitted to an inpatient setting. Many causes of AMS, including delirium, have high mortality rates, and other causes may require advanced diagnostic imaging or a long period of observation.

SYNCOPE

23. **What is syncope?**
Syncope is defined as sudden, brief loss of consciousness due to transient global cerebral hypoperfusion with spontaneous complete recovery.

24. **How does one differentiate between syncope and seizure?**
A syncopal episode can sometimes be confused with seizure. Fortunately, some features of the episode can help differentiate the two (Table 51.8).

25. **What is a "standard" workup for syncope?**
There is no "standard" workup for a patient presenting with syncope. Most guidelines recommend a thorough history, physical examination, and ECG. If an etiology for syncope is found, the patient should be managed according to the causal condition.

26. **How does one best risk stratify a patient who presents with syncope?**
Multiple risk stratification tools have been developed and tested. However, none have been proven to perform better than clinical judgment. Nevertheless, there are some features that are considered high or low risk (Table 51.9).

27. **What is the disposition for a patient presenting with syncope?**
The disposition for the patient should take into account the clinical gestalt, perceived risk, cost, potential adverse events, and clinical utility of hospitalization, as well as patient preference. Patients who are considered low risk, with one or more low-risk features without any high-risk characteristics, can be discharged with outpatient follow-up, assuming no concerning etiology of symptoms is found. Anyone who is at intermediate risk (without any high- or low-risk features, or only low-risk features with significant comorbidities) or high risk (at least one high-risk feature) should be transferred to the nearest emergency department.

RESPIRATORY DISTRESS

28. **What are the top priorities in the approach to a patient presenting in respiratory distress?**
Perform head tilt/chin lift and/or jaw thrust to ensure an open airway. Remove any obvious material obstructing the airway but avoid blind finger sweep. Apply oxygen via nonrebreather, and place the patient in recovery position according to Basic Life Support principles.

29. **What physical exam findings, if present, can help identify the etiology of respiratory distress?**
Table 51.10 lists the physical exam findings.

Table 51.9. Low- and High-Risk Features of Syncope

LOW-RISK FEATURES	HIGH-RISK FEATURES
Age <40 years	
Characteristics of syncope: • Only while standing • Standing from supine/sitting • Nausea/vomiting before syncope • Feeling warm before syncope • Triggered by stress/pain • Triggered by cough/defecation/micturition	• During exertion • In supine position • New onset chest discomfort • Palpitations before syncope • Associated with shortness of breath
Past history: • Prolonged history of recurrent syncope similar to current episode	• Family history of sudden death • Congestive heart failure • Aortic stenosis • Left ventricular outflow tract disease • Dilated cardiomyopathy • Hypertrophic cardiomyopathy • Arrhythmogenic right ventricular cardiomyopathy • Ejection fraction <35% • Ventricular arrhythmias • Coronary artery disease • Congenital heart disease • Previous myocardial infarction • Pulmonary hypertension • Previous ICD implantation
	Vitals and labs: • Anemia (Hb <9 g/dL) • Systolic blood pressure <90 mm Hg • Sinus bradycardia (<40 bpm)
	ECG features: • New (or previously unknown) left bundle branch block • Bifascicular block ± first-degree AV block • Brugada pattern • Ischemic changes • New nonsinus rhythm • Prolonged QTc (>450 ms)

Table 51.10. Physical Exam Findings Pertinent to Respiratory Distress

Bilateral wheezing, prolonged expiratory phase	Asthma or COPD exacerbation
Decreased/absent breath sounds on one side	Pneumothorax, pleural effusion
Crackles/rales	Pulmonary edema, acute decompensated heart failure, pneumonia

30. What potentially life-threatening diagnoses must be considered for a patient in respiratory distress presenting to an urgent care center and their associated interventions?

    Cannot miss diagnoses are listed in Table 51.11.

Table 51.11. Cannot Miss Diagnoses and Treatments in Respiratory Distress

DIAGNOSIS	TREATMENT
Asthma exacerbation	Albuterol, ipratropium, prednisone po if patient can tolerate; if not, methylprednisolone IV
COPD exacerbation	Albuterol, ipratropium, prednisone po if patient can tolerate; if not, methylprednisolone IV
Tension pneumothorax	14-gauge angiocath perpendicular to the chest wall at the second intercostal space in the anterior midclavicular line until whoosh of air is expressed
Pulmonary edema, acute decompensated heart failure	Nitroglycerin, furosemide if blood pressure can tolerate
Pneumonia	Antibiotics
Pulmonary embolism	Anticoagulation

Table 51.12. Diagnostic Criteria for Anaphylaxis

Anaphylaxis is likely when one of the following criteria is fulfilled	
Acute onset symptoms with involvement of the skin, mucosal tissue, or both AND AT LEAST ONE OF THE SIGNS TO THE RIGHT:	• Respiratory compromise (e.g., dyspnea, bronchospasm, stridor, hypoxemia) • Hypotension or symptoms of end-organ dysfunction (e.g., hypotonia, syncope)
Two or more of the signs to the right with rapid onset after exposure to a likely allergen for that patient:	• Cutaneous or mucosal involvement (e.g., urticaria, angioedema, pruritus) • Respiratory compromise (e.g., dyspnea, bronchospasm, stridor, hypoxemia) • Hypotension or symptoms of end-organ dysfunction (e.g., hypotonia, syncope) • Persistent gastrointestinal symptoms (e.g., abdominal pain, vomiting)
Hypotension after exposure to known allergen for that patient:	• Infant and children: hypotension for age or >30% decrease in SBP • Adults: SBP <90 mm Hg or >30% decrease from patient baseline

ANAPHYLAXIS

31. What is anaphylaxis?
Anaphylaxis is a serious allergic reaction that is rapid in onset and potentially life threatening. It is a multisystem disorder that involves symptoms from cutaneous, respiratory, cardiovascular, gastrointestinal, and central nervous systems.

32. What are the most common causes of anaphylaxis?
Food (e.g., nuts, fish, shellfish, dairy, eggs), medications (e.g., penicillins), and insect stings and bites (e.g., bees, vespids, stinging ants) are the most common causes.

33. What are the diagnostic criteria for anaphylaxis?
Diagnostic criteria are listed in Table 51.12.

34. What are the main treatment priorities for a patient in anaphylaxis?
Epinephrine 0.01 mg/kg of 1:1000 solution (up to 0.5 mg for adults, 0.3 mg for children) into intramuscular space of midanterolateral thigh repeated every 5–15 minutes as needed. Large bore intravenous line with crystalloid fluids (5–10 mL/kg) should be given even if patient is not yet hypotensive. Oxygen should be given for patient in respiratory distress.

Box 51.2. SIRS Criteria

Systemic Inflammatory Response Syndrome (SIRS): Two or more of
Temperature >38°C or <36°C
Heart rate >90/min
Respiratory rate >20/min or $PaCO_2$ <32 mm Hg
White blood cell count >12,000/mm^3 or <4,000/mm^3 or >10% immature bands

Table 51.13. Updated Definitions for Sepsis and Septic Shock

SEPSIS	SEPTIC SHOCK
Suspected or documented infection with an acute increase of ≥2 SOFA Score points (http://www.mdcalc.com/sequential-organ-failure-assessment-sofa-score/)	Sepsis and vasopressor therapy needed to elevate mean arterial pressure (MAP) ≥65 mm Hg and lactate >2 mmol/L despite adequate fluid resuscitation

Box 51.3. qSOFA Criteria

Respiratory rate ≥22/min
Altered mental status
Systolic blood pressure ≤100 mm Hg

35. **What are the second-line medications that can be considered for a patient in anaphylaxis?**

Second-line medications such as albuterol should be given for a patient in bronchospasm. Diphenhydramine 25–50 mg IV with the addition of ranitidine can be given for cutaneous symptoms. Corticosteroids have not been shown to improve outcomes in anaphylaxis. Nevertheless, methylprednisolone (1–2 mg/kg) can be given as needed.

36. **How does the disposition differ between patients with anaphylaxis compared to those with a less severe allergic reaction?**

Patients with anaphylaxis should be transferred as soon as possible to the nearest emergency department with critical care capability. Patients with mild allergic reactions without meeting criteria for anaphylaxis, with stable or improving symptoms, can be discharged with close follow-up with their primary care doctor for referral to an allergist. They should always be discharged with strict return precautions and a self-injectable dose of epinephrine. They should be taught how to use the device and demonstrate how to do so before discharge.

SEPSIS

37. **What is the definition of sepsis?**

Sepsis is a syndrome shaped by host and pathogenic factors that is amplified by dysregulated host response to infection leading to life-threatening organ dysfunction.

38. **What are the clinical criteria for the diagnosis of sepsis?**

Traditionally, sepsis was defined as two or more systemic inflammatory response syndrome (SIRS) criteria (Box 51.2) with suspected or documented infection.

However, considering significant advances in the understanding of underlying pathophysiology of sepsis, the Society of Critical Care Medicine and the European Society of Intensive Care Medicine recently refined the clinical criteria for the diagnosis of sepsis as shown in Table 51.13.

Appreciating the fact that many data points may not be available in the initial evaluation of the patient, especially in the urgent care setting, the quick Sequential Organ-Failure Assessment (qSOFA) can be used to identify adult patients with suspected infection who are likely to have poor outcomes (Box 51.3).

39. Why is it important to recognize sepsis?

With an increasing incidence, sepsis is the primary cause of death from infection and one of the leading causes of mortality and critical illness worldwide. It accounted for more than nearly $24 billion in annual U.S. hospital costs in 2013. Those who survive sepsis often have long-term physical, psychological, and cognitive morbidities leading to persistent health and social implications.

40. What are the main management priorities in the urgent care setting when caring for a patient with suspected sepsis?

The urgent care provider can help improve patient outcomes by quickly establishing intravenous access, obtaining cultures in order to initiate early broad spectrum antibiotics, and performing crystalloid fluid resuscitation. Transportation to the nearest hospital with available intensive care capability is crucial.

KEY POINTS

1. In any patient presenting with chest pain, quickly ruling out STEMI on a 12-lead ECG must be a priority.
2. A patient with a suspected stroke or TIA with last known normal within 4.5 hours should be transported to the closest emergency department or stroke center as soon as possible for consideration of thrombolytic therapy.
3. Checking a fingerstick glucose early can rule out hypoglycemia as a treatable cause of any patient presenting with stroke-like symptoms, seizure, and altered mental status.
4. While the differential diagnosis for syncope or altered mental status is broad, there is no "standard workup" for either chief complaint. A thorough focused history and physical exam are crucial to making the diagnosis.
5. Benzodiazepines are the first-line treatment for an actively seizing patient.
6. Rapid recognition, initiation of intravenous fluids and antibiotics after obtaining cultures, and transportation to the nearest hospital with available intensive care capability are the main priorities in caring for patients with sepsis.
7. The mainstay of treatment for anaphylaxis is epinephrine 0.01 mg/kg of 1:1000 solution (up to 0.5 mg for adults, 0.3 mg for children) into intramuscular space of midanterolateral thigh repeated every 5–15 minutes as needed.

BIBLIOGRAPHY

American College of Emergency Physicians; American Academy of Neurology. Clinical policy: use of intravenous tPA for the management of acute ischemic stroke in the emergency department. *Ann Emerg Med*. 2013;61(2):225–243.

American Heart Association. *Advanced Cardiovascular Life Support (ACLS) Provider Manual 2015 Guidelines*; 2016.

American Heart Association. *Basic Life Support (BLS) Provider Manual*; 2016.

American Stroke Association. Stroke Warning Signs and Symptoms. <http://www.strokeassociation.org/STROKEORG/WarningSigns/Stroke-Warning-Signs-and-Symptoms_UCM_308528_SubHomePage.jsp>; 2016.

American Stroke Association. Types of Stroke. <http://www.strokeassociation.org/STROKEORG/AboutStroke/TypesofStroke/Types-of-Stroke_UCM_308531_SubHomePage.jsp>; 2016.

Costantino G, Sun BC, Barbic F, et al. Syncope clinical management in the emergency department: a consensus from the first international workshop on syncope risk stratification in the emergency department. *Eur Heart J*. 2015;(i):ehv378.

Easton JD, Saver JL, Albers GW, et al. Definition and evaluation of transient ischemic attack. *Stroke*. 2009;40(6):2276.

Fanaroff AC, Rymer JA, Goldstein SA, Simel DL, Newby LK. Does this patient with chest pain have acute coronary syndrome? The rational clinical examination systematic review. *JAMA*. 2015;314(18):1955–1965.

Han JH, Wilber ST. Altered mental status in older patients in the emergency department. *Clin Geriatr Med*. 2013;29(1):101–136.

Huff JS, Fountain NB. Pathophysiology and definitions of seizures and status epilepticus. *Emerg Med Clin North Am*. 2011;29(1):1–13.

Kline JA, Mitchell AM, Kabrhel C, Richman PB, Courtney DM. Clinical criteria to prevent unnecessary diagnostic testing in emergency department patients with suspected pulmonary embolism. *J Thromb Haemost*. 2004;2(8):1247–1255.

Koita J, Riggio S, Jagoda A. The mental status examination in emergency practice. *Emerg Med Clin North Am*. 2010; 28(3):439–451.

Opal SM, Rubenfeld GD, van der Poll T, Vincent J, Angus DC. *The Third International Consensus Definitions for Sepsis and Septic Shock (Sepsis-3)*. 2016;315(8):801–810.

Ouyang H, Quinn J. Diagnosis and evaluation of syncope in the emergency department. *Emerg Med Clin North Am*. 2010;28(3):471–485.

Shah AM, Vashi A, Jagoda A. Review article: convulsive and non-convulsive status epilepticus: an emergency medicine perspective. *Emerg Med Australas*. 2009;21(5):352–366.

Zilberstein J, McCurdy MT, Winters ME. Anaphylaxis. *J Emerg Med*. 2014;47(2):182–187.

CHAPTER 52

PEDIATRIC EMERGENCIES PRESENTING TO URGENT CARE CENTERS

Jennifer Dunnick, MD, MPH, Bruce Herman, MD, Jerri A. Rose, MD

ALTERED MENTAL STATUS

1. **Given that the differential diagnosis for altered mental status is quite broad, how can the major categories of potential etiologies be quickly recalled?**
Remember the "tips on vowels." The mnemonic AEIOU TIPS (Box 52.1) is a useful tool for recalling the major categories of causes that should be considered in children presenting with altered mental status.

2. **What are the most common causes of altered mental status in children?**
The potential causes of altered mental status in children are numerous, including both structural brain disorders and systemic diseases. Trauma, infections, intoxications, and metabolic abnormalities are among the most common etiologies in children.

3. **What are the signs of altered mental status in infants and young children?**
Crying, inconsolability, irritability, lethargy, and/or poor feeding are common manifestations for patients in this age group.

4. **What tools can be used to quantify a child's mental status?**
The Glasgow Coma Scale (GCS) and Alert, Voice, Pain, Unresponsive (AVPU) scale (Table 52.1 and Box 52.2) are widely used and accepted tools that can be used to quantify and communicate a child's neurologic status. These scales allow for the standardized evaluation, documentation, and communication of a child's changing neurologic status over time.

5. **What elements of the medical history are particularly critical to obtain for children presenting with altered mental status?**
Focused, goal-directed questions pertaining to suspected etiologies are key to pinpointing the underlying cause of altered mental status. Caregivers should be asked specifically about the child's current medications; medications and potentially toxic substances accessible in his/her environment; as well as any history of seizures, fever, headache, irritability, vomiting, changes in gait, and/or recent changes in behavior. Inquiring about a history of recent head trauma is extremely important. The absence of a history of trauma does not rule it out as an etiology, however, since many cases may be unwitnessed and/or unreported (including in cases of nonaccidental injury).

6. **What is the initial approach for managing a child with altered mental status?**
The initial management of any child presenting with altered mental status should begin with rapid assessment and support of the airway, breathing, and circulation. Oxygen (100% by nonrebreather face mask) should initially be administered to all patients until adequate oxygenation is assured. Because many of the causes of altered mental status in children require treatments with intravenous (IV) fluids or medications, intravenous access should be established in the vast majority of patients. A focused history and careful physical examination must be completed and should guide the selection of laboratory and imaging studies. Prompt transfer to the closest emergency department is of paramount importance.

7. **What laboratory study should be obtained in all children with altered mental status?**
A rapid bedside test for serum glucose should be performed in all children presenting with altered mental status. Additional laboratory studies—including arterial blood gas, serum electrolytes, and toxicology screens—may be useful, depending upon the patient's history and physical examination findings.

8. What is the neuroimaging study of choice in a child with altered mental status?

Noncontrasted computed tomography (CT) of the brain is generally the initial neuroimaging study of choice for evaluating children with unexplained altered mental status. CT brain images can be obtained rapidly and reveal most structural abnormalities that may cause altered mental status, such as intracranial hemorrhage and mass lesions. Although magnetic resonance imaging (MRI) may provide higher-quality, more detailed pictures of the brain than CT, MRI scans are generally more difficult to obtain emergently, take longer to obtain, and often require sedation for young children.

Box 52.1. Potential Etiologies of Altered Mental Status—the "AEIOU TIPS"

A: Alcohol, Abuse of substances
E: Epilepsy, Encephalopathy, Electrolyte disturbances, Endocrine disorders
I: Infection, Intussusception, Ischemia
O: Overdose, Oxygen deficiency
U: Uremia (and other metabolic causes)
T: Trauma (both known and abusive), Temperature abnormality, Tumor
I: Infection, Increased intracranial pressure, Insulin-related problems
P: Poisoning, Psychiatric conditions, blood Pressure (e.g., hypertension or hypotension)
S: Shock, Stroke, Space-occupying CNS lesion, Shunt problems

Table 52.1. Glasgow Coma Scale (GCS) for Infants and Children

	SCORE	INFANT	CHILD
Eye opening	4	Spontaneous	Spontaneous
	3	To speech	To speech
	2	To pain	To pain
	1	None	None
Best verbal response	5	Coos and babbles	Oriented, appropriate
	4	Irritable, cries	Confused
	3	Cries in response to pain	Inappropriate words
	2	Moans in response to pain	Incomprehensible sounds
	1	None	None
Best motor response	6	Moves spontaneously and purposefully	Obeys commands
	5	Withdraws to touch	Localizes painful stimulus
	4	Withdraws to pain	Withdraws to pain
	3	Abnormal flexion to pain	Flexion in response to pain
	2	Abnormal extension to pain	Extension in response to pain
	1	None	None

Box 52.2. AVPU Scale

A: Alert
V: Responsive to Verbal stimuli
P: Responsive to Painful stimuli
U: Unresponsive

9. **What clinical clues should raise suspicion for toxic ingestion as the cause of altered mental status in a child?**

Ingestion of a toxic substance should be strongly considered in children presenting with altered mental status of sudden onset without a preceding history of trauma or illness. A lack of close adult supervision, a chaotic home environment, as well as a history of previous ingestions by the child should raise a clinician's suspicion for intoxication as the underlying etiology of altered mental status.

ANAPHYLAXIS

10. **What is the most common cause of anaphylaxis in children?**

Food allergens represent the most common triggers of anaphylactic reactions among children, teens, and young adults. Other triggers may include medications, insect stings, blood products, immunotherapy, and radiocontrast media. In a significant proportion of cases, the cause is unidentified.

11. **What are the signs and symptoms of anaphylaxis?**

Anaphylaxis is a clinical syndrome that is highly likely when a patient meets any one of three diagnostic criteria listed in Box 52.3.

12. **What features of anaphylaxis are potentially life threatening?**

Anaphylaxis has the potential to result in significant morbidity and even death. Upper airway obstruction (due to edema of the tongue, larynx, and other upper airway structures), cardiovascular collapse, and respiratory compromise due to bronchospasm are potential life-threatening complications.

13. **What immediate interventions are required for patients with anaphylaxis?**

Anaphylaxis is a medical emergency requiring immediate assessment and simultaneous aggressive support of the airway, breathing, and circulation. Intramuscular epinephrine is the first-line treatment for anaphylaxis; it should be given as early as possible (in the anterolateral thigh) to all patients presenting with the characteristic signs and symptoms. Any known or suspected trigger(s) (such as an intravenous medication or blood product) should be discontinued immediately. Patients with circulatory compromise should be placed in the supine position (or position of comfort if vomiting or in respiratory distress).

14. **Can antihistamines and/or corticosteroids be used as an alternative to epinephrine in children with anaphylaxis?**

Neither H_1-receptor antihistamines (such as diphenhydramine) nor corticosteroids are first-line agents for treating anaphylaxis, due to a lack of evidence supporting their efficacy. While these medications are commonly used and may be beneficial for specific symptoms, they are *not* replacements for epinephrine and should serve only as adjuncts in treating anaphylaxis. Treatment with epinephrine should not be withheld or delayed due to the administration of these medications.

Box 52.3. Clinical Criteria for the Diagnosis of Anaphylaxis

Acute onset (within minutes to several hours) of signs/symptoms involving the skin, mucosal tissue, or both (e.g., generalized urticaria, itching or flushing of skin, swollen lips/tongue/uvula) AND at least one of the following:

- Respiratory compromise (e.g., dyspnea, wheeze/bronchospasm, stridor, hypoxia)
- Decreased blood pressure or associated symptoms of end-organ dysfunction (e.g., fainting, dizziness, incontinence)

At least two of the following occurring acutely after exposure to a likely allergen:

- Involvement of the skin and/or mucosal tissue
- Respiratory compromise
- Decreased blood pressure or associated symptoms of end-organ dysfunction
- Persistent gastrointestinal symptoms (e.g., crampy abdominal pain, nausea, vomiting, diarrhea)

Decreased blood pressure following exposure to a known allergen (low age-specific systolic blood pressure or a decrease in systolic blood pressure by 30% or more in infants/children)

15. **What laboratory studies are required to confirm the diagnosis of anaphylaxis?**
None! Anaphylaxis is a clinical diagnosis, based primarily on a thorough history (including recent exposures) and recognition of the characteristic signs and symptoms. While elevated serum tryptase and histamine levels may support the diagnosis in some patients, these tests are not universally available, not useful in all patients, not performed emergently, and not specific for anaphylaxis. Their role in the diagnosis of anaphylaxis is limited and should never delay treatment.

16. **What are the main benefits and contraindications to epinephrine use in patients with anaphylaxis?**
Epinephrine use has been shown to decrease both hospitalizations and death among patients presenting with anaphylaxis. There is no absolute contraindication to its use in anaphylaxis. Therefore, it should be administered as the first-line agent for all patients presenting with anaphylaxis.

17. **Can repeat epinephrine doses be given to children with anaphylaxis?**
Yes! Intramuscular epinephrine doses may be repeated every 5–15 minutes for persistent or recurrent symptoms. In children with circulatory compromise and/or for those in whom multiple intramuscular doses have been ineffective, administration of intravenous epinephrine may be indicated.

18. **How long should children be observed after being treated for anaphylaxis?**
There is no "standard" time period for observing children after treatment for anaphylaxis. Length of observation should be determined for each child based upon factors including severity of illness at presentation, underlying risk factors, and ability of the family to access care. Children with mild to moderate symptoms resolving after treatment may be able to be discharged safely after 4–6 hours of observation, while those with more severe reactions should be monitored for a longer duration (8–24 hours, or even longer in particularly severe and/or complicated cases).

RESPIRATORY DISTRESS
ASTHMA

19. **What is the best initial treatment for an acute asthma exacerbation?**
The mainstays of acute asthma exacerbation therapy are inhaled short-acting beta agonists, corticosteroids, and oxygen. Severity of the exacerbation, however, will ultimately dictate treatment. Patients presenting with a moderate to severe exacerbation require continuous or repetitive inhaled bronchodilators in the first hour. If using a metered-dose inhaler (MDI), give a dose every 20 minutes. Oxygen as needed to maintain SaO_2 >90% should be provided to all patients. Corticosteroids should be given within the first hour for children presenting with a severe exacerbation.

20. **In a patient with asthma, when should a chest x-ray be obtained?**
Chest x-rays should not be routinely ordered during the evaluation of an asthma exacerbation, as they do not change clinical management. Imaging should be ordered if you are concerned about pneumothorax, concomitant bacterial pneumonia, or foreign body aspiration.

21. **When should steroids be administered? IV or oral?**
In patients presenting with a mild to moderate exacerbation, give oral corticosteroids if the patient does not have an immediate response to inhaled beta-agonists or if there is a history of recent steroid use. All patients with a severe exacerbation should receive oral corticosteroids, preferably within the first hour of presentation. IV steroids should be reserved for those patients with respiratory arrest or failure. Oral steroids have been found to be equally effective to IV steroids in several studies.

22. **What are the indications for endotracheal intubation and mechanical ventilation during an asthma exacerbation?**
Patients presenting with an asthma exacerbation are very difficult to mechanically ventilate. As such, pharmacologic treatment should be maximized. Failure of maximal treatment, inability to oxygenate, worsening hypercarbia, or declining mental status is an indication for intubation.

BRONCHIOLITIS

23. **A 9-month-old boy presents with a fever, congestion, hypoxia, and diffusely coarse breath sounds. What is the most likely diagnosis?**
The infant most likely has bronchiolitis, the most common lower respiratory infection in children under the age of 2 years. Respiratory syncytial virus (RSV) is the most common pathogen and

is responsible for up to 80% of cases. Bronchiolitis is marked by fever, nasal congestion, and rhinorrhea, typically followed by a dry cough. As the inflammation progresses to the lungs, there is an increase in mucous production and often the development of tachypnea, rales, wheezing, and hypoxia.

24. How is bronchiolitis diagnosed?
Diagnosis should be clinical, based on history and physical exam. If the diagnosis of bronchiolitis is made, imaging and laboratory studies are not needed.

25. What is the primary treatment for bronchiolitis?
Treatment is largely supportive as bronchiolitis is typically a self-limited disease. Supportive care measures include suctioning, hydration, and supplemental oxygen if needed. The disease process peaks between 3 and 5 days of symptoms, and symptom resolution usually occurs within 2–3 weeks. Since bacterial coinfection is uncommon, antibiotics should not be routinely given.

26. Should bronchodilators be given to children with bronchiolitis?
Numerous studies have investigated the efficacy of bronchodilators for the treatment of bronchiolitis. Most randomized controlled trials have failed to show a benefit. While beta-agonists may improve symptoms and clinical scores, they do not change the progression of the disease or outcomes. There is no decrease in need for hospitalization or length of stay. Therefore, there is no indication for trialing or scheduling bronchodilators for patients with bronchiolitis.

27. Are corticosteroids useful in bronchiolitis?
Many large studies have shown that there is no benefit of giving steroids. Further, steroids may prolong viral shedding. As such, it is strongly recommended that steroids not be administered to patients with bronchiolitis.

CROUP

28. What is croup?
Croup is a viral upper airway infection, typically laryngotracheitis. It is often caused by a parainfluenza virus and is the most common cause of stridor in children greater than 6 months of age. The hallmark presentation is a barky cough, hoarseness, and stridor. These may also be accompanied by coryza and fever. Treatment should include a single dose of dexamethasone, preferably given orally or intramuscularly.

29. When should racemic epinephrine be given and what must occur after its administration?
Racemic epinephrine is reserved for moderate to severe croup, such as children with biphasic stridor, stridor at rest, retractions, decreased air entry, or hypoxia. Racemic epinephrine is given via nebulizer and is effective within 30 minutes of administration. However, racemic epinephrine does not alter the disease course, so patients must be monitored closely for a "rebound effect" after the medication wears off. The recommended monitoring time is 2–4 hours after treatment.

30. Why is hypoxia with croup an emergency?
Since croup is an upper airway obstructive disease, gas exchange at the level of the alveoli is preserved. Therefore, hypoxia is a sign of impending respiratory failure due to severe upper airway obstruction.

31. What is the differential diagnosis for a child who is presenting with fever and stridor?
See Table 52.2.

SEIZURES

32. What is the definition of status epilepticus?
Status epilepticus is defined as a continuous seizure or recurrent seizure activity lasting greater than 5 minutes without regaining consciousness in that time. It is a medical emergency and should be anticipated in any patient presenting with an acute seizure.

33. What are the first-line medications for treating status epilepticus?
See Table 52.3.

Table 52.2. Differential Diagnosis and Clinical Criteria for a Child with Fever and Stridor

CRITERIA	CROUP	EPIGLOTTITIS	RETROPHARYNGEAL ABSCESS	BACTERIAL TRACHEITIS
Anatomy	Subglottic	Supraglottic	Retropharyngeal lymph nodes	Trachea
Etiology	Viral (parainfluenza)	Bacterial (HIB, staph, strep)	Bacterial (oral flora)	Bacterial (staph)
Age	6 mo–5 yr	Any	6 mo–4 yr	Any
Onset	1–3 days	Hours	1–3 days	3–5 days
Toxicity	Mild–moderate	Marked	Moderate	Marked
Drooling	No	Yes	Yes	No
Hoarseness	Yes	No	No	No
Cough	Barky	No	No	Painful, productive
X-ray	"Steeple" sign (anteroposterior)	"Thumb" sign (lateral)	Widened prevertebral soft tissues	"Shaggy" trachea

Adapted from: Kost, S: Stridor. In *Pediatric Emergency Medicine Secrets*, ed 6, Philadelphia, 2015, Elsevier, pp 179-183.

Table 52.3. Usual First-Line Antiepileptic Medications for the Treatment of Status Epilepticus

DRUG	ROUTE	DOSE	MAXIMUM DOSE
Lorazepam	IV, IN	0.05–0.1 mg/kg	4 mg
Midazolam	IV, IM, IN	0.2 mg/kg	10 mg
	Buccal	0.5 mg/kg	
Diazepam	IV	0.2–0.4 mg/kg	10 mg
	PR	0.5–1 mg/kg	

Data from: Chiang VW: Seizures. In *Textbook of Pediatric Emergency Medicine*, ed 6, Philadelphia, 2010, Lippincott Williams & Wilkins, pp 564-570; Mikati MA, Hani AJ: Seizures in Childhood. In *Nelson Textbook of Pediatrics*, ed 20, Philadelphia, 2016, Elsevier, pp 2823-2857.

34. What is a febrile seizure?

A febrile seizure is seizure activity in the setting of a temperature of 38ºC or greater and in the absence of other causes of seizure. They are very common, occurring in 3%–4% of children between the ages of 6 months and 5 years. There is a 30% risk of recurrence for febrile seizures but only a small increase in the risk of developing epilepsy.

35. How can you differentiate between a simple and complex febrile seizure?

In order to meet criteria for a simple febrile seizure, the seizure must be less than 15 minutes in duration and the child can have no more than one seizure in a 24-hour period. Simple febrile seizures are characterized by generalized tonic-clonic activity. Focal seizure activity is a complex febrile seizure.

36. A 3-year-old boy is brought to urgent care after having a 4-minute generalized seizure. He has never had a seizure before. His mom tells you that he felt warm before he started shaking. Now he is back to his baseline mental status. His neurologic exam is normal, but you note that he is febrile. What tests should be performed?

This boy has had a simple febrile seizure. Diagnostic testing should be aimed at determining the cause of the fever. Brain imaging or electroencephalography (EEG) is not needed.

37. How do infantile spasms present?
Infantile spasms occur between the ages of 2 months and 1 year. They are characterized by 1- to 2-second bursts of flexion of the extremities and head. The movements can look like an exaggerated Moro reflex, but they typically cluster and occur during periods of drowsiness or upon awakening during the day. Infants presenting with these spasms need to see neurology and have an EEG performed, as this can be part of the West Syndrome triad (infantile spasm, hypsarrhythmia, and developmental regression).

38. What is a concussive convulsion?
Concussive convulsions are generalized tonic-clonic activity occurring within seconds of head impact. They are also called "impact seizures," though there is controversy as to whether they are truly epileptic activity. A concussive convulsion does not increase a patient's risk of epilepsy and does not require treatment. Focus medical management and evaluation on the concussion.

39. What is Todd paralysis?
Todd paralysis is a transient paresis or paralysis in the postictal period. Symptoms typically resolve within 24 hours after the seizure.

40. What are the indications for ordering urgent brain imaging after a first-time seizure?
While MRI is the preferred imaging technique, it may not be available or feasible immediately following a seizure. An urgent CT scan should be obtained in the following situations:
- Focal neurologic deficits that are not resolving
- Persistent decreased level of consciousness
- Signs of increased intracranial pressure
- Posttraumatic seizures not consistent with concussive convulsions
- In cases where nonaccidental trauma is a concern, especially in children less than 1 year of age

41. After a nonfebrile seizure, when can brain imaging be scheduled as an outpatient?
A nonurgent MRI is necessary in patients less than 1 year old, patients with focal seizures, or if there are unexplained abnormalities on neurologic exam including cognitive function. Patients with a known seizure disorder should have an MRI if they present with a change in their typical seizure pattern.

SEPSIS

42. What is SIRS?
SIRS stands for systemic inflammatory response syndrome. Two of the following criteria are necessary, one of which must be temperature instability or abnormal leukocyte count:
- Temperature >38.5°C or <36.0°C
- Tachycardia (>2 standard deviations [SD] above the mean for age)
- Tachypnea (>2 SD above the mean for age)
- Abnormal leukocyte count or >10% immature cells

Remember that SIRS is not specific to infection and can be present in settings such as trauma, burns, leukemia, and other diseases. Many children presenting with fever will meet SIRS criteria.

43. How do you differentiate between sepsis, severe sepsis, and septic shock?
Sepsis is SIRS with an infectious source, either presumed or proven.

Severe sepsis is sepsis plus organ dysfunction or hypoperfusion. This must be cardiovascular dysfunction, acute respiratory distress syndrome (ARDS), or two other organ systems. Signs of organ dysfunction include hypotension, acute change in mental status, or creatinine over two times the upper limit of normal.

Septic shock is a subset of severe sepsis where cardiovascular compromise is evident. A child with sepsis and any of the following criteria is in septic shock.
- Altered mental status
- Flash capillary refill or capillary refill >2 seconds
- Bounding or weak peripheral pulses
- Wide pulse pressure
- Hypotension
- Urine output <1 mL/kg/hr

44. What vital sign abnormality can be a sign of early septic shock?

Unexplained tachycardia. As stroke volume decreases, due to capillary leak and third spacing, heart rate increases to maintain cardiac output.

45. Is blood pressure a reliable tool to diagnose early septic shock in a child?

Unlike in adults, hypotension is a late sign of septic shock in children. Pediatric patients can typically compensate through tachycardia and vasoconstriction as a response to endogenous catecholamines. Hypotension indicates uncompensated shock and should be a warning to you that your patient is in a prearrest phase.

46. What physical exam findings can you use to tell the difference between warm and cold shock?

See Table 52.4.

47. You have diagnosed a child with septic shock. What should your initial management include?

Always start with ABCs. The first hour is critical, and a patient in shock requires emergency medical care. After establishing that the patient has an adequate airway and is breathing, begin oxygen and obtain vascular access. Patients in septic shock have intravascular volume depletion and require rapid fluid resuscitation with isotonic saline or colloid. Give 20-mL/kg boluses over 5–10 minutes until capillary refill normalizes or until rales and hepatomegaly develop. If present, correct hypoglycemia and hypocalcemia. Start empiric antibiotics. Obtaining blood cultures prior to starting antibiotics is ideal but should not delay antibiotic administration.

48. What are the empiric antibiotics that should be used for neonates and children presenting in septic shock?

See Table 52.5.

49. A 14-day-old infant presents with a temperature of 38.5°C rectally. Her parents report that she has been a little more fussy, but you find her to be otherwise well appearing. What is the risk of serious bacterial illness (SBI) in this infant?

In febrile infants (1–90 days old), studies demonstrate that approximately 7%–11% will have an SBI. The risk increases to 11%–25% in infants less than 28 days old. Of infants with an SBI, one study documented that 67% had a urinary tract infection, 16% were bacteremic, and 2% were diagnosed with meningitis. Keep in mind that bacteremic infants are clinically well appearing nearly half of the time.

Table 52.4. Physical Exam Findings to Differentiate Warm and Cold Shock

	WARM SHOCK	COLD SHOCK
Capillary Refill	Flash	Delayed (>2 seconds)
Peripheral Pulses	Bounding	Weak
Skin Appearance	Flushed and dry	Mottled, extremities cool to touch
Cardiac Output	Increased	Decreased

Table 52.5. Empirical Antibiotic Therapy for Septic Shock

AGE	BACTERIAL ETIOLOGY	ANTIBIOTIC CHOICE
Neonate	Group B streptococcus (GBS), gram-negative enteric organisms, *Listeria* species	Ampicillin + gentamicin or third-generation cephalosporin (cefotaxime) • Add vancomycin for nosocomial infection or late-onset sepsis
Child	*Staphylococcal pneumoniae, Neisseria meningitidis, Haemophilus influenzae* type b, *Staphylococcus aureus*, group A streptococcus (GAS)	Third-generation cephalosporin + vancomycin • Add aminoglycoside if concerned about nosocomial or gram-negative infection • Add clindamycin for toxic shock syndrome

SYNCOPE

50. **What is syncope?**

Syncope is sudden but transient loss of consciousness and muscle tone caused by inadequate cerebral blood flow. Unconsciousness is typically less than 1–2 minutes in length. Most syncope occurs during early adolescence, and up to 25% of people will have had a syncopal event by early adulthood.

51. **What are the common causes of syncope in children?**

The most common cause in children is neurocardiogenic syncope (also known as vasovagal syncope). Dysautonomia, such as orthostatic hypotension, is also common. There are also several situational causes to consider: prolonged standing, pain, breath-holding spells, and Valsalva.

52. **Most causes of syncope in children are benign. However, what life-threatening causes must be ruled out?**

- Long QT syndrome
- Cardiomyopathy (hypertrophic cardiomyopathy)
- Wolff-Parkinson-White syndrome
- Coronary artery anomalies
- Complete atrioventricular block
- Seizures
- Intracranial hemorrhage
- Drug ingestion
- Carbon monoxide poisoning

53. **How can you determine whether the etiology of a syncopal event is benign or potentially fatal?**

The most important step in diagnosis is a thorough history. Ask specifics about the prodromal event and what the patient was doing leading up to the syncopal event. Family history of similar events, cardiac diseases, or sudden death is also essential to obtain. Obtain orthostatic blood pressures and perform a complete cardiac and neurologic exam. Every patient presenting with an initial episode of syncope should also receive an electrocardiogram (ECG).

54. **What are the red flags in the history and physical exam of a syncope patient?**

- Syncope during exercise
- Syncope while supine
- Syncope preceded by a loud noise
- No presyncopal symptoms
- Chest pain or dyspnea
- Murmur
- Abnormal blood pressure
- Cyanosis
- Family history of sudden death or arrhythmia

55. **You have completed an ECG on a 13-year-old girl who "passed out" at soccer practice. You note that her QTc is 0.600 second. She takes no medications but does have a family history of arrhythmias. What should you do next?**

Consult cardiology immediately. This patient has several red flags including syncope during exercise, an abnormal ECG, and a positive family history.

56. **When should cardiology or neurology be consulted?**

Patients presenting with any of the red flags listed in question 54, those with a positive family history of arrhythmia or sudden death, and those with an abnormal ECG should be seen by cardiology. Neurology referrals should be made for patients with a focal neurologic exam or with a history concerning for seizure.

KEY POINTS

1. The mnemonic AEIOU TIPS is a useful tool for recalling the major categories of causes that should be considered in children presenting with altered mental status.
2. Immediate priorities in the management of children with anaphylaxis include assessment and support of the ABCs, along with prompt administration of intramuscular epinephrine.

3. The mainstays of acute asthma exacerbation therapy are inhaled short-acting beta agonists, cortico-steroids, and oxygen.
4. Status epilepticus is defined as a continuous seizure or recurrent seizure activity lasting greater than 5 minutes without regaining consciousness in that time.
5. Hypotension is a late sign of shock in children.

BIBLIOGRAPHY

Avner JR. Altered states of consciousness. *Pediatrics in Review.* 2006;27:331. http://dx.doi.org/10.1542/pir.27-9-331.
Bell LM. Shock. In: *Textbook of Pediatric Emergency Medicine.* 7th ed. Baltimore: Lippincott Williams & Wilkins; 2015:46–57.
Chiang VW. Seizures. In: *Textbook of Pediatric Emergency Medicine.* 7th ed. Philadelphia: Lippincott Williams & Wilkins; 2015:564–570.
Dellinger RP, et al. Surviving sepsis campaign: international guidelines for management of severe sepsis and septic shock. *Critical Care Medicine.* 2012;41(2):2013.
Dudley NC. Central nervous system emergencies. In: *Pediatric Emergency Medicine Secrets.* 6th ed. Philadelphia: Elsevier; 2015:228–235.
Glissmeyer EW, Nelson DS. Coma. In: Shaw KN, Bachur RG, eds. *Textbook of Pediatric Emergency Medicine.* 7th ed. Philadelphia: Lippincott Williams & Wilkins; 2015:99–108.
Kost S. Stridor. In: *Pediatric Emergency Medicine Secrets.* 6th ed. Philadelphia: Elsevier; 2015:179–183.
Lieberman P, et al. Anaphylaxis—a practice parameter update 2015. *Ann Allergy Asthma Immunol.* 2015;115:341–384.
Ralston SL, et al. Clinical practice guideline: the diagnosis, management, and prevention of bronchiolitis. *Pediatrics.* 2015;136(4):782.
Stevenson MD, Ruddy RM. Allergic emergencies. In: *Textbook of Pediatric Emergency Medicine.* 7th ed. Philadelphia: Lippincott Williams & Wilkins; 2015:616–620.

CHAPTER 53

OFFICE EMERGENCY AND DISASTER PREPAREDNESS

Robert P. Olympia, MD, Chadd E. Nesbit, MD, PhD, FACEP

1. **A 4-year-old boy presents to your urgent care center after falling from monkey bars 1 hour prior. He sustained a blunt head injury, but there was no loss of consciousness. While in your waiting area he proceeds to have a generalized tonic-clonic seizure, has multiple episodes of vomiting, turns blue, and stops breathing. You detect no peripheral pulses. How often do serious emergencies occur in urgent care centers?**

   Although not meant to replace emergency departments (EDs), urgent care centers may need to provide the acute assessment and management of moderately to severely ill or injured infants and children. While studies examining the etiology of pediatric emergencies, including those considered life threatening, that present to urgent care centers have not been published, retrospective studies have found that the rate of emergencies in primary care practices that provide care to children range from less than 1 per office per year to more than 30 per office per year, with the most common reported emergencies being respiratory distress, severe dehydration, seizures, severe trauma, abdominal pain, syncope, and behavioral/psychiatric disorders. A recently published study of urgent care centers in the United States showed that 71% of respondents reported that their center has contacted 911 or community EMS to transport a critically ill or injured child to a definitive care facility.

2. **Do emergencies occur more or less frequently in the adult urgent care setting?**

   Emergencies in the adult population are frequently encountered in outpatient offices and in the urgent care setting. A Canadian study from the Ottawa area recorded more than 3,000 calls for "life-threatening" emergencies to family practice offices over the 3-year period of the study. In addition, an Australian study found that 95% of family practice offices had seen an emergency in the preceding 12 months. Although these studies were conducted in the primary care office settings, they may help to give us an estimate of the frequency of emergencies in the urgent care center setting. The Urgent Care Association of America notes that 4% of patients are either "directed or transferred from an urgent care center to an emergency department."

3. **What types of adult emergencies are seen in the urgent care setting?**

   Almost any kind of emergency could conceivably present to an urgent care center. The patient who presents with "indigestion" may experience a cardiac arrest as his complaint is really a myocardial infarction. The patient who presents with a headache or weakness may be having a stroke. Allergic reactions may rapidly progress to airway obstruction. One must also consider that patients may be brought into the urgent care center from traumatic events such as motor vehicle collisions that occur in close proximity to the center. A Canadian study found that general illness and cardiovascular, respiratory, neurologic, and endocrine problems were the five most common reasons for adult life-threatening emergencies to occur in the outpatient office setting.

4. **What kind of equipment should be readily available in the urgent care setting in the event of a life-threatening emergency?**

   The urgent care center must be prepared to act in emergency situations involving both adult and pediatric populations. Therefore it is important to have equipment that is appropriate for all age ranges from neonate to adult populations. Box 53.1 lists emergency equipment that should be maintained in the urgent care setting. In some emergency situations airway management is necessary. Often this can be achieved by use of airway adjuncts and effective bag-valve mask ventilation. If the center is staffed by physicians who are certified in endotracheal intubation, having the equipment needed for placing an endotracheal tube is a consideration.

Box 53.1. Suggested Office Equipment for Adult and Pediatric Emergencies

Automatic external defibrillator (AED) or a cardiac monitor with defibrillator
Bag-valve mask ventilators in multiple sizes with masks for infants through adults
Blood pressure cuffs of various sizes
Color-coded resuscitation tape (pediatrics)
Gloves, masks, and eye protection
Glucometer
IV access equipment (IV catheters, butterfly needles)
IV tubing
Nasopharyngeal airway set
Oropharyngeal airway set
Nebulizer sets
Oxygen delivery devices (nasal cannula, simple mask, nonrebreather masks) in appropriate sizes
Oxygen tank(s) for portable use
Portable suction device with catheter
Pulse oximeter, adult and pediatric sizes

> ***Additional Equipment to Consider***
> Laryngoscope with curved and straight blades of various sizes
> Endotracheal tubes, various sizes
> Magill forceps
> Cervical collars and backboards

Box 53.2. Suggested Medications for Adult Emergencies

Drugs and Fluids
Acetaminophen
Albuterol (MDI or nebulized)
Aspirin, chewable 81 mg
Ceftriaxone IM or IV
Corticosteroids (IV and po)
Dextrose (25% and 50% for IV use)
Diazepam, IV (Valium)
Diphenhydramine (IV and po) Benadryl
Epinephrine (EpiPen)
Epinephrine (cardiac 1:10,000)
Naloxone
Nitroglycerin (spray or sublingual tablets)
Saline (IV fluid)

Other Medications to Consider
Narcotics, such as morphine
Lidocaine
Glucagon
Atropine
Flumazenil (Romazicon)

5. **What emergency medications should an urgent care center stock for use in an office emergency?**
Box 53.2 and Table 53.1 list recommended medications that should be readily available in the event of an adult or pediatric emergency. The Joint Commission recommends that, whenever possible, emergency medications are available in unit-dose, age-specific, ready-to-administer forms.

6. **What kind of training should the office staff have, to deal with emergencies?**
The Urgent Care Association of America notes that approximately 80% of urgent care centers employ a combination of physicians, physician assistants, and nurse practitioners. The remaining 20% are

Table 53.1. Essential (E) and Suggested (S) Emergency Medications as per the American Academy of Pediatrics

DRUGS/FLUIDS	RECOMMENDATION
Oxygen source	E
Nebulized/inhaled β-agonist	E
Epinephrine (1:1000)	E
Activated charcoal	S
IV/IM ceftriaxone	S
IV lorazepam	S
Rectal diazepam	S
IV methylprednisolone	S
IV dextrose	S
Epinephrine (1:10,000)	S
Atropine	S
Naloxone	S
Normal saline	S
IM midazolam	S

staffed by physicians only. They recommend that all providers and staff in urgent care centers be trained to provide Basic Life Support in emergency situations until EMS arrives. Furthermore, the most senior clinical provider in the office on a given day should additionally be trained in Advanced Cardiac Life Support (ACLS) and Pediatric Advanced Life Support (PALS). Additional certification for the stabilization of trauma victims, such as the Advanced Trauma Life Support (ATLS) course, may be helpful. If possible, advanced practice clinicians, nurses, and technicians ideally should be certified in lifesaving courses as well. Maintenance of certification is imperative as the standards for these courses are frequently updated to reflect the latest basic science findings and may change significantly from one version to the next.

7. **Your office manager would like to develop a quality improvement initiative, developing written emergency plans for adult and pediatric emergencies and performing monthly mock codes. What should this initiative be based on?**
As outlined above, there are a number of emergencies that may occur in the urgent care setting, and your office staff must be prepared to handle medical and traumatic emergencies that may present or occur at your facility. Simulation of emergencies has been shown to improve performance in the office and outpatient settings. Simulations should take place on a regular basis but ideally should not be announced to staff so as to be more realistic. Following these simulations or mock codes, quality improvement strategies should be discussed and changes implemented to ensure patient safety and to improve morbidity and mortality outcomes.

8. **An adult patient presents to your center with expressive aphasia. His spouse tells the secretary that this started as they were shopping in a nearby store. Does your staff have assigned roles in emergency situations?**
Having the office staff assigned to particular tasks may help to reduce confusion during an emergency in the urgent care setting. A staff member should be assigned to alert the physician of the problem. Alternatively, the office may have a panic button to summon personnel to a predesignated location in the event of an emergency. The physician or senior clinician should be the team leader, assisted by advanced practice clinicians depending on the office staff model. Nurses should be assigned to gather equipment, prepare medications, and document during the emergency. A secretary should be assigned to call 911 and lead EMS to the room where the patient is located. Records of any procedures or medications given should be sent with the patient to the ED.

9. **Your staff has just resuscitated a patient from a cardiac arrest after he had a heart attack. How are patients transported from the center to the local hospital?**

   It is important to understand the capabilities of the EMS agency that provides service to the locale where the urgent care is located. If the center is in an urban area, it is likely that it is covered by an Advanced Life Support (ALS) service staffed by paramedics who are ACLS and PALS trained and have a relatively short response time. More remote locations may only be served by an ambulance staffed by EMTs providing Basic Life Support services. ALS, if available, may be available only with a delayed response time. Staff may need to be prepared to take care of the patient for a longer period of time prior to EMS arrival. Staff should also be familiar with the capabilities of local hospitals regarding specialty designations such as trauma, pediatric trauma, stroke, or cardiac catheterization centers to ensure that patients are transferred to an appropriate facility. Local EMS is generally very aware of these designations.

10. **Your patient is on the stretcher and ready to be transported. What information should staff send to the emergency department along with the patient?**

    A recent paper revealed that ED physicians want to know the reasons a patient is being referred from the urgent care center to the emergency department. They would also like to receive a copy of the urgent care center chart. A phone call from the center, and having contact information for the center that the patient was being sent from were additional pieces of information that receiving ED physicians would like to have.

11. **Besides medical emergencies, are there other emergencies that the urgent care office should anticipate and prepare for?**

    The Joint Commission has standards for urgent care centers relative to disaster preparedness. This is an "all hazards" type of approach to disasters that may be internal (loss of power, loss of water, infrastructure failure) or external (storms, flooding, snow) causing disruptions in service. A survey of centers published in 2016 shows that only 27% of centers had a disaster plan involving their centers and the surrounding community. Less than 25% of centers took part in local disaster drills. Less than half of the centers had a disaster plan that they practiced more than once a year. Suggested areas for improvement included developing and practicing disaster plans, familiarization with community disaster plans and shelters, providing surveillance for chemical and biological acts of terrorism, and assisting in the community with disaster planning.

12. **I've heard about syndromic surveillance. What is this and why is it important? Do urgent care centers do this?**

    Syndromic surveillance is defined by the World Health Organization as "the continuous, systematic collection, analysis and interpretation of health-related data needed for the planning, implementation, and evaluation of public health practice." It is an early warning system for public health events such as the spread of disease. It may also serve as a means of detection of biological or chemical attacks. The Public Health Information Network of the CDC is one such program that collects real-time data from a variety of acute and urgent care settings. A 2016 paper found that 17% of urgent care centers that returned the survey participated in some type of syndromic surveillance.

13. **Are there signs that might be suspicious for a covert biological or chemical attack?**

    Covert biological and chemical attacks are very difficult to detect. The presentation of large numbers of patients to a facility with similar complaints may be suggestive of such an attack. Large numbers of patients presenting with fevers, cough, and myalgias may be nothing unusual in mid-January, but if this is happening in August it may be something that needs to be investigated. Maintaining a high degree of suspicion is your best defense against this kind of activity. Participation in a syndromic surveillance network helps to strengthen the safety net for detection of these events. Table 53.2 lists common presenting signs and symptoms for the CDC class A biological weapons.

KEY POINTS

1. Urgent care centers must be able to rapidly recognize, assess, stabilize, and transfer patients presenting to their center with medical and traumatic emergencies beyond the capability of the center.
2. Communication among staff, local EMS, and the receiving hospital is important when dealing with an office emergency and arranging patient transfer.
3. Consistent oversight, planning, and quality improvement/management are crucial in emergency and disaster preparedness.

Table 53.2. Common Presenting Signs and Symptoms of Class A Biological Agents

AGENT	INFLUENZA-LIKE ILLNESS	RAPIDLY PROGRESSIVE PNEUMONIA	BLOODY DIARRHEA	FEVER, RASH, MENINGITIS	HEPATITIS
Anthrax	50%–90%	10%–20%		10%–50%	
Botulism (see note)	Not seen	Not seen	Not seen	Not seen	Not seen
VHF	>90%	10%–50%	50%–100%	Highly variable	Variable
Pneumonic plague	10%–50%	100%		<10%	Not seen
Smallpox	50%–90%	<10%	10%–50%	>90%	
Pneumonic tularemia	25%–50%	100%			

VHF, Viral hemorrhagic fever (Ebola, Marburg).
Botulism classically presents with the triad of bulbar nerve palsy and descending paralysis, lack of fever, and a clear sensorium. The signs listed above are typically not seen with botulism.

BIBLIOGRAPHY

Committee on Pediatric Emergency Medicine. Pediatric care recommendations for freestanding urgent care facilities. *Pediatrics.* 2014;133(5):950–953.

Dunnick J, Olympia RP, Wilkinson R, Brady J. Low compliance of urgent care centers in the United States with recommendations for office-based disaster preparedness. *Pediatr Emerg Care.* 2016;32(5):298–302.

Gardener R, Choo EK, Gravenstein S, Baier RR. Why is this patient begin sent here? Communication from urgent care to the emergency department. *J Emerg Med.* 2016;50:416–421.

LaVelle BA, McLaughlin JJ. Simulation-based education improves patient safety in ambulatory care. In: Henriksen K, Battles JB, Keyes MA, et al., eds. *Advances in Patient Safety: New Directions and Alternative Approaches (Vol. 3: Performance and Tools).* Rockville, MD: Agency for Healthcare Research and Quality (US); 2008. Available from http://www.ncbi.nlm.nih.gov/books/NBK43667/.

Liddy C, Dreise H, Gaboury I. Frequency of in-office emergencies in primary care. *Can Fam Physician.* 2009;55(1004-1005):e1–e4.

Scaramuzzo LA, Wong Y, Voitle KL, Gordils-Perez J. Cardiopulmonary arrest in the outpatient setting: enhancing patient safety through rapid response algorithms and simulation teaching. *Clin J Onc Nursing.* 2014;18:61–64.

Shamji H, Baier RR, Gravenstein S, Gardner RL. Improving the quality of care and communication during patient transitions: best practices for urgent care centers. *Jt Comm J Qual Patient Safety.* 2014;40:319–324.

Toback S. Medical emergency preparedness in office practice. *Am Fam Physician.* 2007;75:1679–1684.

Wilkinson R, Olympia RP, Dunnick J, Brady J. Pediatric care provided at urgent care centers in the United States: compliance with recommendations for emergency preparedness. *Pediatr Emerg Care.* 2016;32(2):77–81.

CHAPTER 54

DIAGNOSTIC ULTRASOUND

Steven Kleinman, DO, Joni Rabiner, MD

INTRODUCTION TO ULTRASOUND

1. What is point-of-care (POC) ultrasound (US)?

US examinations performed at the bedside by practitioners, interpreted in real time, and used to answer specific clinical questions in order in improve or expedite patient care. Most US applications have a higher specificity than sensitivity, meaning that US is better as a "rule-in" tool for pathology.

2. What are the advantages of US in the urgent care setting?

When available to the trained provider, US is noninvasive, dynamic, and easy to repeat at the bedside. It has no radiation and does not require sedation. It has also been found to be cost-effective. It may be useful for augmenting the physical examination findings and for enhancing performance with procedures.

3. What common terminology is used to describe US images?

- Anechoic: complete absence of returning sound waves, appears black
- Isoechoic: structure has similar appearance to the surrounding tissue
- Hypoechoic: structure appears darker than the surrounding tissue
- Hyperechoic: structure appears brighter than the surrounding tissue

    Fluids, including water and blood, are anechoic or hypoechoic (black or dark gray), and bone and air are hyperechoic (white) on US images. Soft tissue and muscle have echotextures with varying shades of gray.

4. What are the four main types of US probes and for what are they typically used?

- Phased Array: FAST, cardiac, abdominal imaging
- Linear: Thoracic, musculoskeletal, ocular, procedural guidance
- Curvilinear: Abdominal imaging, transabdominal obstetrical and gynecological imaging, cardiac
- Intracavitary probe: Transvaginal obstetrical and gynecological imaging, peritonsilar abscess evaluation

FAST

5. What is the purpose of the focused assessment with sonography for trauma (FAST) examination?

The FAST examination can provide quick and reliable information on potential bleeding into the peritoneal, pericardial, or pleural spaces and can identify clinically significant injury requiring operative intervention.

6. How do you perform the FAST examination?

There are four basic views:

- Right upper quadrant: Looking for fluid between the liver and kidney in Morison's pouch. This is the most common site of fluid accumulation in adults. The probe is placed in the right mid-axillary line in the seventh to ninth intercostal spaces with the indicator toward the patient's head.
- Left upper quadrant: Looking for fluid around the spleen and kidney. The probe is placed in the left posterior axillary line in the fifth to seventh intercostal spaces with the indicator toward the patient's head.
- Suprapubic: To evaluate for fluid in the rectovesical pouch in male patients or pouch of Douglas in female patients. Two perpendicular views should be obtained, with the probe superior to the symphysis pubis and angled toward the patient's feet, with the indicator oriented toward the patient's head and to the patient's right side.
- Subxiphoid: To evaluate for pericardial effusion and cardiac activity. The probe is placed almost flat on the patient's abdomen just inferior to the xiphoid process, directed toward the patient's left shoulder, with the indicator toward the patient's right side.

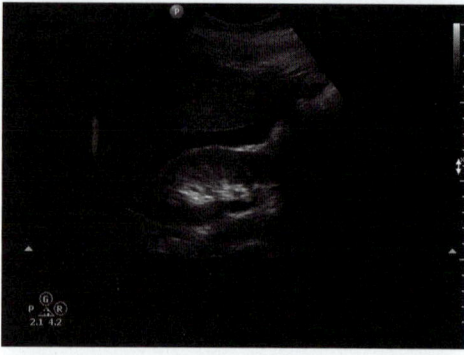

Fig. 54.1. Free Fluid in Morrison's Pouch in a Right Upper Quadrant (RUQ) FAST View.

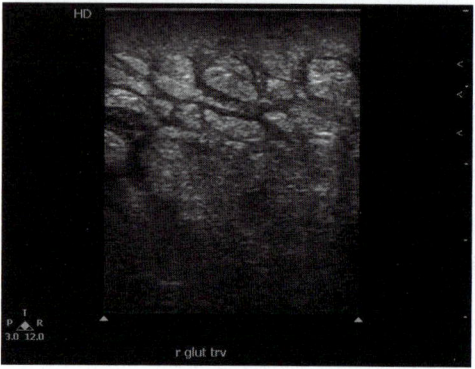

Fig. 54.2. Cobblestoning.

7. **What are the limitations of the FAST examination?**

The FAST examination is not reliable for solid organ, retroperitoneal, or hollow viscous injuries.

8. **What does blood look like on US?**

Acute hemorrhage appears as an anechoic fluid collection, but as blood clots, may appear complex, hypoechoic, or even isoechoic to surrounding structures (Fig. 54.1).

SOFT TISSUE/MUSCULOSKELETAL US

9. **What utility does POC US have for soft tissue infections?**

POC US improves the ability to detect the presence of drainable abscesses in the setting of soft tissue infections better than a physical examination. It also helps to identify important surrounding structures to aid in procedure planning and execution.

10. **Describe how cellulitis and abscess appear on US.**

In cellulitis on US, there is fluid in the subcutaneous tissue, which appears as "cobblestoning" when hyperechoic fat lobules are separated by hypoechoic fluid (Fig. 54.2). An abscess on US is a collection of hypoechoic fluid that has absence of internal vascular flow (Fig. 54.3). The abscess size and depth can be measured, which can facilitate the drainage procedure.

11. **Describe how skin foreign bodies appear on US.**

Skin foreign bodies are hyperechoic structures in the subcutaneous tissue and may have artifacts associated with them such as shadowing (wood, plastic) or reverberation/comet tail artifact (metal) (Fig. 54.4).

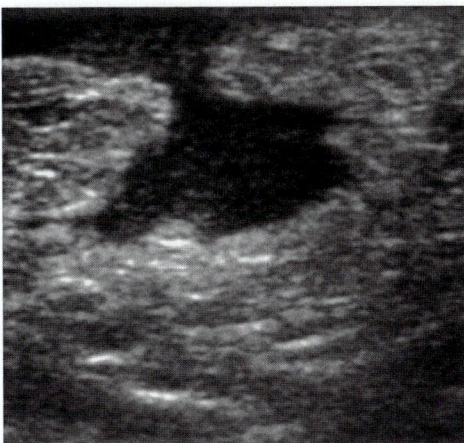

Fig. 54.3. Abscess.

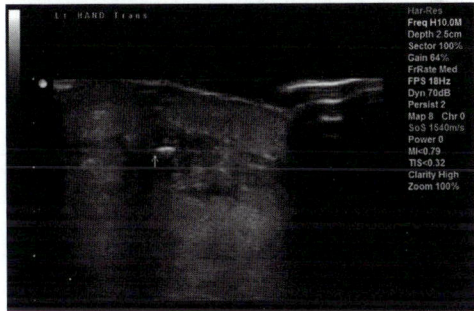

Fig. 54.4. Foreign Body.

RENAL

12. What are the indications for renal POC US?
Clinical suspicion for renal colic, urinary retention, trauma.

13. What are you looking for on renal POC US in a patient presenting with signs and symptoms of urolithiasis?
POC renal US is used primarily to identify the presence of hydronephrosis in patients for whom urolithiasis is suspected. Its presence and degree of hydronephrosis can be a predictor for the presence and size of a ureteral stone.

14. How does one calculate bladder volume in the setting of acute urinary retention?
The bladder is scanned in transverse and sagittal planes measuring the height, width, and length. Width is measured in the transverse plane. Height is obtained in the sagittal plane, and length can be measured in either plane. Using the volume formula L × W × H × 0.75, most machines will calculate the bladder volume.

PULMONARY

15. What utility does POC pulmonary US have?
This modality can be used in many clinical scenarios to evaluate the patient with acute dyspnea and look for pathologies such as pneumothoraces, pulmonary edema, pleural effusions, and pneumonia.

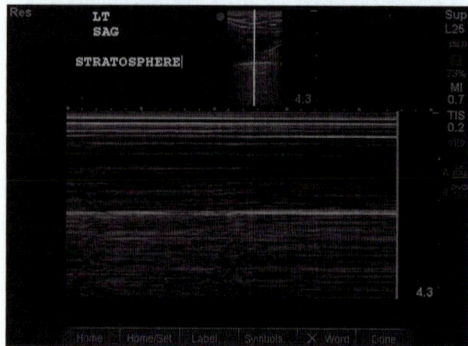

Fig. 54.5. Stratosphere Sign.

16. **How does normal lung appear on US?**
Unlike other US applications, pulmonary US relies heavily on artifacts for imaging. Normal lung exhibits sliding or movement between the parietal and visceral pleura, a "seashore sign" or "waves on a beach sign" on M-mode, and reverberation artifacts referred to as "A-lines."

17. **What are findings associated with pneumothorax?**
A pneumothorax will exhibit lack of pleural sliding and loss of the normal appearance of A and B lines. M-mode will show a "barcode sign" or "stratosphere sign" (Fig. 54.5). One may also see a lung point or the point of interface between normal lung appearance and absence thereof.

18. **Describe the US appearance of pulmonary edema.**
Simply, pulmonary edema exhibits an excess of B-lines on US. B-lines are reverberation artifacts that look like spotlights arising from the pleural line and extend to the bottom of the screen without fading. Pulmonary edema exhibits three or more simultaneous B-lines in a single view in two or more different areas.

19. **What does a pleural effusion look like on US?**
Pleural effusions are typically gravity dependent and appear as anechoic fluid collections in the costophrenic spaces of the thorax.

GALLBLADDER

20. **What is the primary goal of POC right upper quadrant ultrasound (RUQ US)?**
To evaluate for evidence of acute cholecystitis.

21. **Briefly, describe how to perform a POC RUQ US.**
Typically performed in the lateral decubitus or supine position using a low-frequency curvilinear probe, one should obtain views of the gallbladder (GB) in two orthogonal planes. Attention should be paid to the contents of the gallbladder and its neck as well as the diameter of the common bile duct (CBD); secondary signs of cholecystitis should be noted.

22. **What is the "WES" sign?**
The "WES" (wall, echo, shadow) sign is a phenomenon caused when the gallbladder is contracted around a large or multiple stones obliterating the lumen. All that is visible is the echogenic gallbladder wall anterior to the strongly hyperechoic gallstone(s) and the posterior shadow behind it.

23. **What findings are considered to be suspicious for acute cholecystitis?**
Presence of gallstones, biliary sludge, thickened GB wall (>3 mm), sonographic Murphy's sign, enlarged CBD (>6 mm), pericholecystic fluid, GB wall edema, dilated GB (>4 cm in transverse and >8 cm in sagittal), air in the gallbladder wall.

PEDIATRIC ABDOMINAL ULTRASOUND

24. **Which probe should be used for abdominal US?**
Start with the high-frequency linear probe, which has higher resolution and is sufficient for abdominal imaging in most children.

25. How does appendicitis appear on US?

Appendicitis on US is a blind-ending, tubular structure that has a diameter >6 mm (from outer wall to outer wall), is noncompressible, connects to the cecum, and has no peristalsis. Evaluate the area of maximal tenderness. If the patient is unable to localize the pain, the appendix normally lays on the psoas muscle, adjacent to the external iliac vessels, landmarks that can be used to locate the appendix. Graded compression may be needed to displace bowel gas.

26. How is intussusception diagnosed by US?

Using the linear transducer probe, scan from the right lower quadrant to the right upper quadrant, across the transverse colon to the left upper quadrant, and down to the left lower quadrant. Intussusception is most often ileocecal, and it appears as a "target sign" in cross-sign in longitudinal view from the layers of one section of bowel invaginating into another section of bowel.

27. How do you evaluate for pyloric stenosis on US?

Feed the child Pedialyte during the US evaluation and place the patient in the right decubitus position to facilitate visualization of liquids entering the pylorus. Using the linear transducer probe, locate the pylorus to the right of the midline. In pyloric stenosis, the pyloric muscle wall thickness is >3 mm, the pyloric channel length is >12 mm, and gastric contents fail to pass through the pylorus.

KEY POINTS

1. US is better used as a "rule-in" tool.
2. The FAST examination should be used as a screening tool in trauma, not for definitive diagnosis of pathology.
3. US can be used to differentiate cellulitis from abscess.

BIBLIOGRAPHY

Blackbourne LH, Soffer D, McKenney M, et al. Secondary ultrasound examination increases the sensitivity of the FAST exam in blunt trauma. *J Trauma.* 2004;57:932.

Branney SW, Wolfe RE, Moore EE, et al. Quantitative sensitivity of ultrasound in detecting free intraperitoneal fluid. *J Trauma.* 1995;39:375.

Cohen HL, Langer J, McGahan JP, et al. AIUM Practice Guideline for the Performance of the Focused Assessment With Sonography for Trauma (FAST) Examination. *J Ultrasound Med.* 2014;33:2047–2056.

Dalziel P, Noble VE. Bedside ultrasound and the assessment of renal colic: a review. *Emerg Med J.* 2013;30:3–8.

Dickman E, Tessaro MO, Arroyo AC, et al. Clinician-performed abdominal sonography. *Eur J Trauma Emerg Surg.* 2015;41:481.

Eckert K, Ackermann O, Janssen N, et al. Accuracy of the sonographic fat pad sign for primary screening of pediatric elbow fractures: a preliminary study. *J Med Ultrasonics.* 2014;41(4).473.

Fritz DA. Emergency Bedside Ultrasound. In: Stone C, Humphries RL, eds. *Current Diagnosis & Treatment Emergency Medicine.* 7th ed. New York, NY: McGraw-Hill; 2011. http://accessmedicine.mhmedical.com/content.aspx?bookid=385&Sectionid=40357219. Accessed June 26, 2016.

Grechenig W, Clement HG, Fellinger M, Seggl W. Scope and limitations of ultrasonography in the documentation of fractures—an experimental study. *Arch Orthop Trauma Surg.* 1998;117:368.

Kendall JL, Shimp RJ. Performance and interpretation of focused right upper quadrant ultrasound by emergency physicians. *J Emerg Med.* 2001;21:7–13.

Lichtenstein DA, Lascols N, Meziere G, Gepner A. Ultrasound diagnosis of alveolar consolidation in the critically ill. *Intensive Care Med.* 2004;30(2):276.

Nance ML, Mahboubi S, Wickstrom M, Prendergast F, Stafford PW. Pattern of abdominal free fluid following isolated blunt spleen or liver injury in the pediatric patient. *J Trauma.* 2002;52:85.

Ma JO, Mateer JR, et al. *Ma and Mateer's Emergency Ultrasound.* 3rd ed. China, 2014: McGraw Hill; 2014.

Rabiner JE, Khine H, Avner JR, et al. Accuracy of point-of-care ultrasonography for diagnosis of elbow fractures in children. *Ann Emerg Med.* 2013;61:9.

Shackford SR, Rogers FB, Osler TM, et al. Focused abdominal sonogram for trauma: the learning curve of nonradiologist clinicians in detecting hemoperitoneum. *J Trauma.* 1999;46:553.

Stengel D, Bauwens K, Sehouli J, et al. Discriminatory power of 3.5 MHz convex and 7.5 MHz linear ultrasound probes for the imaging of traumatic splenic lesions. *J Trauma.* 2001;51:37.

Squire BT, Fox JC, Anderson C. ABSCESS: applied bedside sonography for convenient evaluation of superficial soft tissue infections. *Acad Emerg Med.* 2005;12(7):601–606.

Volpicelli G, Elbarbary M, Blaivas M, et al. International evidence-based recommendations for point-of-care lung ultrasound. *Intensive Care Med.* 2012;38(4):577.

Zenobii MF, Accogli E, Domanico A, et al. Update on bedside ultrasound (US) diagnosis of acute cholecystitis (AC). *Intern Emerg Med.* 2016;11:261.

CHAPTER 55

MENTAL HEALTH URGENCIES

Jodi Brady-Olympia, MD

1. **A 14-year-old male with no significant past medical history presents to your urgent care center with a 6-month history of daily headaches and poor appetite. His parents are concerned because he has become more "withdrawn" recently, spending much of his day in his room alone, playing on his computer. On exam, he is sullen, unengaging, and says he "doesn't want to talk about it." His vital signs and physical exam are unremarkable. What signs and symptoms may lead you to consider depression in a child or adolescent?**
   - Isolation or withdrawing from friends and family
   - Loss of interest in things he/she previously enjoyed
   - Changes in sleep patterns (i.e., hypersomnia or insomnia)
   - Decline in school grades or performance
   - Somatic complaints: headaches, abdominal pain, chest pain
   - Change in appetite: loss of appetite, weight loss or weight gain
   - Irritability

2. **What other conditions must be considered when suspecting a diagnosis of depression?**
   - Psychiatric conditions: anxiety, eating disorders, ADHD, substance or alcohol use
   - Endocrine: hypo- or hyperthyroidism, Addison disease, Cushing disease
   - Hematologic: anemia, oncologic process
   - Insomnia

3. **What is an essential element to obtaining a psychosocial history in an adolescent?**
   In talking with an adolescent it is necessary to discuss confidentiality. When a medical provider has a discussion about confidentiality at the onset of the visit, adolescents are more likely to disclose information about sensitive topics. In addition, when confidentiality is not discussed, the adolescent is more likely to forgo care, or not disclose the information.

4. **What is a "conditional" discussion of confidentiality?**
   Confidentiality is best discussed with the adolescent and family/guardian at the start of the encounter. The idea that confidentiality is "conditional" means that there are situations in which confidentiality will be breached. Under these circumstances, disclosure is required by law such as abuse or homicidal ideation, or when the provider has concern for risk or harm to the adolescent such suicidal ideation or high-risk behavior.

5. **What are some of the risk factors for suicide attempt in adolescents?**
   - Male gender
   - Age >16 years
   - Homosexual orientation
   - Parental mental health problems
   - Family history of suicide or suicide attempts
   - History of physical or sexual abuse
   - Previous suicide attempt
   - Mood disorder
   - Substance use
   - Pathologic internet use
   - Access to firearms or lethal means
   - Poor social support
   - Bullying
   - Recent psychosocial stressor

6. **What questions can be asked to screen for suicide risk?**
The Ask-Suicide Screening Questions (ASQ), which have a sensitivity of 96.9% and specificity of 87.6% in patients presenting to a pediatric emergency department. Answering yes to one or more of the four questions is considered a positive screen.
1. In the past few weeks, have you ever felt that your family would be better off if you were dead?
2. In the past few weeks, have you wished you were dead?
3. In the past week, have you been having thoughts about killing yourself?
4. Have you ever tried to kill yourself?

7. **An 11-year-old female is brought to the urgent care clinic by her mother. The daughter has been complaining of stomachaches over the past 2 weeks since starting school. She is eating very little at lunch and cries every morning before leaving for school. She has never expressed any concerns about body image but says she is just not hungry. What signs may a child present with when exhibiting anxiety?**
- School avoidance or refusal
- Avoidance of social situations or activities
- Somatic complaints (headache, chest or abdominal pain)
- Restlessness, nail biting, or hair pulling
- Declining school performance, inattentiveness
- Decreased appetite

8. **What should your differential diagnosis include when considering a child presenting with anxiety?**
- Psychiatric conditions: separation anxiety disorder, childhood-onset social phobia or social anxiety disorder, generalized anxiety disorder, agoraphobia and specific phobias, selective mutism, post-traumatic stress disorder, panic disorder, psychosis
- Acute painful conditions
- Central nervous system: trauma, tumor, meningitis/encephalitis
- Cardiac: dysrhythmias, shock states/dehydration
- Respiratory: acute asthma, hypoxia
- Endocrine: hyperthyroid
- Ingestions and exposures

9. **What toxidromes may present as acute psychiatric conditions?**
- Anticholinergic toxidrome: "Red as a beet, dry as a bone, blind as a bat, mad as a hatter, and hot as a hare."
  - Fever, tachycardia, cardiac arrhythmias
  - Hypertension
  - Delirium, psychosis, convulsions, coma
  - Mydriasis
  - Flushed, dry skin
- Amphetamine/cocaine toxidrome: fever, tachycardia, hypertension; hyperactive, delirious; tremors, myoclonus, psychosis; seizures; mydriasis; sweaty
- Opiate toxidrome: bradycardia, bradypnea, hypotension, hypothermia, euphoria to coma, hyporeflexia, pinpoint pupils
- Organophosphate toxidrome:
  - Bradycardia to tachycardia
  - Tachypnea
  - Confusion, coma, convulsion, muscle fasciculations, weakness to paralysis
  - Miosis, blurry vision, lacrimation
  - Sweating
  - Salivation, bronchorrhea, bronchospasm, urinary frequency, diarrhea
- Neuroleptic malignant syndrome: fever, axial muscular rigidity, autonomic instability/shock, altered consciousness
- Serotonin syndrome: use of SSRI, agitation, stupor, myoclonus, hyperreflexia, diaphoresis, shivering, tremor, diarrhea, incoordination, fever

10. **A 15-year-old female presents to your urgent care center with her mother because of a 3-month history of daily abdominal pain. She denies fever, vomiting, or diarrhea. She has lost approximately 15 pounds over the past 3 months, admitting that she has "no appetite." She has been seen by her pediatrician several times and has an extensive workup, including blood tests and computed tomography (CT) scans, all reported as normal. She was healthy prior to the onset of pain. Social history reveals that her parents are recently divorced. Her physician exam is unremarkable. You have a suspicion for an eating disorder. In addition to your physical exam, what initial studies should be ordered?**
    - Comprehensive metabolic panel (including electrolytes, blood urea nitrogen [BUN], creatinine, glucose, and liver function tests [LFTs])
    - Calcium, magnesium, and phosphorus levels
    - Complete blood count
    - Thyroid function testing (thyroid-stimulating hormone [TSH] and free thyroxine [free T4])
    - Electrocardiogram (EKG)
        Hypokalemic, hypochloremic metabolic alkalosis may be seen with vomiting while hypophosphatemia may be seen with refeeding syndrome. A complete blood count may demonstrate anemia or leukopenia. An EKG may demonstrate significant sinus bradycardia. Normal lab and EKG results do not exclude the diagnosis of an eating disorder.

11. **What other conditions should be considered in an adolescent presenting to the urgent care with weight loss?**
    - Endocrine: hyperthyroidism, glucocorticoid insufficiency, diabetes mellitus
    - Gastrointestinal: inflammatory bowel disease, celiac disease, peptic ulcer disease
    - Neoplastic: central nervous system tumor or other malignancies

12. **What are the medical indications for direct referral to the emergency department and consideration of inpatient hospitalization for eating disorders and other psychiatric conditions?**
    - Acute food refusal
    - Acute medical complications such as syncope or seizures
    - Uncontrolled binging and purging
    - Failure of outpatient treatment
    - <75% mean BMI for age and gender
    - Physiologic instability
        - Heart rate <40 bpm
        - Orthostatic blood pressure changes
        - High or low respiratory rate
        - Poor extremity perfusion with prolonged capillary refill
        - Weak/thread or strong/bounding pulses
    - Acute mental status changes or focal neurologic findings
    - EKG abnormalities
    - Electrolyte disturbances: hypophosphatemia, hypokalemia, hypoglycemia
    - Moderate to severe dehydration
    - Psychiatric emergencies: homicidal or suicidal ideations, significant psychosis, severe depression
    - Concern for toxic ingestion or exposure
    - Social or family instability

13. **A 17-year-old female presents to your urgent care center with her 16-year-old sister with complaints of lower abdominal pain and vaginal bleeding. She admits to having unprotected sex and is worried that she may be pregnant or have a sexually transmitted infection. Do you need to contact her guardian?**
    Circumstances that an adolescent can consent to his or her own health care in most states include:
    - Testing and treatment for sexually transmitted infections, including human immunodeficiency virus (HIV)
    - Contraceptive counseling and services
    - Prenatal care
    - Evaluation and treatment for substance use

- Evaluation and treatment for mental health care
- Life-threatening emergency care
- Judicial bypass

Keep in mind that laws may vary from state to state such as the minimal age necessary for an adolescent. Remember to check the laws governing your specific state of practice.

14. **A 16-year-old female presents to your urgent care center with a 1-month history of headache. While in the waiting room, she begins to have shaking of her arms and legs, despite being able to follow commands and nod "yes" and "no" to questions. You are able to stop the seizure by merely holding the extremity. When you place her arm over her face, she avoids hitting herself when you drop her arm. What is likely going on?**

She is most likely exhibiting a pseudoseizure. Associated with a conversion disorder, pseudoseizures are commonly seen in adolescent females and are typically nonrhythmic and prolonged. Pseudoseizures may be generalized or focal. The adolescent may be able to communicate with words or sounds, follow commands, and have purposeful movements during the event. Injury to the patient, urinary and bowel incontinence, and postictal states are rare. Anticonvulsants are unnecessary in the management of pseudoseizures.

Conversion disorder is an involuntary, stress-related condition where the patient presents with an alteration of physical functioning that does not correspond to a recognizable medical condition. Examples of conversion disorder include pseudoseizures, syncope, psychogenic cough, and paralysis/ paresthesia of the extremities.

KEY POINTS

1. Underlying medical conditions must be considered in a child or adolescent presenting to the urgent care with depression or anxiety.
2. In most circumstances, adolescents are able to consent for themselves when presenting for testing and treatment of sexually transmitted infections.
3. Normal labs, weight, and EKG do not exclude the diagnosis of an eating disorder.
4. Substance abuse, medication overdose, and alcohol intoxication must be considered in a child or adolescent presenting with a change in mental status.
5. There are certain circumstances in which confidentiality may be breached, including when disclosure is required by law such as with abuse or homicidal ideation or when the provider has concern for risk or harm to the adolescent such with suicidal ideation or high-risk behavior.

BIBLIOGRAPHY

American Psychiatric Association. *Diagnostic and Statistical Manual of Mental Disorders.* 5th ed. (DSM-5). Arlington, VA: APA; 2013.
Berlan ED, Bravender T. Confidentiality, consent, and caring for the adolescent patient. *Curr Opin Pediatr.* 2009;21(4):450–456.
Ford CA, Millstein SG, Halpern-Felsher BL, Irwin CE. Influence of physician confidentiality assurances on adolescents' willingness to disclose information and seek future health care: a randomized controlled trial. *JAMA.* 1997;278:1029–1034.
Golden NH, Katzman DK, Sawyer SM, et al. Update on the medical management of eating disorders in adolescents. *J Adolesc Health.* 2015;56(4):370–375.
Horowitz LM, Bridge JA, Teach SJ, et al. Ask Suicide-Screening Questions (ASQ): a brief instrument for the pediatric emergency department. *Arch Pediatric Adolesc Med.* 2012;166(12):1170–1176.
Kennedy SP, Baraff LJ, Suddath RL, Asarnow JR. Emergency department management of suicidal adolescents. *Ann Emerg Med.* 2004;43(4):452–460.
Levine SB. In brief: adolescent consent and confidentiality. *Pediatr Rev.* 2009;30(11):457–458.
Mairs R, Nicholls D. Assessment and treatment of eating disorders in children and adolescents. *Arch Dis Children (June 28).* 2016. [Epub ahead of print].
Maslow GR, Dunlap K, Chung RJ. Depression and suicide in children and adolescents. *Pediatr Rev.* 2015;36(7):299–310.
Morreale M, Stinnett AJ, Dowling EC, eds. *Policy Compendium on Confidential Health Services for Adolescents.* 2nd ed. Chapel Hill, NC: Center for Adolescent Health and the Law; 2005. <http://www.cahl.org/PDFs/PolicyCompendium/Policy Compendium.pdf>.
Shain B. Committee on adolescence: suicide and suicide attempts in adolescents. *Pediatrics (June).* 2016.

CHAPTER 56

TRAVEL MEDICINE

Sandra K. Schumacher, MD, MPH, CTropMed, Jeffrey I. Campbell, MD

1. **What are VFRs, and why is this population at particular risk of acquiring travel-related illness?**

   VFRs (visiting friends and relatives) are individuals who travel to visit relatives or friends, which often involves return to the individuals' country of origin. VFRs tend to have a higher prevalence of travel-related infectious diseases (e.g., VFRs are eight times more likely to be diagnosed with malaria than are tourist travelers). Many VFRs assume immunity against infectious diseases in their home countries; however, immunity has often waned by the time of travel. Also, ≤30% of VFRs have a pretravel health care encounter, so these travelers may lack awareness of risk. Furthermore, many may travel to higher risk destinations while staying in homes that lack health amenities frequently available to foreign tourists, such as bed nets and safe food and water.

2. **In a returning traveler who is sick, what illnesses might you suspect based on duration of time since travel?**

   Time since potential exposure can help identify illness in returning travelers. Chikungunya, dengue, Japanese encephalitis, enteric fever, influenza, and spotted fever Rickettsial illnesses often have an incubation period of <2 weeks. Hepatitis A and E often have an incubation of 2 to 6 weeks; enteric fever may also be seen during this time period. Hepatitis B, amebic liver abscesses, schistosomiasis, leishmaniasis, and tuberculosis often have an incubation of >6 weeks. Although malaria typically presents within 2 weeks of travel, symptoms may not develop for up to months after return (98% of *Plasmodium falciparum* infections present within 3 months of travel; however, almost 50% of *P. vivax* infections present after 30 days of travel and may not be seen until 12 months after return). Human immunodeficiency virus (HIV) may present at any time.

3. **What special concerns do health care workers face when practicing abroad?**

   Health care workers who spend time abroad in health care settings may face health risks less prevalent in the United States, as well as decreased access to effective treatment while abroad. Risk is largely dependent upon the specific environment in which the health care worker operates. Specific considerations include increased exposure to bloodborne pathogens such as hepatitis B and HIV, highly contagious diseases such as measles and tuberculosis, and epidemics such as cholera. Health care workers should consider bringing postexposure prophylaxis antiretrovirals with them for potential HIV exposure. Health care workers also may experience unique psychological stress related to their work.

4. **What causes cholera and how is it treated?**

   The bacterium causing cholera, *Vibrio cholerae,* is typically acquired from untreated, contaminated water, but it can also be transmitted on food, especially seafood. The characteristic symptom is a diffuse, "rice-water" secretory diarrhea that may lead rapidly to hypovolemia. Treatment focuses on rehydration with oral rehydration solution and/or intravenous fluids; antibiotics, including macrolides, fluoroquinolones, or tetracyclines, may reduce symptom duration and fluid requirements but do not obviate the need for aggressive rehydration. In mid-2016, the FDA approved Vaxchora, a live, attenuated vaccine for the prevention of cholera caused by serogroup O1 in adults 18–64 years old.

5. **What is the meningitis belt?**

   The meningitis belt is an area of sub-Saharan Africa where meningococcal meningitis is hyperendemic (Fig. 56.1), most notably during the dry season (December–June). Although meningococcal outbreaks are most common in the meningitis belt, outbreaks can occur worldwide (notably, the Hajj pilgrimage to Saudi Arabia has been associated with outbreaks). Transmission occurs person-to-person by close contact with saliva or respiratory secretions. The six major *Neisseria meningitidis* serogroups are A, B, C, W, X, and Y; serogroup A predominates in the meningitis belt. At-risk travelers are recommended to receive a quadrivalent meningitis vaccine, which protects against serogroups A, C, W, and Y.

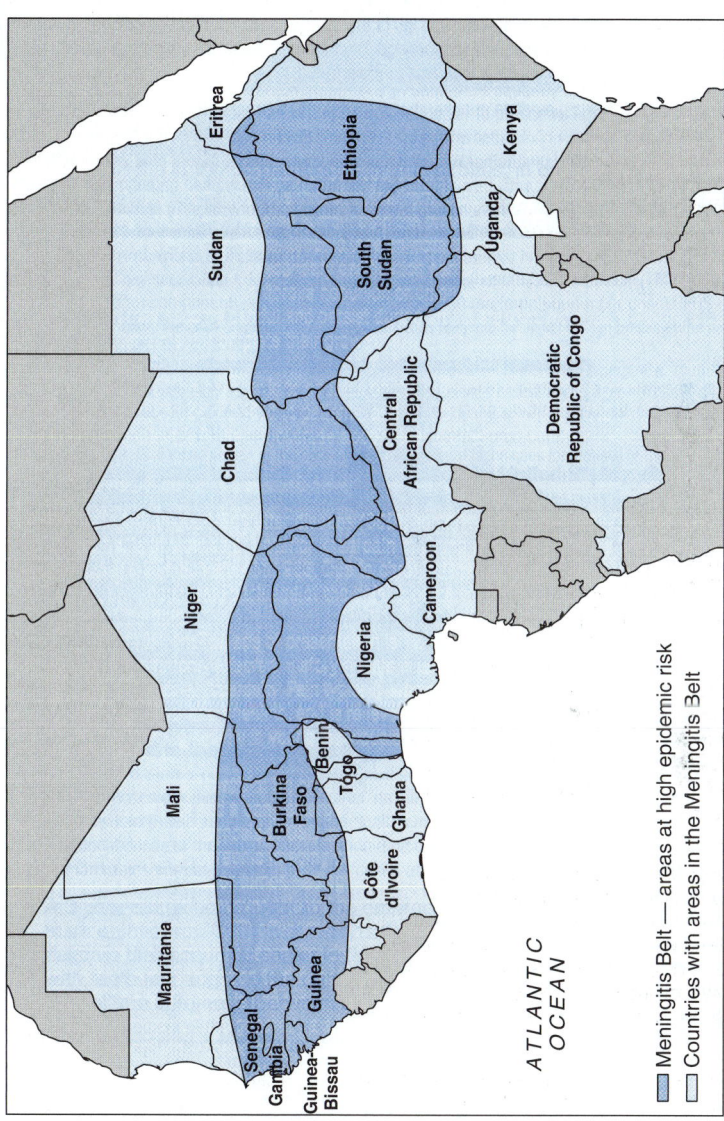

Fig. 56.1. The Meningitis Belt. *(http://wwwnc.cdc.gov/travel/yellowbook/2016/infectious-diseases-related-to-travel/meningococcal-disease)*

Meningitis Belt — areas at high epidemic risk

Countries with areas in the Meningitis Belt

6. **What causes travelers' diarrhea, and how can it be prevented and treated?**

Travelers' diarrhea is the most common travel-related illness and occurs worldwide, especially in most of Asia, Mexico, Central and South America, Africa, and the Middle East. Bacterial pathogens are the typical cause, led by enterotoxigenic *Escherichia coli*. Prevention centers on good hand hygiene, avoiding ice and tap water in endemic areas, and eating foods that are well prepared. Oral hydration is key in treatment of travelers' diarrhea. Indications for antibiotic use include more than four unformed stools daily, fever, or blood or mucus in the stool. In adults, a fluoroquinolone is often prescribed empirically; azithromycin is recommended for children, pregnant women, and travelers to Asia (where quinolone-resistant *Campylobacter* is prevalent).

7. **What causes ciguatera, and what are the symptoms of ciguatera?**

Reef fish (such as barracuda) predate on ciguatoxin-producing dinoflagellates. These fish may then accumulate the toxin and pass it to humans when eaten. Ciguatera typically presents with gastrointestinal symptoms starting 3–24 hours after eating a toxin-laden fish but may include more severe symptoms such as hypotension and bradycardia as well as neurologic and psychiatric symptoms such as paresthesias, hot/cold reversal, and hallucinations. Symptoms usually last a few days but may persist up to 4 weeks; treatment is primarily supportive. Ciguatera toxin–containing fish do not smell or appear unusual, and neither cooking nor freezing destroys the toxin. There is no clinical testing for ciguatera.

8. **A patient presents to urgent care with facial flushing, diarrhea, and respiratory distress shortly after eating at a sushi restaurant. What likely caused this acute illness?**

Scombroid, also known as histamine toxicity from fish, causes up to 40% of seafood-related, foodborne illness in the United States and is common worldwide. Illness occurs when bacteria, proliferating in poorly refrigerated fish, convert the amino acid histidine into histamine. Symptoms result from consuming histamine and present like an allergic reaction, starting between 5 and 60 minutes after eating contaminated fish. Classically, patients may describe contaminated fish as tasting bitter, peppery, or metallic, but concentrations of histamine needed to produce symptoms are much lower than concentrations needed to affect taste. Treatment is usually not necessary, although antihistamines may be helpful and possibly epinephrine if anaphylaxis is a concern.

9. **What vector-borne diseases should travelers be wary of, and what transmits them?**

Vector-borne diseases are infections transmitted by the bite of infected arthropods, such as mosquitoes, ticks, triatomine bugs, and fleas. They account for more than 17% of all infectious diseases. Vector-borne illnesses worldwide include malaria (*Anopheles* mosquitoes); dengue, chikungunya, yellow fever, Rift Valley fever, and Zika (*Aedes* mosquitoes); Japanese encephalitis, lymphatic filariasis, and West Nile fever (*Culex* mosquitoes); Rickettsial diseases and Lyme (ticks); American trypanosomiasis (triatomine bugs); African trypanosomiasis (tsetse flies); leishmaniasis (sandflies); and onchocerciasis (blackflies). Many of these diseases are preventable by limiting exposures to their respective vectors.

10. **An adult who returned to the United States from Kenya 1 week ago presents to your office with an intermittent fever, headaches, and body aches. He did not seek travel counsel before traveling and said he had multiple mosquito bites during his trip. You find he is anemic as well. What potentially life-threatening infectious illness should you be certain to exclude?**

Malaria is found in over 100 countries, is caused by the *Plasmodium* parasite, and is transmitted by *Anopheles* mosquitoes, which bite humans (thereby transmitting the parasite) at dusk and during the night. An experienced laboratorian can distinguish between the four most common disease-causing *Plasmodium* species—*P. falciparum, P. vivax, P. malariae,* and *P. ovale*—based on their appearance on a blood smear. *P. falciparum* is typically associated with severe malaria, and *P. vivax* and *P. ovale* can develop dormant liver stages. Most cases of malaria are curable. However, malaria causes more than 400,000 annual deaths globally, primarily among children <5 years old.

11. **How can malaria be prevented?**

Travelers to malaria-endemic areas can reduce the chances of infection by taking prophylactic medications before, during, and after their trip. Prophylactic medications include doxycycline, mefloquine, and atovaquone-proguanil; choice of which medication to take should account for local resistance patterns in the traveler's destination. Other methods of prevention include sleeping under bed nets, staying in well-screened areas at night, properly using mosquito spray, avoiding standing water, and wearing long-sleeved shirts and long pants at night to cover skin and avoid mosquito bites.

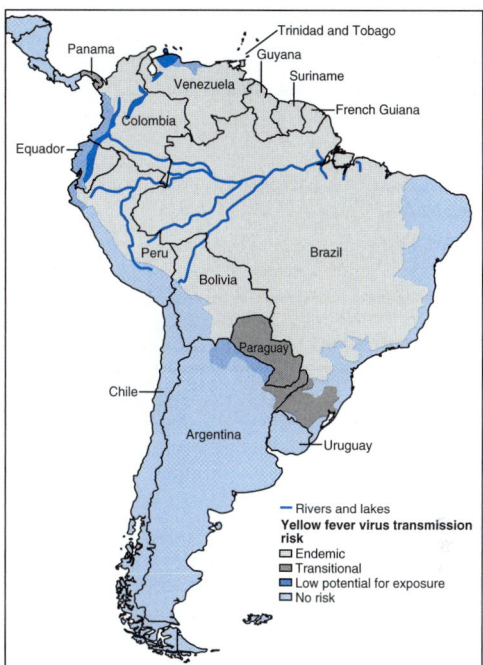

Fig. 56.2. Areas with Risk of Yellow Fever Virus Transmission in South America. *(*http://www.cdc.gov/yellowfever/maps/southamerica.html*)*

12. **What is yellow fever?**
    Yellow fever is a syndrome caused by the yellow fever virus, which is found in certain parts of South America and Africa (Figs. 56.2 and 56.3) and spread via bites of infected *Aedes* mosquitoes. Yellow fever can cause fever and flu-like symptoms, jaundice, hemorrhage, multiple organ failure, and death (in 20%–50% of serious cases).

13. **What are the indications and contraindications for yellow fever vaccination?**
    The yellow fever vaccine is a live, attenuated virus vaccine that is given in a single injection to people 9 months to 59 years old traveling to an area of risk (as outlined in the CDC's *Yellow Book*) or traveling to a country with an entry requirement for the vaccination. Anyone <6 months old or with a life-threatening allergy to any component of the vaccine, including eggs, should not get the vaccine. Additional relative contraindications to yellow fever vaccination include ages 6–9 months old, ≥60 years old, having a weakened immune system, having had a thymectomy or thymic disorder, being pregnant, or breastfeeding. Protection against yellow fever lasts for a lifetime after vaccination.

14. **What is Japanese encephalitis, and who should be vaccinated against it?**
    Japanese encephalitis virus (JEV) is a *Culex* mosquito–transmitted arbovirus and is the primary cause of encephalitis in East Asia. The majority of individuals infected with JEV are asymptomatic, and fewer than 1% of JEV infections result in symptomatic neuroinvasive disease. However, when neurologic disease does occur, it is usually quite severe, with a high case fatality rate and neurologic sequelae occurring in 30%–50% of survivors. The CDC recommends JEV vaccination for long-term (≥1 month) travel to endemic areas or short-term travel if the traveler is visiting an endemic area and participating in activities that will increase exposure to JEV-bearing mosquitoes (e.g., camping, hiking, or farming).

15. **What postexposure prophylaxis steps should be taken after a potential rabies exposure?**
    After a potential rabies exposure, bite wounds should be cleaned thoroughly with soap and water; suturing should be avoided if possible unless required for hemostasis. For exposed individuals who did not receive pre-exposure vaccination, postexposure prophylaxis consists of rabies immune globulin

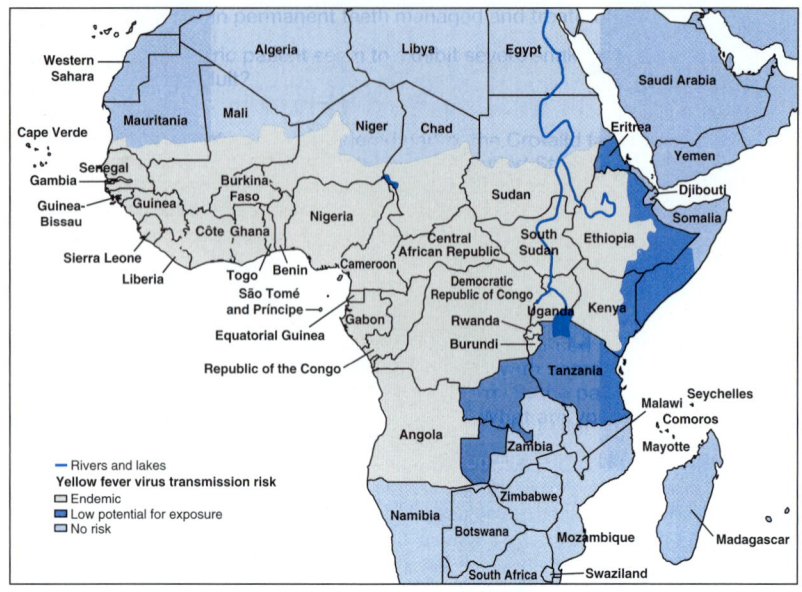

Fig. 56.3. Areas with Risk of Yellow Fever Virus Transmission in Africa. (http://www.cdc.gov/yellowfever/maps/africa.html)

injected at the wound site (prior to suturing, if closure is required) and intramuscularly, as well as four doses of the rabies vaccine. Individuals who completed the three-dose pre-exposure rabies vaccination series should receive two additional booster doses of the vaccine if exposed.

16. How can travelers protect themselves from tetanus?

Tetanus typically occurs when wounds are contaminated with dirt or soil containing the bacterium *Clostridium tetani*. The CDC recommends tetanus booster vaccinations prior to travel to areas where access to health services may be limited. When a potential exposure occurs (e.g., a laceration or a dog bite), the patient should receive a booster vaccine if the last booster was ≥5 years prior and at least three previous tetanus doses were obtained, if the patient received an unknown amount of doses, or if the patient received less than three doses regardless of time since the last dose.

17. When should infant travelers be vaccinated against measles, mumps, and rubella (MMR), and how does MMR vaccination affect the timing of other vaccinations?

The first dose of the MMR vaccine is typically administered to children between 12 and 15 months old. However, infants between the ages of 6 and 11 months who travel to areas where these diseases remain prevalent should receive the first MMR dose prior to departure. Children ≥12 months old should receive two doses of the vaccine, separated by 28 days. If the MMR vaccine is given prior to 12 months of age, this dose typically does not count toward the MMR series, and the child must get two doses of MMR after turning 1 year old. The MMR vaccine is a live vaccine, and administration of another live vaccine should occur either on the same day as MMR or ≥28 days later (≥30 days later if yellow fever vaccine) to ensure immunogenicity.

18. Where is polio found, and when is vaccination indicated?

Although most people infected with polio are asymptomatic, this enterovirus can famously cause paralysis. Despite massive global polio vaccination campaigns, polio has not been eradicated. Only two countries (Afghanistan and Pakistan) continue to have endemic polio. However, wild poliovirus still circulates in a number of countries. The CDC recommends that travelers to any country where wild-type polio was found to be circulating in the previous 12 months protect themselves by being fully vaccinated against polio, including a single lifetime polio vaccine booster for adults. The World Health Organization posts up-to-date booster recommendations for countries with wild poliovirus.

19. **In addition to handwashing and consuming only well-prepared foods, how can travelers protect themselves from hepatitis A?**

Hepatitis A virus is transmitted fecal–orally via contaminated water and food or from close contact with someone who is infected. Young children infected with the virus are often spared severe symptoms but can shed the virus. Because of lack of exposure in the United States, many older children and adults born in the United States lack natural immunity to the virus, and so can acquire this infection if exposed. The CDC recommends the two-dose series hepatitis A vaccination for travelers to endemic areas. Contraindications to the vaccine include age <12 months and allergy to a component of the vaccine. Individuals who cannot or opt not to receive the vaccine, including travelers <12 months old, can instead receive immune globulin, which confers protection against the virus for up to 5 months, although this duration depends upon the dose of immune globulin given.

20. **What vaccines protect against typhoid, and how effective are they?**

Enteric fever (also known as typhoid fever) is caused by *Salmonella* serovar Typhi bacteria and is transmitted fecal–orally by consumption of contaminated food or water. Two typhoid vaccines, an oral version (Ty21a, a live, attenuated vaccine) and an injected version (ViCPS, an inactivated vaccine), are available commercially in the United States. The oral vaccine is administered in four doses (1 pill every other day for a week), is approved for children ≥6 years old, and requires redosing after 5 years. The injected vaccine is approved for children ≥2 years old and requires redosing after 2 years. Studies of these vaccines have shown efficacy rates of 50%–80%; vaccination therefore does not eliminate the need to avoid potentially contaminated food or water.

21. **How can altitude sickness be prevented?**

Altitude sickness is divided into three syndromes: acute mountain sickness, high-altitude cerebral edema, and high-altitude pulmonary edema. Individuals with a history of altitude sickness and those who rapidly ascend to 2,500 meters or higher are at particular risk for altitude sickness. To help prevent altitude sickness, individuals should be advised to ascend gradually, avoiding going directly from low altitude to more than 2,750 meters sleeping altitude in a single day. Once above 2,750 meters, individuals should increase sleeping altitude no more than 500 meters per day and plan an extra day for acclimatization every 1,000 meters. Acetazolamide may assist acclimatization, potentially by acidifying blood, which results in compensatory increased respirations and oxygenation.

22. **What are useful websites that provide accurate, current information about travel-related health risks?**

Regularly updated online resources that are of particular relevance are:
- The CDC's *Health Information for International Travel* (the *Yellow Book*) provides detailed assistance for health care providers, and comprehensively summarizes pre-, during, and posttravel health concerns and their management.
  http://wwwnc.cdc.gov/travel/page/yellowbook-home-2014
- The U.S. State Department publishes travel notifications and travel-related policies that are up to date and country specific.
  https://travel.state.gov/content/travel/en.html

KEY POINTS

1. VFRs (visiting friends and relatives) tend to have a higher prevalence of travel-related infectious diseases than other tourists.
2. Health care workers face special concerns when working abroad.
3. Many illnesses, mostly infectious in origin, are associated with travel but can often be prevented.
4. It is crucial to inquire about the countries traveled to, time of travel, travel activities, and basic health status to determine what illnesses need to be considered in a returning traveler who is sick.
5. There are many websites that provide accurate, current information about travel-related health risks.

BIBLIOGRAPHY

Centers for Disease Control and Prevention. Vaccines. Medicines. Advice. <http://wwwnc.cdc.gov/travel/>; Accessed 22.06.16.
Centers for Disease Control and Prevention. *Yellow Book*. <http://wwwnc.cdc.gov/travel/page/yellowbook-home-2014>; Accessed 22.06.16.
Kimberlin DW, Brady MT, Jackson MA, Long SS, eds. *Red Book*. 30th ed. Elk Grove Village, IL: American Academy of Pediatrics; 2015.
World Health Organization. <http://www.who.int/en/>; Accessed 22.06.16.

CHAPTER 57

THE BUSINESS OF URGENT CARE

Michael C. Bachman, MD, MBA

1. **What are the key components of a business plan?**
   When developing a business plan for a new urgent care (UC) business, it is important to include the following components: concept (description of the project, problem you are solving, benefits to customers, and why it will succeed), market assessment (industry overview, target market, competition, potential market size, and expected penetration), strategy, operations, marketing activities, corporate structure, financial data, and risks involved.

2. **What expenses should be considered prior to opening a new UC center?**
   Cost of the build-out, furniture, fixtures, equipment, opening supplies, software and training, attorney fees, deposits, architect and filing fees.

3. **What expenses should be considered after the opening of a new UC center?**
   It is very important to calculate the expected ramp-up losses. These should include personnel expenses (salary, payroll taxes, benefits, malpractice coverage), rent and related costs, marketing expenses, supplies, billing and collections, miscellaneous fees, and accounts receivable.

4. **Is urgent care a variable or fixed cost business?**
   Urgent care is primarily a fixed cost business. The only true variable cost is supplies. Personnel are semifixed, because as volume grows, new staff need to be added incrementally. Because urgent care is a fixed cost business, profitability is volume driven. Once fixed costs are covered, a very high percentage of additional revenue will increase profits. It is important for an urgent care business to determine its initial breakeven volume and then recalculate as staffing increases.

5. **What are the different sources of capital to fund an urgent care business?**
   Sources of capital include friends and family, bank loans, finance companies, landlord contribution, equipment leasing, angel investors, venture capital, and private equity. For a newer company, the best sources of funding are investment by the founders, banks loans, and landlord contribution. As the company grows to a multiple site practice, the other funding sources may become better options.

6. **You figure out how much cash you need until you expect to break even and are able to secure the funds from friends and family. Should you be ready to take the leap?**
   No, you need to anticipate issues that may arise and increase your costs. Examples include permit or construction delays that result in a delayed opening even while paying rent, unanticipated capital or operating expenses, a slower ramp-up than predicted, and delays in reimbursement from insurance companies. It is essential to have contingency funds to cover these unexpected expenses, as much as 50% more than your calculated needs.

7. **What demographic data are essential to determine the ideal site for a new UC center?**
   Important demographics to consider are total population within your catchment area, population trends (i.e., is the local population growing?), average age of population, income levels, and population density (i.e., people per square mile). It is important to determine your catchment area—that is, where patients will come from, driving distance, and ease of travel to get to your site. Local behaviors are important to consider, such as if the local population drives, relies on public transportation, walks to destinations, etc. Sources of demographic data include real estate brokers, commercial real estate web listings, and the U.S. Census Bureau.

8. **After deciding on the location of your new UC center, what specific site characteristics should you evaluate?**
   Key characteristics include accessibility, visibility from major roads, adequate parking, and the size and shape of available space. The condition of the building should be considered to determine if there will

be exterior work needed and if there are adequate utilities. Based on your business model, you need to determine if your business should be placed in a freestanding building, retail shopping center, or medical office building. If you choose a retail center, consider your co-tenants and the customer activity in the center. Local zoning and use laws should be reviewed to determine if your use is permitted in the space, if any variances will be required, and what types of building signage are allowed.

9. What are the important leasing considerations for a new UC site?

It is important to consider the desired term of the lease. If investing in the space build-out, you want to benefit from that investment as long as possible, but you don't want to be locked in for too long if things don't work out. Termination rights for the lease need to be determined as well as a guarantee to reimburse the landlord for their investment in the deal. Rent will also include a proportionate share of real estate tax and common area maintenance and often increases over time by a predetermined percentage. Rent start should be delayed until after building and sign permits are issued and ideally until after build-out and outfitting are complete and the business is ready to open. Construction allowances from the landlord should also be negotiated and can be delivered in the form of cash or free rent and may be rolled into the base rent.

10. What is EBITDA?

EBITDA stands for earning before interest, taxes, depreciation, and amortization. It serves as a common measure of a company's profitability before deductions that are considered superfluous to the business decision-making process.

11. Are profits all that matter?

Profits = Revenue − Expenses. Revenue is the amount of money earned, but it is not necessarily the money collected. It is important to understand that being profitable does not mean the business is guaranteed to succeed. Cash is extremely important to help cover capital expenditures, accounts payable, loan repayments, etc. Profits may not be realized until accounts receivable are realized and expenses are covered.

12. What are the important business metrics to be followed?

- Visit patterns: determine monthly growth, hourly volumes, seasonal patterns, and zip code analysis
- Revenue: average revenue per visit, average time to collect
- Expenses: personnel costs per visit, supply cost per visit
- Marketing: advertising effectiveness

13. Describe the different ways of contracting reimbursement with payers.

UC businesses can contract with payers as fee for service or at a case rate. With fee for service, each service provided is paid for separately. A case rate provides a flat amount per visit, covering a group of procedures and services. While fee for service may generate higher reimbursements, case rates provide ease of coding and billing and lower risk of audits. In certain markets, UC businesses may not participate with insurance companies and may offer various self-pay rates.

14. What are the legal considerations for an urgent care business?

Legal considerations include malpractice and liability coverage, licensing requirements, the corporate practice of medicine, and local laws regarding medication dispensing and e-prescribing. It is very important to understand the state and local laws where your UC center is located. Many states have "no surprise billing laws" that require patients be notified if the UC center is part of a hospital and will charge an additional facility fee if out of network, and of any extra fees that may be charged for certain procedures or diagnostic tests.

15. Does your UC business need a compliance program?

Any UC center that gets reimbursements from Medicare or Medicaid must have a compliance program. They should have a Code of Conduct that provides rules for all employees to follow, to comply with fraud and abuse laws and other legal mandates. The compliance program should provide ongoing employee education on fraud and abuse laws as they may change over time.

16. What are the important methods for marketing your UC business?

Marketing methods include branding the UC business with an identifiable logo, signage, print advertising, direct mail, web and social media, grassroots and community outreach, and public relations. Increasing numbers of customers seek health care providers online, so it is important to have a modern and easy-to-navigate website that is an extension of the brand. Equally important is for the website to have a mobile-friendly format. The website should be developed with search engine optimization in mind. The social media landscape is rapidly growing and becoming a low-cost effective marketing tool for UC businesses.

17. **What are drivers of customer satisfaction in urgent care?**

It is essential to understand what urgent care customers' values include: convenient and clean locations, speed of service, attention and empathy of staff, and excellent care. The design and appearance of the physical space impacts the customers' first impressions, and site layout must be conducive to efficient treatment and facilitate effective communication between staff and patients. All staff should understand the mission of the company and the values and priorities of the company. Staffing with the right people who receive the right training will help ensure excellent service. Staff should be happy and motivated and always willing to go above and beyond customer expectations.

KEY POINTS

1. Develop a thorough business plan, consider both upfront expenses and ongoing expenses that will occur after opening, and make sure to have contingency funds to cover unexpected expenses that may arise.
2. Choose your location wisely, taking into account local demographics, travel habits, ease of access, and characteristics of the specific site.
3. Your UC business must practice in accordance with state and federal laws including meeting all the licensure, insurance, compliance, billing, and credentialing requirements.
4. The success of an urgent care business is dependent on providing top-notch customer service. Locations must be convenient, clean service must be fast and efficient, staff must be attentive and empathetic, and the level of care must be excellent.

INDEX

Pages followed by *b, t,* or *f* refer to boxes, tables, or figures, respectively.

C

Contrast —
No   Bones
        Kidney stones
Yes ✓ cmp
        soft tissue abscess

        IV for vascular   AAA
                            carotids

        Disc & bone   MRI's

    Diverticulosis — CT Abd pelvis c̄ contrast
    Gall bladder — US
                    Hida.
                    MRCP or ERCP

Sutures   Kids
Facial — 5-7 days
Scalp — 6-8-10
Eyelid — 3-5   5-7
Ear —   4-5   3-5
Nose —   3-5   3-5
Neck   7   3-5
Trunk/Upr 10-14
        Ext
Lower Ext 14-21